TEXTBOOK OF REMEDIAL **Massage**

Sandra Grace PhD, MSc, Grad Cert Sports Chiro, Cert Clinical Chiro Paediatrics, Dip Acup, DBM, DO, DC, Dip Ed, BA

Senior Lecturer in Osteopathic Medicine, Southern Cross University
Adjunct Research Associate, The Education for Practice Institute, Charles Sturt University

Mark Deal BSc, DC, DO, Dip Ed (Technical)

Chiropractor, Osteopath, Acupuncturist and Educator
Independent Contractor to Noosa Parade Medical Centre

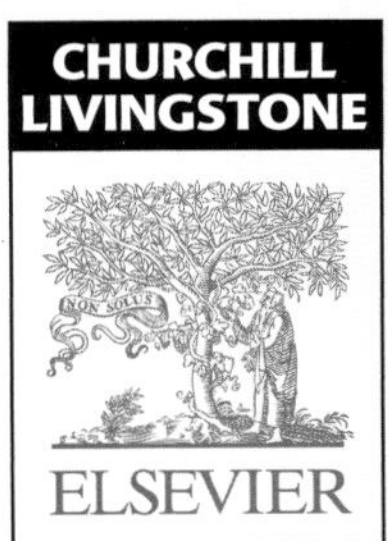

Sydney Edinburgh London New York Philadelphia St Louis Toronto

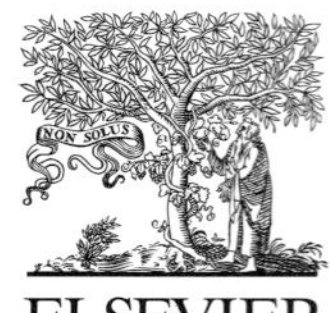

Churchill Livingstone
is an imprint of Elsevier

Elsevier Australia. ACN 001 002 357
(a division of Reed International Books Australia Pty Ltd)
Tower 1, 475 Victoria Avenue, Chatswood, NSW 2067

National Library of Australia Cataloguing-in-Publication Data

---

Grace, Sandra.

Textbook of remedial massage / Sandra Grace, Mark Deal.

1st ed.

9780729539692 (pbk.)
Includes index.

Massage.
Massage therapy.

Deal, Mark Philip.

615.822

Publisher: Luisa Cecotti
Developmental Editor: Neli Bryant
Project Coordinator: Natalie Hamad and Karthikeyan Murthy
Edited by Jo Crichton
Proofread by Tim Learner
Picture research by Copperleife
Photography by Diverze Photography
Cover design by Lisa Petroff
Illustrated by Gaul Designs
Index by Robert Swanson
Typeset by Toppan Best-set Premedia Limited
Printed by CTPS

TEXTBOOK OF REMEDIAL Massage

Contents

Preface

The aim of this book is to present a comprehensive practical guide for students, practitioners and educators of remedial massage. It is framed in the context of current evidence for practice and emphasises the values of critical appraisal and life-long learning, both of which are served by maintaining conversancy with current research.

It assumes mastery of the knowledge and skills required for therapeutic relaxation massage (Certificate IV level). Safe practice is a key focus of the book. Remedial massage practitioners treat a broad range of conditions, often as first contact practitioners. Safe practice requires a sound knowledge of red and yellow flags and a willingness to collaborate with other healthcare practitioners in co-managing clients.

STRUCTURE OF THE BOOK

The book is presented in three sections. The first discusses the scope of practice of remedial massage, its place within the Australian healthcare system, and its potential role in the key field of integrative health. It presents a comprehensive and evidence-based approach to assessment and principles of treatment. The approach to short- and long-term treatment planning prioritises client safety and the use of current research, and highlights the important role of client education.

The second section deals with some of the most important and widely used techniques of remedial massage. The exposition of each technique is accompanied by a rationale based on current supporting evidence and an explanation of contraindications and precautions. Applications of techniques are illustrated by photographs and drawings. A demonstration of integrated techniques is also presented on the DVD accompanying the book.

The final section of the book is divided into regions of the body. Each chapter contains an exposition of common conditions of the region, relevant assessment procedures and a range of remedial massage techniques that can safely be applied in treatment. A distinctive feature of this book is its approach to treatment: it presents techniques as they are often integrated in practice and clearly articulates the clinical reasoning that supports treatment choices. Summary tables illustrating a range of remedial massage techniques for specific muscles are included in each chapter.

The final chapter of the book focuses on remedial massage assessment and treatment considerations for specific population groups.

This is the first remedial massage text that aligns itself with Australian Health Training Package requirements. Competencies in the Training Package for remedial massage were developed by educators, curriculum designers and professional association representatives and are regularly peer-reviewed for accuracy and currency. The content of the book is also highly applicable to other jurisdictions where remedial massage is practised. This book clarifies what constitutes remedial massage and what separates it from other manual therapies like relaxation massage, osteopathy and physiotherapy. Such clarification is necessary if the benefits of remedial massage are to be recognised in their own right and the safety and competence of its practitioners are to be assured. Remedial massage would then be assured of its rightful place within the healthcare system.

Acknowledgements

I would like to thank my colleagues Jane Graves, Catrin Jonsson and Yolanda Paino for their unstinting support. Their expertise and flair were indispensable to the relevance and currency of content. Thanks also to Mark Deal, Peter Thompson, Julie Harm, Patricia Farnsworth and Allan Hudson who have enriched the book with their expertise in particular content areas.

Thanks are also due to Sophie Kaliniecki, Neli Bryant and Natalie Hamad from Elsevier who guided the project from inception to publication and to Greg Gaul who drew the high-quality illustrations, to our photographers Dianne and Veronique from Diverze Photography and Sarah Craig, and to Dragan Dimitrovski from Mak Video who shot the videos.

Jane, Catrin and Mark were outstanding demonstrators. I am also deeply indebted to our models, Aynur Aksu, Umit Aksu, Yavus Aksu, Hannah Temby, and Jeremy Clarke Eleanor Nurse whose stamina and good humour got us through some long days.

Thanks to my editors Stephen Clarke, who brought his formidable skills to imposing precision and clarity wherever they were needed, and to Jo Crichton who copy edited the manuscript. Many skilled and experienced therapists and teachers gave their expert knowledge and time to reviewing sections of the book. I am extremely grateful for their insights, which contributed so much to the final form of the book.

This also gives me an opportunity to acknowledge the inspiration I have had over thirty years of practice and pedagogy from the teachings of many leading lights in the field of manual therapies, none more cherished than Leon Chaitow and such pioneers as Janet Travell and Vladimir Janda.

Foreword

There are a finite number of ways in which force (load) can be applied to the tissues of the body. These can be listed as compression, shear (shunt), torsion, tension (stretch) and bend.

Apart from the particular clinical situation, the physiological effects of such load application appears to depend on:

- the degree of surface contact
- the degree and direction of load applied – light, heavy, variable, etc.
- whether forces are direct or indirect, i.e. towards or away from restriction barriers, or in other directions
- the velocity and amplitude of force application (slow, rapid, varied) involving small or large areas
- whether the application of manual force is sustained, gliding, rhythmic or variable
- the duration or length of these applications
- what combinations of forces are selected, e.g. compression plus rapid variable shear leads to friction, which might be combined with isometric, isotonic or isolytic contractions – depending on the desired outcome
- how frequently and how many repetitions of the selected elements are employed
- whether the patient/client is active or passive.

Additional features might include simultaneous, preceding or subsequent use of heat, cold, exercise – or other modalities. The use of all or any of these multiple interacting variables are determined by why they have been selected and designed. Is it:

- to tone, to modify circulation, to lengthen tissues?
- to stimulate, sedate, mobilise, or to have reflexive physiological effects?
- to have other effects altogether – such as inducing relaxation?

Such choices depend to a large extent on the current state of the individual receiving attention – the age, vitality, history and current medical condition.

A further, primary consideration involves the degree of evidence existing in relation to potential benefit. Is there evidence of such benefit in similar situations – or are the choices being made from a background of clinical experience?

And, what are the risks and precautions that might apply?

And of course, the expectations of the client/patient need to merge with these interacting features and factors, summarised above, as clinical reasoning evolves towards a therapeutic plan.

Remedial massage can be seen, therefore, to be anything but a 'fluff and buff' exercise. It is – as this book explains and demonstrates – a highly complex and effective, science-based approach to healthcare, that incorporates both physical (neurological, circulatory, lymphatic and biomechanical features) as well as psychological considerations – with a vast evidential base of effectiveness, in a range of conditions too varied to list.

This excellent book sets out to describe the foundations for the delivery of safe and effective remedial massage – and it succeeds in doing so via clearly expressed text combined with crisp and effective illustrations.

This is a highly recommended text, suitable for students, educators and therapists/practitioners alike.

Leon Chaitow ND DO
Honorary Fellow, University of Westminster, UK
Editor-in-Chief, Journal of Bodywork & Movement Therapies

Contributors

Patricia Farnsworth, DRM, RCST
Founder of The Craniosacral Therapy Academy and the Myofascial Release Centre; Executive Member of the Craniosacral Therapy Association of Australia; Member of ATMS

Jane Graves, (B.Sc., M. Chiropractic)
Naturopathy Head of Program, School of Biomedical and Health Sciences, University of Western Sydney Campbelltown, NSW, Australia

Julie Harm, BAppSc (Human Movement), Grad Dip VET, Ass Dip Health Sc (Massage Therapy)
Massage Course Coordinator, TAFE NSW – Illawarra Institute

Allan Hudson, ND, Dip Acup, DRM, LMT, Member of ATMS
Head of Faculty Tactile Therapies and Continuing Education Nature Care, Care College NSW Australia

Catrin Jonsson, B Health Sc (Complementary Medicine), Ass Dip In Health Sc (Massage Therapy) MEx Sport Sc
Registered Exercise Professional with Fitness Australia, Member of Association of Massage Therapists (AMT)

Peter Thompson, DC, DO, Dip Acup, MSc.
Lecturer in Chiropractic Science, Macquarie University, Lecturer, TAFE, Sydney, Australia.

Reviewers

Kurt Edmonds Certificate IV
Australian Association of Massage Therapists, Flow Again Massage & Wellness Centre, Safety Bay, WA

Michael Ferguson Bohs Dip Rem Massage, Dip Sport/Recreation
Lecturer Dip/CIV Massage
Wide Bay TAFE, Hervey Bay, QLD

Jill Harrison Diploma of Remedial Massage, Diploma of Anatomy Physiology & Body Massage (ITEC), Diploma of Reflexology
Lecturer in Anatomy & Biomechanics and Remedial Massage, Australian Institute of Holistic Medicine

Glenn Jones Bachelor of Education, Advanced Diploma in Applied Science (Remedial Massage), Cert IV OHS
Member of AMT
Soft Tissue & Sports Massage Teacher, Canberra Institute of Technology

Shelley Keating Bachelor of Exercise Science and Rehabilitation, Hon-1 Masters of Exercise and Sport Science (Clinical Exercise Science) Diploma of Remedial Massage
Program Director, Manual Therapies, Australasian College of Natural Therapies

Pauline Kelly
Programme Coordinator – Natural Therapies, Kangan Institute, Kangan Batman TAFE

Sandie Leong Bachelor of Health Science, Advanced Diploma in Remedial Massage, Bachelor of Business (Marketing)
Chronic Pain Clinic, Eight Mile Plains, QLD

Catherine Traynor Diploma of Remedial Massage, Cert IV TAA04 Training and Assessment
Kit Laughlin P&F Stretch Therapist and Stretch Teacher, Diploma of Bodywork and Aromatherapy, Myofascial Release and related techniques, Teacher of Remedial Massage techniques (Diploma); Anatomy and physiology Cert IV; Communications; Business Skills; Personal Development; Stretching at Tropical North Queensland Institute of TAFE, Cairns, QLD, Member of Australian Natural Therapists Association, Member of Cairns Remedial Therapists

Remedial massage in Australian healthcare

1

The content of this chapter relates to the following Unit of Competency:
HLTCOM502C Develop professional expertise

Health Training Package HLT07

Learning Outcomes

- Define remedial massage and describe the difference between remedial massage and other levels of massage training including relaxation massage.
- Demonstrate an understanding of the context of remedial massage practice including the extent of public use of remedial massage and attitudes of other healthcare practitioners towards remedial massage.
- Demonstrate an understanding of the evidence base for remedial massage.

DEFINING REMEDIAL MASSAGE

Many authors writing about massage therapy fail to distinguish between different types of massage, differences in training requirements for practitioners and varying levels of recognition by professional associations, medical benefit funds and WorkCover authorities.[1–3] In particular, there is confusion between what constitutes relaxation or Swedish massage and remedial massage, the terms often being used interchangeably.[4] The Australian Standard Classification of Occupations (ASCO)[5] described only one massage occupation, that of massage therapist, who 'performs therapeutic massage and administers body treatments for relaxation, health, fitness and remedial purposes' and in 2001, in the Australian Standard Classification of Education, massage therapy was described as 'the study of treating disorders through massage of the soft tissue'.[6] Moreover, Australian professional associations often use definitions of massage and set levels of practice that they develop independently.[7–9]

Most Australian training institutions refer to two levels of massage therapy: a basic level (Certificate IV) for relaxation massage; and a more advanced level (Diploma) for diagnosing and treating musculoskeletal and other conditions. Recent years have seen the development of a third and more comprehensive level of massage therapy.[10, 11] Consensus on curricula for Advanced Diplomas, Associate Degrees in massage and Bachelor's Degrees in musculoskeletal therapy is yet to be reached. Furthermore, the difference between the ways osteopaths and remedial massage therapists apply the same soft tissue techniques needs to be clarified.

In Australia, the Health Training Package, first developed in 2002 and revised in 2007, described two levels of massage therapy practice (Certificate IV in Massage Therapy Practice and Diploma of Remedial Massage) which clearly delineate between the scope of two levels of massage practice: *massage therapy* and *remedial massage* (see Table 1.1). The consensus among practitioners and educators of massage therapy, as reflected in the Health Training Package, is that remedial massage therapists assess and treat musculoskeletal and other system disorders.

Diploma-qualified therapists are expected to demonstrate a level of analysis, judgment, problem-solving skills, responsibility for their own work and the work of others, and self-evaluation capabilities in practice. (A diploma is the minimum qualification required for most Australian medical benefit funds.) Massage therapists with more basic levels of training, on the other hand, require sufficient knowledge and skills to determine the suitability of their clients for treatment using a contraindications checklist, and to perform a massage therapy routine with a limited range of variations. Any definition of remedial massage must reflect not only the level of technical skills required for this qualification, but also the level of analysis, evaluation and responsibility required for assessing and treating musculoskeletal and other conditions amenable to massage therapy. A common practice of training institutions is to interpret curriculum purely in terms of the range of content to be included. Such an interpretation is not only prone to misuse of the graduate capabilities outlined in Table 1.1, but also runs the risk of ignoring other important aspects of curriculum, including hidden or implicit ones (e.g. acculturation that occurs in student training clinics).

In this book we define remedial massage as:

i) the application of a range of diagnostic techniques[a] to identify clients and their conditions as suitable for remedial massage therapy and to enable adaptation of remedial massage therapy techniques to suit the needs of individual clients;

[a]The terms diagnosis/diagnostic techniques refer to assessment practices accepted as falling within the scope of remedial massage. They are to be understood solely as remedial massage diagnosis/diagnostic techniques whenever they are used in this book.

Table 1.1 Comparison between Certificate IV and Diploma qualifications

	Certificate IV	Diploma
Purpose	The Certificate IV qualifies individuals who apply a broad range of specialised knowledge and skills in varied contexts to undertake skilled work and as a pathway for further learning.	The Diploma qualifies individuals who apply integrated technical and theoretical concepts in a broad range of contexts to undertake advanced skilled or paraprofessional work and as a pathway for further learning.
Knowledge	Graduates of a Certificate IV will have broad factual, technical and theoretical knowledge in a specialised field of work and learning.	Graduates of a Diploma will have technical and theoretical knowledge and concepts, with depth in some areas within a field of work and learning.
Skills	Graduates of a Certificate IV will have: • cognitive skills to identify, analyse, compare and act on information from a range of sources • cognitive, technical and communication skills to apply and communicate technical solutions of a non-routine or contingency nature to a defined range of predictable and unpredictable problems • specialist technical skills to complete routine and non-routine tasks and functions • communication skills to guide activities and provide technical advice in the area of work and learning.	Graduates of a Diploma will have: • cognitive and communication skills to identify, analyse, synthesise and act on information from a range of sources • cognitive, technical and communication skills to analyse, plan, design and evaluate approaches to unpredictable problems and/or management requirements • specialist technical and creative skills to express ideas and perspectives • communication skills to transfer knowledge and specialised skills to others and demonstrate understanding of knowledge.
Application of knowledge and skills	Graduates of a Certificate IV will demonstrate the application of knowledge and skills: • to specialised tasks or functions in known or changing contexts with responsibility for own functions and outputs, and may have limited responsibility for organisation of others • with limited responsibility for the quantity and quality of the output of others in a team within limited parameters.	Graduates of a Diploma will demonstrate the application of knowledge and skills: • with depth in some areas of specialisation, in known or changing contexts • to transfer and apply theoretical concepts and/or technical and/or creative skills in a range of situations • with personal responsibility and autonomy in performing complex technical operations with responsibility for own outputs in relation to broad parameters for quantity and quality • with initiative and judgment to organise the work of self and others and plan, coordinate and evaluate the work of teams within broad but generally well-defined parameters.
Volume of learning	The volume of learning of a Certificate IV is typically 0.5–2 years. There may be variations between short duration specialist qualifications that build on knowledge and skills already acquired and longer duration qualifications that are designed as entry level requirements for work.	The volume of learning of a Diploma is typically 1–2 years.

(Qualification descriptors reproduced with permission of the Australian Qualifications Framework Council[12])

and

ii) the use of a range of basic and advanced massage techniques (e.g. trigger points, myofascial release and lymphatic drainage) to treat a variety of musculoskeletal and other system conditions.

THE CONTEXT OF REMEDIAL MASSAGE: USE OF COMPLEMENTARY AND ALTERNATIVE MEDICINE IN AUSTRALIAN HEALTHCARE

Remedial massage is one of the many modalities that are encompassed by the term *complementary and alternative medicine* (CAM). One study puts the number of Australians using CAM as high as 70% at an estimated annual cost of about $4 billion.[13] Further information on the specific use of touch therapies or body work in South Australia was collected in three surveys between 1993 and 2004.[14–16] The surveys included categories for reflexologists and aromatherapists but not specifically for remedial massage therapists (see Table 1.2). The surveys found that chiropractic was the most commonly used CAM.

THE REMEDIAL MASSAGE WORKFORCE IN AUSTRALIA

Little information is available about the remedial massage workforce in Australia. The total CAM workforce represents only 1.9% of all health occupations, according to the Australian Government Productivity Commission 2005.[17] However, between 1996 and 2001, the growth in complementary health occupations represented the second highest increase (29.6%) of all health occupations. The Australian Bureau of Statistics reported 8533 CAM practitioners in 2001.[18] However, in 2003 the combined membership of the Australian Traditional Medicine Society (ATMS) and the Australian Natural Therapists' Association (ANTA), reportedly together representing 75% of the CAM workforce (excluding chiropractic and osteopathy), was reported at approximately 12,000[19] and by July 2010 the membership of ATMS alone had reached 11,472 financial members.[20]

There have been few attempts to collect data on the number of remedial massage therapists working in Australia. Such a task is confounded by the lack of a central register or government registration and because many remedial massage therapists work part-time or casually and may not report remedial massage as their occupation. Most graduates of colleges and courses accredited with professional associations seek membership with their respective associations.[21–23] There are at least nine massage therapy associations for remedial massage therapists in Australia (see box below). Practitioners who have trained overseas, trained with a non-accredited college, who have not undertaken any formal training or who have not sought professional association membership may also be in practice. It is possible that the number of remedial massage therapists in Australia is considerably higher than the official professional association figures. An estimate based on 2009 information from professional massage associations in the box below put the number of massage therapists working in Australia at that time at just over 22,000.[24] (Note: Members of the Australian Kinesiology Association, Bowen Association, International Federation of Aromatherapists and Reflexology Association of Australia do not require qualifications in remedial massage and have not been included in the tally.)

Three national surveys of CAM practitioners, funded by the Department of Health and Ageing, were conducted in Australia in 2000.[23, 25, 26] At the time the remedial massage workforce was predominantly female, part time and sole practice (see Table 1.3).

Table 1.2 Comparison of choices of CAM practitioners

CAM practitioner	Percentage of respondents' choices 1993	2000	2004
Chiropractor	15.0	16.7	16.7
Naturopath	5.0	6.0	5.7
Acupuncturist	2.0	2.8	2.1
Homeopath	1.2	1.2	0.5
Iridologist	0.8	1.2	0.8
Reflexologist	0.7	1.2	1.0
Aromatherapist	0.6	1.3	1.1
Herbalist	0.4	0.9	1.9
Osteopath	0.2	0.4	0.4
Other	1.8	1.2	4.8

(MacLennan et al 1996,[14] 2002[15] and MacLennan et al 2006[16])

Massage therapy associations in Australia

Australian Association of Massage Therapists
Australian Kinesiology Association*
Association of Massage Therapists
Australian Natural Therapists Association
Australian Traditional Medicine Society
Association of Remedial Masseurs
Bowen Association*
International Federation of Aromatherapists*
Massage Association Australia
Massage Australia
Queensland Association of Massage Therapists
Reflexology Association of Australia*
South Australia Massage Therapists Association

*Members do not require qualifications in remedial massage.

Table 1.3 Comparison of three national CAM workforce surveys[23, 25, 26]

	Remedial therapists[23]	Naturopaths, Western medical herbalists, acupuncturists[26]	Naturopaths, Western medical herbalists[25]
Average age (range)	26–55 years	34–45 years	44 years
Gender	76%: female	74.8%: female	76%: female
Practice location: metropolitan/rural	54%: metropolitan	57%: metropolitan	Twice as many metropolitan as rural practices
Type of practice	64%: sole practitioner 18%: group practice	59%: sole practices 28%: group practice	30%: group practice
Length of training (full-time equivalent)	41%: one year 37%: two year	42%: four years (7.8%: bachelor degree)	6 months–6 years
Average number of consultations per week	12	15.7	22.3
Income	91% less than $50,000 per annum	53% less than $30,000 per annum	
Length of time in practice	64%: 1–5 years	39%: 1–5 years	Average 6.7 years

ATTITUDES TOWARDS CAM BY MEDICAL AND OTHER HEALTHCARE PRACTITIONERS

There appears to be growing tolerance and endorsement of CAM among members of the medical profession and other non-CAM healthcare providers.[27, 28] The Australian Medical Association's position statement on complementary medicine recognised that scientific evidence-based aspects of complementary medicine are part of the repertoire of client care and might have a role in mainstream medical practice.[29] In the USA, 70–90% of family doctors who responded to a survey considered such therapies as diet advice, exercise therapy, behavioural medicine, counselling and hypnotherapy to be legitimate medical practice.[30] In Canada, acupuncture, chiropractic and hypnosis were considered the most useful complementary therapies[31] and in the UK, chiropractic, acupuncture and osteopathy were rated most effective.[32] In Australia, acupuncture, massage, meditation, hypnosis and spinal manipulation were the complementary therapies most commonly chosen for client referral.[33–35] In practice, members of the medical profession are more likely to refer to, and to share practices with, practitioners of CAM occupations that have wider acceptance, such as acupuncture, chiropractic and massage, and less likely to do so with lower-profile CAM occupations such as Reiki and flower essences.

EVIDENCE FOR REMEDIAL MASSAGE PRACTICE

The willingness of Western medicine to embrace CAM is conditional on increasing its evidence base,[36–38] that is, evidence based on Western science's gold standard (randomised controlled trials) or on systematic reviews and meta-analyses where data from randomised controlled trials is statistically pooled.

Many early attempts at clinical trials had serious methodological flaws associated with lack of randomisation and failure to identify appropriate placebo interventions.[39] Some authors have argued that biomedical science methodology is not suitable for CAM research.[40, 41] Fundamental differences between the underlying philosophies of Western medicine and CAM have been cited as the main barrier to high-quality scientific research in CAM.[39, 42, 43] These differences may not be as clear-cut in contemporary healthcare as mainstream medicine and CAM tend to become more integrated. Historically, differences between the two approaches have been described in broad terms as:

- the reductionist, mechanistic approach of biomedicine as opposed to the biocultural approach of CAM
- Western medicine's focus on eliminating the disease-producing agent as opposed to CAM's focus on encouraging the innate ability of the human body to restore itself to health
- Western medicine's traditional focus on illness as opposed to CAM's focus on wellness.

However, despite the complexities of finding or developing suitable methodologies for CAM research, it is possible to design research studies for CAM that generate evidence capable of informing clinical practice. The Cochrane Complementary Medicine Field[b] was established in 1996 to meet the need for scientific evidence-based research in CAM practices.[40] In 2004 there were over 7000 randomised controlled trials of the effectiveness of CAM.[44] A study by Ernst et al[45] compared the evidence base of massage therapy in 2000 with that of 2005 as reported in two editions of their book *The Desktop Guide to Complementary and Alternative Medicine*. The authors reported that the evidence for the effectiveness of massage therapy in several areas had become more solid and for anxiety and back pain it had become more positive.

A summary of systematic reviews for massage therapy is presented below. It shows that there is little high-quality evidence for many of the claims made about the effectiveness of massage therapy. It is important to remember that insufficient evidence means just that: that there have been insufficient high-quality trials to draw conclusions about whether massage therapy is effective or ineffective for particular conditions or groups.[46] Most systematic reviews have reported insufficient evidence (i.e. insufficient number of high-quality trials) to be able to draw conclusions; a few have reported evidence of benefit (see Appendix 1.1 for further details).

EVIDENCE FOR THE EFFECTIVENESS OF MASSAGE THERAPY

Evidence of benefit

- Antenatal perineal massage helps reduce both perineal trauma during birth and pain afterwards.[47, 48]
- Massage and aromatherapy reduce anxiety and increase psychological wellbeing in the short term in patients with cancer.[49]
- Massage has been shown to reduce short-term anxiety[50–52] but there is limited evidence for any long-term effects.

Inconclusive (some promising results)

- Aromatherapy massage had mild transient effects in reducing anxiety, based on six trials with hospital patients.[53]
- Massage gives some relief from back pain that has continued for many weeks or months and its benefit may last at least a year after massage treatments cease. There is still not enough evidence to make claims about the benefit of massage therapy for acute back pain.[54] Massage may be especially beneficial when combined with exercises and education.[55]
- Massage may be effective in reducing labour pain.[56]
- Aromatherapy may benefit people with dementia but more studies are required.[57]
- Infant massage may be useful for mother–infant interaction, infant sleeping and crying, and reducing the production of stress hormones, but further research is needed.[58, 59]
- There is weak evidence that massage is of benefit for preterm infants.[60]
- Abdominal massage for treating chronic constipation has shown some promising results.[61]

[b]The Cochrane Collaboration is an international organisation which prepares, maintains and promotes the accessibility of systematic reviews of the effectiveness of healthcare interventions.[44]

Inconclusive evidence (further research needed)

- There is insufficient evidence to draw any conclusions about the effectiveness of massage therapy for lymphoedema.[62] Although results from case studies and pilot studies are promising, manual lymphatic drainage techniques remain based on hypothesis, theory and preliminary evidence.[63]
- No conclusions can be drawn from trials into the effectiveness of deep transverse friction massage for treating tendinitis.[64]
- No recommendations for practice can be made for the effectiveness of massage for neck pain.[65, 66]
- There is insufficient evidence to draw any conclusions about the effectiveness of massage therapy for reducing pain in tension-type headaches.[67]
- The small amount of evidence currently available is in favour of massage and touch interventions, but is too limited in scope to allow for general conclusions about the effectiveness of massage therapy on dementia.[59]
- There is no evidence that therapeutic touch promotes healing of acute wounds.[68]
- There is insufficient evidence to draw any conclusions about the effectiveness of massage for treating asthma.[69]

There have been urgent calls for more high-quality research to support the increasing prevalence and use of CAM.[70, 71] Such research is hampered by lack of funding and suitably qualified CAM researchers. The National Centre for Complementary and Alternative Medicine (NCCAM) in the USA was allocated US$117.7 million in 2004 for CAM research, part of which was used to establish a sustainable research infrastructure by the creation of research centres.[72–74] Funding for CAM research in Australia is very scant by comparison, although it received a substantial boost in November 2006 when the National Health and Medical Research Council allocated up to $5 million towards CAM research.[75]

FUTURE DIRECTIONS

The escalating costs associated with the healthcare needs of ageing populations have focused attention on the role of healthcare strategies for chronic health conditions and for preventive healthcare.[76] Remedial massage has relevance for many Australians, including those with chronic non-life-threatening conditions. An increasing number of clients will rely on remedial massage to minimise or eliminate pain and other symptoms that return when massage treatment stops for a period of time. Without a maintenance program, these clients report increased difficulties with activities of daily living and absenteeism from work.[c] Remedial massage therapists can also make an important contribution to preventive healthcare through their capacity for identifying sub-clinical indicators of musculoskeletal problems.

Given the increasing use of CAM in modern Western societies, it is reasonable to expect an increasing acceptance of remedial massage as a legitimate part of Australian healthcare by the public and other healthcare workers. From the perspectives of medical and other healthcare workers, acceptance will inevitably be linked to an increasing evidence base for CAM. High-quality research in remedial massage therapy depends on both available funding and training for those interested in CAM research. Increasing research literacy of remedial massage students and practising therapists is likely to influence the effectiveness of clinical practice by providing a strong evidence base. More consistent and better clarified levels in massage therapy training and graduate attributes linked to those levels, and stronger links between private colleges, TAFEs and university courses, will secure pathways and support for students and practitioners who are interested in remedial massage research projects. As research into remedial massage continues to emerge, some of the claims about its efficacy will be confirmed and some will be refuted. A robust remedial massage profession will want to be involved in, or at least kept abreast of, current research findings. It will be able to critique those findings, adjust education programs and inform its practitioners to ensure safe and competent remedial massage practice.

[c] The role of remedial massage therapy in maintaining health status and/or delaying expected progressive deterioration of clients' conditions has been recognised by WorkCover NSW.

APPENDIX 1.1
Massage therapy: systematic reviews

Evidence of benefit

Systematic review	Author(s)	Author(s)' Conclusion
Antenatal perineal massage for reducing perineal trauma	(Beckmann & Garrett, 2006)[47]	Antenatal perineal massage reduces the likelihood of perineal trauma (mainly episiotomies) and the reporting of ongoing perineal pain and is generally well accepted by women. As such, women should be made aware of the likely benefit of perineal massage and provided with information on how to massage.
Preventing perineal trauma during childbirth: a systematic review	(Eason et al, 2000)[48]	Factors shown to increase perineal integrity include avoiding episiotomy, spontaneous or vacuum-assisted rather than forceps birth, and in nulliparas, perineal massage during the weeks before childbirth. Second-stage position has little effect. Further information on techniques to protect the perineum during spontaneous delivery is sorely needed.

Continued

Evidence of benefit—cont'd

Systematic review	Author(s)	Author(s)' Conclusion
Aromatherapy and massage for symptom relief in patients with cancer	(Fellowes et al, 2008)[49]	Massage and aromatherapy massage confer short-term benefits on psychological wellbeing, with the effect on anxiety supported by limited evidence. Effects on physical symptoms may also occur. Evidence is mixed as to whether aromatherapy enhances the effects of massage. Replication, longer follow-up and larger trials are need to accrue the necessary evidence.
A meta-analysis of massage therapy research	(Moyer et al, 2004)[77]	Single applications of massage therapy reduced state of anxiety, blood pressure and heart rate but not negative mood, immediate assessment of pain and cortisol level. Multiple applications reduced delayed assessment of pain. Reductions of trait anxiety and depression were massage therapy's largest effects, with a course of treatment providing benefits similar in magnitude to those of psychotherapy. No moderators were statistically significant, though continued testing is needed. The limitations of a medical model of massage therapy are discussed, and it is proposed that new massage therapy theories and research use a psychotherapy perspective.

Inconclusive evidence – some promising results

Systematic review	Author(s)	Author(s)' Conclusion
Aromatherapy: a systematic review	(Cooke & Ernst, 2000)[53]	These studies suggest that aromatherapy massage has a mild, transient anxiolytic effect. Based on a critical assessment of the six studies relating to relaxation, the effects of aromatherapy are probably not strong enough for it to be considered for the treatment of anxiety. The hypothesis that it is effective for any other indication is not supported by the findings of rigorous clinical trials.
Abdominal massage therapy for chronic constipation: a systematic review of controlled clinical trials	(Ernst, 1999)[61]	The results imply that massage therapy could be a promising treatment for chronic constipation. Future, more rigorous, trials should evaluate its true value.
Massage therapy for low-back pain: a systematic review	(Ernst, 1999)[55]	Massage seems to have some potential as a therapy for low-back pain. More investigations of this subject are urgently needed.
Massage for low-back pain	(Furlan et al, 2008)[78]	Massage might be beneficial for patients with subacute and chronic non-specific low-back pain, especially when combined with exercises and education. The evidence suggests that acupuncture massage is more effective than classic massage, but this needs confirmation. More studies are needed to confirm these conclusions and to assess the impact of massage on return-to-work, and to measure longer-term effects to determine cost-effectiveness of massage as an intervention for low-back pain.
Preventing occupational stress in healthcare workers	(Marine et al, 2006)[79]	Limited evidence is available for the effectiveness of interventions to reduce stress levels in healthcare workers. Larger and better-quality trials are needed.
Nonpharmacological relief of pain during labour: systematic reviews of five methods	(Simkin & O'Hara, 2002)[56]	The five methods included continuous labour support, baths, touch and massage, maternal movement and positioning and intradermal water blocks for back pain relief. An extensive search of electronic databases and other sources identified studies for consideration. Critical evaluation of controlled studies of these five methods suggests that all five may be effective in reducing labour pain and improving other obstetric outcomes, and they are safe when used appropriately. Additional well-designed studies are warranted to further clarify their effect and to evaluate their cost-effectiveness.
Aromatherapy for dementia	(Holt et al, 2003)[57]	Aromatherapy showed benefit for people with dementia in the only trial that contributed data to this review, but there were several methodological difficulties with this study. More well-designed large-scale RCTs are needed before conclusions can be drawn on the effectiveness of aromatherapy. Additionally, several issues need to be addressed, such as whether different aromatherapy interventions are comparable and the possibility that outcomes may vary for different types of dementia.

Inconclusive evidence – some promising results—cont'd

Systematic review	Author(s)	Author(s)' Conclusion
Massage intervention for promoting mental and physical health in infants aged under six months	(Underdown et al, 2006)[58]	The only evidence of a significant impact of massage on growth was obtained from a group of studies regarded to be at high risk of bias. There was, however, some evidence of benefits on mother–infant interaction, sleeping and crying, and on hormones influencing stress levels. In the absence of evidence of harm, these findings may be sufficient to support the use of infant massage in the community, particularly in contexts where infant stimulation is poor. Further research is needed, however, before it will be possible to recommend universal provision.
Massage for promoting growth and development of preterm and/or low birth-weight infants	(Vickers et al, 2004)[60]	Evidence that massage for preterm infants is of benefit for developmental outcomes is weak and does not warrant wider use of preterm infant massage. Where massage is currently provided by nurses, consideration should be given as to whether this is a cost-effective use of time. Future research should assess the effects of massage interventions on clinical outcome measures, such as medical complications or length of stay, and on process-of-care outcomes, such as caregiver or parental satisfaction.
Massage and touch for dementia	(Hansen et al, 2006)[59]	Massage and touch may serve as alternatives or complements to other therapies for the management of behavioural, emotional and perhaps other conditions associated with dementia. More research is needed, however, to provide definitive evidence about the benefits of these interventions.

Inconclusive – further research needed

Systematic review	Author(s)	Author(s)' Conclusion
Deep transverse friction massage (DTFM) for treating tendinitis	(Brosseau et al, 2002)[64]	DTFM combined with other physiotherapy modalities did not show consistent benefit over the control of pain, or improvement of grip strength and functional status for patients with iliotibial band friction syndrome or for patients with extensor carpi radialis tendonitis. These conclusions are limited by the small sample size of the included RCTs. No conclusions can be drawn concerning the use or non-use of DTFM for the treatment of iliotibial band friction syndrome. Future trials, utilising specific iliotibial band friction syndrome methods and adequate sample sizes, are needed before conclusions can be drawn regarding the specific effect of DTFM on tendinitis.
Iliotibial band friction syndrome: a systematic review	(Ellis et al, 2007)[80]	There seems limited evidence to suggest that the conservative treatments that have been studied offer any significant benefit in the management of iliotibial band friction syndrome. Future research will need to re-examine those conservative therapies, which have already been examined, along with others, and will need to be of sufficient quality to enable accurate clinical judgments to be made regarding their use.
Massage for mechanical neck disorders: a systematic review	(Ezzo et al, 2007)[65]	No recommendations for practice can be made at this time because the effectiveness of massage for neck pain remains uncertain. Pilot studies are needed to characterise massage treatment (frequency, duration, number of sessions and massage technique) and establish the optimal treatment to be used in subsequent larger trials that examine the effect of massage as either a stand-alone treatment or part of a multimodal intervention. For multimodal interventions, factorial designs are needed to determine the relative contribution of massage. Future reports of trials should improve reporting of the concealment of allocation, blinding of outcome assessor, adverse events and massage characteristics. Standards of reporting for massage interventions, similar to Consolidated Standards of Reporting Trials, are needed. Both short- and long-term follow-up are needed.
Are manual therapies effective in reducing pain from tension-type headache? A systematic review	(Fernandez-de-Las-Penas et al, 2006)[67]	The most urgent need for further research is to establish the efficacy beyond placebo of the different manual therapies currently applied in patients with tension-type headache.

Continued

Inconclusive – further research needed—cont'd

Systematic review	Author(s)	Author(s)' Conclusion
Massage and touch for dementia	(Hansen et al, 2006)[59]	Massage and touch interventions have been proposed as an alternative or supplement to pharmacological and other treatments to counteract anxiety, agitated behaviour and depression, and if possible to slow down cognitive decline in people with dementia. This review provides an overview of existing research on the use of massage for people with dementia. Eighteen studies of the effects of massage interventions were located, but only two small studies were of a sufficient methodological rigour to count as evidence to answer the question of effect. The small amount of evidence currently available is in favour of massage and touch interventions, but is too limited in scope to allow for general conclusions.
Massage for mechanical neck disorders	(Haraldsson et al, 2006)[66]	No recommendations for practice can be made at this time because the effectiveness of massage for neck pain remains uncertain. Pilot studies are needed to characterise massage treatment (frequency, duration, number of sessions and massage technique) and establish the optimal treatment to be used in subsequent larger trials that examine the effect of massage as either a stand-alone treatment or part of a multimodal intervention. For multimodal interventions, factorial designs are needed to determine the relative contribution of massage. Future reports of trials should improve reporting of the concealment of allocation, blinding of outcome assessor, adverse events and massage characteristics. Standards of reporting for massage interventions, similar to CONSORT, are needed. Both short- and long-term follow-up are needed.
Manual therapy for asthma	(Hondras, Linde & Jones, 2005)[69]	The review found there is not enough evidence from trials to show whether manual therapies can improve asthma symptoms, and more research is needed.
Therapeutic touch for healing acute wounds	(O'Mathuna & Ashford, 2003)[68]	There is no evidence that therapeutic touch promotes healing of acute wounds.
Physical therapies for reducing and controlling lymphoedema of the limbs	(Preston et al, 2004)[62]	All three trials have their limitations and have yet to be replicated, so their results must be viewed with caution. There is a clear need for well-designed, randomised trials of the whole range of physical therapies if the best approach to managing lymphoedema is to be determined.
Therapeutic touch for anxiety disorders	(Robinson et al, 2007)[81]	Given the high prevalence of anxiety disorders and the current paucity of evidence on therapeutic touch in this population, there is a need for well-conducted, randomised, controlled trials to examine the effectiveness of therapeutic touch for anxiety disorders.

REFERENCES

1. Ernst E. The safety of massage therapy. Rheumatology 2003;42:1101–6.
2. Peters D, Chaitow L, Harris G, et al. Integrating complementary therapies in primary care. Edinburgh: Churchill Livingstone; 2002.
3. House of Lords Select Committee on Science and Technology. Complementary and Alternative Medicine 2000. Online. Available: www.publications.parliament.uk/pa/ld199900/ldselect/ldsctech/123/12302.htm; 2002.
4. Cox C. Remedial massage. J Complement Med 2003;2(1):24–9.
5. Australian Standard Classification of Occupations. 349-11 Massage Therapist. Online. Available: http://www.abs.gov.au/Ausstats/ABS@.nsf/0/C96E19BE6C3FB351CA25697E0018502C?opendocument; 1997.
6. Australian Standard Classification of Education. 061711 Massage Therapy. Available from: http://www.abs.gov.au/AUSSTATS/ABS@.NSF/0/DE3341F1D2B22D28CA256AAF001FCAA0?opendocument; 2001.
7. Association of Massage Therapists Ltd. Membership Levels. Online. Available: http://www.amt-ltd.org.au/index.php?Page=Join%20AMT_Membership%20Levels_1.php; 2009.
8. Australian Association of Massage Therapists. Membership Structure. Online. Available: http://www.aamt.com.au/page.php?pgname=MemberStruct; 2009.
9. Australian Traditional Medicine Society. Membership Qualifications. Online. Available from: http://www.atms.com.au/membership/Membership_Qual.asp; 2009.
10. Gordon Institute of TAFE. Advanced Diploma of Remedial Massage (Myotherapy). Online. Available: http://www.gordontafe.edu.au/index.cfm?action=5&secAction=1&terAction=1&Search; 2009.
11. Endeavour College of Natural Health. Bachelor of Health Science (Musculoskeletal Therapy). Online. Available: http://www.endeavour.edu.au/courses/musculoskeletal-therapy/; 2009.
12. Australian Qualifications Framework Council. AQF Qualifications. Online. Available: http://www.aqf.edu.au/AbouttheAQF/AQFQualifications/tabid/98/Default.aspx; 2009.
13. Xue C, Zhang A, Lin V, et al. Complementary and alternative medicine use in Australia: a national population-based survey. J Altern Complement Med 2007;13(6):643–50.
14. MacLennan AH, Wilson DH, Taylor AW. Prevalence and cost of alternative medicine in Australia. Lancet 1996;437:569–73.
15. MacLennan AH, Wilson DH, Taylor AW. The escalating cost and prevalence of alternative medicine. Prev Med 2002;35:166–73.
16. MacLennan AH, Myers SP, Taylor AW. The continuing use of complementary and alternative medicine in South Australia: costs and beliefs in 2004. Med J Aust 2006;184(1):27–31.
17. Australian Government Productivity Commission. Australia's Health Workforce 2005. Online. Available: www.pc.gov.au/study/healthworkforce/finalreport/html; 2006.
18. Australian Institute of Health and Welfare. Health and community services labour force, 2001.

Canberra: Australian Institute of Health and Welfare; 2003.
19. Khoury R. Introduction to the Australian Traditional Medicine Society 2004; Online. Available: www.atms.com.au; 2006 (30/09).
20. Australian Traditional Medicine Society. Welcome to the Australian traditional medicine society. Online. Available: http://www.atms.com.au/index.asp; 2010.
21. Australian Natural Therapists' Association. Practitioner Search. Online. Available: www.anta.com.au; 2005.
22. Australian Traditional Medicine Society. Qualified natural therapists membership directory 2007. Sydney: Australian Traditional Medicine Society; 2007.
23. Hale A. 2002 National Survey of Remedial Therapists. J Aust Tradit Med Soc 2003;9(3):119–24.
24. Grace S. Integrative medicine in Australian health care. Rotterdam: Sense; 2009.
25. Bensoussan A, Myers S, Wu SM, et al. A profile of naturopathic and western herbal medicine practitioners in Australia. Sydney: CompleMED, University of Western Sydney; 2003.
26. Hale A. 2002 Survey of ATMS: acupuncturists, herbalists and naturopaths. Journal of the Australian Traditional Medicine Society 2002;8(4):143–9.
27. Martin JB. Historical and professional perspectives of complementary and alternative medicine with a particular emphasis on rediscovering and embracing complementary and alternative medicine in contemporary Western society. J Altern Complement Med 2001;7(Supplement 1):11–18.
28. Perry R, Dowrick C. Complementary medicine and general practice: an urban perspective. Complement Ther Med 2000;8(2):71–5.
29. Australian Medical Association. Position Statement: Complementary Medicine 2001. Online. Available: http://www.ama.com.au/web.nsf/doc/SHED-5FK4U9; 2001.
30. Berman B, Singh BK, Lao L, et al. Physicians' attitudes toward complementary or alternative medicine: a regional survey. J Am Board Fam Pract 1995;8(5):361–6.
31. Verhoef M, Sutherland LR. Alternative medicine and general practitioners. Can Fam Physician 1995;41: 1005–11.
32. White A, Resch K-L, Ernst E. Complementary medicine: use and attitudes among GPs. Fam Pract 1997;14:302–6.
33. Easthope G, Tranter B, Gill G. Normal medical practice of referring patients for complementary therapies among Australian general practitioners. Complement Ther Med 2000;8:226–33.
34. Easthope G, Tranter B, Gill G. General practitioners' attitudes towards complementary therapies. Soc Sci Med 2000;51:1555–61.
35. Hall K, Giles-Corti B. Complementary therapies and the general practitioner: a survey of Perth GPs. Aust Fam Physician 2000;29(6):602–6.
36. Cohen M. CAM practitioners and 'regular' doctors: is integration possible? Med J Aust 2004;180(12): 645–6.
37. Dwyer JA. Good medicine and bad medicine: science to promote the convergence of 'alternative' and orthodox medicine. Med J Aust 2004;180(12): 647–8.
38. Phelps K. Speech to the Natural and Complementary Healthcare Summit 2001; 2006 (25 January). Online. Available: www.ama.com.au/web.nsf/doc/WEEN-5GB44J.
39. Nahin RL, Straus SE. Research into complementary and alternative medicine: problems and potential. BMJ 2001;322(7279):161–4.
40. Archer C. Research issues in complementary therapies. Complement Ther Nurs Midwifery 1999;5(4):108–14.
41. Teicher LA. Nursing the human: not the machine. Aust J Holist Nurs 1996;3(1):41–4.
42. Black D. Pigs in the dirt: how a little common sense can help resolve the healthcare mess. Health & Wellness Report 1993;3(9):1–6.
43. Capra F. Turning point. London: HarperCollins; 1983.
44. Green S, editor. The Cochrane collaboration ten years on: achievements of the past, challenges for the future and the relevance to integrative medicine. Holistic Solutions for Sustainable Healthcare Tenth International Holistic Health Conference. Coffs Harbour: Australian Integrative Medicine Association; 2004.
45. Ernst E. Massage therapy: is its evidence-base getting stronger? Complement Health Pract Rev 2007;12(3):179–83.
46. Grace S. The evidence for massage therapy. In: Casanelia L, Stelfox D, editors. Foundations of massage. 3rd edn. Chatswood, NSW: Elsevier; 2010.
47. Beckmann MM, Garrett AJ. Antenatal perineal massage for reducing perineal trauma. Cochrane Database Syst Rev 2006;(1)CD005123.
48. Eason E, Labrecque M, Wells G, et al. Preventing perineal trauma during childbirth: a systematic review. Obstet Gynecol 2000;95(3):464–71.
49. Fellowes D, Barnes K, Wilkinson S. Aromatherapy and massage for symptom relief in patients with cancer. Cochrane Database Syst Rev 2008;(4) CD002287.
50. Brattberg G. Connective tissue massage in the treatment of fibromyalgia. Eur J Pain 1999;3: 235–45.
51. Field T, Grizzle N, Scafidi F, et al. Massage relaxation therapies' effects on depressed adolescent mothers. Adolescence 1996;31:903–11.
52. Hernandez-Reif M, Martinez A, Field T. Premenstrual symptoms are relieved by massage therapy. J Psychosom Obstet Gynaecol 2000;18: 238–45.
53. Cooke B, Ernst E. Aromatherapy: a systematic review. Br J Gen Pract 2000;50:493–6.
54. Furlan A, van Tulder M, Cherkin D, et al. Acupuncture and dry-needling for low back pain. Cochrane Database Syst Rev 2005;(1)CD001351.
55. Ernst E. Massage therapy for low back pain: a systematic review. J Pain Symptom Manage 1999;17(1):65–9.
56. Simkin PP, O'Hara M. Nonpharmacologic relief of pain during labor: systematic reviews of five methods. Am J Obstet Gynecol 2002;186(5 Suppl Nature):S131–59.
57. Holt FE, Birks TPH, Thorgrimsen LM, et al. Aromatherapy for dementia. Cochrane Database Syst Rev 2003;(3)CD003150.
58. Underdown A, Barlow J, Chung V, Stewart-Brown S. Massage intervention for promoting mental and physical health in infants aged under six months. Cochrane Database Syst Rev 2006;(4)CD005038.
59. Hansen NV, Jørgensen T, Ørtenblad L. Massage and touch for dementia. Cochrane Database Syst Rev 2006;(4)CD004989.
60. Vickers A, Ohlsson A, Lacy J, Horsley A. Massage for promoting growth and development of preterm and/or low birth-weight infants. Cochrane Database Syst Rev 2004;(2)CD000390.
61. Ernst E. Abdominal massage therapy for chronic constipation: a systematic review of controlled clinical trials. Forsch Komplementmed 1999;6(3): 149–51.
62. Preston NJ, Seers K, Mortimer PS. Physical therapies for reducing and controlling lymphoedema of the limbs. Cochrane Database Syst Rev 2004;(4) CD003141.
63. Vairo G, Sayers J, McBrier N, et al. Systematic review of efficacy for manual lymphatic drainage techniques in sports medicine and rehabilitation: an evidence-based practice approach. J Man Manip Ther 2009;17(3):e80–9.
64. Brosseau L, Casimiro L, Milne S, et al. Deep transverse friction massage for treating tendinitis. Cochrane Database Syst Rev 2002;(4)CD003528.
65. Ezzo J, Haraldsson BG, Gross AR, et al. Massage for mechanical neck disorders: a systematic review. Spine 2007;32(3):353–62.
66. Haraldsson B, Gross A, Myers CD, Ezzo J, Morien A, Goldsmith CH, Peloso PMJ, Brønfort G, Cervical Overview Group. Massage for mechanical neck disorders. Cochrane Database of Systematic Reviews 2006;(3)CD004871.
67. Fernandez-de-Las-Penas C, Alonso-Blanco C, Cuadrado ML, et al. Are manual therapies effective in reducing pain from tension-type headache? A systematic review. Clin J Pain 2006;22(3):278–85.
68. O'Mathuna DP, Ashford RL. Therapeutic touch for healing acute wounds. Cochrane Database Syst Rev 2003;(4)CD002766.
69. Hondras MA, Linde K, Jones AP. Manual therapy for asthma. Cochrane Database Syst Rev 2005;(2) CD001002.
70. Berman B. Cochrane Complementary Medicine Field. Online. Available: http://compmed.umm.edu/compmed/cochrane/cochrane.htm; 2003.
71. NHS Research and Development Centre for Evidence-Based Medicine. Teaching Materials. Oxford: NHS Research and Development Centre for Evidence-Based Medicine; [cited 1999 13/04]. Online. Available: cebm.jr2.ox.ac.uk/index.extras; 1999.
72. Chesney MA. International research conference highlights progress, new directions. Edmonton, Alberta: CAM at the NIH. Focus on Complementary and Alternative Medicine; 2006 [updated 29/10/2006; cited XIII 2].
73. Harlan WR. Research on complementary and alternative medicine using randomized controlled trials. J Altern Complement Med 2001;7(Supplement 1):S-45–52.
74. Chesney MA, Straus SE. Complementary and alternative medicine: the convergence of public interest and science in the United States. Med J Aust 2004;181(6):335–6.
75. National Health and Medical Research Council. Special Call for Research Applications into Complementary and Alternative Medicine. Canberra: Australian Government National Health and Medical Research Council. Online. Available: http://www.nhmrc.gov.au/funding/types/granttype; 2006 [cited 2007 17 March].
76. Australian Government Department of Health and Ageing. Australian Better Health Initiative: Promoting Good Health, Prevention and Early Intervention. Canberra: Department of Health and Ageing. Online. Available: www.health.gov.au/internet/wcms/publiching.nsf/Content/feb2006coag03.htm; 2006 [cited 2007 31 January].
77. Moyer CA, Rounds J, Hannum JW. A meta-analysis of massage therapy research. Psychol Bull 2004;130(1):3–18.
78. Furlan AD, Imamura M, Dryden T, Irvin E. Massage for low-back pain. Cochrane Database Syst Rev 2008;(4)CD001929.
79. Marine A, Ruotsalainen J, Serra C, Verbeek J. Preventing occupational stress in healthcare workers. Cochrane Database Syst Rev 2006;(4) CD002892.
80. Ellis R, Hing W, Reid D. Iliotibial band friction syndrome: a systematic review. Manual Therapy 2007;12(3):200–8.
81. Robinson J, Biley FC, Dolk H. Therapeutic touch for anxiety disorders. Cochrane Database Syst Rev 2007;(3)CD006240.

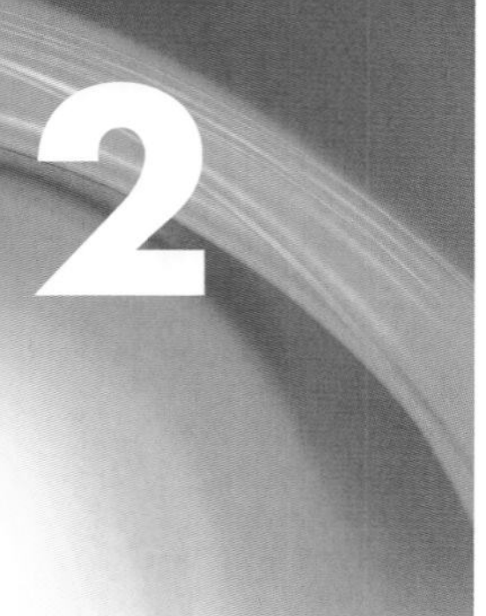

2 Assessment procedures for remedial massage: an evidence-based approach

The content of this chapter relates to the following Units of Competency:

HLTAP501B Analyse health information
HLTREM504C Apply remedial massage assessment framework
HLTREM505C Perform remedial massage health assessment

Health Training Package HLT07

Learning Outcomes

- Demonstrate an understanding of the role of assessment in remedial massage practice.
- Demonstrate an understanding of the current evidence-based approach to musculoskeletal assessment.
- Identify red and yellow flags when conducting remedial massage assessment.
- Perform appropriate remedial massage assessments (case histories, outcome measures, postural observation, gait analysis, functional assessments and palpation) on a range of clients.
- Analyse and interpret assessment findings to guide the assessment process.

INTRODUCTION

As primary care practitioners, remedial massage therapists are required to make clinical judgments including identifying those clients whose treatment lies outside their scope of practice. It is estimated that between 34% and 40% of clients who visit complementary medicine practitioners have not been previously assessed by a general medical or other health practitioner.[1,2] It is, therefore, a key safety requirement of remedial massage training to adequately prepare practitioners for their primary contact role. Moreover, remedial massage is not entirely risk free, even though adverse events appear to be rare.[3] Competent performance and analysis of appropriate remedial massage assessments, including the selection of appropriate assessment procedures for individual clients, is essential for safe and effective remedial massage practice.

PRINCIPLES OF ASSESSMENT IN REMEDIAL MASSAGE PRACTICE

- Remedial massage should always be performed in conjunction with appropriate and ongoing assessment.[a]
- A definitive assessment is not always possible or necessary for many musculoskeletal problems. It is essential, however, that clients requiring referral to other healthcare practitioners are identified (red and yellow flags).
- A holistic approach to assessment considers all aspects of a client's biopsychosocial health.
- Remedial massage assessments are conducted in a logical order, usually beginning with a case history. Interpretations of assessment findings progressively guide the need for further assessments.
- Findings of individual assessments should always be interpreted cautiously and correlated with findings from other assessments.
- Assessment findings guide remedial massage practice: negotiating treatment plans with clients, monitoring responses to treatment, adjusting treatments and reviewing plans as required.
- Strategies for assessing remedial massage clients may change with emerging evidence about the efficacy of individual assessments.

PURPOSE OF ASSESSMENTS

The purpose of remedial massage assessment is to:

- identify indicators of serious conditions (red flags)
- identify the presence of psychosocial factors that may influence presenting symptoms and response to treatment (yellow flags)
- assess clients' functional limitations
- guide treatment and management options
- monitor clients' responses to treatment so that treatment plans can be adjusted if required
- assess treatment effectiveness.

[a]This is the current view of educators and professional associations of remedial massage in Australia. However, remedial massage, particularly seated massage, corporate massage and post-event sports massage is frequently performed without full assessment of clients.

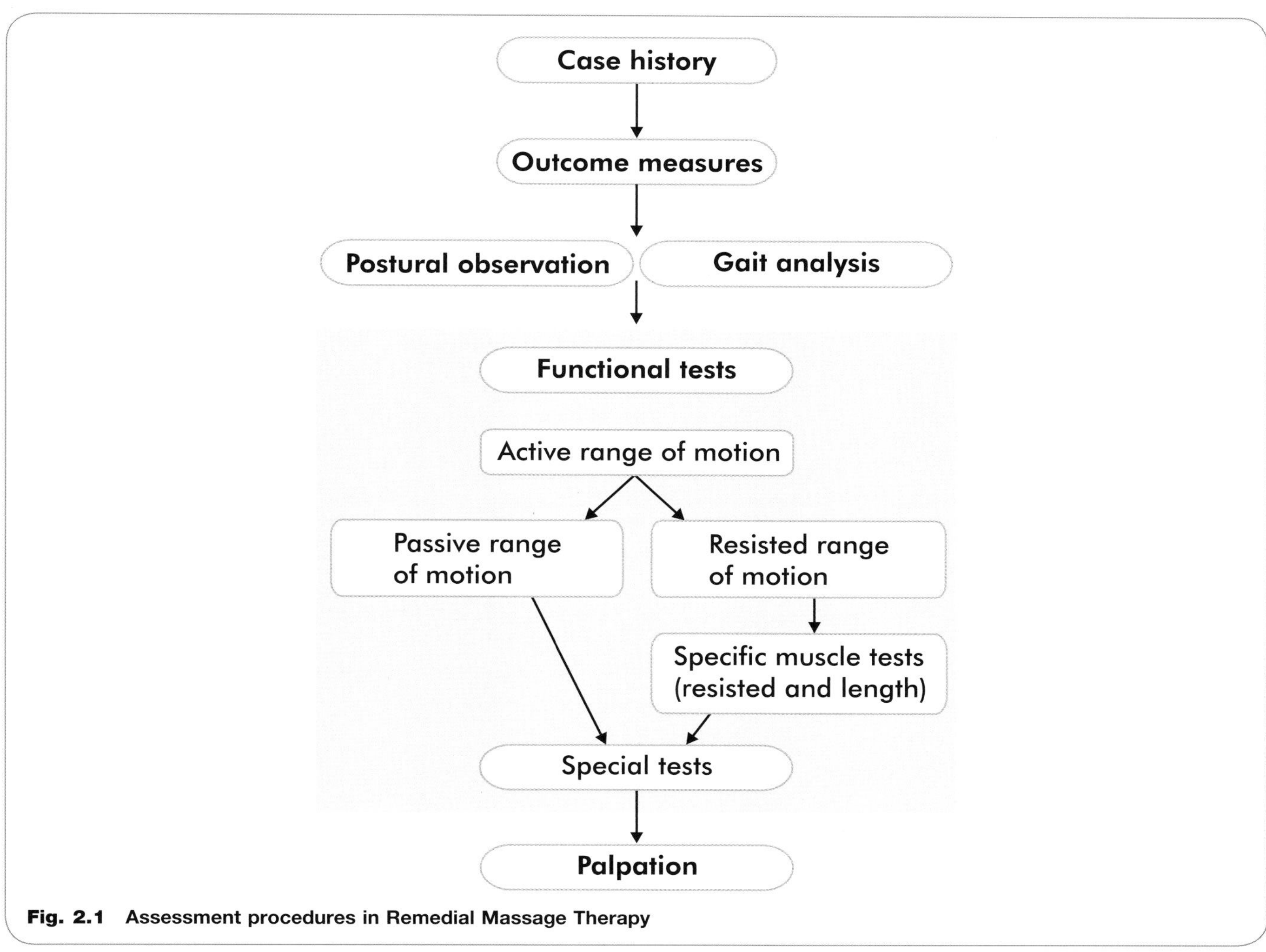

Fig. 2.1 Assessment procedures in Remedial Massage Therapy

DEMONSTRATING TREATMENT EFFECTIVENESS

To monitor clients' responses to treatment, remedial massage therapists must first collect suitable baseline data, including information collected from case histories and observed or measured by practitioners. The pain scale is commonly used for this purpose. Repeated collection of pain scale data enables changes in clients' perceptions of pain to be recorded and may demonstrate the perceived effectiveness of treatment. The amount of medication that clients require to manage symptoms can also be used in this way. Recording details of medication at the initial consultation and changes in medication use over the ensuing period of treatment provides evidence of progress towards treatment goals.

ASSESSMENT PROCEDURES

The most commonly used assessment tools in remedial massage therapy are presented below in the order in which they are usually applied and easiest to learn. In reality, assessments are overlapping and ongoing throughout the consultation from first encounters with clients in waiting rooms to the continual assessments and adjustments that are required when applying any technique (e.g. for pain tolerance, for age, to meet clients' expectation). A flowchart of remedial massage assessments is illustrated in Figure 2.1.

CLIENT HISTORY

Taking a comprehensive client history is one of the most important assessment tools of healthcare practitioners. It is an important opportunity to establish relationships with clients that enhance positive outcomes of treatment.[4,5] It also enables the practitioner to learn about the biopsychosocial influences on the client's health. The first responsibility of remedial massage therapists is to determine clients' suitability for remedial massage or for referral to another healthcare practitioner. The term *red flag* refers to clinical features (signs or symptoms) that may indicate the presence of serious underlying medical conditions requiring further investigation. Such conditions include cancers, fractures and infections (see Table 2.1 on p 12). Clients who choose to complement medical treatment of serious conditions with remedial massage therapy require supervision by their medical practitioner and liaison between practitioners (or at the very least awareness of the entirety of their clients' treatment). Clients should always be encouraged to disclose their remedial massage treatment to

NAME .... DATE OF BIRTH ....

ADDRESS ....

.... POSTCODE ....

PHONE B/H ________________ A/H ________________ Mobile ________________

FAX __________ ____________ EMAIL ________________________________

OCCUPATION

SPORTS / HOBBIES

REFERRED BY

PRESENTING SYMPTOMS *How can I help you?* Record nature of complaint and duration. Inquire and record: nature of pain, frequency and intensity of symptoms, first occurrence, mode of onset. If recurrent, previous treatment. Associated symptoms. Aggravating and relieving factors. Any other symptoms. IDENTIFY POSSIBLE RED AND YELLOW FLAGS.

PAST HISTORY *Have you ever had any major illnesses or diseases? Any hospitalisations? Any major accidents?* IDENTIFY POSSIBLE RED AND YELLOW FLAGS.

FAMILY HISTORY *Has any member of your family had a major illness or disease?*

OBSTETRICS HISTORY Ask any female client about pregnancies and births.

SOCIAL HISTORY *Do you drink or smoke? Recreational drugs?*

MEDICATION *Are you taking any medication?* Record all details.

ALLERGIES *Do you have any allergies?* Record all details.

SYSTEMS REVIEW Either by questionnaire or orally, ask a few questions relating to each system as required. (Central nervous: headaches, dizziness, numbness. Cardiovascular: chest pain, shortness of breath. Respiratory system: shortness of breath, wheezing, cough. Alimentary: nausea, vomiting, indigestion, abdominal pain, change in bowel habit. Urogenital: pain on urination, frequency of urination. Endocrine: Heat or cold intolerance, change in sweating, excessive thirst.)

Fig. 2.2 **A typical case history form for remedial massage**

Table 2.1 Red and yellow flags

Red flags	**Yellow flags**
Clinical features that may be associated with the presence of a serious physical condition.	Psychosocial and occupational factors that may influence presenting symptoms, treatment approach and outcomes.

their doctor. However, many remedial massage clients do not have serious medical conditions. If there are no signs or symptoms associated with specific diseases or serious conditions, further investigations (such as X-rays, MRIs or blood tests) are generally not indicated.[6, 7]

Once practitioners have dismissed the likelihood of serious conditions, they gather information to guide further assessments: identifying likely contributing factors, types of tissues that could be involved, clients' responses to previous treatments, aggravating and relieving factors and psychosocial factors that could affect clients' responses to treatment (yellow flags). Questions should proceed logically and presenting conditions prioritised. A sound grounding in physiology, pathology and symptomatology is required for analysing the health information collected and for recognising deviations from normal findings and signs and symptoms of common pathophysiologies. Practitioners are not required to read X-rays, MRIs or other diagnostic imaging but they are expected to interpret their reports. Figure 2.2 is a typical remedial massage case history.

Assessing the well client

Remedial massage has long played a role in health maintenance and preventive medicine. Assessment of the well client is based on lifestyle history, postural and gait observations, functional tests, particularly those for muscle and joint function, and palpation. Clients who present for massage therapy without symptoms are sometimes surprised when massage elicits pain or tenderness or when they feel the ropiness of fibrotic tissues or the tightness of a muscle being stretched.

They are being made aware of potential muscle imbalances that could lead to future problems (sub-clinical indicators). Early interventions (e.g. correcting posture, improving manual handling techniques, or modifying an exercise program) may divert many potential problems.

THE NATURE OF PAIN

Pain is a common presenting symptom of remedial massage clients. Perceptions of pain are complicated by its multi-dimensional nature and its changing nature over time. Questioning clients about pain helps determine their suitability for remedial massage and possible sources of pain. Ask clients about:

- the location of the pain
- the character of the pain, e.g. sharp shooting pain in a relatively narrow band (radicular pain), a dull ache that is hard to localise (referred pain), burning pain (from trauma to sympathetic and somatic sensory nerves)
- the severity of the pain
  - A number of pain intensity measures are available although the validity and reliability of such measures continues to be debated.[8] A simple procedure is to ask clients to rate their pain on a pain scale from 0 to 10, where 0 is no pain and 10 is extreme pain. Alternatively, practitioners can use a Visual Analogue Scale of Pain Intensity (VAS), a 10 cm line on which clients are asked to put a mark to show their current pain level.
- the onset of the pain
- the duration of the pain
- the course of the pain, e.g. intermittent, constant, episodic
- aggravating and relieving factors.

Questions designed to distinguish between pain of local origin and pain referred from a distant site (in particular, from a spinal segment) are useful in directing treatment to the source of pain. As a guide for determining the nature of pain, consider the following:

- local pain
  - usually sharp
  - well localised
- referred pain
  - dull
  - poorly localised
  - often refers in a predetermined pattern (e.g. nerve impingement at the spinal segment will refer pain in dermatomal patterns, trigger points refer in predictable patterns).

If a client reports numbness in an area of skin, the nerves supplying that dermatome[b] could be damaged. Similarly, if a client reports weak muscles in a particular myotome, the motor neuron in that spinal segment may be damaged. Knowing the spinal cord segment which supplies each dermatome and myotome can help locate the source of pain (see Figure 2.3).

[b]Every spinal nerve contains both sensory and motor neurons. Somatic sensory neurons carry impulses from the skin to the spinal cord and brain stem. A dermatome is the area of skin that provides sensory input to one pair of spinal nerves. Somatic motor neurons carry impulses from the spinal cord to skeletal muscles. All muscles innervated by the motor neurons in a single spinal segment constitute a myotome. In general, dermatomes overlie corresponding myotomes.

Table 2.2 (p 15) is designed to assist practitioners identify red flags associated with pain of the lumbar, thoracic and cervical regions.

Identifying yellow flags

Yellow flags are indicators of psychosocial and occupational factors that may affect clients' presenting symptoms and responses to treatment. Identifying the presence of yellow flags may prompt early interventions and better outcomes for clients. For example, clients with high stress levels may benefit from referral to a counsellor; clients with concern about job security after extended absences from work may benefit from reassurance from their employer. The presence of yellow flags is not a contraindication for remedial massage. Rather, yellow flags alert the practitioner to possible complicating factors which may prompt referral to other health practitioners or delay the normal recovery process.

Yellow flags include:[6]

- belief that pain and activity are harmful
- sickness behaviours (e.g. extended rest)
- low or negative moods, social withdrawal
- problems with claims and compensation
- overprotective or unsupportive family
- apportioning blame
- overt anxiety or depression
- non-compliance with rehabilitation program
- long time between injury and referral.

Informed consent

As part of the initial interview clients need to have proposed assessments and treatments and any associated risks fully explained. Informed consent must be obtained for all assessment and treatment procedures.[9]

OUTCOME MEASURES

Outcome measures are standardised questionnaires in which clients record perceived changes to their health status. They are used to assess clients' perceived health status and also to demonstrate the benefits of treatment. Three common outcome measures for musculoskeletal pain and disability are the Oswestry Disability Index, the Vernon Mior Neck Disability Questionnaire, and the Patient Specific Scale which can be used for disability in any region of the body. Research into the use of Outcome Measures demonstrate high validity[c] and reliability[d, 10–12] for some questionnaires which may account for their increasing use in clinical trials and in clinical practice. They are simple to administer and their standardised scoring systems allow comparisons of clients' responses over time. They are also readily interpreted by healthcare practitioners from other disciplines.

Completing questionnaires takes time and clients with low levels of English literacy will need assistance. Appointment times may need to be adjusted accordingly or clients invited to come to the clinic a few minutes before their scheduled appointment to complete the questionnaires. Outcome

[c]Validity is the extent to which a measure estimates the true nature of what it purports to measure.
[d]Reliability is the consistency of repeated applications of a measurement.

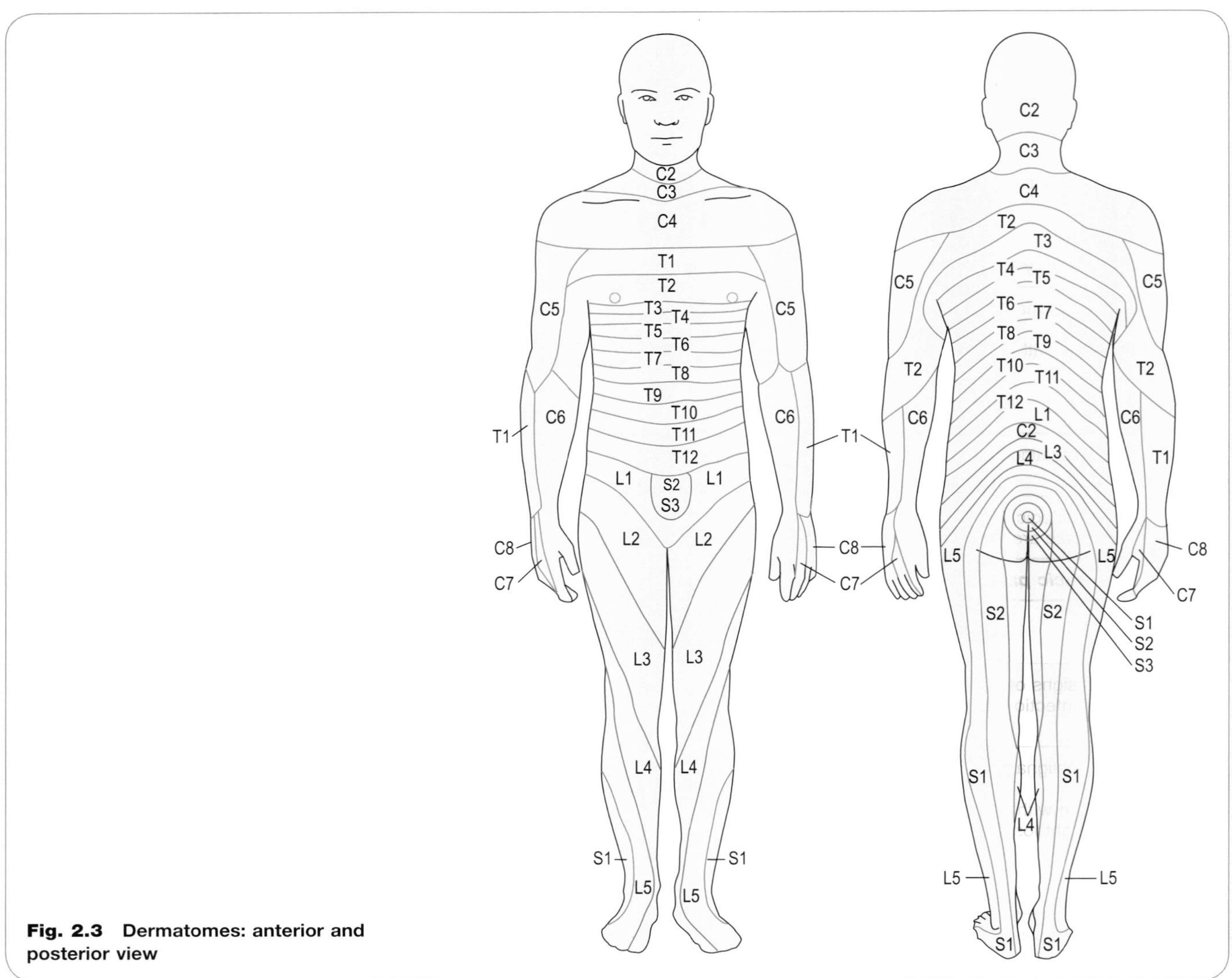

Fig. 2.3 Dermatomes: anterior and posterior view

measures should be used at every opportunity by remedial massage therapists to demonstrate perceived effectiveness of their treatments.

POSTURAL ANALYSIS

Postural observation forms an important part of the physical assessment of clients. It involves observing clients standing erect to assess structural and habitual postures and their associated muscle imbalances. Observing the whole client, regardless of the complaint, is consistent with the holistic approach of complementary medicine. Postural observation is not an exact science. However, findings from postural observation, along with case history and other assessment findings, can contribute useful information to the development of treatment plans.

By observing erect postures from the posterior and lateral aspects, practitioners can compare one side of the body with the other, the upper half with the lower half, the left foot with the right foot and so on to identify postural patterns and/or factors that could contribute to presenting conditions or predispose to future symptoms. Postural observation can provide information about the effects on the musculoskeletal system of right or left dominance, of regular sports and hobbies, of work-related activities and of adaptations to diseases and traumas. For example, cervicogenic headaches can be perpetuated by a scoliosis and without postural observation this connection could remain undetected. Failing to take such predisposing factors into account could result in short-lived treatment effects. Moreover conditions and postural tendencies identified (sometimes incidentally) can prompt appropriate advice from therapists. For example, advising a client with bilateral pes planus about appropriate footwear, or a client who works at a computer all day about the importance of regular pectoralis major stretches, may prevent compensatory muscle imbalances and reduce susceptibility to injury.

Identifying anatomical landmarks

To accurately describe and record postural observations, practitioners should be familiar with the following anatomical landmarks (see Figure 2.4 on p 16):

Table 2.2 Red flags of serious conditions associated with acute low back, thoracic and neck pain

Red flags	Possible condition
For acute low back pain	
Symptoms and signs of infection (e.g. fever) Risk factors for infection (e.g. underlying disease, immunosuppression, penetrating wound)	Infection
History of trauma Minor trauma (if >50 years, history of osteoporosis, taking corticosteroids)	Fracture
Past history of malignancy Age >50 years Failure to improve with treatment Unexplained weight loss Pain at multiple sites Pain at rest	Cancer
Absence of aggravating factors	Aortic aneurysm Other serious condition
Widespread neurological symptoms and signs in the lower limb (e.g. gait abnormality, saddle area numbness) ± urinary retention, faecal incontinence	Cauda equina syndrome (a medical emergency and requires urgent hospital referral)
For acute thoracic pain	
Minor trauma (if >50 years, history of osteoporosis, taking corticosteroids) Major trauma	Fracture
Symptoms and signs of infection (e.g. fever, night sweats) Risk factors for infection (e.g. underlying disease, immunosuppression, penetrating wound)	Infection
Past history of malignancy Age >50 years Failure to improve with treatment Unexplained weight loss Pain at multiple sites Pain at rest Night pain	Cancer
Chest pain or heaviness Movement/change in posture has no effect on pain Abdominal pain Shortness of breath, cough	Other serious condition
For acute neck pain	
Symptoms and signs of infection (e.g. fever, night sweats) Risk factors for infection (e.g. underlying disease, immunosuppression, penetrating wound)	Infection
History of trauma Minor trauma (if taking corticosteroids)	Fracture
Past history of malignancy Age >50 years Failure to improve with treatment Unexplained weight loss Dysphagia, headache, vomiting	Cancer
Neurological symptoms in the limbs	Neurological condition
Cerebrovascular symptoms or signs, anticoagulant use	Cerebral or spinal haemorrhage
Cardiovascular risk factors; transient ischaemic attack	Vertebral or carotid aneurysm

Note that acute pain in this context refers to pain of less than three months' duration.
Adapted from the New Zealand Guidelines Group[6] and the Acute Musculoskeletal Pain Guidelines Group[7].

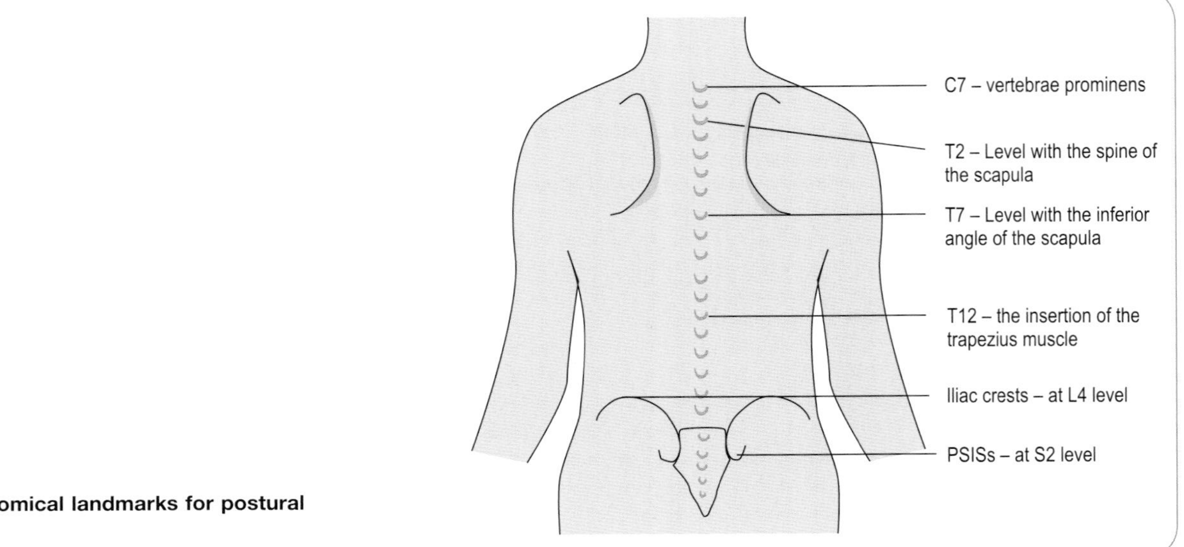

Fig. 2.4 Anatomical landmarks for postural observation.

ANTERIOR AND LATERAL

- The nipple line is approximately level with the 5th rib or 4th intercostal space.
- The umbilicus is approximately level with the L3/4 disc.
- The iliac crests are approximately level with L4.

POSTERIOR

- The spine of the scapula is approximately level with T2 spinous process.
- The inferior angle of the scapula is approximately level with T7.
- The insertion of the trapezius muscle is approximately level with T12.
- The PSISs are approximately level with S2.

Performing postural observation

Clothing that does not obscure posture is required for the most accurate postural assessments. Swimwear or sportswear are suitable. Alternatively clients may disrobe to their underwear and wear a gown that opens at the back. Stand two or three metres behind the client. Ask the client to walk up and down on the spot a few times with their eyes closed and then to open their eyes, and stand comfortably, hands by their sides.

A plumb line (either real or imaginary) is used to project a centre of gravity line onto the external surface of the body. In the ideally aligned erect posture, the plumb line should pass as follows (see Figure 2.5).

In the posterior view:

- equidistant through the heels, ankles, calves, knees and thighs
- through the midline of the trunk
- through the midline of the neck and head.

In the lateral view:

- anterior to the lateral malleolus[e]
- anterior to the axis of the knee joint
- posterior to the hip joint
- through the bodies of L1 and L5
- bisecting the shoulder joint
- bisecting the ear.

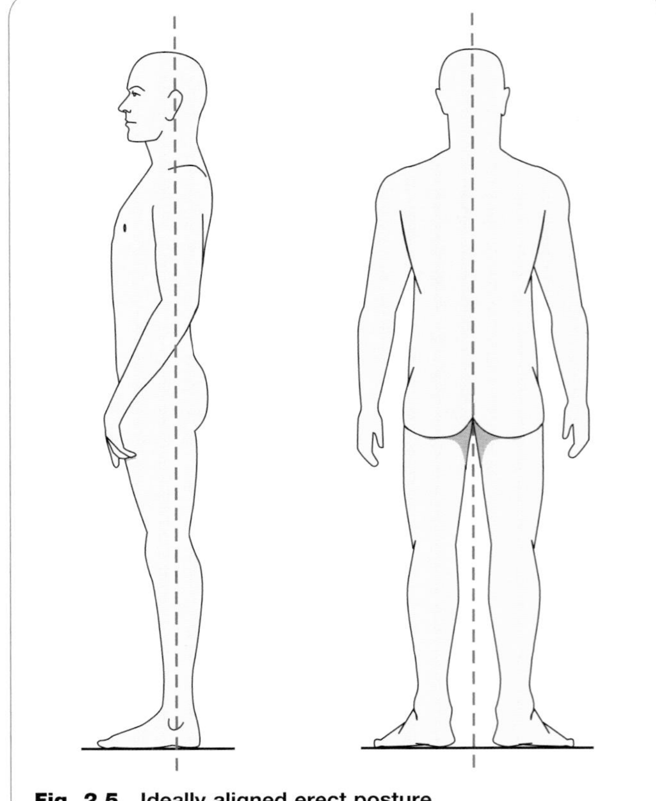

Fig. 2.5 Ideally aligned erect posture

[e]Some controversy exists among authors about the exact location of the centre of gravity line in the lateral view. It is sometimes said to bisect the lateral malleolus, rather than pass anteriorly to it.

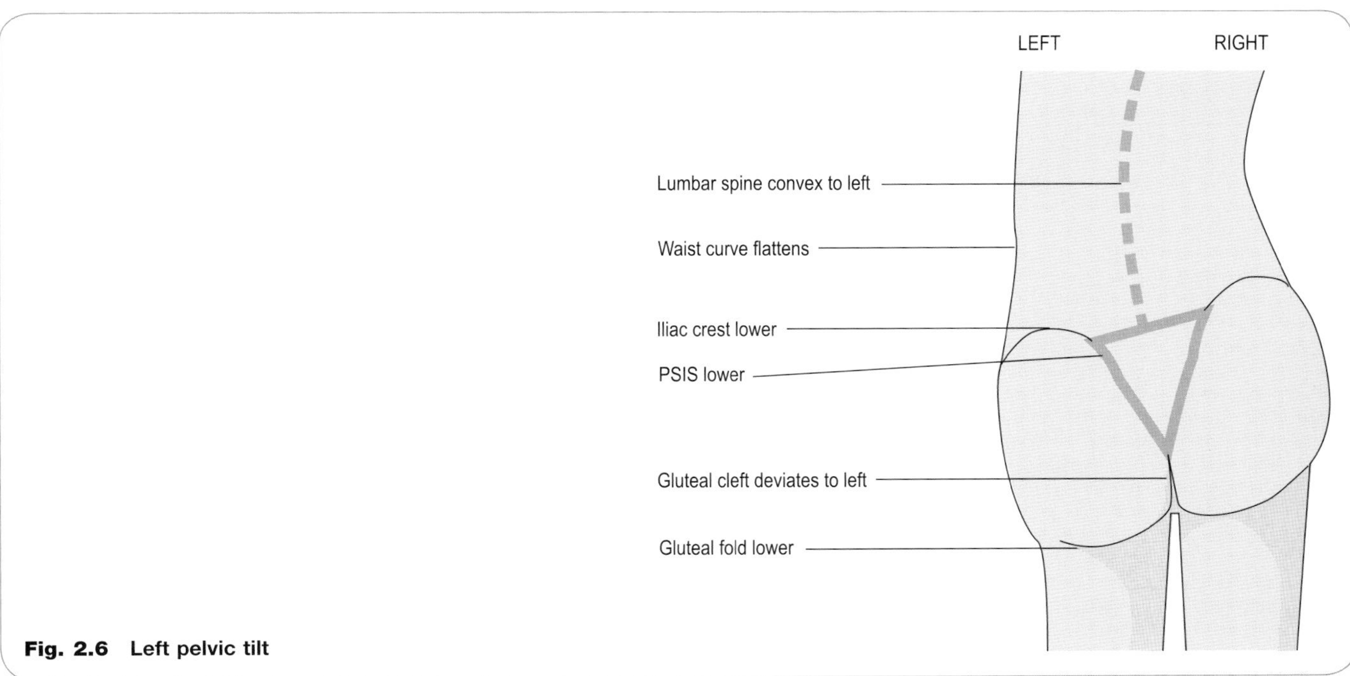

Fig. 2.6 Left pelvic tilt

General observations

A common reason that remedial massage therapists find postural observation difficult is that they look for detail before making general observations. Always begin by asking, 'What stands out? Are there any regions of the body that appear to be overloaded, under stress or very different from normal?' Next, focus on pelvic alignment which is useful for identifying common posture deviations like hyperlordosis or scoliosis. Learning to observe details like colour changes (e.g. the pallor of poor circulation, butterfly rash across the cheeks in rheumatoid conditions, a hairy tuft in the lumbosacral area in spondylolisthesis[f]), and unusual skin markings (e.g. petechiae, surgical scars, stretch marks, moles[g]) can be developed after the basics of postural observation have been mastered. Remember that postural observations are never definitive. They only indicate possibilities. In most cases clients present with minor deviations from normal standing alignment and communication with clients about postural observations should always make this clear.

In the posterior view, observe:

1. The level of the pelvis. One of the most important findings of postural observation is the level of the pelvis, as many treatment plans address imbalances associated with pelvic tilt. The pelvis comprises two ilia which articulate with each other at the symphysis pubis anteriorly and with the sacrum at the sacroiliac joints. Observe the level of the gluteal folds, PSISs, iliac crests, deviation of the gluteal cleft, the waist curvature and the distance between arms and trunk. To assist your determination of the level of the pelvis, the following describes the pattern of postural changes most often observed when the pelvis tilts. In this example, the client's pelvis is lower on the left than the right (see Figure 2.6). (For a client whose pelvis tilts lower on the right, the reverse would follow.) For a client whose pelvis is lower on the left than the right:
   - the PSIS is usually lower on the left
   - the gluteal fold is usually lower on the left
   - the gluteal cleft usually deviates to the left
   - the iliac crest is usually lower on the left
   - the waist curve usually flattens on the left
   - the lumbar scoliosis is usually convex on the left
   - the left foot is usually anterior and everted.

   If the level of the pelvis is not easily determined by observation, palpate the pelvis by placing your thumbs on the PSISs and fingers (held horizontally) on the iliac crests. Use your palpatory findings to confirm the presence (or absence) of a pelvic tilt.
2. The level of the shoulders
   Look at the contour of the trapezius muscle between the neck and the acromion and compare both sides.
3. Determine the nature of the scoliosis.
   The exact nature of scolioses can only be determined by diagnostic imaging. However, estimates of the shape of the curve can be ascertained from the presence of pelvic or shoulder tilt. Figure 2.7 illustrates common C-shaped and S-shaped spinal curvatures. Most thoracic scolioses are convex to the right (see Chapter 11).
4. Any other features of the back, neck or head that stand out (e.g. hypertonic muscles mid thoracic area, asymmetrical development from sports, work, or right or left dominance, muscle wasting).
5. Any lower limb features (e.g. ankle pronation, genu valgus or varus, oedema, feet everted) (see Figure 2.8).

[f]Spondylolisthesis is the anterior displacement of a vertebra in relation to the vertebra below (see Chapter 10).

[g]Massage therapists can play an important role in the detection of skin cancers among their clients. See Appendix 2.1 for a useful checklist.

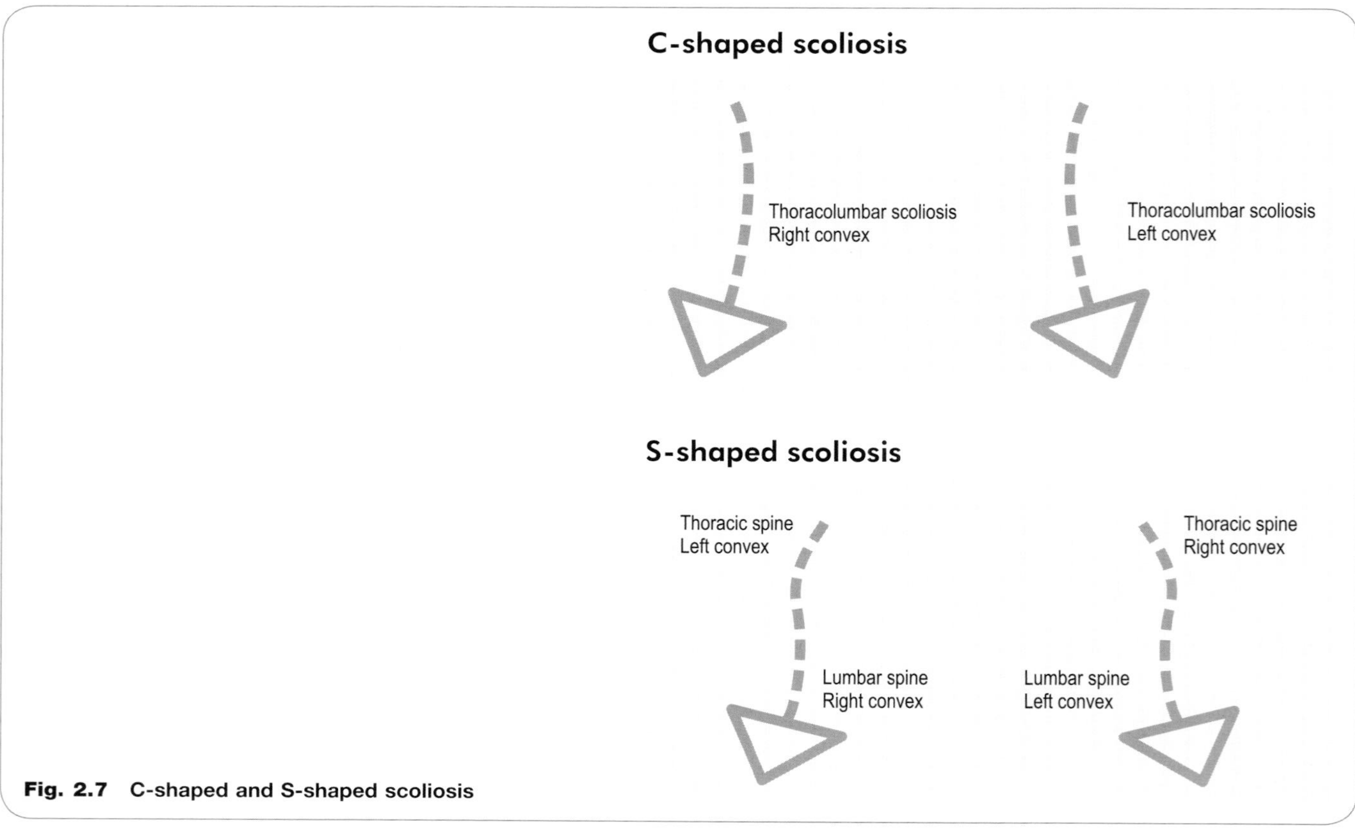

Fig. 2.7 C-shaped and S-shaped scoliosis

In the lateral view, note:

1. the relation of the body to the centre of gravity line: assess the alignment of the ear, shoulder, hips and lateral malleoli
2. the level of the pelvis (e.g. hyperlordosis, hypolordosis)
3. the shape of the kyphosis (e.g. hyperkyphosis, flattened thoracic curvature)
4. the position of the head (ear position in relation to shoulder, cervical hyper or hypolordosis)
5. the position of shoulders (rounded), arms and hands
6. any lower limb features (e.g. genu recurvatum, pes planus, pes cavus, hallux valgus, claw and hammer toes).

Method of recording

Postural observations are most easily recorded by marking diagrams of the posterior and lateral aspects of the erect body. A standardised recording system is yet to be developed for remedial massage. Only the most obvious and important findings need be recorded. These include the level of the pelvis, any major posture distortion (e.g. scoliosis, hyperlordosis), and any possible factors that could predispose to current or future symptoms. In the following section ways of recording common posture observations are presented. Figure 2.8 on p 19 shows how common posture observations of the lower limb can be recorded.

COMMON POSTURE OBSERVATIONS

In the posterior view:

Scoliosis

Scoliosis refers to a lateral curvature of the spine, observed when the client is viewed anteriorly or posteriorly. Diagnostic imaging is required to determine the exact nature and degree of spinal curvature. Postural observation enables practitioners to estimate large changes in spinal curvature and to suggest postural factors that may contribute or predispose to symptoms.

There are two major types of scoliosis:

- **Structural (idiopathic) scoliosis.** This is a curvature of the spine of unknown cause. It is relatively fixed and does not straighten on forward bending of the trunk (Adam's test) (see Figure 2.9 on p 20). It is often associated with vertebral and rib abnormalities and in severe cases can require bracing and surgery. Scoliosis screening tests in schools are designed to detect severe idiopathic scolioses that require such medical interventions. As a general rule, refer any child under 16 with a moderate or severe rib hump on forward flexion (Adam's test) who has not been previously screened by a medical practitioner, chiropractor, osteopath, physiotherapist or in a school screening program.
- **Functional scoliosis.** This is a compensatory curvature that may be associated with pelvic tilt and imbalance of muscles due to work and sport activities. This type of scoliosis usually straightens on forward bending of the trunk (i.e. Adam's test is negative). It is usually correctable with such interventions as exercise programs, remedial massage, spinal manipulation, and the use of orthotics in shoes.

Scoliosis is recorded on a posterior posture diagram by drawing three lines: i) a straight line at the level of the iliac crests angled

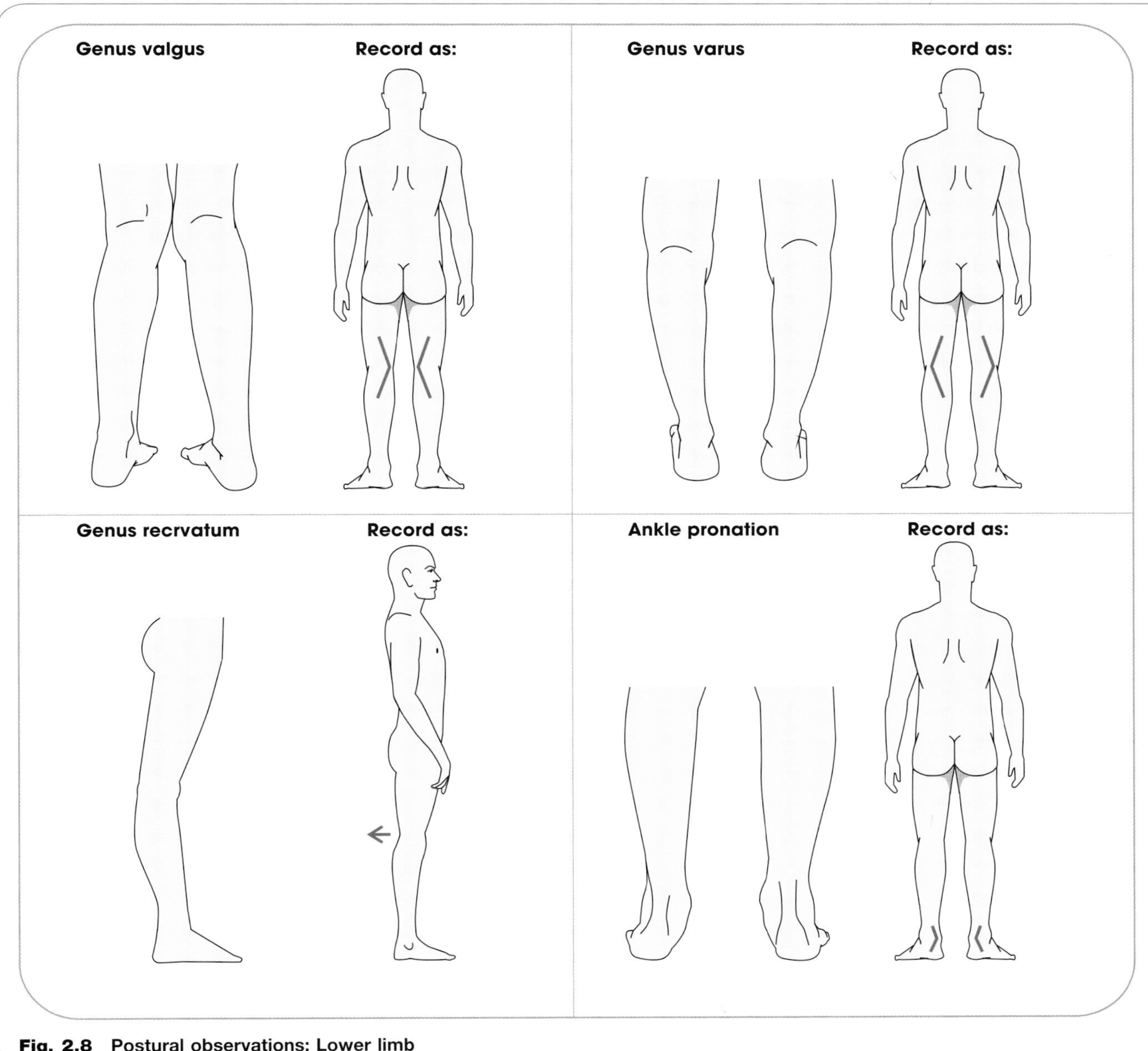

Fig. 2.8 Postural observations: Lower limb

to indicate the pelvic tilt. Try to make the angle of the straight line indicate the degree of pelvic tilt: an almost horizontal line would represent a small degree of pelvic tilt; a more diagonal line would represent a greater degree of pelvic tilt; ii) a straight line indicating the level of the shoulders; and iii) a curved line estimating the scoliosis. (see Figure 2.10 on p 20)

In the lateral view:

Lumbar hyperlordosis

This is a commonly observed posture (see Figure 2.11). Its causes include an anteriorly tilted pelvis and muscular imbalance such as weak abdominal muscles relative to tight erector spinae muscles, and/or weak hamstring muscles relative to tight hip flexor muscles. Hyperlordosis is commonly associated with lower crossed syndrome (see Chapter 10).

Standing hyperlordosis test

Another quick test for hyperlordosis: The client removes their shoes and stands with their shoulders, buttocks and heels against a wall. Without adjusting the position, the client places one hand into the space between their waist and the wall. One flat palm in the space between the back and the wall is usual. Any more than this could indicate lumbar hyperlordosis. (Some clients can fit two fists placed one on top of the other.)

(Note: There could be other reasons for excessive space between the wall and the client's body, such as overdeveloped gluteus maximus muscles.)

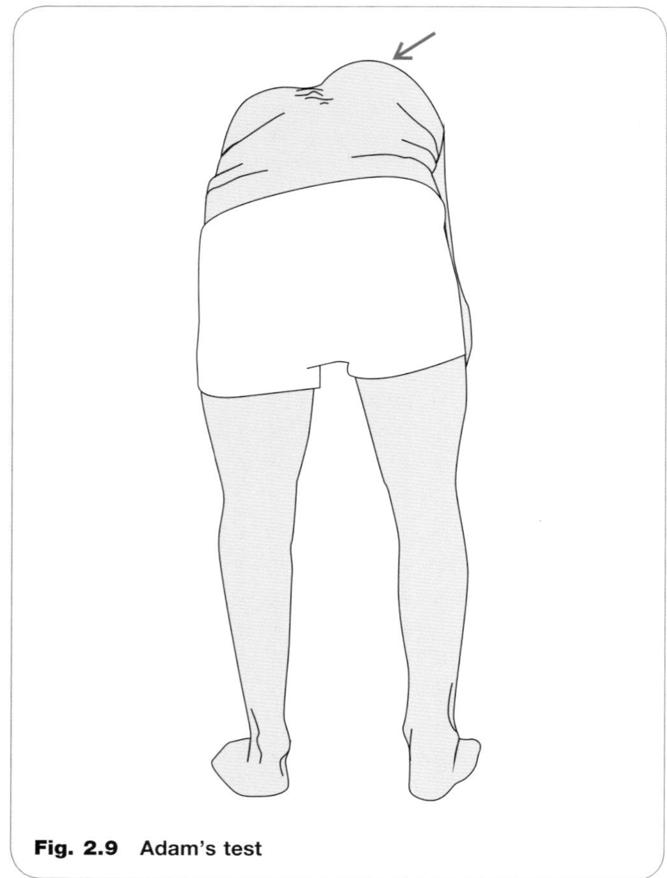

Fig. 2.9 Adam's test

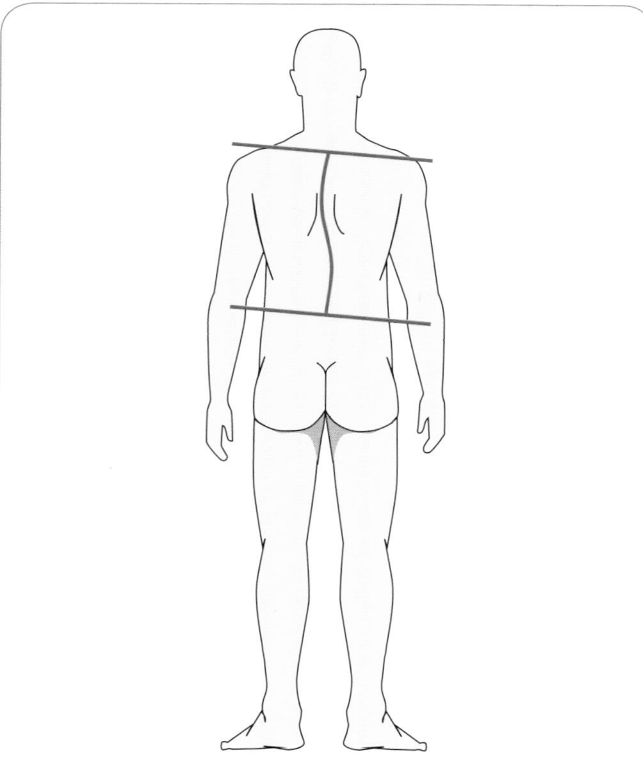

Fig. 2.10 Method of recording scoliosis

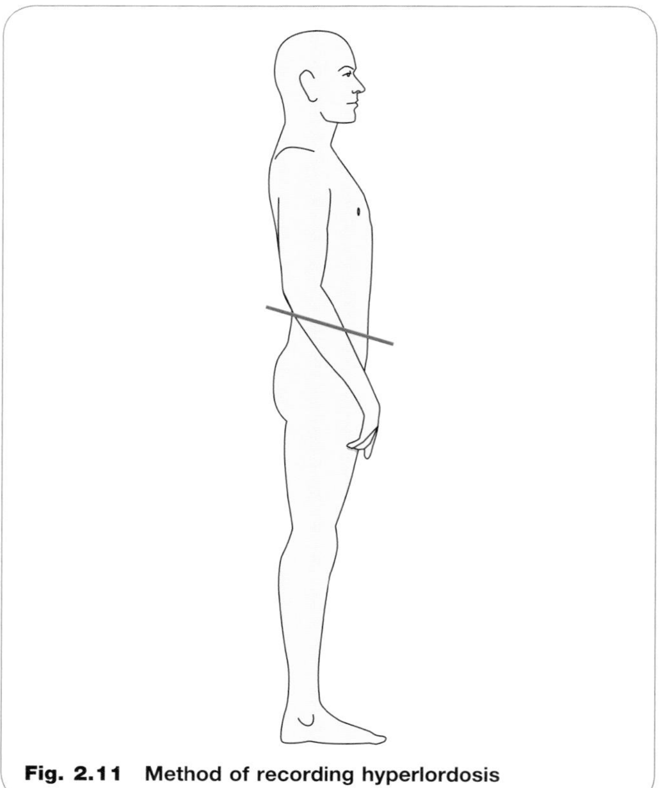

Fig. 2.11 Method of recording hyperlordosis

Hyperlordosis is recorded on a lateral posture diagram by a straight line indicating the level of the sacral base. Try to indicate the degree of anterior pelvic tilt with the angle of the line.

Decreased lumbar curvature

Spinal curvatures that appear to flatten or reverse may indicate a serious underlying condition.[h] For example, decreased lumbar lordosis is sometimes observed in clients with acute lumbar disc herniation. The symptoms may be severe and the client may be unable to stand upright, adopting an antalgic lean to reduce their level of pain (see Chapter 10 and Figure 2.12 on p 21). Such clients require referral to a medical practitioner, chiropractor, osteopath or physiotherapist.

Hypolordosis is recorded on a lateral posture diagram by a straight line indicating the level of the sacral base. Try to indicate the degree of pelvic tilt with the angle of the line.

Increased thoracic kyphosis

Increased thoracic kyphosis is commonly observed in people with sedentary jobs as a result of prolonged sitting and is associated with upper crossed syndrome (see Chapter 12 and Figure 2.13 on p 21). Another important cause is Scheuermann's disease which produces a fixed kyphosis, often in the thoracolumbar area. It occurs in 3–8% of the population and in males more than females. Clients may become round shouldered and find it difficult, if not impossible, to stand with shoulders in good alignment. Early intervention (ideally before

[h]An exception is the adaptation that sometimes occurs in pregnancy when the centre of gravity shifts posteriorly to accommodate the growing foetus.

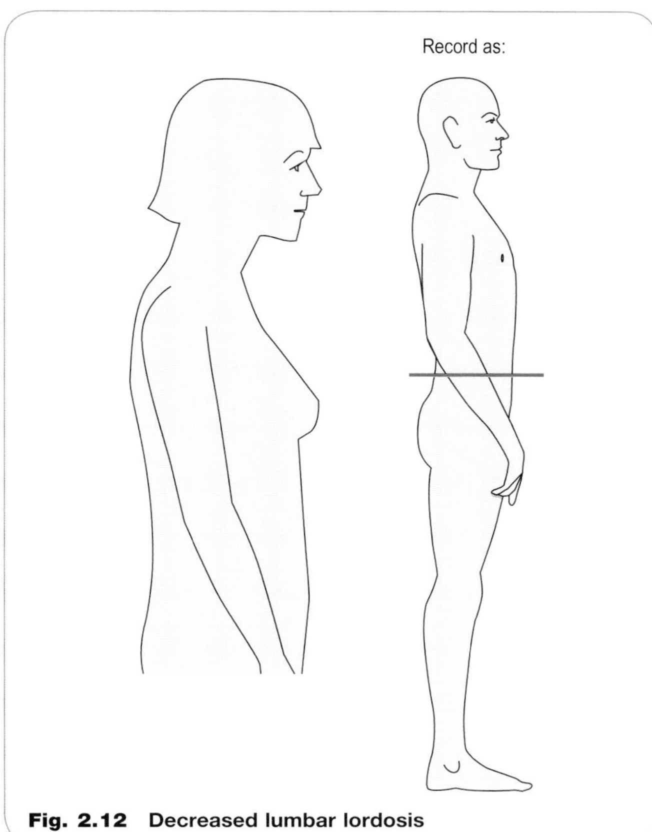

Fig. 2.12 Decreased lumbar lordosis

late teens or early twenties) with massage and exercise may help reduce the hypomobility associated with this condition (see Chapter 11).

Hyperkyphosis and hypokyphosis are recorded on a lateral posture diagram by drawing a curve to represent the position and degree of curvature of the thoracic spine.

Decreased thoracic kyphosis

A flattened thoracic kyphosis, also called 'dishing' or 'saucering', may be observed in the thoracic spine, particularly between the level of T2 and T7 (between the shoulder blades). This postural deviation appears to be becoming more common and may be related to prolonged sitting (see Figure 2.14 below).

Increased cervicothoracic curvature

This kyphotic curve of the cervicothoracic spine (C7 to T3), also called a 'dowager's hump', is most commonly observed in postmenopausal women and is associated with osteoporotic compression fractures and low levels of oestrogen (see Chapter 12 and Figure 2.15 on p 22).

Cervicothoracic hyperkyphosis is recorded on a lateral posture diagram by drawing a curve to represent the position and degree of curvature of the cervicothoracic spine.

Sway back

Sway back is distinguished from hyperlordosis by the relationship of the body to the centre of gravity line. In sway back the pelvis is tilted posteriorly but the pelvis is anterior to the centre of gravity line. The upper body extends backwards as

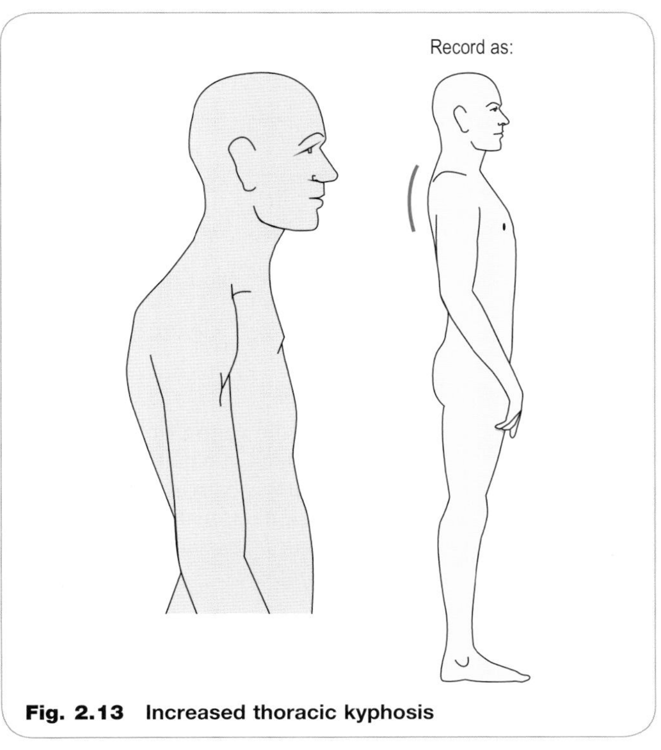

Fig. 2.13 Increased thoracic kyphosis

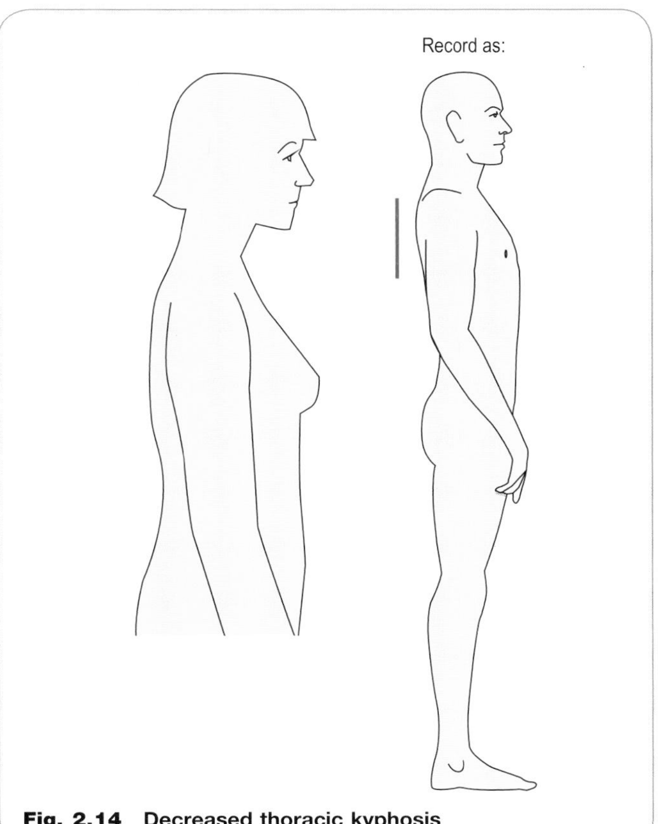

Fig. 2.14 Decreased thoracic kyphosis

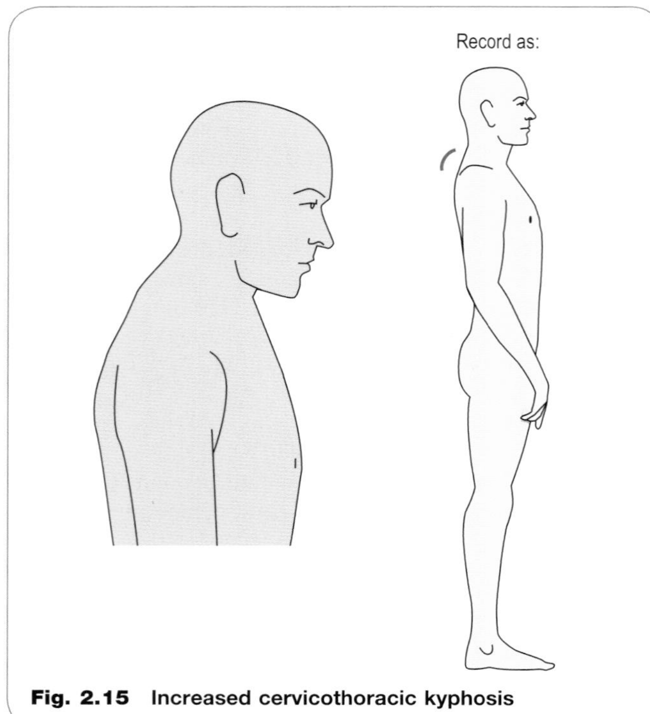

Fig. 2.15 Increased cervicothoracic kyphosis

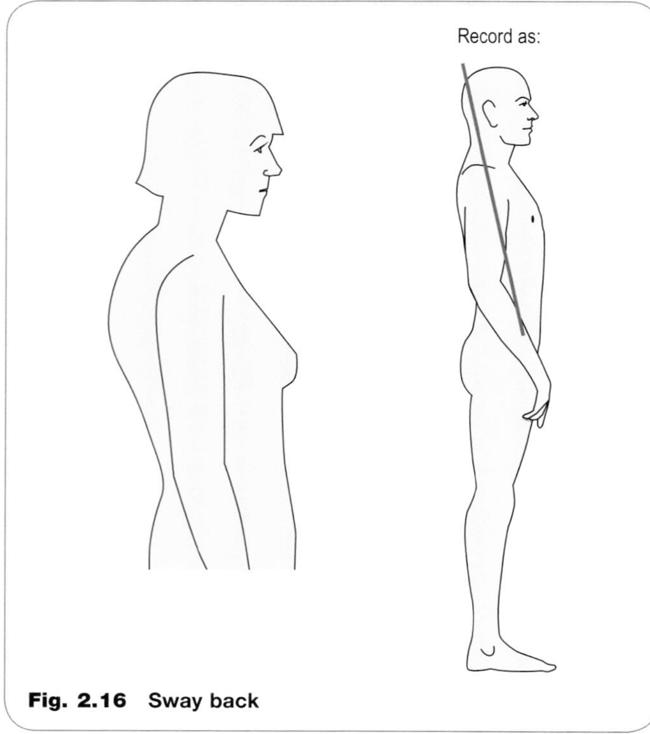

Fig. 2.16 Sway back

a counterbalance. The lumbar erector spinae and hamstrings are short and tight; the hip flexors and thoracic erector spinae are lengthened (Figure 2.16).

GAIT ANALYSIS

Gait analysis, although not widely used by remedial massage therapists, can contribute useful information to treatment plans and can be performed simply, efficiently and without recourse to expensive equipment. Gait disturbances can arise from upper motor neuron lesions, disorders of the cerebellar, vestibular and proprioceptive systems, and dysfunctions of the musculoskeletal system. Many gait and other movement abnormalities are easily observed as clients enter the clinic. Remedial massage therapists will recognise the festinating gait of Parkinson's disease (short, shuffling steps with knees, trunk and neck held in flexion), the hemiplegic gait that results from upper motor neuron lesions (leg abducted in a semicircle with each step, shoulder adducted, elbow flexed, wrist flexed and pronated), and the staggering ataxic gait of cerebellar disease or diminished sensation in the extremities (wide base of support and exaggerated movements).[13]

Less pronounced disturbances in the symmetry, rhythm and speed of gait are also easily detected. Of particular interest to remedial massage therapists is the influence of joint and muscle function on normal gait. Common musculoskeletal causes of gait disturbance include functional short leg, sore feet, muscle shortness and weakness, and hypomobility or hypermobility of joints.[14] A range of remedial massage techniques can be used to release muscle contractures, increase the mobility of hypomobile joints and, in some cases, to normalise muscle firing patterns and gait reflex patterns through muscle energy techniques.[14]

Normal gait has two phases:

- stance phase which accounts for 60% of the cycle
- swing phase which takes up the remaining 40%.

These two phases can be further subdivided (see Table 2.3):

Stance phase

HEEL STRIKE

When the heel first strikes the ground the foot is approximately 90° to the leg. The knee is extended but not locked.

FOOT FLAT

In this phase the ankle plantarflexes under the control of anterior and posterior leg muscles, especially the eccentric contraction of tibialis anterior. The foot arch flattens slightly as it takes the load of the body and the foot pronates to absorb shock. The quadriceps and gluteal muscles stabilise the hip and knee.

MIDSTANCE

As the body moves over the foot the centre of gravity shifts to the weight-bearing limb. Gluteus medius and minimus control the hip as it internally rotates, adducts slightly and the pelvis drops on the opposite side. The pronated foot moves to slight supination and body weight is transferred to the lateral aspect of the foot. The ankle dorsiflexes.

PUSH-OFF

Weight is transferred to the ball of the foot and the gastrocnemius strongly contracts to plantarflex the ankle to about 20°. Tibialis posterior inverts the heel and the foot supinates. The metatarsophalangeal joints passively extend and the knee flexes to about 35°. Continued toe extension is controlled by the plantar fascia and eccentrically contracting toe flexors. The hip and knee extend and externally rotate.

Swing phase

ACCELERATION

In the acceleration phase, the knee flexes and the ankle dorsiflexes to shorten the limb to clear the ground. The forward swing of the leg is initiated by the quadriceps muscle.

MIDSWING

The hip flexors and knee extensors move the limb forward. The ankle is slightly dorsiflexed and the toes extended to clear the ground. Next, the hip extensors (especially gluteus maximus) and knee flexors (hamstrings) eccentrically contract to slow the forward motion. The hip internally rotates.

DECELERATION

The hamstrings contracting eccentrically and the quadriceps contracting concentrically stop the forward motion of the limb.[15]

Gait assessment: the procedure

Observe the client walking without shoes at their normal walking pace from the front, from the side and from behind. As with static postural observation, begin with general observations about the symmetry, rhythm and speed of gait.

1. GENERAL OBSERVATIONS

Note any changes in the smooth coordinated pattern of normal gait.

- Step length is the distance between the point of first contact of one foot to the point of first contact of the other foot. In a study by Latt et al[16] involving 10 healthy adults (four male and six female) with ages ranging from 17 to 31 years, the average step length was 73 ± 3 cm. Step length decreases with age, fatigue, pain and pathology in the lower limb. (Note: Stride length is the distance between the first point of contact of one foot to the first point of contact with the same foot, i.e. two steps.)
- Adults walk at an average cadence of 90–120 steps per minute.[16, 17] The rate decreases with age, fatigue, pain and if footing is uncertain (e.g. if the surface is slippery or uneven).
- The width of the base (i.e. the distance between the feet) is usually 5–10 cm in adults.[18] Clients widen their base if they have cerebellar problems, decreased sensation in the soles of their feet, or if they feel dizzy or unsteady on their feet.
- In normal gait the body oscillates vertically usually no more than 5 cm with each step.[17]
- The pelvis makes a figure-eight movement, alternately shifting laterally over the weight-bearing limb in stance phase and then rotating forward approximately 40° in swing phase.[14]

2. IDENTIFY THE PHASE OF GAIT THAT IS DISRUPTED AND THE PARTS AFFECTED

A useful strategy for identifying gait disturbances that arise from local musculoskeletal problems is to locate the phase of gait that is affected. Common problems arising in each phase and possible causes are listed in Table 2.4 on p 25.

Stance phase

Most gait problems are apparent in stance phase. Clients who experience pain in stance phase when the single weight-bearing limb is loaded with the entire body weight may shorten the normal duration of the phase or adopt an antalgic gait (e.g. walking on the ball of the foot). Footwear as a source of pain should always be considered when symptoms occur in stance phase.

Heel strike

Pain from a heel spur, bruise or retrocalcaneal bursitis may cause the client to hop onto the foot to avoid heel strike. Normal knee extension may be prevented by a joint fused in flexion or weak quadriceps muscles. In the latter case, the client may push their knee into extension with their hand. If the hip extensors are weak, the client may increase their lumbar lordosis to compensate.[19] Weak hip adductors may result in abnormal rotation of the pelvis and lower limb.

Foot flat

Weak or non-functioning dorsiflexors (tibialis anterior, extensor digitorum longus, extensor hallucis longus) may cause the foot to slap down after heel strike. If the ankle joint is fused, the client may not reach foot flat until midstance.

Midstance

The foot supports the entire body weight and the hip and knee move into extension. Degenerative joint disease, pes planus or plantar fasciitis may cause pain in the weight-bearing ankle or foot. Painful calluses may develop over the metatarsal heads, often as a result of fallen transverse arches of the foot. If gluteus medius is weak, the pelvis drops on the non-weight-bearing side (gluteus medius or Trendelenburg or abductor gait).Weak quadriceps may cause excessive knee flexion.

Push off

If gluteus maximus is weak the client may thrust their trunk backwards to maintain hip extension (gluteus maximus or hip extensor gait). If the knee extensors are weak the knee may buckle. Weak gastrocnemius, soleus or flexor hallucis longus may lead to flat-footed (calcaneal) gait. Degenerative joint disease or hallux rigidus may interrupt normal push off which requires extension of the metatarsophalangeal joint. Clients with hallux rigidus push off from the lateral aspect of their foot. Calluses on the metatarsal heads and corns can also cause pain during push off.

Swing phase

Acceleration

In the acceleration phase the ankle dorsiflexors help shorten the lower limb so it can clear the ground. Weak ankle dorsiflexors may cause foot drop. The hip flexes and medially rotates as the knee flexes to a maximum of 65° to shorten the leg. If the quadriceps muscles are weak the leg is swung forward with an exaggerated anterior pelvic rotation.

Midswing

If ankle dorsiflexors are weak in mid swing, the client may flex the hip excessively to bend the knee to avoid scraping the toe on the ground (steppage gait).

Table 2.3 Phases of gait

Phases of gait

Stance phase				Swing phase		
Heel strike	***Foot flat***	***Midstance***	***Push off***	***Acceleration***	***Mid swing***	***Deceleration***
The foot makes first contact with the ground and the limb decelerates. A closed kinetic chain for the lower limb is initiated.	Foot adapts to surface and takes the weight of the body. The pelvis is stabilised. Trunk is carried forward by momentum.	The knee remains stabilised. Momentum continues to carry the body forward.	The body is accelerated into forward motion.	The lower limb is shortened and swung forward. The innominate moves anteriorly.	The foot clears the ground. On the weight-bearing side the innominate moves posteriorly; the sacrum tilts laterally towards the side of loading.	Decelerate the limb, and prepare for first contact with the ground.
Major muscle groups						
Concentric Ankle dorsiflexors ***Eccentric*** Hip extensors Tibialis anterior	***Concentric*** Knee extensors Ankle plantar flexors Isometric Hip abductors ***Eccentric*** Hip extensors Quadriceps Tibialis anterior	***Isometric*** Ankle plantar flexors Hip abductors ***Eccentric*** Plantar flexors	***Concentric*** Ankle plantar flexors ***Eccentric*** Toe flexors	***Concentric*** Hip flexors Knee flexors Ankle dorsiflexors	***Concentric*** Hip flexors Ankle dorsiflexors ***Eccentric*** Hip extensors	***Concentric*** Quadriceps Ankle dorsiflexors ***Eccentric*** Knee flexors Hip extensors

Table 2.4 Common gait problems

Stance Phase	
Antalgic gait (often minimising the duration of stance phase)	Any condition causing pain, especially in the weight-bearing limb or lower back (e.g. shoe problems, DJD ankle, knee, hip, lumbar disc herniation)
Avoiding heel strike (e.g. hopping onto flat foot)	Heel spurs, bruise, bursitis
Drop foot gait	Weak tibialis anterior
Trendelenburg gait The pelvis drops and the trunk lurches to the unaffected side to maintain balance	Weak gluteus medius
Hip extensor gait Immediately after heel strike, the hip is thrust forward and the trunk thrown into extension	Weak gluteus maximus
Back knee gait to lock the knees into extension, pushing knee into extension with hand	Weak quadriceps
Unstable knee which may suddenly buckle into flexion	Dislocating knee cap, torn menisci, torn collateral ligaments
Walking on the balls of the feet	Gastrocnemius/soleus shortening or tear; heel or foot pain (antalgic gait)
Flat foot gait, no forceful toe-off	Weak gastrocnemius/soleus; hallux rigidus
Swing Phase	
Steppage gait (lifting knee high)	Weak dorsiflexors
Abnormal hip rotation in acceleration	Weak quadriceps
Heavy heel strike	Weak hamstrings

Deceleration

If the hamstrings are weak heel strike can be excessively hard and the knee may hyperextend (back knee gait).

Findings from gait analysis should be correlated with findings from other assessments, particularly length and strength tests for specific muscles which are detailed in Chapters 10–20 and assessment of the sacroiliac joints, and hip, knee, ankle and foot regions (Chapters 10, 18, 19 and 20 respectively). Further assessments such as muscle firing patterns (see Fritz et al[14]) and neuromuscular treatments like muscle energy techniques (see Chaitow[20]) are beyond the scope of this book but will be of interest to remedial massage therapists who use advanced soft tissue techniques.

FUNCTIONAL TESTS

As part of their assessment procedures, remedial massage therapists use a range of functional tests. These include active and passive range of motion, resisted muscle tests and other tests of functional limitation (e.g. tests for the strength of specific muscles, muscle length tests and other special tests including straight leg raising, Valsalva, Adam's test), and less commonly vital signs (blood pressure, temperature, pulse rate). Active, passive and resisted tests are usually performed before more specific tests.

Although functional tests are widely used by physical therapists including physiotherapists, chiropractors and osteopaths, several studies have found that many tests lack validity and reliability. The Australian Acute Musculoskeletal Pain Guidelines Group[7] has urged practitioners to interpret clinical signs elicited during physical assessment cautiously. 'Eyeballing' a client's active range of motion (i.e. measuring by eye without the use of a goniometer or other measuring tool) is particularly unreliable in clinical practice. Many functional tests have not been fully researched; however, increasingly, information about their diagnostic accuracy is becoming available. Measures of sensitivity (the probability of a positive test among clients with the condition) and specificity (the probability of a negative test among clients who don't have the condition) are available for some tests, however such measures are really only useful when they are very high (≥95%) to help rule a condition in or out.[15]

Likelihood ratios (LRs) are another measure of the usefulness of diagnostic tests. LRs greater than 1 indicate an increased probability that a condition is present. LRs of 10 or more usually rule in a condition. LRs less than 1 indicate a decreased probability that a condition is present. LRs of 0.1 or less usually rule out a condition.[21] Figure 2.17 summarises common measures used to rate the diagnostic accuracy of functional tests.

The decision to perform diagnostic tests is based on client history and other findings that indicate the likelihood of a condition and also whether it is important to have a definitive diagnosis. Remember that in many cases it is not possible or necessary to have a definitive diagnosis of the cause of acute musculoskeletal pain to have effective management of the condition.[7] Where diagnostic tests are appropriate, tests with the highest diagnostic accuracy are preferred. However,

Validity
Degree to which a test measures what it is intended to measure
Reliability
Degree of consistency with which an instrument or rater measures a particular attribute (expressed as a percentage or decimal e.g. 80% or 0.8)
Sensitivity
Ability of a test to detect people who actually have a condition (usually recorded as a percentage: sensitivity ≥ 95% rules in a condition)
Specificity
Ability of a test to correctly identify people who do not have a condition (usually recorded as a percentage: specificity ≥ 95% rules out a condition)
Likelihood ratios
LR >1 increased probability that a condition is present (the higher the number the better: LR >10 rules in the condition)
LR < 1 decreased probability that a condition is present (the lower the number the better: LR ≤ 0.1 rules out the condition)

Fig. 2.17 Measuring the diagnostic accuracy of functional tests

even results of functional tests with good ratings for diagnostic accuracy are best interpreted as indicators of possible conditions, such as hamstring strain, tennis elbow or degenerative joint disease and used to guide treatment planning (see Table 2.6 on page 27). Physical testing demonstrates clients' functional limitations and suggests the types of tissues involved, the range of treatment options likely to benefit clients, and guides the application of techniques (e.g. depth and duration).

Active range of motion (AROM) tests

LOCATING THE REGION

Active tests require the client to move the body through ranges of motion. Muscles are activated and joints move so active movements are not specific to the types of tissues involved. They are useful in locating regions of the body that are likely sources of symptoms. For example, active range of motion tests of a client with posterior thigh pain will help determine if the lumbar spine, hip or knee regions are likely sources of pain and guide the choice of further assessments and treatment options.

SAFE PRACTICE

Safe practice is based on assessing functional limitations and making realistic interpretations of verbal and non-verbal information from clients. AROM testing has an important safety function. It precedes all other functional assessments. Observing clients' active movements helps practitioners determine appropriate pressure, speed and range for passive range of motion (PROM) and other tests. For example, if a client reports pain at 30° active lumbar flexion, all further assessment and treatment procedures must take this into account. In this case, bilateral knee to chest stretches of the erector spinae muscles are likely to reproduce painful lumbar flexion and should be avoided. As a general rule, observe clients and watch them move before making any physical contact.

SEE	MOVE	TOUCH[22]
Observation	*AROM*	*PROM*

Regularly ask clients for feedback and always be alert to non-verbal cues about discomfort or pain.

Passive and resisted tests: Determining tissue types

Active, passive and resisted tests are used initially to help determine the types of tissues that are injured. They also guide decisions about the need for more specific testing. The results of all functional testing are general guides only (see Table 2.6) and must be interpreted in the light of other assessment findings and of individual responses.

Active tests indicate the region of the body which is a likely source of symptoms. Next passive range of motion (PROM) and resisted range of motion (RROM) tests are carried out to help identify the likely types of tissue involved.

PASSIVE RANGE OF MOTION TESTS (PROM)

PROM tests are performed by the therapist, who moves the joint or body part through its range of motion. Pain and other symptoms reproduced during PROM testing may be related to inert structures including articulating cartilage, joint capsules or ligaments. Muscles are not actively recruited during PROM testing. However, they are passively stretched and RROM and palpation may be required to help differentiate the involvement of contractile or inert tissue. PROM tests help detect ligament laxity, joint hypermobility or hypomobility, crepitus and end-feel (the practitioner's interpretation of the feeling of the available movement in the client's tissues at the end of their range of motion). For example, compare the soft end-feel of elbow flexion when muscles are brought together, the hard (bony) end-feel of elbow extension when the olecranon fossa restricts the movement of the ulna, the muscular end-feel of a fully stretched hamstring muscle, and the boggy end-feel when movement is restricted by oedema. Some remedial massage techniques, such as passive joint articulation, are performed near the end of normal physiological range to stretch joint capsules and other tissues around the joint, to prevent the formation of scar tissue and to improve mobility. Stretching beyond the normal physiological limit may result in tissue damage. Sensitivity to tissue tightening near the limits of normal physiological movement is important for safe practice. Remedial massage therapists are strongly urged to observe AROM before PROM and other assessment and treatment procedures (See-Move-Touch) to determine broad parameters of clients' comfortable movement ranges. Crepitus is sometimes heard and felt and, when related to joint movement, can indicate cartilage wear in the joint space.

Many texts describe capsular patterns of joint limitations in clients with degenerative joint disease or joint inflammation (see Table 2.5). They are included here because they are commonly reported in clinical practice. However, the concept of capsular pattern does not appear to be supported by research evidence.[23, 24]

RESISTED RANGE OF MOTION TESTS (RROM)

RROM tests are used to test contractile tissue in specific ranges of motion. Position the client's body region or joint (usually in mid-range) and instruct them to hold the position against your resistance. Resistance normally lasts for 3–5 seconds. RROM tests help locate muscle groups according to their actions. For example, performing an RROM test of knee extension tests the integrity of the knee extensor muscles as a group but will not differentiate between the rectus femoris, vastus medialis, intermedialis or lateralis muscles. Further testing, such as resisted tests for specific muscles and palpation, are required to help identify individual muscles.

Tests for specific muscles

Resisted tests and length tests for specific muscles are of particular interest to remedial massage therapists who often focus their treatments on assessing and treating muscle imbalances (e.g. relationships between agonists and antagonists, patterns of kinetic dysfunction, muscle tightness or weakness, impacts on postural alignment, and compensatory patterns). Muscle imbalances have been associated with the development of almost all musculoskeletal pain and dysfunction. Muscles can be classified as mobilisers and stabilisers. Mobilisers tend to be superficial, span two joints and contain fast twitch fibres for power rather than endurance. Stabilisers, on the other hand, are usually deep, cross one joint and are made up of slow twitch fibres for endurance; they contribute to habitual postures. Mobilisers tend to become short and tight and can inhibit the action of stabilisers that may have become weak and long. Commonly shortened muscles include upper trapezius, pectoralis major, sternocleidomastoid, erector spinae, quadratus lumborum, iliopsoas, hamstring muscles

Table 2.5 Capsular patterns

Joint	Limitation of range of motion
Cervical spine	Lateral flexion = rotation > extension
Thoracic spine	Lateral flexion = rotation > extension
Lumbar spine	Lateral flexion = rotation > extension
Shoulder	Lateral rotation > abduction > medial rotation
Elbow	Flexion > extension
Wrist	Flexion = extension
Metacarpophalangeal	Flexion > extension
Distal interphalangeal	Flexion > extension
Proximal interphalangeal	Flexion > extension
Hip	Flexion, abduction, medial rotation > extension
Knee	Flexion > extension
Ankle	Plantarflexion > dorsiflexion
Subtalar	Inversion > eversion
2nd–5th metatarsophalangeal	Flexion > extension
1st metatarsophalangeal	Extension > flexion

Table 2.6 Direction of treatment following active, passive and resisted range of motion tests

Type of test	Indications	Implications for treatment
Active range of motion (AROM)	Helps locate musculoskeletal region that is the likely source of symptom, e.g. helps determine if symptoms in the upper limb emanate from the cervical spine or shoulder joint	Long-term management usually involves treatment of the source of symptoms. Client education about the likely source of symptoms
Passive range of motion (PROM)	Inert tissue (e.g. the articulation itself, ligaments, joint capsule, bursae) (Note: muscles are also passively stretched during PROM testing)	Treatment focuses on inert structures: Swedish massage, thermotherapy, passive joint articulation, myofascial release, range of motion exercises for joint mobility, joint stabilisation, etc
Resisted range of motion (RROM)	Contractile tissue (e.g. major muscles performing a movement tested as a group) Normally followed by specific muscle testing to isolate involved muscle(s)	Treatment focuses on muscle function: Swedish massage, thermotherapy, deep transverse friction, trigger point therapy, soft tissue releasing techniques, muscle stretching and strengthening

and hip adductors. Shortened hamstrings, adductors and hip flexors are often associated with weakened and lengthened transversalis abdominis and posterior gluteal muscles.

Specific muscle testing to identify correctable abnormalities of muscle strength and length may be prompted by (1) postural observation (e.g. hyperlordotic posture may prompt testing bilateral iliopsoas muscles for shortness), or (2) resisted muscle testing (RROM) in an initial screening that suggests contractile tissue as a source of symptoms.

RESISTED TESTS FOR SPECIFIC MUSCLES

Resisted tests are used by many healthcare professionals to test muscle strength, and grading systems, such as the one described in the box below, have been developed. However, in remedial massage, resisted tests for specific muscles are more commonly used to locate possible lesions in specific muscles. Grading muscle strength is often restricted to bilateral comparisons or judgments based on clinical experience.

A typical grading system rates muscle strength on a scale from 5 to 0:

5 Normal strength: movement is possible against maximum resistance by the examiner
4 Good: movement is possible against gravity and some resistance by the examiner
3 Fair: movement is possible against gravity but not against resistance by the examiner
2 Poor: movement is possible when gravity is eliminated (i.e. testing joint in its horizontal plane)
1 Trace: muscle tightens but no movement
0 Zero: no contraction

In the following example, resisted testing is used to isolate the specific muscles that are likely sources of the presenting symptoms in a client with shoulder pain.

▼ The client would be tested for shoulder range of motion (AROM, PROM, RROM). AROM tests help identify the region of the body that is the likely source of symptoms. If active shoulder abduction reproduces the pain, the injury is likely to be related to the shoulder joint or associated muscles (and not referred from the cervical spine, for example). PROM and RROM tests are required to help determine the likely tissues involved. If PROM tests do not reproduce the pain (i.e. inert structures are probably not involved) but RROM testing for shoulder abduction does, then contractile tissue is implicated. The client's injury is probably related to the shoulder abductor muscles. Further resisted testing is required to discriminate between the two abductor muscles (deltoid and supraspinatus muscles) (see Figure 2.18).

Isolating the injured muscle(s) enables practitioners to develop targeted treatment plans which are likely to produce faster and better outcomes for clients. Resisted tests for muscles implicated in commonly occurring conditions are detailed in Chapters 10–20. (For further information see Kendall McCreary et al[25] and Hislop and Montgomery[26].)

MUSCLE LENGTH TESTS

Muscle length and flexibility both refer to the ability of a muscle to be lengthened to the end of its range of motion.[27] There are many reasons why muscles become shortened, including maintaining postures for excessively long periods (e.g. hip flexors may become shortened after prolonged periods of sitting), adaptive responses to other conditions (e.g. the presence of a trigger point, scoliosis or a leg length discrepancy) and ageing. When a shortened muscle is identified, muscle-stretching techniques are usually applied to restore its normal length. Stretching can be performed as part of consultation and/or prescribed as home exercises. For example, the length of the hamstring muscles can be assessed by straight leg raising when the client is supine. Shortness is assessed by comparison to population norms (normal hamstring length permits approximately 65–80° straight leg raising) and/or by bilateral comparison. A range of stretching techniques can be applied to the posterior thigh after Swedish massage or heat application has warmed the area (see Chapter 5). Length tests of some of the major muscles of the body are included in Table 2.7.

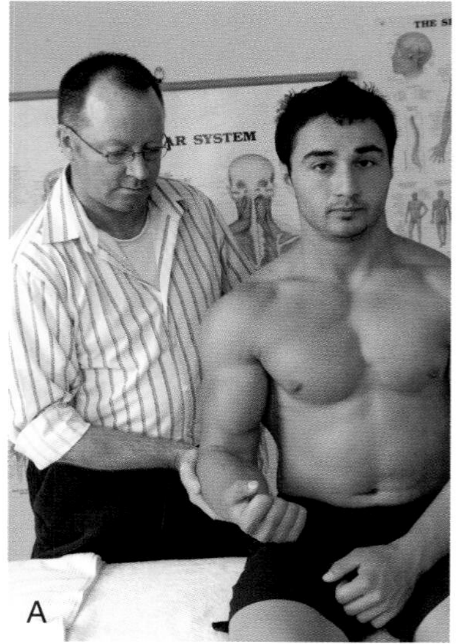

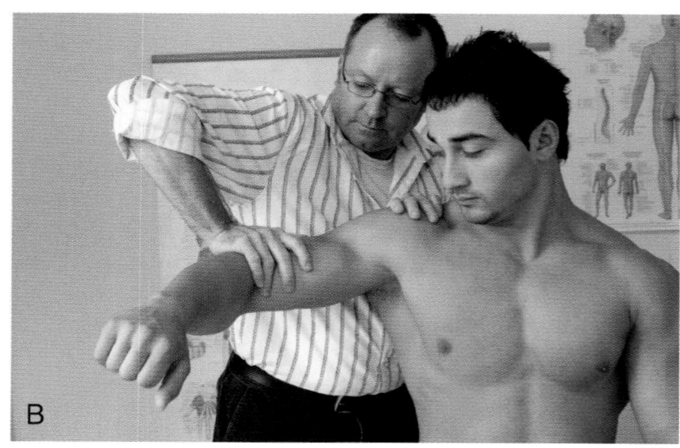

Fig. 2.18 Differentiating (a) supraspinatus and (b) middle deltoid strains

Positioning the client

- Muscle should be placed in the fully elongated position.
- As far as possible isolate the muscle across one joint.
- Bony landmarks used to measure should be palpable and in proper alignment.

Table 2.7 Length tests of major muscles[27, 28]

Muscle – upper extremity	Length test	
Levator scapulae	The client lies supine. The practitioner stabilises the client's shoulder with one hand and flexes, sidebends and rotates the occiput to the opposite side.	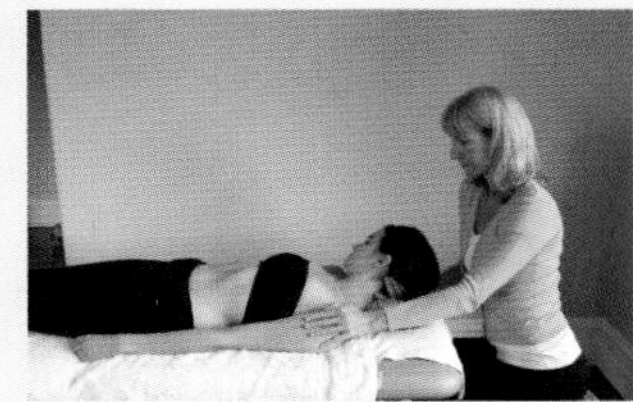
Upper trapezius	The client lies supine. The practitioner stabilises the client's shoulder with one hand. With the other the occiput is laterally flexed to the opposite side and rotated to the side of testing.	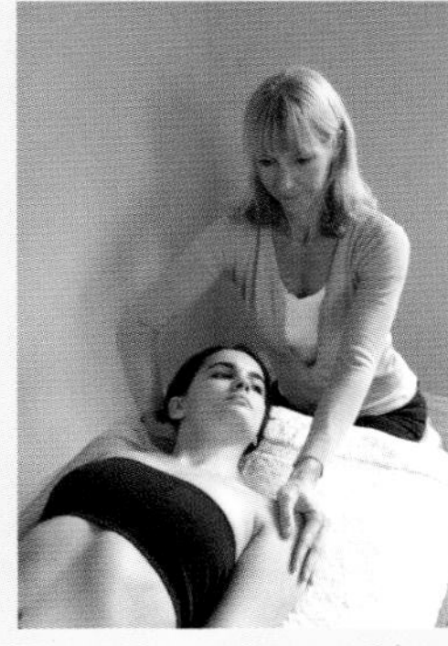
Latissimus dorsi	The client lies supine and fully flexes the extended arm. Observe the distance between the extended arm and the table.	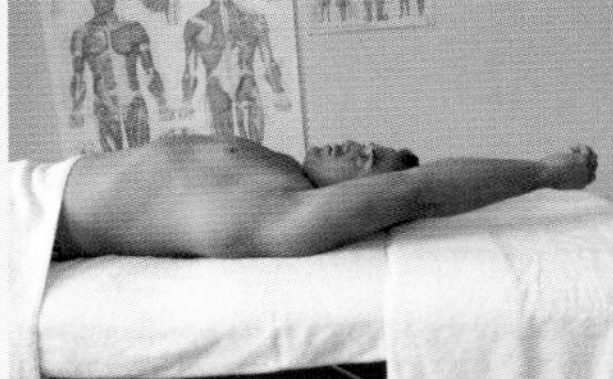
Pectoralis major	The client lies supine with hand behind head. Observe the distance between the elbow and the table.	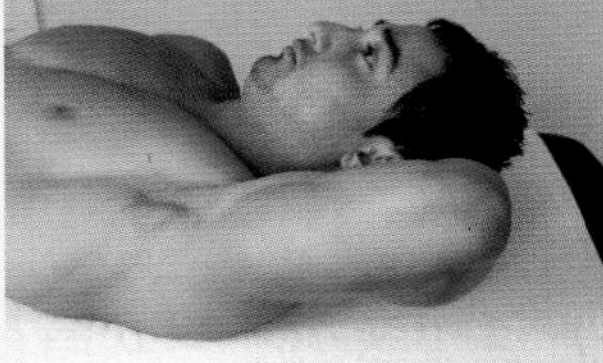
Pectoralis major – sternal (lower) portion	The client lies supine and abducts the extended arm to about 135°. The arm is allowed to fall into maximum horizontal abduction.	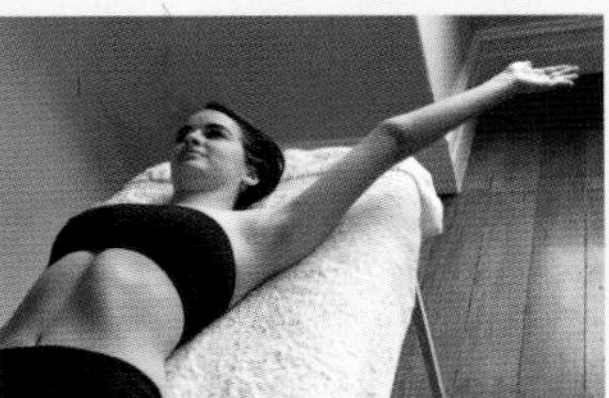
Pectoralis major – clavicular (upper portion)	As above except that the arm is abducted to 90°.	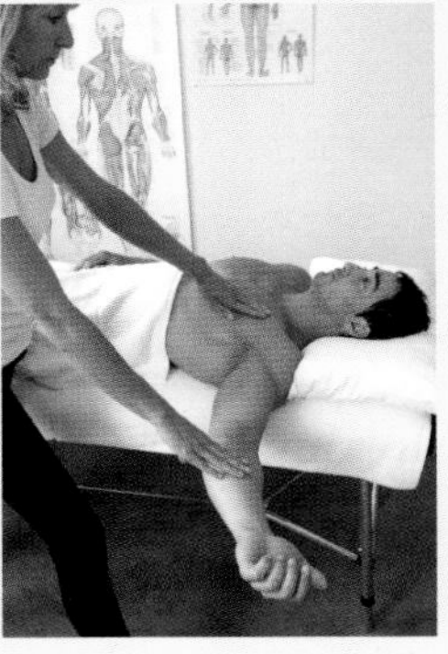

Continued

Table 2.7 Length tests of major muscles—cont'd

Muscle – upper extremity	Length test	
Pectoralis minor muscle	The client lies supine with arms by sides. Observe the distance between the shoulders and the table.	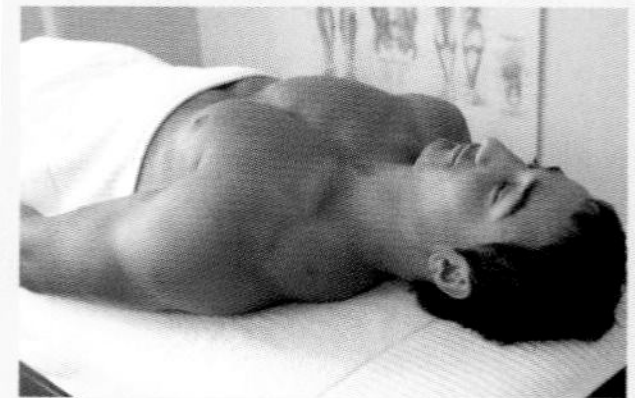
Triceps brachii	The client is seated and tries to touch the back of their shoulder with their hand keeping their humerus fully flexed.	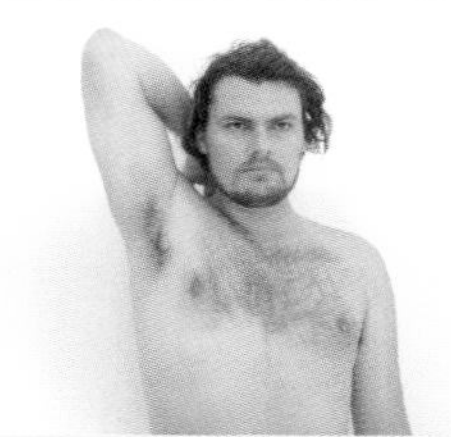
Biceps brachii	The client lies supine with their shoulder level with the edge of the table, elbow extended and forearm pronated. The client extends their shoulder to their comfortable limit, keeping their elbow fully extended.	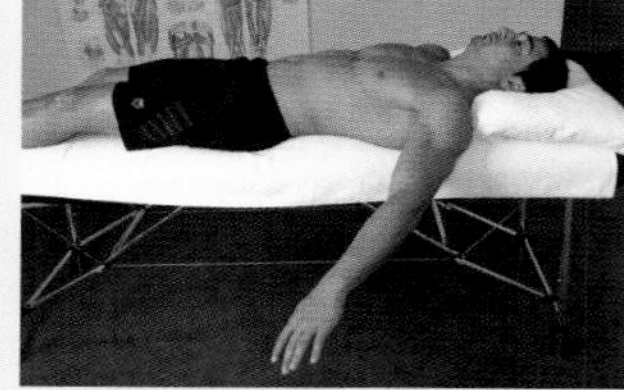
Flexor digitorum superficialis, flexor digitorum profundus, flexor digiti minimi	The client lies supine with shoulder abducted to 70–90°, elbow extended, forearm supinated and fingers extended. The practitioner fully extends the client's wrist.	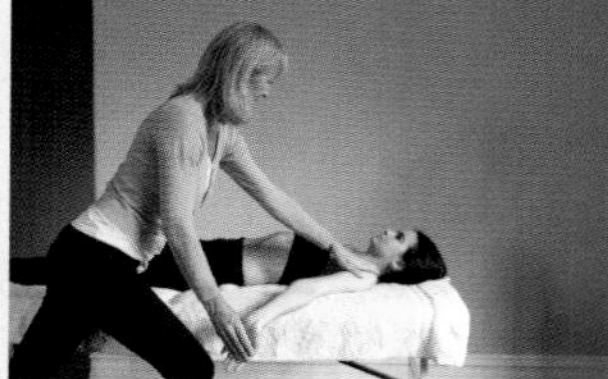
Extensor digitorum, extensor indicis, extensor digiti minimi	The client lies supine with shoulder abducted to 70–90°, elbow extended, forearm pronated and fingers flexed. The practitioner fully flexes the client's wrist.	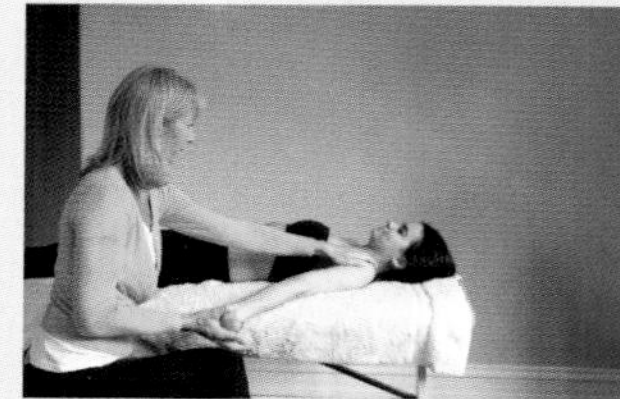
Trunk		
Lumbar erector spinae	The client is seated on the table, keeping the pelvis as vertical as possible. The client bends forward as far as possible from the lumbo-pelvic region.	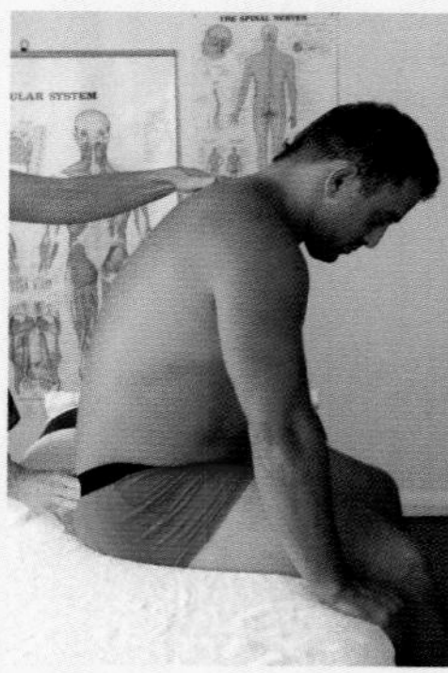

Table 2.7 Length tests of major muscles—cont'd

Trunk	**Length test**	
Quadratus lumborum	The client lies on their side with their back near the edge of the table. The client bends their lower leg slightly and holds on to the table for stability. The client extends the upper leg beyond the edge of the table letting the leg drop towards the floor.	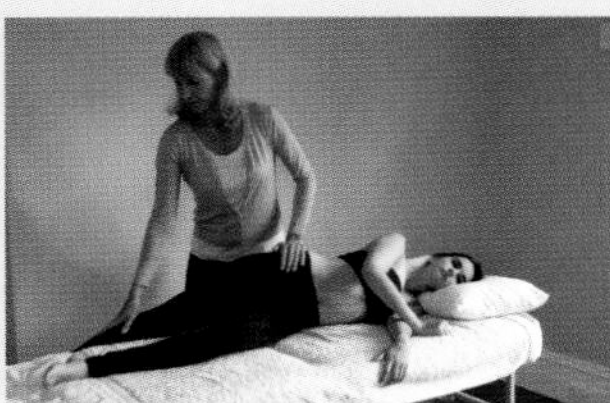
Muscle – lower extremity		
Iliopsoas – supine	The client lies supine at the end of the table so that the hips can fully extend. The client fully flexes one knee. Observe the distance between the extended thigh and the level of the table.	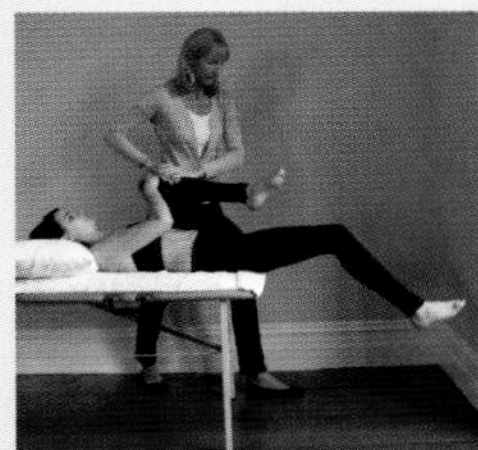
Iliopsoas – prone	The client lies prone with knee flexed to 90°. The practitioner stabilises the pelvis with one hand. The practitioner lifts the client's thigh as far as possible without moving the pelvis.	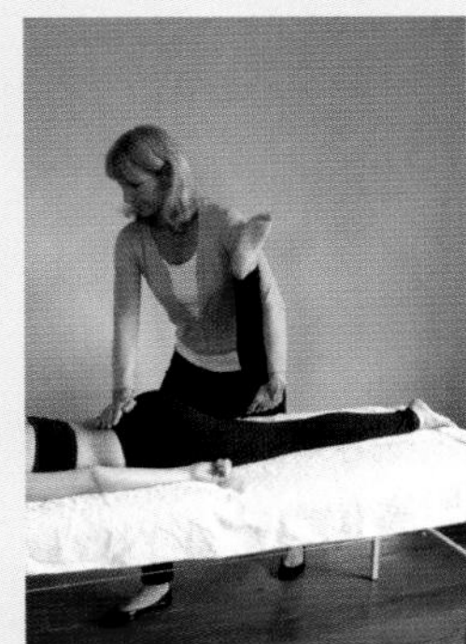
Rectus femoris – supine	The client's position is the same as for the supine ilio psoas test. Observe the degree of knee flection on the side of the extended thigh.	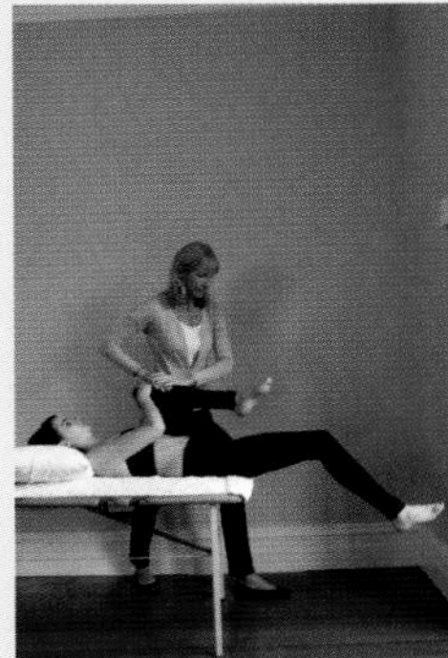
Rectus femoris – prone	The client lies prone, knee flexed and the foot is taken towards their buttock.	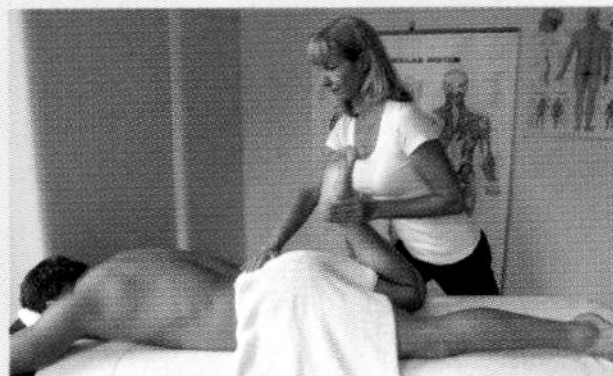
Hamstring	The client lies supine and the extended leg is raised. The test may also be performed with the knee slightly flexed.	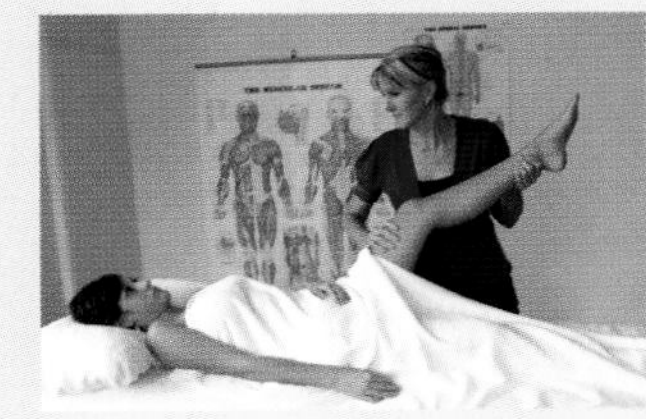

Table 2.7 Length tests of major muscles—cont'd

Muscle – lower extremity	Length test	
Hip external rotators	The client lies prone, knee flexed to 90°. The client's leg drops laterally as far as possible.	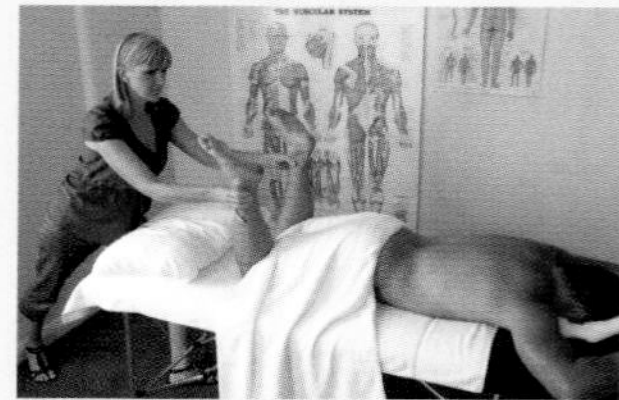
Hip internal rotators	As above, except that the client's leg drops medially as far as possible.	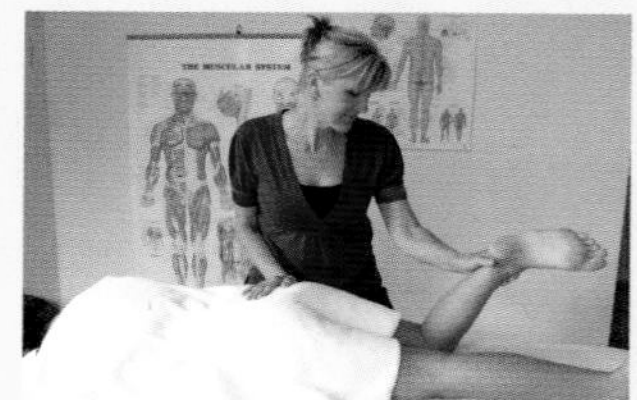
Iliotibial band and tensor fasciae latae muscle length (Ober's test)	The client lies on their side, lower knee slightly flexed. The upper knee is flexed to 90°. The practitioner abducts and slightly extends the upper thigh. The client then allows the upper leg to drop towards the table. A shortened iliotibial band prevents the leg from reaching the table.	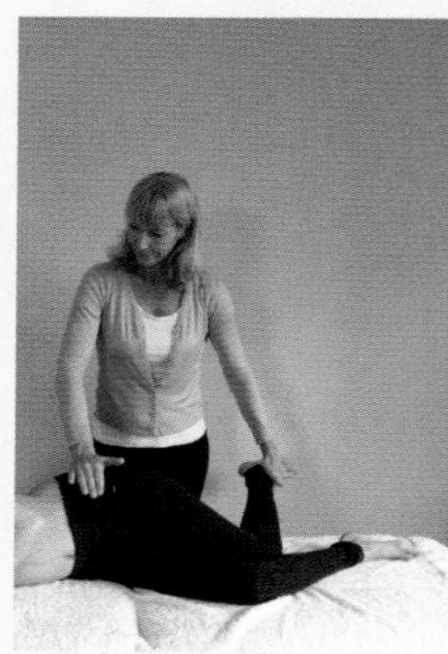
Hip adductors	The client lies supine with knees bent and feet flat on the table. The practitioner stabilises the pelvis on one side as the opposite knee drops to the side as far as possible.	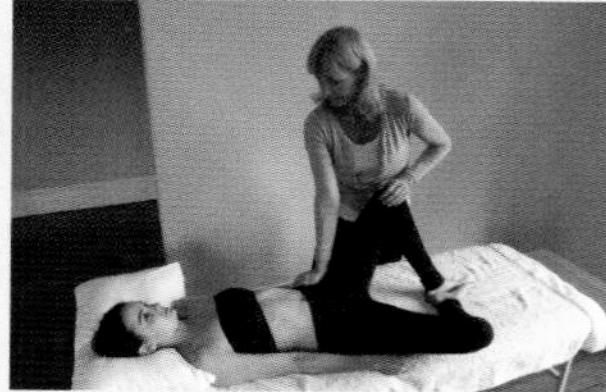
Gastrocnemius	The client lies supine, knees extended. The practitioner dorsiflexes the client's ankle.	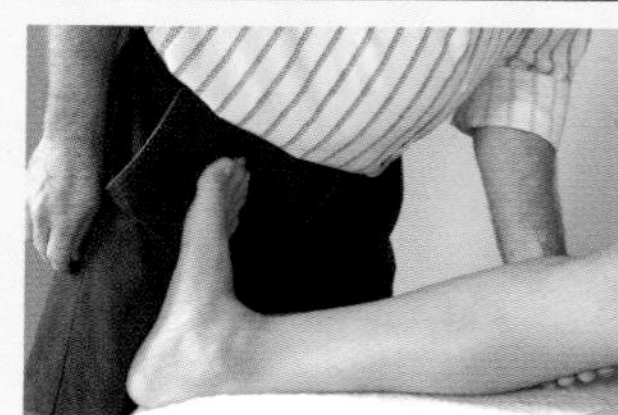
Soleus	The client lies prone, knee flexed to 90°. The practitioner dorsiflexes the client's ankle.	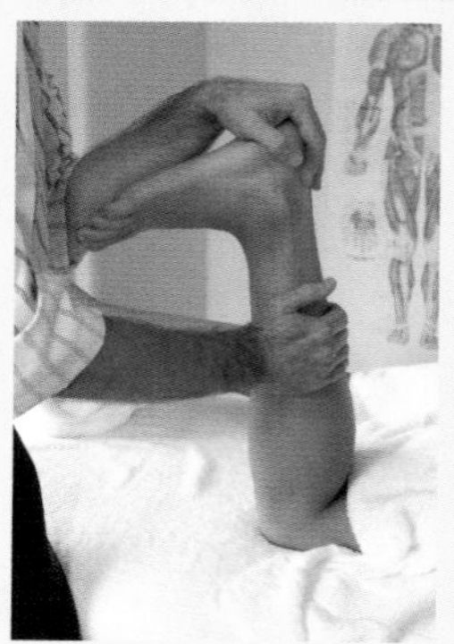

- Movement should not be blocked by external supports or pillows.
- Client must be able to assume the position.

Stabilisation of proximal bony segment of the associated joint

- Required to isolate intended motion.
- Avoids the client substituting another muscle to perform the motion.

Note the end-feel

- Bony (e.g elbow extension).
- Capsular (e.g. medial hip rotation).
- Muscular (e.g. knee extension with hip flexion).
- Soft tissue (e.g. knee flexion).

Special (orthopaedic) tests

A range of special (orthopaedic) tests can be used by remedial massage therapists to help identify specific conditions. Remember that findings from special tests should be interpreted cautiously, especially where the specificity or sensitivity of the tests are less than 95%, or where likelihood ratios (LR) are in the range $0.1 \geq LR \geq 10$.

Some commonly used special tests are listed in Table 2.8. Details of relevant tests will be discussed in Chapters 10–20.

PALPATION

Palpation is considered by many to be the most important assessment tool of massage therapists. Palpatory assessment continues throughout the treatment as an inherent function of manual therapy. Beginning students can rapidly learn to detect differences in muscle tone as they massage. With practice, palpation can be used to identify specific tissues (see Table 2.9) and to assess tissues for pathological states and stages of healing using the following indicators:

- Temperature: use the dorsum of the hand just above or lightly touching the skin to identify changes in temperature (e.g. increased temperature in acute inflammation, decreased temperature in impaired circulation).
- Changes in normal tissue (e.g. fibrotic cords in muscles, hard pea-shaped painful trigger points, muscle flaccidity, microtears in musculotendinous junctions and muscle bellies).
- Presence of oedema (e.g. sponginess of tissues in acute inflammation, pitting and non-pitting[i]).

The chiropractic, osteopathic and physiotherapy literature contains a number of studies on the efficacy of palpation. One annotated bibliography found only slight interexaminer reliability and moderate intraexaminer reliability for palpation.[30] Inter- and intraexaminer discrepancies were also found in a small study in which two physiotherapists identified 12 anatomical landmarks that enabled measurement of eight joint angles.[31] Joensen et al[32], on the other hand, found strong agreements between palpation for tendon hypertrophy. As with many other aspects of massage assessment practices, further research is needed to confirm the efficacy of palpation as an assessment strategy for remedial massage practice.

Palpatory findings must also be recorded on clients' files. There have been several attempts at categorising palpatory findings but none has been widely taken up. Recording the tissue type and any abnormal temperature, tissue quality or water content is usually sufficient (e.g. fibrotic left upper trapezius, hot swollen right lateral ankle joint, trigger point right supraspinatus muscle).

[i]Pitting oedema results when a swollen area is pressed and an indentation persists after the pressure is released. This is the most common form of oedema. It is caused by any form of pressure (e.g. from tight socks). In non-pitting oedema pressure applied to a swollen area does not create a persistent indentation. Non-pitting oedema occurs in disorders of the lymphatic system (e.g. lymphoedema after lymph-node surgery or congenitally). It is usually observed in the arms or legs. It can also be associated with hyperthyroidism.

LEGAL AND ETHICAL REQUIREMENTS FOR REMEDIAL MASSAGE ASSESSMENT

Issues of privacy, confidentiality, child protection and the safe and efficient use of equipment and resources are of paramount importance in all aspects of remedial massage practice, including assessment. Remedial massage assessments must be recorded accurately and in a well-organised manner so as to be easily interpreted by others. Lack of standard abbreviations of key terms and recordings of remedial massage assessments confounds the transparency of record keeping. SOAP[j] and other similar charting methods are useful guides for massage therapists, however they often lack the capacity for recording the range of assessments commonly used in remedial massage practice. Practice management software can often be used to record assessments, copies of X-ray and CT scans and other medical reports and correspondence.

Figure 2.19 is an extract from a sample client assessment form which accommodates commonly used remedial massage assessments.

Another simple method for recording trunk ranges of motion involves drawing a star diagram to represent cervical, thoracic or lumbar motion as if observed from above (see Figure 2.20). Each line represents normal ROM for the movement. Restrictions in ranges of motion are indicated by drawing dashes, and pain is indicated by recording P on the lines of the star diagram. The closer to the centre of the star, the more marked the restriction or the earlier the onset of pain.

KEY MESSAGES

Remedial massage assessments determine the suitability of clients for remedial massage through screening for red flags. Those deemed suitable for remedial massage undergo further assessments to identify potential sources of symptoms, to understand clients' perceptions of their own functional impairments and to develop effective therapy plans.

For safe practice, all assessments should adhere to the following principles:

1. See-Move-Touch; that is, clients should be observed and perform active range of motion tests first before any physical contact is made with clients.
2. Assessments should be performed slowly and carefully especially when using tests that can reproduce symptoms.

[j]SOAP charting encourages therapists to record subjective (S) and objective (O) assessments, assessment or analysis (A) and their therapy plan (P).[34]

Table 2.8 Special tests commonly used by remedial massage therapists (see Chapters 10–20 for specific regional orthopaedic tests)

Adam's test	Test to discriminate idiopathic and functional scoliosis
Anterior draw (knee)	Test for integrity of anterior cruciate ligament of the knee (SN 18–95, SP 86–100, LR+ 1.8–8.3, LR– 0.1–0.5)
Anterior draw (ankle)	Test for anterior talofibular instability (SN 78–95, SP 74–84, LR+ 3.1, LR– 0.29)
Apley's test	Test for meniscal tear in the knee (R 0.95, SN 13–16, SP 86–100, LR+ 0.8–5.9, LR– 0.63–1.1)
Cervical compression test	Test for pressure on a nerve root (increased peripheral pain), joint damage or ligament strain (increased local pain)
Cervical distraction	Pressure on a nerve root relieved by distraction. Increased local pain suggests muscle, ligament or joint capsule damage (R 0.82, SN 40–50, SP 80–100, LR+ 4.4; LR– 0.62)
Drop arm test	Useful to rule in rotator cuff tear (R 0.28–0.66, SN 8–27, SP 88–100, LR+ 2.6–5 LR– 0.83–0.94)
Elbow extension test	Useful to rule out bony or joint injury (SN 97, SP 69, LR+ 3.1, LR– 0.04)[29]
Elevated arm stress test (Roo's test)	Test for thoracic outlet syndrome (SN 82, SP 100)
Empty can test	Pain or weakness suggests supraspinatus damage (SN 44–89, SP 50–90, LR+ 1.8–4.2, LR– 0.22–0.63)
Finkelstein's test	Test for tenosynovitis of the abductor pollicis longus and extensor pollicis brevis (SN 81, SP 50, LR+ 1.6, LR– 0.38)
Iliac compression test	Test for sacroiliac lesion
Impingement test	Test for shoulder impingement syndrome: shoulder impingement suggested if pain during active flexion; supraspinatus impingement suggested if pain when shoulder internally rotated; biceps long head implicated if pain when shoulder externally rotated.
Kemp's/quadrant test	Leg pain suggests nerve root compression or radiculopathy; low back pain suggests local sprain/strain or facet syndrome
Morton's test	Test for Morton's neuroma, metatarsal joint arthritis, fracture of the metatarsal heads or metatarsalgia
Painful arc	Test for impingement syndrome, rotator cuff or AC pathology (SN 33–98, SP 10–81, LR+ 1.1–3.9, LR– 0.2–0.82)
Patella apprehension test	Test for dislocation or subluxation of the patella (SN 7–37, SP 86–100, LR+ 0.9–2.3, LR– 0.8–1.0)
Patellofemoral grind test	Test for patellofemoral syndrome, DJD, osteochondritis of the patella, patella fracture (SN 29–49, SP 67–75, LR+ 0.9–1.9, LR– 0.7–1.1)
Patrick's/FABERE test	Test for hip joint pathology, DJD, sprain/strain, fracture, tight hip adductors (SN 88)
Phalen's test	Test for carpal tunnel syndrome (compression of median nerve) (R 0.79, SN 10–88, SP 33–100, LR+ 0.7–41.5, LR– 0.1–1)
Posterior draw (knee)	Test for the integrity of the posterior cruciate ligament (SN 22–100, SP 99, LR+ 90, LR– 0.1)
Posterior draw (ankle)	Test for the integrity of the posterior ankle ligaments
PSIS asymmetry	Test for sacroiliac lesion, anatomical variation (R 0.7, SN 69)
Shoulder (anterior) apprehension test	Test for anterior glenohumeral instability (SN 53, SP 99, LR+ 53, LR– 0.47)

Table 2.8 Special tests commonly used by remedial massage therapists—cont'd

SI compression test	Test for SI sprain, fracture, joint dysfunction (R 0.64–0.79, SN 25–69, SP 63–100, LR+ 1.6–2.2, LR– 0.4–0.63)
SI distraction test	Test for anterior SI or pubic symphysis sprain, pelvic fracture (R 0.36–0.94, SN 11–60, SP 74–100, LR+ 1.1–3.2, LR– 0.5–0.98)
Sign of the buttock	Test to distinguish whether pain on straight leg raising arises from SI joint dysfunction, bursitis, gluteal muscle strain or from lumbar spine pathology, nerve root pressure or hamstring tension
Slump test	Leg symptoms suggest nerve root tension, radiculopathy, disc herniation. Local lumbosacral pain suggests lumbosacral sprain or strain (SN 83, SP 55, LR+ 1.8, LR– 0.3)
Straight leg raising	Test to distinguish sciatic nerve impingement, disc herniation, piriformis syndrome from SI/lumbar strain or sprain (R 0.92, SN 78–98, SP 11–64, LR+ 1.03–2.2, LR– 0.05–0.86)
Thomas test	Test for hip contracture, tight hip flexors (R 0.91)
Tinel's sign	Test for neuropathy Tinel's sign at elbow (SN 70, SP 98, LR+ 35, LR– 0.31) Tinel's sign at wrist (R 0.5–0.8, SN 23–97, SP 53–100, LR+ 0.7–11, LR– 0.03–1.0)
Trendelenburg test	Test for gluteus medius weakness or paralysis, Legg-Calve-Perthes disease, poliomyelitis, hip dislocation, fracture (R 0.68, SN 73, SP 77, LR+ 3.15, LR– 0.36)
Valgus/varus elbow stress test	Test for medial/lateral collateral ligament sprain
Valgus/varus stress test (knee)	Test for medial/lateral collateral ligament sprain (R 0.16, SN 86–100, SP 100)
Valsalva	Test for space occupying lesion, disc herniation, IVF encroachment (R 0.69, SN 22, SP 94, LR+ 3.67, LR– 0.82)
Yergason's test	Test for biceps brachii tendonitis or strain, glenoid labrum pathology, torn transverse humeral ligament (SN 9–50, SP 79–93, LR+ 1.3–3.0, LR– 0.72–0.94)

(R) = reliability, (SN) = sensitivity, (SP) = specificity, (LR) = likelihood ratios
Adapted from Visniak[15]

Table 2.9 Palpating tissue layers

Epidermis	Place dorsum of hands lightly on the skin and compare the temperature of different parts of the body. Slide hand over the skin and note the dryness/moistness and texture of the skin. Slide fingers over the skin so that it wrinkles and note any resistance between the epidermis and the underlying tissue.
Muscle	Muscle tissue feels firmer than subcutaneous tissue. Postural muscles often palpate as tight bundles of fibres. Fibrotic tissue feels ropey.
Tendons	Tendons feel like thin firm movable cords.
Ligaments	Ligaments feel like flat bands of tissue, less mobile and elastic than tendons.
Joint capsules	Not palpable unless thickened. Articular disorders are often associated with joint line tenderness.
Peripheral nerves	Peripheral nerves feel like small threads, thinner and less elastic than tendons, often fairly mobile.
Lymph glands	Small soft rubbery nodes, rarely bigger than 0.5 cm.
Blood vessels	Superficial blood vessels feel like soft tubes, pulses are often detected.

Adapted from Chaitow[33]

Postural observation

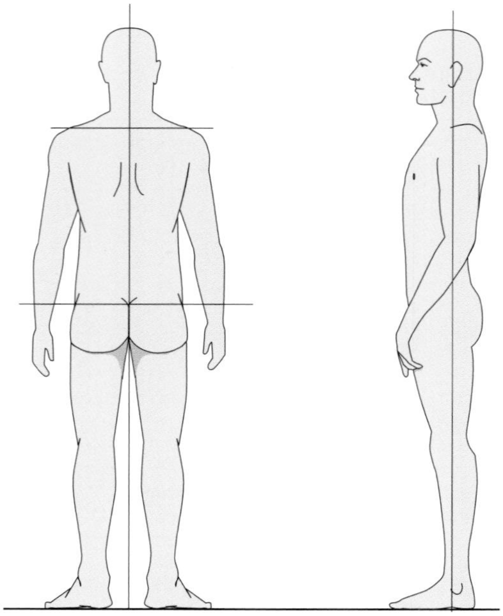

Gait assessment

Rate Rhythm Symmetry

Phase

	Heel strike	Foot flat	Midstance	Push off	Acceleration	Mid Swing	Deceleration
Joint Muscle							

Palpatory findings

____

____

____

____

Cervical

AROM	**Flexion**	**Extension**	**R lat flexion**	**L lat flexion**	**R rotation**	**L rotation**
PROM	**Flexion**	**Extension**	**R lat flexion**	**L lat flexion**	**R rotation**	**L rotation**
RROM	**Flexion**	**Extension**	**R lat flexion**	**L lat flexion**	**R rotation**	**L rotation**
Specific muscle tests						
Special tests	**Compression**		**Distraction**		**Valsalva**	

Fig. 2.19 Sample client assessment form

Thoracic

AROM	Flexion	Extension	R lat flexion	L lat flexion	R rotation	L rotation
PROM	Flexion	Extension	R lat flexion	L lat flexion	R rotation	L rotation
RROM	Flexion	Extension	R lat flexion	L lat flexion	R rotation	L rotation
Specific muscle tests						
Special tests	Adam's test		Deep breathing		Elevated arm stress test	

Shoulder

AROM	Flexion		Extension		Abduction		Horiz adduc		Med rot		Lat rot	
	L	R	L	R	L	R	L	R	L	R	L	R
PROM	L	R	L	R	L	R	L	R	L	R	L	R
RROM	L	R	L	R	L	R	L	R	L	R	L	R
Specific muscle tests												
Special tests	Apley's scratch L R				Impingement L R				Apprehension L R			
	Drop arm L R				Yergason's L R				Empty can test L R			

Elbow

AROM	Flexion		Extension		Supination		Pronation		
	L	R	L	R	L	R	L	R	
PROM	L	R	L	R	L	R	L	R	
RROM	L	R	L	R	L	R	L	R	
Specific muscle tests									
Special tests	Valgus stress L R				Varus stress L R				Extension test L R
	Resisted wrist flexion L R						Resisted wrist extension L R		

Wrist

AROM	Flexion		Extension		Abduction		Adduction		Supination		Pronation	
	L	R	L	R	L	R	L	R	L	R	L	R
PROM	L	R	L	R	L	R	L	R	L	R	L	R
RROM	L	R	L	R	L	R	L	R	L	R	L	R
Specific muscle tests												
Special tests	Phalen's test L R				Tinel's test L R				Finkelstein's test L R			

Fig. 2.19, cont'd

Continued

Lumbar

AROM	Flexion	Extension	R lat flexion	L lat flexion	R rotation	L rotation
PROM	Flexion	Extension	R lat flexion	L lat flexion	R rotation	L rotation
RROM	Flexion	Extension	R lat flexion	L lat flexion	R rotation	L rotation
Specific muscle tests						
Special tests	Kemp's test L R		Valsalva		SLR L R	
	Centralisation peripheralisation		Patrick's test L R		SI compression L R	
	SI distraction L R		Short leg L R			

Hip

AROM	Flexion		Extension		Abduction		Adduction		Med rot		Lat rot	
	L	R	L	R	L	R	L	R	L	R	L	R
PROM	L	R	L	R	L	R	L	R	L	R	L	R
RROM	L	R	L	R	L	R	L	R	L	R	L	R
Specific muscle tests												
Special tests	Patrick's test L R				Thomas test L R				Trendelenburg L R			
	Ober's test L R											

Knee

AROM	Flexion		Extension		Med rot		Lat rot	
	L	R	L	R	L	R	L	R
PROM	L	R	L	R	L	R	L	R
RROM	L	R	L	R	L	R	L	R
Specific muscle tests								
Special tests	Patellofemoral grind L R		Patella apprehension L R		Valgus stress test L R			
	Varus stress test L R		Anterior draw L R		Posterior draw L R			
	Apley's compression L R							

Fig. 2.19, cont'd

Ankle and foot

AROM	Flexion		Extension		Inversion		Eversion	
	L	R	L	R	L	R	L	R
PROM	L	R	L	R	L	R	L	R
RROM	L	R	L	R	L	R	L	R
Specific muscle tests								
Special tests	Anterior draw L R		Posterior draw L R		Lat stability L R			
	Morton's test L R							

Fig. 2.19, cont'd

Star diagram

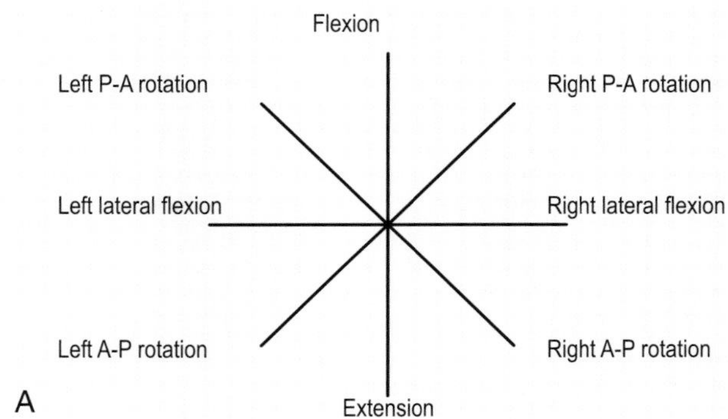

Lumbar: mildly restricted flexion, moderately restricted right lateral flexion

Cervical: severely restricted extension moderately restricted left rotation and lateral flexion

B

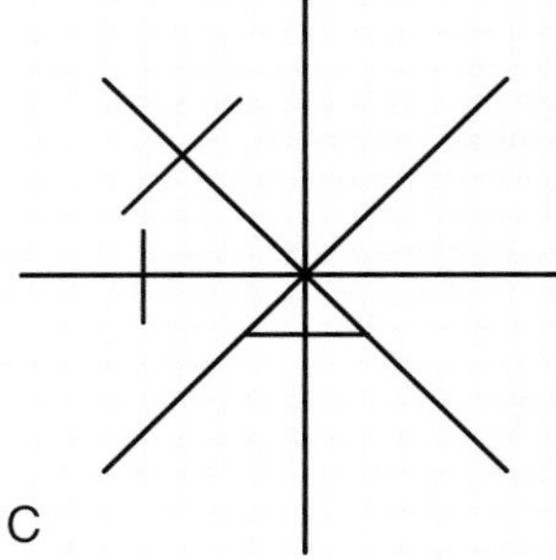

Fig. 2.20 Recording trunk ranges of motion: (a) the star diagram, (b) and (c) are examples showing how to use the star diagram.

Remedial massage assessments include:

- Case history
  - Identify red and yellow flags
  - Is the client's condition mild, moderate or severe?
- Outcome measures
  - Monitor progress towards treatment goals
- Postural observation
  - Look for underlying predisposing factors to presenting symptoms
- Gait assessment
  - Observe disturbances of symmetry, rate and rhythm of normal gait
- Functional tests
  - Active range of motion (AROM)
    – to locate source of lesion
  - Passive range of motion (PROM)
  - Resisted tests (RROM)
  - Specific muscle tests (where appropriate)
    – Resisted tests and length tests for specific muscles
  - Special (orthopaedic) tests
- Palpation
  - Identify tissues involved, stage of healing

Review questions

1. Complete the following sentences with a word or phrase:
   a) Red flags are ______________________________
   b) A common cause of increased kyphosis of the cervicothoracic spine is ______________________________
   c) Passive range of motion tests are used to test __________
   d) A dermatome is ______________________________
   e) __________ test is used to discriminate between idiopathic and functional scoliosis.
2. What would you do if a client came to your clinic for assessment and treatment of pain in the upper thoracic spine, bilateral shoulders and hands, and with a history of night sweats?
3. Circle the correct answer:
   A client is observed to have a mild scoliosis with the right iliac crest lower than the left. It is likely that:
   a) the right gluteal fold is lower/higher on the right
   b) the gluteal cleft deviates to the left/right
   c) the left PSIS is lower/higher than the right PSIS
   d) the right foot is anterior/posterior to the left foot
   e) the left/right knee is slightly flexed
   f) the waist curve on the right appears to increase/decrease
4. Indicate True or False for each of the following statements.
   a) Using the principle of See-Move-Touch, passive tests are conducted before active tests. True/False
   b) The centre of gravity passes anterior to the lateral malleolus in the ideally aligned erect posture. True/False
   c) Referred pain is sharp and poorly localised. True/False
   d) The inferior angle of the scapula is approximately at the level of T5 spinous process. True/False
5. What type of tissue is implicated if active shoulder flexion is positive and resisted shoulder flexion is positive but passive shoulder flexion is not?
   What further testing, if any, is required?
6. What type of tissue is implicated if active hip abduction is positive and passive hip abduction is positive but resisted hip abduction is not?
   What further testing, if any, is required?
7. How would you interpret the following assessment findings for the lumbar spine: active right lateral flexion positive, resisted right lateral flexion positive, and passive right lateral flexion positive?
   What further testing, if any, is required?
8. Describe a test for the length of the hamstring muscle.
9. What type of tissue is suggested by the following palpatory findings:
   a) Soft, rubbery, pea-shaped, less than 0.5 cm diameter
   b) Tight cord
   c) Small threads
   d) Small pulsing tubes
10. Name a possible cause for the following observations of gait:
    a) steppage gait
    b) heavy heel strike
    c) back knee gait
    d) excessive hip rotation in acceleration phase
11. What are the implications for practice of using a functional test with a sensitivity of 95%?
12. How would you interpret the lumbar ranges of motion indicated by the following star diagram?

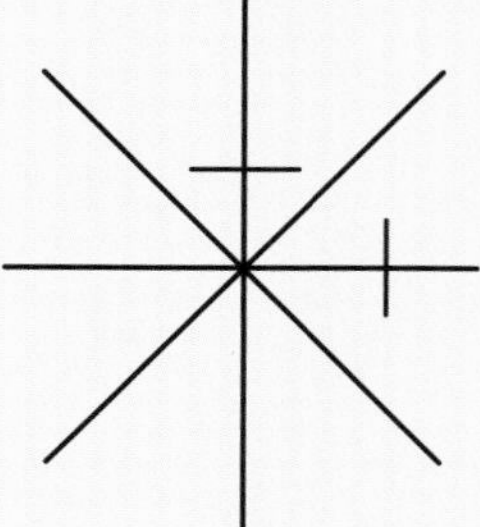

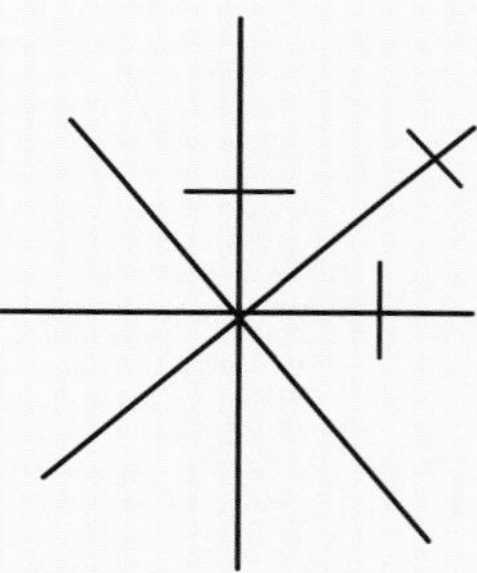

APPENDIX 2.1

Skin cancer

In Australia 70–80% of all skin cancers are basal cell carcinomas, 15–20% are squamous cell carcinomas and less than 5% are melanomas.[35]

Basal cell carcinomas usually occur in people over 40 years of age, although they may occur in younger people. They are slow growing and present as either small, raised pearly tumours with small blood vessels on the surface or a red plaque. The latter is more common on the trunk.

Squamous cell carcinomas may develop as a slowly enlarging, scaly nodule or an ulcerated sore with raised, rolled edges or a red, scaly plaque.

Malignant melanoma is a malignant change in the pigment cells of the skin. It can develop in normal skin as a flat, coloured spot or appear as a change in an existing pigmented lesion such as a mole. They can appear anywhere on the body. In the early stages, a melanoma is a flat, coloured spot.

Encourage clients to seek medical attention for pigmented lesions which are either new or changing, especially if their size, colour or shape is changing.

The following checklist may be useful:[36]

a. Asymmetry – one half of the lesion is dissimilar to the other
b. Border irregularity – lack of distinct edge, spread of pigmentation into apparently normal skin
c. Colour change – red, white, blue, sudden darkening, particularly shades of brown or black
d. Changes in surface – scaliness, erosion, bleeding, oozing, crusting
e. Diameter enlarging

Seborrhoeic keratoses are raised, pigmented lesions which are common benign tumours occurring in people over 40 years old. **Solar keratoses** are scaly lesions which may come and go. They occur on the sun-exposed areas of the body and are seen in 40–50% of people over 40 years old. These lesions are often confused with melanomas. However, their presence indicates that a person has had sufficient sun exposure to be at high risk of having either a basal cell or squamous cell carcinoma somewhere on the sun-exposed areas of their body.

What to look for

Any mole or freckle that has:

1. changed colour. Melanomas often develop a blue or black colour. Sometimes areas may become lighter and many different colours such as reds, greys, blues may be found.
2. changed shape or increased in size. The change in shape is usually from an oval or round mole to an irregular 'coastline' appearance. The increase in size can be overall or simply an elevation above surrounding skin. React quickly to a flat mole that becomes elevated, especially if the elevation is dark or a different colour from the original mole.
3. an irregular border. Most harmless moles have smooth, regular borders. Melanomas often have irregular borders.
4. become itchy or bleeds. A mole that bleeds without any significant injury should be examined by a doctor. Itch may be an important symptom but only if there are other changes.
5. appeared recently from normal-looking skin, especially if it is dark or is rapidly growing.

Any pigmented lesion that looks different from the others on an individual's skin should be examined closely and biopsied if diagnosis is uncertain. (Most moles or pigmented spots on an individual resemble each other – show a family resemblance.)

Clinical features suggestive of malignancy

- size greater than 6 mm
- irregular shape
- variation in colour within the mole
- noticeable increase in size over 3–18 months
- unexplained inflammation in and around the mole (redness and/or tenderness around a mole for longer than two months is suspicious)
- bleeding and itching (repeated bleeding with minor injury is unusual)

REFERENCES

1. Chow R. Complementary medicine: impact on medical practice. Curr Ther 2000;41(7):76–9.
2. Grace S, Vemulpad S, Beirman R. Training in and use of diagnostic techniques among CAM practitioners: an Australian study. J Altern Complement Med 2006;12(7):695–700.
3. Ernst E. The safety of massage therapy. Rheumatology 2003;42:1101–6.
4. Anderson T, Ogles B, Patterson C, et al. Therapist effects: facilitative interpersonal skills as a predictor of therapist success. J Clin Psychol 2009;65(7):755–68.
5. Weiss L, Blustein J. Faithful patients: the effect of long-term physician-patient relationships on the costs and use of health care by older Americans. Am J Public Health 1996;86(12):1742–7.
6. New Zealand Guidelines Group. New Zealand acute low back pain guide. Online. Available: www.nzgg.org.nz/guidelines/0072/acc1038_col.pdf; 2004.
7. Australian Acute Musculoskeletal Pain Guidelines Group. Evidence-based management of acute musculoskeletal pain: a guide for clinicians. Bowden Hills, Qld: Australian Academic Press; 2004.
8. WorkCover NSW. Training manual for providers of remedial massage therapy to injured workers. Gosford: WorkCover NSW; 2010.
9. Weir M. Complementary Medicine: ethics and law. Ashgrove: Prometheus Publications; 2000.
10. WorkCover NSW. Delivering Physical Treatment to Injured Workers – using evidence-based practice and treatment outcomes. Sydney: WorkCover NSW; 2005.
11. Bayar K, Bayar B, Yakut E, et al. Reliability and construct validity of the Oswestry Low Back Pain Disability Questionnaire in the elderly with low back pain. The Pain Clinic 2003;15(1):55–9.
12. Harcourt B, Wijesinha M, Harcourt G. Subjective and Objective Numerical Outcome Measure Assessment. A combined outcome measure tool: findings on a study of reliability. J Manipulative Physiol Ther 2003;26(8):481–92.
13. Beirman R. Handbook of clinical diagnosis. Sydney: R. Beirman; 2003.
14. Fritz S, Chaitow L, Hymel GM. Clinical massage in the healthcare setting. St Louis, MI: Mosby Elsevier; 2008.
15. Vizniak N. Physical assessment. Burnaby, B.C.: Professional Health Systems; 2008.
16. Latt M, Menz H, Fung V, et al. Walking speed, cadence and step length are selected to optimize the stability of head and pelvic accelerations. Exp Brain Res 2008;184:201–9.
17. Hoppenfeld S. Physical examination of the spine and extremities. 2nd edn. Upper Saddle River, NJ: Prentice Hall; 2010.
18. Magee D. Orthopedic Physical Assessment. 5th edn. Philadelphia: Saunders; 2008.
19. Rattray F, Ludwig L. Clinical massage therapy: Understanding, assessing and treating over 70 conditions. Elora, Ont: Talus; 2000.
20. Chaitow L. Muscle energy techniques. 2nd edn. Edinburgh: Churchill Livingstone; 2001.
21. McGee S. Simplifying likelihood ratios. J Gen Intern Med 2002;17(8):646–9.
22. Esposito S, Phillipson S. Spinal adjusting technique: The chiropractic art. Sydney: Well-Adjusted Publishing; 2005.
23. Klassbo M, Harms-Ringdahl K, Larsson G, et al. Examination of passive ROM and capsular patterns in the hip. Physiother Res Int (Research Support, Non-U.S. Gov't) 2003;8(1):1–12.
24. Bijl D, Dekker J, van Baar ME, et al. Validity of Cyriax's concept capsular pattern for the diagnosis of osteoarthritis of hip and/or knee. Scand J Rheumatol (Clinical Trial Randomized Controlled Trial Research Support, Non-U.S. Gov't) 1998;27(5):347–51.
25. Kendall McCreary E, Provance P, McIntyre Rodgers M, et al. Muscles, testing and function, with posture and pain. 5th edn. Philadelphia, PA: Lippincott Williams and Wilkins; 2005.
26. Hislop H, Montgomery J. Daniels and Worthingham's muscle testing: Techniques of manual examination. 8th edn. Oxford: Saunders Elsevier; 2007.
27. Reese N, Bandy W. Joint range of motion and muscle length testing. Philadelphia: W.B. Saunders; 2002.
28. Reiman M, Manske R. Functional testing in human performance. Champaign, IL: Human Kinetics; 2009.
29. Cleland J, Koppenhaver S. Netter's orthopaedic clinical examination: an evidence-based approach. 2nd edn. Philadelphia: Saunders; 2011.
30. Haneline M, Cooperstein R, Young M, et al. An annotated bibliography of spinal motion palpation reliability studies. J Can Chiropr Assoc 2009;53(1):40–58.
31. Moriguchi C, Carnaz L, Silva L, et al. Reliability of intra- and inter-rater palpation discrepancy and estimation of its effects on joint angle measurements. J Can Chiropr Assoc 2009;53(1):40–58.
32. Joensen J, Couppe C, Bjordal J. Increased palpation tenderness and muscle strength deficit in the prediction of tendon hypertrophy in symptomatic unilateral shoulder tendinopathy: an ultrasonographic study. Physiotherapy 2009;95:83–93.
33. Chaitow L. Palpatory literacy: they complete instruction manual for the hands on therapist. London: Thorsons Element; 1991.
34. Fritz S. Mosby's Fundamentals of Therapeutic Massage. 4th edn. St Louis, MI: Mosby Elsevier; 2009.
35. Australian Cancer Council. Cancer types 2009: Online. Available from: www.cancer.org.au.
36. Berwick M, Begg C, Fine J, et al. Screening for cutaneous melanoma by skin self-examination. J Natl Canc Inst 1996;88(1):17–23.

Useful Websites

http://www.pennchiro.org/files/clinical/doctor/Oswestry.pdf

3 Planning remedial massage therapy

The content of this chapter relates to the following Units of Competency:

HLTREM503C Plan remedial massage treatment strategy
HLTREM504C Apply remedial massage assessment framework
HLTREM502C Provide remedial massage treatment

Health Training Package HLT07

Learning Outcomes

- Prioritise client safety when planning treatment by using information from assessment findings (See-Move-Touch principle).
- Develop short- and long-term treatment plans to address presenting symptoms and predisposing factors.
- Develop treatment plans that progressively increase the self-help component of therapy.
- Use the best available evidence to inform treatment plans.
- Take clients' preferences into account when formulating treatment plans.
- Use treatment protocols based on tissue type, stage of inflammation and severity of injury to guide treatment.
- Use cryotherapy and thermotherapy safely and effectively in treating clients.
- Regularly monitor and review treatment plans.

PRINCIPLES OF TREATMENT

Treatment plans are co-produced by practitioners and clients from negotiations between them: the practitioner informing the client of the assessment findings, the range of available approaches and their rationale and the client negotiating options that fit their preferences and values. A broad range of techniques is available within the scope of remedial massage therapy, and practitioners individualise treatments based on their preferred techniques and personal treatment style. Client safety and treatment effectiveness are always priorities. Strategies to ensure safe treatment include warming the area to be treated with Swedish massage before applying deeper techniques, and working within the client's pain tolerance.[1] Treatment effectiveness derives from treatment protocols based on the best available evidence, the type of tissue(s) to be treated, the severity of the condition and the stage of inflammation.

PRIORITISING CLIENT SAFETY

Practitioners have a duty of care to promote their clients' wellbeing and to keep them from harm. The following strategies are used by remedial massage therapists to ensure their clients' safety.

SWEDISH MASSAGE BEFORE REMEDIAL MASSAGE

Most remedial massage begins with Swedish or basic massage to the area to be treated. This practice enables the targeted area to be warmed in preparation for deeper techniques. It also relaxes the client and alerts the practitioner to the client's responses to pressure. In some cases Swedish massage constitutes the whole treatment. This may be because the practitioner and client decide to focus on relaxation therapy or because the practitioner is unsure of the underlying condition and chooses to take a conservative approach.

ACTIVE MOVEMENTS BEFORE PASSIVE

As discussed in Chapter 2, the guiding principle, See-Move-Touch, underpins safe practice; that is, observation and active movements precede any physical contact in assessment or treatment. In treatment this principle dictates that active muscle stretches precede passive muscle stretches, that active soft tissue releasing techniques precede passive soft tissue releasing techniques and so on.

TREATING WITHIN PAIN TOLERANCE

Assessments often aim to locate the source of symptoms and to achieve this clients are asked to perform movements that could reproduce symptoms. The See-Move-Touch principle helps practitioners assess and treat clients within a pain-free or tolerable pain range and minimises the risk of aggravating symptoms. Range of motion assessments, in particular, guide the application of techniques. For example, if a client reports pain when they turn their head 30° to the right, techniques that involve passive rotation of the cervical spine to the right to 30° or beyond may reproduce or aggravate symptoms. There are many remedial massage techniques, including muscle energy and assisted stretching techniques, that could be used to treat limited cervical rotation within the client's pain-free range.

Techniques like trigger points rely on reproducing symptoms to locate their source and to treat the condition. Pain elicited during trigger point and other deep techniques is monitored by using a pain scale to ensure that the practitioner works within the client's tolerable pain range (usually not beyond 7 or 8 out of 10).

OVERVIEW OF A REMEDIAL MASSAGE TREATMENT APPROACH

Remedial massage clients require a course of treatment designed to address presenting conditions and to progressively introduce self-help and health-promotion strategies. Key features of this approach are planning for optimal outcomes for clients in the long term, the central role of educating clients to be active participants in their treatment, and respect for clients' healthcare preferences.

SHORT- AND LONG-TERM TREATMENT PLANS

It is helpful to develop a short-term and a long-term plan for each client. The short-term plan directs treatment to the highest priority (usually determined by symptoms). The long-term plan can be introduced when presenting symptoms have subsided. Treatment then focuses on contributing or predisposing factors such as underlying structural features and lifestyle factors.

CLIENT EDUCATION AND SELF-HELP

An important part of remedial massage treatment involves educating clients about likely causal or aggravating factors and guiding their management of these factors. Clients should become directly engaged in their recovery as soon as possible by taking an active role in rehabilitation and health promotion activities (e.g. regular walks to reduce stress and strengthening and stretching exercises to address muscle imbalances). Most soft tissue injuries resolve within four weeks, although a small number go on to cause permanent disability. Psychosocial factors (yellow flags) influence a return to normal activities. Clients are encouraged to resume normal activities as soon as possible. It is good practice to include a self-help program, such as home exercises, posture correction and lifting advice in all treatments. Transition from more passive care to increased client activity in exercise rehabilitation, postural and ergonomic correction, weight-loss programs and lifestyle modification within 4 to 6 weeks after injury helps prevent long-term disability and time off work.[2] Strategies such as realistic goal setting and enlisting family support may help motivate clients to participate in self-help programs.

CLIENTS' PREFERENCES

Clients are actively involved in discussions about their treatment. Effective communication skills are required to build rapport with clients and to guide the consultation. Attention to the way clients approach the assessment process provides other important information including their psychological states and value systems which must also be taken into account when formulating treatment plans. Clients must be fully informed of proposals for therapy, the reasons for such proposals and their likely prognoses, and they must give their consent to a negotiated plan before treatment begins.

Figure 3.1 is designed as a guide for developing therapy plans. Provisional assessments are based on a synthesis of findings (e.g. from case history, postural observation, functional testing and palpation). Provisional assessments could include stage of injury, severity, affected tissues, condition and likely cause (e.g. acute mild right supraspinatus tendinitis or chronic cervicogenic headache secondary to right C-shaped thoracic scoliosis). Clear aims for both short-term and long-term management help focus the treatment. Short-term aims are usually directed to decreasing or to eliminating symptoms (e.g. decrease pain from 7/10 to 4/10 in two weeks). Long-term aims usually address underlying or predisposing conditions (e.g. correct muscle imbalance associated with hyperlordosis).

TREATMENT PROTOCOLS

The evidence base for remedial massage is discussed in Chapter 1. The efficacy of many assessment and treatment techniques used in clinical practice remains unconfirmed by scientific study, despite an increasing number of high-quality studies in massage therapy. Clinical Guidelines have been developed for some musculoskeletal conditions. They are based on the best available evidence and offer guidelines for the management of these conditions. Massage therapists should use Clinical Guidelines where they exist to inform their treatment practice. (See, for example, *Low back disorders*[3] and *Evidence-based management of acute musculoskeletal pain*.[4]) To keep abreast of recent developments, practitioners should regularly consult professional associations' websites, relevant journals, research websites and attend conferences where current research is presented.

In the absence of evidence-based Clinical Guidelines specifically for remedial massage, therapists rely on treatment protocols derived from clinical practice and based on the best available evidence. Treatment protocols can be modified to suit the needs of individual clients. Treatment protocols for a range of clinical presentations including acute, subacute and chronic inflammatory conditions, grade 1, 2 or 3 injuries, and for a variety of tissue types, are presented in this chapter. For example, a typical remedial massage protocol for a chronic mild or moderate soft tissue injury would be:

- Begin with Swedish or basic massage to the injured site, surrounding or compensatory areas and areas of the spine from which the nerve and blood supply to the injured area emanates.
- Apply specific remedial massage therapy techniques appropriate to the tissue type (e.g. muscle stretching and deep transverse friction for muscle injuries, passive joint mobilisation for joint conditions) and phase of inflammation.
- Make recommendations to clients including self-help activities (e.g. home exercise program and advice about posture) and a schedule for ongoing remedial massage therapy.

Planning Remedial Massage Therapy

1. Provisional assessment

Red or yellow flags? If yes, give details

2. Short-term treatment plan
Massage therapy plan:

Aim:

Techniques:

Recommendations
Home exercise program

Other (e.g. heat/cold, posture correction, lifestyle mdification)

Referral (if required)

Proposed treatment schedule

3. Long-term treatment plan
Massage therapy plan:

Aim:

Techniques:

Recommendations
Home exercise program

Other (e.g. heat/cold, posture correction, lifestyle modification)

Referral (if required)

Proposed treatment schedule

Fig. 3.1 Developing short- and long-term therapy plans

ALIGNING TREATMENT TO ASSESSMENT FINDINGS

Remedial massage therapy plans take into account tissue type, stage of inflammation and severity of the condition when treatment techniques are being considered. It is essential that red and yellow flags[a] are identified (see Chapter 2). A definitive assessment is not always possible or necessary for many musculoskeletal conditions. However, a provisional assessment that directs treatment according to assessment findings (e.g. tissue type, stage of inflammation, severity of injury) is likely to provide effective treatment.

Tissue type

As discussed in Chapter 2, active range of motion (AROM) tests are designed to locate the source of symptoms and the quality and range of movement. For example, clients with shoulder pain could be suffering referred pain from the lower cervical spine (C5 dermatome) or from a local shoulder injury (among other things). If AROM of the cervical spine reproduces the symptoms, but AROM of the shoulder does not, then the source of the problem is likely to be the lower cervical spine and clients are likely to respond to treatments directed to that area. However, active movements do not discriminate between inert and contractile components of the joint complex. Passive range of motion (PROM) and resisted range of motion (RROM) tests usually follow active tests to help identify the type of tissue that could be involved.

PROM tests are designed to test the integrity of joints and non-contractile structures like joint capsules, ligaments and cartilage.[b] If symptoms are reproduced by PROM consider the following treatments for subacute or chronic conditions:

- Swedish massage and/or heat therapy to increase blood flow to the area, to relieve pain and to prepare tissues for more specific techniques.
- Passive joint mobilisation for joint conditions like degenerative joint disease (see Chapter 7).
- Deep transverse friction for ligament sprains (see Chapter 4).
- Myofascial releasing techniques for associated fascial restrictions (see Chapter 8).

RROM tests are designed to test the integrity of contractile tissue. If symptoms are reproduced on resisted muscle tests, consider the following treatments for subacute or chronic conditions:

- Swedish massage and/or heat therapy to increase blood flow to the area, relieve pain, prepare tissues for more specific techniques.
- Muscle-specific techniques including deep gliding, cross-fibre frictions, deep transfers frictions and soft tissue releasing techniques (see Chapter 4), muscle stretching (see Chapter 5) and trigger point therapy (see Chapter 6).

[a]Red flags are indicators of a serious underlying physical condition. Such conditions include tumours, infection, fractures and neurological damage. Yellow flags are indicators of underlying psychosocial and occupational factors that may impede recovery. They include attitudes and beliefs about pain, compensation issues, emotions, family and work.

[b]During passive range of motion tests, muscles are also passively stretched. Resisted tests will usually confirm any specific muscle involvement.

- Myofascial releasing techniques for associated fascial restrictions (see Chapter 8).

Stage of inflammation

Musculoskeletal injuries are often classified as acute, subacute or chronic.[5] Acute injuries are recent, usually occurring within the previous one or two days. They are characterised by the five signs of acute inflammation: redness, heat, pain, swelling and loss of function. A single force, either extrinsic or intrinsic, is usually responsible for the injury. Examples of acute injuries are fractures, joint dislocations and recent strains and sprains. Within 2–4 days of the injury, the subacute repair and healing phase begins and, by 6 weeks, injuries are usually classified as chronic. Examples of chronic injuries include chronic synovitis, tendinitis, tenosynovitis, compartment syndrome and chronic sprains and strains. Each phase of tissue healing requires a specific treatment approach.

ACUTE INJURY MANAGEMENT

The body's response to injury is non-specific and consistent regardless of whether the cause is microbial invasion or tissue damage from a chemical or mechanical source. The inflammatory response is initiated and propagated by several inflammatory chemicals including histamine and kinins that are released from damaged cells. The acute inflammatory response usually lasts 24 to 48 hours. These inflammatory mediators dilate blood vessels and attract neutrophils, monocytes and macrophages to the injury site. Clearing the area of infectious and toxic substances and tissue debris is the main function of the inflammatory response. Within about an hour of the injury, neutrophils migrate from capillaries into interstitial spaces to ingest damaged cells, bacteria and other inflammatory agents. Monocytes which mature into macrophages follow in the next 8 to 12 hours. Released histamine also increases capillary permeability and blood plasma leaks into the interstitial spaces. Plasma proteins such as clotting and anti-clotting factors and proteins in the complement system that are vital for the immune response, also escape to the injury site. The area becomes red, warm and swollen. Pain receptors are activated by inflammatory mediators and by local oedema. Clotting proteins lay down fibrin to wall off the injured area and prevent the spread of pathogens.

The aim of treatment in the acute inflammation phase is to reduce the bleeding and swelling that occur as a normal response to tissue damage. Immediate management of acute injuries usually follows the RICE regimen:

- R rest or restrict movement of the injured area
- I ice the injured area immediately for 10–15 minutes, then every 60 minutes for the rest of the day or until symptoms subside
- C compress the injured area (e.g. using compression bandaging)
- E elevate the injured area preferably above the level of the heart

There is little quality research on the use of ice in musculoskeletal medicine. A Cochrane review on the use of superficial heat and cold could only locate three poor-quality trials and could not draw any conclusions about the effects of cold applications for low back pain.[6] The evidence for the effectiveness of ice applications to reduce oedema is conflicting, some authors suggesting that compression is more important than ice in reducing swelling.[7, 8] Evidence does appear to suggest that ice has a local anaesthetic effect.[9] Given the widespread clinical application of ice, there is a need for further high-quality studies to inform its use.

In current clinical practice all acute soft tissue injuries, regardless of severity, are treated promptly to forestall further damage. Ice is applied immediately to the affected area for 10–15 minutes and every 60 minutes thereafter for the rest of the day or until symptoms subside. Note that many sources recommend different durations and frequencies for ice application. For example, the University of Michigan Health System[10] recommends applying ice for 10 minutes every hour for the first day after an injury and then 10–15 minutes three times a day until the swelling goes away. Carnes and Vizniak[11] recommend applying ice for 20 minutes, removing it for 60 minutes, reapplying for 20 minutes and so on until swelling subsides. However, consistent in all such protocols is the action of applying and removing and re-applying ice.

Massage techniques that promote circulation and heat the region are contraindicated in acute injury management. However, a range of massage techniques including reflexology[c], acupressure, aromatherapy and other complementary therapies (e.g. Reiki, acupuncture, homoeopathy, herbal and nutritional supplementations including vitamin C, bromelain and calcium) may be indicated at this stage. Light lymphatic drainage proximal to the injury site and midrange passive movements may be suitable.[12] The rate of recovery of an injury to soft tissue can be increased by early mobilisation with careful supervision. The nature of the injury determines when mobilisation may begin.[5, 13] Introduce pain-free AROM and/or isometric exercises as soon as possible to assist fibrous repair.

Cryotherapy

Cryotherapy is the local, regional or whole-body application of cold for therapeutic purposes. In remedial massage cryotherapy commonly refers to local applications of ice. The aim of cryotherapy in acute injury management is to reduce the amount of blood flow to the area, swelling and pain. Superficial applications of ice cause vasoconstriction which reduces swelling and the rate of metabolism which in turn reduces the inflammatory response. Lower tissue temperature also increases blood viscosity which further reduces blood flow and leakage of fluid into the interstitial spaces.

Contraindications and precautions

Never apply cold:

- if the client has cold hypersensitivity
- to an open wound
- directly to the skin (unless applying ice massage)
- if the client is taking analgesics
- if the client has circulatory insufficiency (e.g. Raynaud's disease[d], diabetes mellitus)

---

[c]Note that reflexology is contraindicated in acute injuries of the foot and ankle where pressure applied to the injured area is likely to cause further inflammation.

[d]Raynaud's phenomenon (or disease) refers to digital ischaemia brought on by cold or emotional stress. Affected fingers turn white (digital artery spasm or obstruction), blue (deoxygenation of static venous blood) and red (reactive hyperaemia).[14]

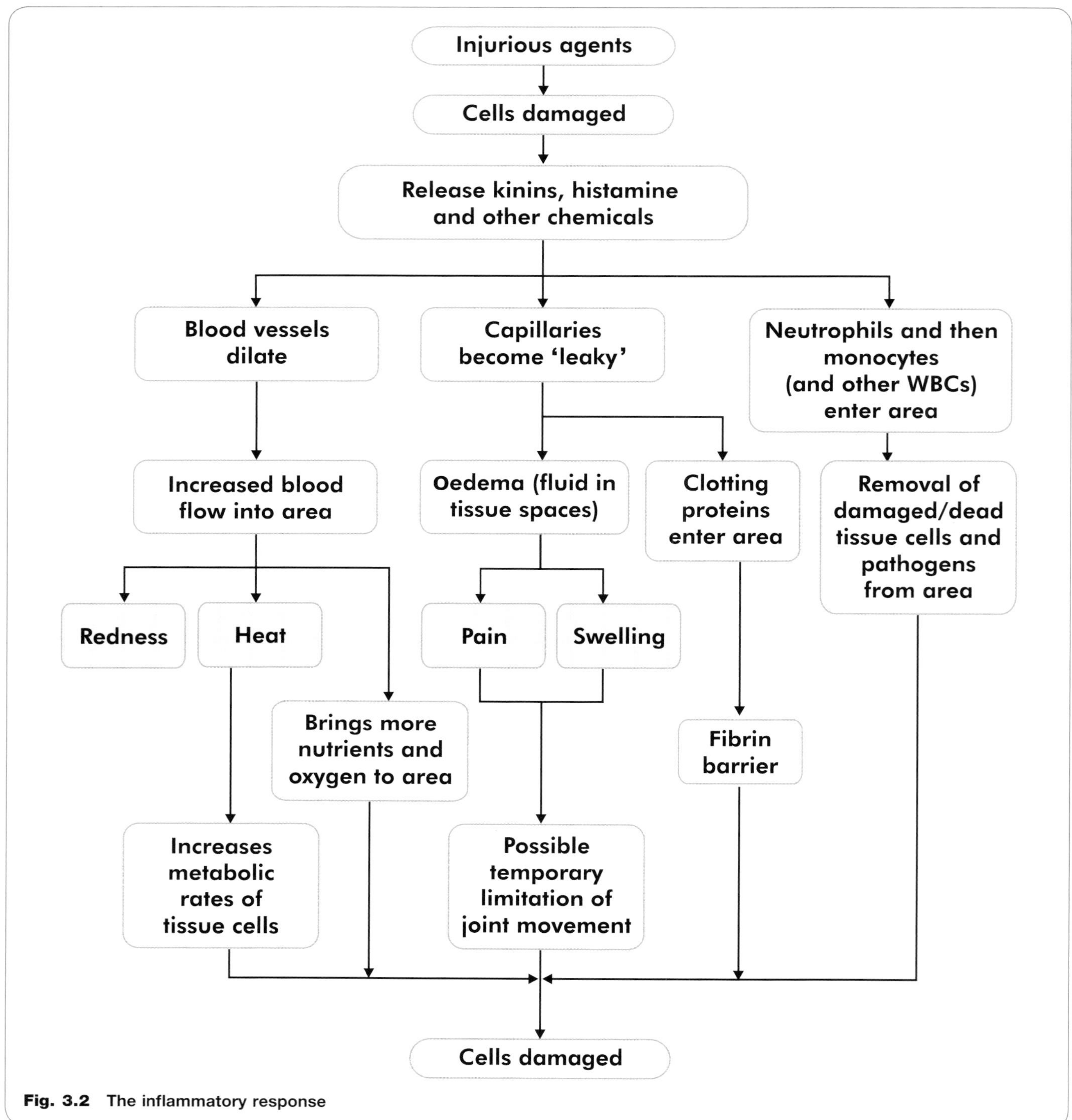

Fig. 3.2 The inflammatory response

Methods of application

Cryotherapy can be applied using immersions in buckets of ice or ice-cold water. The most common applications in remedial massage practice are ice packs and ice massage.

Ice packs Ice packs should be kept refrigerated in the clinic and ready to use. Wrap the ice pack in a towel and apply it to the injured area as soon as possible. If required, use an elastic wrap or tape to keep the ice pack in place. If no ice is available, use a packet of frozen peas, wet cold sponges, cold running water or ice blocks. Apply ice for 10–15 minutes at a time.

Ice massage Ice cups are easily made by freezing a polystyrene drinking cup filled with water. The brim of the cup can be peeled away so that the ice cup resembles an ice-cream cone. As the ice melts, the brim of the cup can be progressively peeled away to expose the ice. (Note: cover the

Table 3.1 Stages of ice massage

	Response	Time after initiation
1	Cold sensation	0–3 minutes
2	Burning, aching	2–7 minutes
3	Local numbness, anaesthesia, pain reflex impulse stops	5–12 minutes

CAUTION: Some clients experience severe pain during ice massage. Check the client's pain tolerance using the pain scale (see Chapter 2) and stop immediately if the pain reaches more than 7 out of 10.

treatment table and client's clothes with towels to keep them dry as the ice melts.) Short applications of ice massage are sometimes used in trigger point therapy. Longer applications may be needed to treat acute inflammation. Table 3.1 shows the stages that usually occur during long applications of ice massage.

SUBACUTE INJURY MANAGEMENT

The subacute phase begins about 2 to 4 days after the injury. In this phase, tissue regeneration and repair begin. As tissues heal, capillary beds grow into the area bringing nutrients and oxygen to the area and removing waste products. New cells rapidly develop to restore normal function. In non-regenerative tissue such as nerve and muscle, injured cells are replaced by scar tissue which is less elastic and less strong than the tissue it replaces. Collagen, the main component of scar tissue, is secreted by rapidly dividing fibroblasts. It is laid down in a random and disorganised way and in this immature form is less dense and more easily injured than the mature collagen that develops over the ensuing two months. Collagen also develops abnormal cross-links, decreasing the flexibility of the tissue. The inflammatory exudate that accumulates at the injury site is slowly removed through the lymph vessels. Any remaining bacteria or tissue debris are destroyed by white blood cells in lymph nodes.

During this phase gentle mobilisation of scar tissue can be commenced. Lymphatic drainage and active and passive range of motion exercises may be beneficial. Rehabilitation exercises during this phase can assist collagen to reorient along lines of stress.

CHRONIC INJURY MANAGEMENT

Chronic inflammation begins 2 to 3 weeks after an injury and can last from 6 weeks to months or years where repeated microtrauma or chronic irritation persists. It is characterised by the presence of mononuclear cells rather than neutrophils at the injury site and by simultaneous destruction and healing of tissue from the inflammatory process. Continued fibroblast activity can lead to excessive scar tissue formation, accompanied by loss of flexibility and strength (scar tissue never achieves more than about 70–80% of the strength of the original tissue).[15]

Most clients of remedial massage have chronic conditions. Treatment for chronic conditions includes such remedial massage techniques as heat application, deep transverse friction (see Chapter 4), myofascial release (see Chapter 8) and exercise therapy, which are designed to produce strong mobile scar tissue. Rehabilitation exercises help realign collagen fibres to make the scar tissue as strong as possible. Remedial massage therapy is also directed to musculoskeletal compensations that are often associated with chronic inflammation (e.g. hypertonic flexor muscles and weakened extensor muscles associated with chronic arthritis of the knee[16]).

Thermotherapy

Thermotherapy is the local or systemic application of heat to the body. It is mainly used for pain relief and psychological relaxation. It accelerates tissue metabolism, increases vasodilation and reduces viscosity of synovial fluid. In remedial massage, thermotherapy commonly refers to local applications of heat. There is scant evidence for the use of superficial heat. One systematic review concluded that heat wrap therapy appears to reduce pain and disability for clients with back pain of less than three months' duration, although the effect is small and only lasts for a short time after the application has been removed.[6]

Contraindications and precautions

Never apply heat:

- immediately after an injury (acute phase)
- where there is loss of sensation (skin test first) or sensitivity to heat (consider skin type: fair-skinned people may be sensitive to heat)
- where there is decreased circulation
- directly to eyes or genitals
- directly to the abdomen during pregnancy or menstruation
- if the client has a fever
- on skin infections, open wounds or if a client has frail skin
- if a client is using analgesics
- if a client has cardiac disease, cancer or hypertension.

Use cautiously where bone is close to the surface (e.g. anterior leg).

Methods of application

A wide range of thermotherapy products are available including:

- hydrocollator or microwave for sandbags, volcanic sand, chemical gel packs, wheat packs and therabead packs
- chemically activated packs
- paraffin wax baths
- oriental methods such as moxa sticks and cupping
- creams, rubs and ointments (e.g. Dencorub, Deep Heat, Capsolin, Tiger Balm, Zheng Gu Shui). Many of these products contain methyl salicylate and camphor.

Do not apply heat packs directly to the skin. Wrap the pack in a pillow case or towel to avoid burning the skin. Heat applications are usually applied for 20–30 minutes. If required, secure the application with an elastic bandage, towel or Velcro belt to ensure that it cannot slip during treatment.

Precautions associated with the use of heat creams

Check the composition of all topical products. Be aware of interactions between creams, rubs and ointments with massage oil and remember that vigorous massage increases surface heat

Table 3.2 Massaging with essential oils: Contraindications and precautions

Major hazardous oils – do not use (potential for dermal toxicity, skin sensitisation and skin irritation)	ajowan, bitter almond, bitter fennel, boldo leaf, buchu, calamus, camphor, cassia, cinnamon bark, costus, elecampane, horseradish, mugwort, mustard, origanum, pennyroyal, rue, thuja, dwarf pine, sassafras, savin, winter savory, summer savory, southernwood, tansy, wormseed, wormwood, clove (leaf, stem and bud), parsley seed, wintergreen
Essential oils that can cause skin reactions (may irritate the skin when used in baths or massage; do not use if client is known to have sensitive skin or is susceptible to reactions)	sweet basil, peppermint, lemon, lemongrass, tea tree, Virginian cedarwood, juniper berry, sweet orange, clary sage
Essential oils that can cause sensitisation (avoid if positive patch test for sensitive skin or history of allergies)	basil, geranium, sweet orange, tea tree, bergamot, lemon expressed, peppermint, ylang ylang, Virginian cedarwood, lemongrass, rose absolute
Essential oils that may cause dermatitis	basil, geranium, damask rose, Virginia cedarwood, bergamot, lemon, rosemary CT2, sweet orange, ylang ylang
Phototoxic essential oils (avoid UV light and sunbeds for 12 hours after application)	bergamot expressed, lemon expressed, bitter orange expressed, Virginia cedarwood, sweet orange expressed
Essential oils which should not be used during pregnancy	aniseed, basil, birch, cajeput, atlas cedarwood, Virginia cedarwood, clary sage, cypress, sweet fennel, frankincense, geranium, jasmine absolute, juniper berry, lemongrass, sweet marjoram, may chang, melissa, myrrh, peppermint, damask rose, rosemary, sage, spearmint, thyme, valerian
Essential oils which should not be used by people with epilepsy	fennel (sweet), hyssop, sage, rosemary, spike lavender, eucalyptus
Essential oils which should not be used by people with high blood pressure	hyssop, rosemary, sage, thyme, spike lavender, sweet basil, eucalyptus

Adapted from Battaglia[17]

which potentiates some heat creams. Note that clients with chronic conditions often suffer long-term pain and may look for relief at any cost. Be especially careful with the home use of practitioner-only products and essential oils (see Table 3.2).

Considerations for applications of heat creams

- Test the area to be warmed with a skin sensation test.
- Warn clients of possible side effects (e.g. burning).
- Some heat creams/gels can be reactivated hours after use (e.g. when showering).
- Warn clients not to touch areas treated with creams to avoid transferring products to eyes, mouth or genitals.
- Check the client's response often.
- Use a wooden stick for individual applications of creams/gels to avoid contaminating stock.
- Transfer ointments and creams to small jars and store the main stock in a dark and cool environment.

Severity of injury

Injuries are often graded according to severity which determines the most appropriate treatment. Characteristics of injuries to muscles, tendons and ligaments according to severity are described in Table 3.3.

Grade 1 and 2 injuries (mild and moderate) are generally suitable for remedial massage therapy. Severe injuries (Grade 3) require referral to a medical practitioner for surgical repair. However, remedial massage can contribute to the treatment of Grade 3 injuries in the rehabilitation phase when techniques like deep transverse friction, resisted stretches and passive joint mobilisation can be applied. Treatment is directed to the injury itself and to compensatory muscle imbalances. Therapists can educate clients about causative and predisposing factors from a remedial massage perspective and develop and/or monitor exercise rehabilitation programs (see Table 3.4).

MONITORING AND REVIEWING TREATMENT PLANS

Initial assessments are important for establishing baseline data against which repeated assessments can be measured. Clients are continually assessed, both during treatments and at the end of a single treatment or a course of treatments. Changes in assessment findings are crucial for monitoring treatment progress and form the basis of regular reviews of treatment plans. An essential part of monitoring and reviewing treatment is explaining to clients the rationale for, and outcomes of, treatment and encouraging clients to ask questions about their treatment. Practitioners also negotiate treatment schedules, from frequent to less frequent consultations as recovery progresses, and the transition from rehabilitation

Table 3.3 Grading injuries: Characteristics of injuries

a) Grading muscle strains

Muscle strains	**Definition**	**Characteristics**
Grade 1	A small number of fibres are torn.	Localised pain. No loss of strength.
Grade 2	A significant number of fibres are torn.	Pain and swelling. Pain is reproduced on muscle contraction. Strength is reduced and movement is limited by pain.
Grade 3	A complete tear of the muscle.	Significant pain and swelling. Significant loss of strength. Most often occurs at the musculotendinous junction.

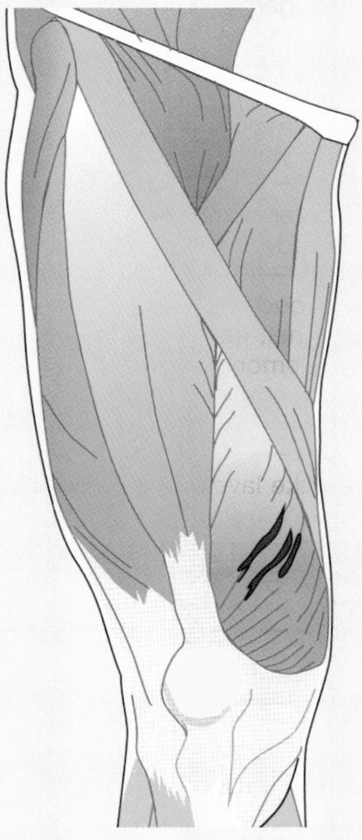

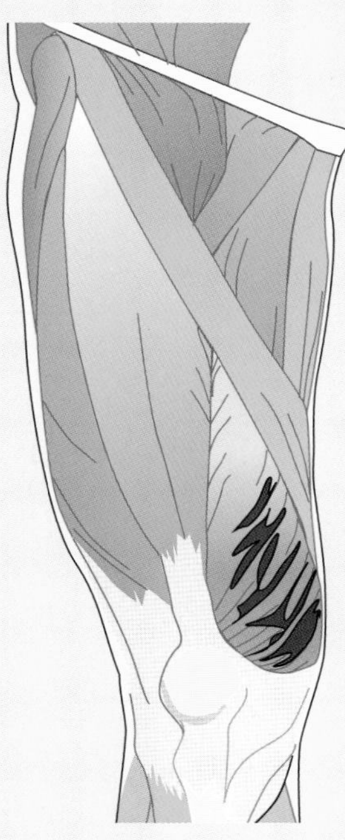

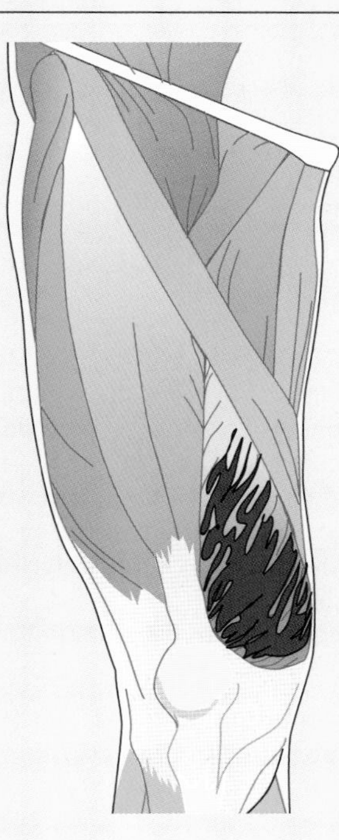

Fig. 3.3 Grades of muscle strain

b) Grading ligament sprains

Ligament sprain	**Definition**	**Characteristics**
Grade 1	A small number of fibres are torn.	Pain is felt on stressing the ligament with no increase in joint laxity.
Grade 2	A significant number of fibres are torn.	Pain is felt on stressing the ligament and joint laxity increases.
Grade 3	A complete tear of the ligament.	Pain may be present with gross joint laxity.

c) Grading tendon injuries

Tendon injury	**Definition**	**Characteristics**
Grade 1	A small number of fibres are torn.	Pain after activity only.
Grade 2	A few fibres are torn.	Pain at start of activity. Pain disappears during activity and returns after activity.
Grade 3	A considerable number of fibres are torn.	Pain at the start of the activity that persists during and after activity. Restriction of activity.
Grade 4	A significant number of fibres are torn.	Pain during everyday activities. Pain progressing and worsening.

Adapted from Brukner and Khan[5]

Table 3.4 Treatment approach according to injury grade

Grade 1 and 2 injuries	Acute injury management	First aid management (e.g. RICE, acupuncture, homoeopathy) Exercise advice
	Subacute/ chronic injury management	Remedial massage therapy Electrophysical therapy Heat therapy Joint mobilisation Exercise rehabilitation and training
Grade 3 injuries	Acute injury management	First aid management (e.g. RICE, acupuncture, homoeopathy) Referral for surgical repair
	Subacute/ chronic injury management	Remedial massage therapy Electrophysical therapy Heat therapy Joint mobilisation Exercise rehabilitation and training

to a health maintenance or promotion plan. As a general guideline, massage for mild or moderate conditions is usually performed weekly; acute conditions could require two or three treatments a week. Most soft tissue injuries recover within 6 weeks.[18] Maintenance treatments become progressively less frequent until a schedule that prevents deterioration and promotes health is determined.

The frequency and duration of treatment ultimately depends on a number of factors including

- how quickly the condition responds to treatment (influenced by age, nature and severity of injury and previous history)
- the client's level of compliance with a self-help program
- the occurrence of any setbacks such as falls, injuries or emotional stress during the course of treatment
- the presence of pre-existing or complicating factors (e.g. underlying disease, yellow flags).

Approximate healing times for soft tissue injuries are illustrated in Table 3.5.

Table 3.5 Approximate healing times[18]

General muscle soreness	24–48 hours
Grade 1 and 2 lesions Mild contusions	Grade 1: 2–3 weeks Grade 2: 3–6 weeks
Severe Grade 2 lesions Grade 3 lesions	2–6 months (Note: muscle scarring can become permanent)
Fractures	3–6 weeks (months for geriatric clients)
Nerve root lesions	6 weeks–2 years

RECORDING REMEDIAL MASSAGE TREATMENTS

Treatment records should include the major techniques used in treatment, the specific locations of their application and recommendations made to clients. Records should also reflect relevant responses to treatment. There are currently no standardised recording procedures. The example in Table 3.6 is a possible model.

Table 3.6 A three-stage method of recording remedial massage treatment

	Record	Treatment technique
1	Swed mass lower back, BL lower limbs	Remedial massage usually begins with a Swedish or basic massage to a region
2	L up traps TP L lev scap XFF distal attach L up traps act rel	List two or three of the major techniques used: • Left upper trapezius; trigger point • Left levator scapulae: cross fibre frictions at the distal attachment • Left upper trapezius active releasing technique
3	Home ex: L up traps, lev scap stretches 3 × 3/24	Self-help program: • Left upper traps and left levator scapulae stretches 3 repetitions, 3 times per day

KEY MESSAGES

- Client safety is a priority. Strategies to ensure client safety include:
  - beginning treatment with Swedish massage before applying deeper more specific remedial techniques
  - using active movements to gauge client's range of motion before applying passive techniques
  - using a pain scale and working within the client's pain tolerance.
- A remedial massage treatment approach involves:
  - planning for both long- and short-term management of clients
    - short-term therapy plans which often focus on presenting symptoms
    - long-term therapy plans which often focus on potential contributing factors (e.g. lifestyle factors, underlying structural features, or underlying disease processes)
  - educating clients about likely causal and predisposing factors
  - over time increasing the client self-help component of treatment wherever possible (to reduce likelihood of recurrence and/or to promote health maintenance and illness prevention)
  - taking the client's preferences and value system into account.
- Consider the best, available evidence (e.g. refer to Clinical Guidelines) when planning therapy. Treatment protocols can be used to guide remedial massage treatment and modified to suit the needs of individual clients. Treatment protocols take into consideration:

- tissue type: assessment findings suggest appropriate techniques for particular tissue types (e.g. passive joint mobilisation for joint conditions, deep transverse friction and other muscle-specific techniques for muscle lesions)
- stage of inflammation:
  - acute soft tissue injuries are treated using the RICE regimen, cautious lymphatic drainage and passive range of movement exercises midrange
  - subacute soft tissue injuries are treated with lymphatic drainage, gentle mobilisation of scar tissue and active and passive range of motion exercises
  - chronic soft tissue injuries are treated with heat application and other remedial massage techniques (e.g. deep transverse friction, cross-fibre frictions, trigger point therapy), myofascial releasing techniques and exercise therapy
- severity of the injury: no referral is required to treat grade 1 and mild to moderate grade 2 injuries; severe grade 2 and grade 3 injuries may be treated after surgical repair.
- Continuously monitor and review treatment plans.

Review questions

1. Match the following descriptions with their injury grade:

Pain may be present with gross joint laxity.	Grade 1 ligament sprain
Significant pain and swelling. Significant loss of strength. Most often occurs at the musculotendinous junction.	Grade 1 muscle strain
Pain is felt on stressing the ligament with no increase in joint laxity.	Grade 2 tendon strain
Pain at start of activity. Pain disappears during activity and returns after activity.	Grade 3 ligament sprain
Pain during everyday activities. Pain progressing and worsening.	Grade 3 muscle strain
Localised pain. No loss of strength	Grade 4 tendon strain

2. List five precautions for the use of ice.
3. A client presents with neck pain. On active cervical flexion and right rotation the client reports pain. The practitioner performs resisted tests for cervical flexion and right rotation. The client reports pain on resisted right rotation of the cervical spine. It is likely that the pain is related to *inert/contractile* tissue.
4. a) How would you identify an acute soft tissue injury?
   b) What is the usual treatment for acute soft tissue injuries?
5. How soon after an injury can exercise rehabilitation start?
6. For client safety, it is recommended that active movements be performed before passive movements. Explain the rationale for this treatment approach.
7. Name three essential oils that could cause skin reactions.
8. Describe a typical treatment schedule for a client who has recently sprained his ankle (grade 1).
9. Complete the following:

When tissue is injured two immediate responses occur in blood vessels near the injury: i) vasodilation and ii) increased __________ of capillaries so that antibodies and clotting factors can enter the injured area. This response is initiated and propagated by several inflammatory chemicals including __________ and __________. Within an hour neutrophils squeeze through the blood vessel walls to reach the injury site. Neutrophils dominate initially, followed by __________ and __________which contribute to phagocytic activity. The main function of the inflammatory response is to ____________________________________. Plasma proteins including __________________ also arrive at the injury site. The area is walled off by __________ laid down by clotting proteins. During the repair phase new blood vessels supply nutrients and oxygen to the area and remove waste products. In muscle tissue new cells form __________which is less dense and more easily injured than the tissue it replaces.

REFERENCES

1. Sherman KJ, Cherkin DC, Deyo RA, et al. The diagnosis and treatment of chronic back pain by acupuncturists, chiropractors, and massage therapists. Clin J Pain 2006;22(3):227–34.
2. WorkCover NSW. Improving outcomes: integrated, active management of workers with soft tissue injury. Lisarow NSW: WorkCover NSW; 2007.
3. US Department of Health and Human Services. Low back disorders; 2010.
4. National Health and Medical Research Council. Evidence-based management of acute musculoskeletal pain. Online. Available: www.nhmrc.gov.au/publications/synopses/cp94syn.htm; 2003.
5. Brukner P, Khan K. Clinical sports medicine. 3rd edn. North Ryde, NSW: McGraw-Hill; 2006.
6. French SD, Cameron M, Walker BF, et al. Superficial heat or cold for low back pain. Cochrane Database Syst Rev 2006;(1):CD004750.
7. Hubbard T, Denegar C. Does cryotherapy improve outcomes with soft tissue injury? J Athlet Train 2004;39(3):278–9.
8. Bleakley C, McDonough S, MacAuley D. The use of ice in the treatment of acute soft tissue injury: a systematic review of randomized controlled trials. Am J Sport Med 2004;32(1):251–61.
9. Nadler S, Weingand K, Kruse R. The physiological basis and clinical applications of cryotherapy and thermotherapy for the pain practitioner. Pain Physician 2004;7(3):395–459.
10. University of Michigan Health System. Use heat or ice to relieve low back pain [updated 2010, cited 2011 Apr 3]. Online. Available: http://www.uofmhealth.org/health-library/hw47901.
11. Carnes M, Vizniak N. Quick reference evidence-based conditions manual. 3rd edn. Burnaby, BC: Professional Health Systems; 2009.
12. Fritz S, Grosenbach M. Mosby's essential sciences for therapeutic massage. 3rd edn. St Louis, MO: Mosby Elsevier; 2009.
13. Handoll HHG, Gillespie WJ, Gillespie LD, et al. Moving towards evidence-based healthcare for musculoskeletal injuries: featuring the work of the cochrane bone, joint and muscle trauma group. J R Soc Health [Review] 2007;127(4):168–73.
14. Munro J, Campbell I, editors. Macleod's clinical examination. Edinburgh: Churchill Livingstone; 2000.
15. Halloran C, Slavin J. Pathophysiology of wound healing. Surgery 2002;20(5):i–v.
16. Fritz S, Chaitow L, Hymel GM. Clinical massage in the healthcare setting. St Louis, MO: Mosby Elsevier; 2008.
17. Battaglia S. The complete guide to aromatherapy. 2nd edn. Virginia, Qld: Perfect Potion; 2004.
18. WorkCoverSA. Recovery timeframes for common injury types. Online. Available: http://www.workcover.com/site/treat_home/guidelines_by_injury_type/recovery_timeframes_for_common_injury_types.aspx?str=Recovery%20timeframes; 2009.

4 Remedial massage techniques for muscles

The content of this chapter relates to the following Units of Competency:
HLTREM503C Plan remedial massage treatment strategy
HLTREM504C Apply remedial massage assessment framework
HLTREM502C Provide remedial massage treatment
HLTREM505C Perform remedial massage health assessment

Health Training Package HLT07

Learning Outcomes

- Assess clients for muscle injuries and imbalances.
- Describe the current evidence for the effectiveness of specific remedial massage techniques on muscle function.
- Apply specific remedial massage techniques to muscles effectively and safely on a range of clients.
- Advise and resource clients who have been assessed and treated with specific remedial massage techniques for muscles.

INTRODUCTION

Just about everyone will experience a muscle strain at some time in their life. Any sport that involves high-intensity sprinting efforts (e.g. football, tennis, cricket) will have a high incidence of muscle strains.[1] Muscle strains also have high recurrence rates: for example, 12% in professional soccer players and 30% in Australian football players.[2, 3] Such conditions as a quadriceps contusion incurred on a football field, a fibrotic tangle of muscle left years after a bone fracture, muscles and joints aching from postural distortion or a triceps head strained during a motorcycle accident are common presentations to remedial massage therapists. Much can be done to assist restoration of normal muscle function. One of the roles of remedial massage therapists is to assess and treat muscle strains and imbalances and to work with other health professionals to achieve the best outcomes for clients.

The aim of this chapter is to explore some approaches to the assessment of muscle lesion and dysfunction and to examine techniques which are often incorporated into treatment regimens. Techniques presented in this chapter are based on the best available research.

ASSESSING MUSCLE FUNCTION

Several approaches to the assessment of muscles are presented in this chapter:[4-9]

- functional deficit demonstration (active functional range of motion)
- postural assessment
- muscle length testing
- muscle strength testing
- palpation.

FUNCTIONAL DEFICIT DEMONSTRATION

During the history-taking interview, ask the client if their pain or restriction stops them from doing anything that they want or need to do.[6] The inability to bend far enough to tie shoes or to reach high enough to wash and dry one's hair can be significant problems for clients. The therapist can interpret the functional deficit more accurately by observing the movements it affects. Range of motion examination should be familiar to the reader. The joints of the body can move through various planes of motion and through certain ranges within those planes. Normative data has been collected for joint range of motion and can be used when assessing clients. In active range of motion (AROM) tests, the client performs the movements to their comfortable limit, which necessarily involves the use of muscles. AROM tests are usually performed in single planes. However, some tests like Apley's scratch test (see Figure 15.21 on page 270) and the standing ankle AROM tests assess multiplanar movements that mimic everyday functions which are rarely performed in only one plane (see Figure 4.1). It should also be noted that AROM or active functional deficit tests may need to be repeated a number of times to reproduce symptoms.

POSTURAL ASSESSMENT

A common cause of soft tissue dysfunction and pain is postural distortion.[10] Our bodies are often required to maintain positions for extended periods, sometimes due to occupational demands. Our responses to these demands are reflected in our musculoskeletal framework and an assessment of posture is a vital part of clinical examination.

A common postural distortion is forward carriage of the head, rounded shoulders, increased thoracic kyphosis, elevated and protracted scapulae, internally rotated glenohumeral joints, and hyperextended cervical spine to raise the eyes. These positions are maintained by muscular effort (cervical extensor muscles, sternocleidomastoid, levator scapulae, pectoralis major, possibly pectoralis minor and others), and permitted by muscular weakness (rhomboids, middle and lower trapezius, infraspinatus, deep flexors of the cervical spine and others). This postural distortion is referred to as upper-crossed syndrome (see Figure 12.21 on page 219).[11, 12] Other occupational distortions include the externally rotated femurs of a long-distance driver or dancer, and the spinal rotation and lateral flexion of a sedentary worker whose work station is positioned to the side (see Figure 4.2). It has been estimated that, on average, we take more than 20 million steps in a decade.[13] With such heavy demands on the body, even a small distortion or compensation to normal gait or posture amplifies over time.

Muscle imbalances involve a muscle or functional group of muscles which become structurally shortened either as a result of spasm or contracture (*locked short*), and a muscle or functional group of muscles, often antagonistic, which are overstretched (*locked long*) and are usually functionally weak.[10, 14, 15] There has been some discussion between researchers regarding the tendency of certain muscles to become hypertonic when overstressed (e.g. upper trapezius, levator scapulae, quadratus lumborum, rectus femoris, iliopsoas, hamstrings), while others typically tend towards hypotonicity under the same conditions (e.g. middle and lower trapezius, serratus anterior, rhomboids, rectus abdominis, gluteals).[15-17] These muscles have been categorised as *postural* (or *antigravity*) and *phasic* respectively[5, 15] although there is disagreement about classifications of some muscles, including the scalenes.[15] Each muscle or muscle group should be assessed to determine its functional state which may differ in different individuals. Figure 4.3 shows major postural and phasic muscles.

Case study: The forklift driver (part 1)

Consider John, 34 years of age with no significant injury history. He played soccer and cricket (mainly as a batsman) until his early twenties when he married and had children. Since then he has worked in various jobs, mostly assisting in warehouses and workshops, with no major physical complaints.

Over the past 2–3 months, John has been experiencing headaches, neck stiffness, some upper back discomfort and sometimes a feeling of tightness across the chest. He also reports that taking deep breaths is not as easy as it used to be. He has seen his doctor and had stress tests for his heart, which showed nothing unusual. He has had his eyes tested at an optometrist and his vision is fine. The doctor prescribed some NSAIDs for his neck and back pain and referred him to you for treatment.

On questioning you learn that John obtained his forklift ticket about four months ago and secured a full-time position in a warehouse about a month later. This was about the time when his symptoms began.

Do some research on forklift driving. Are there occupational or ergonomic conditions that could contribute to John's symptoms?

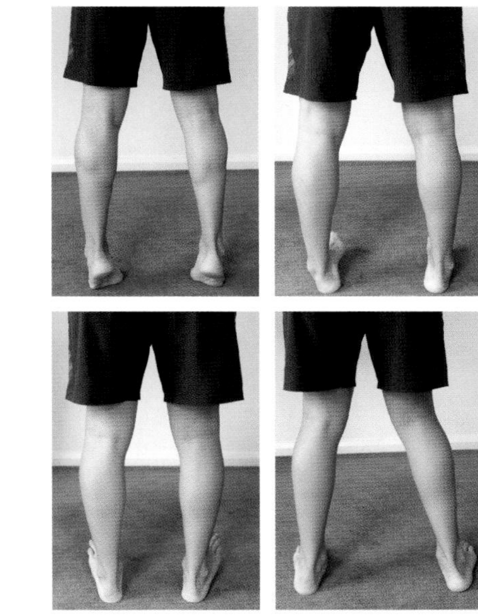

Fig. 4.1 Functional multiplanar tests for ankle range of motion

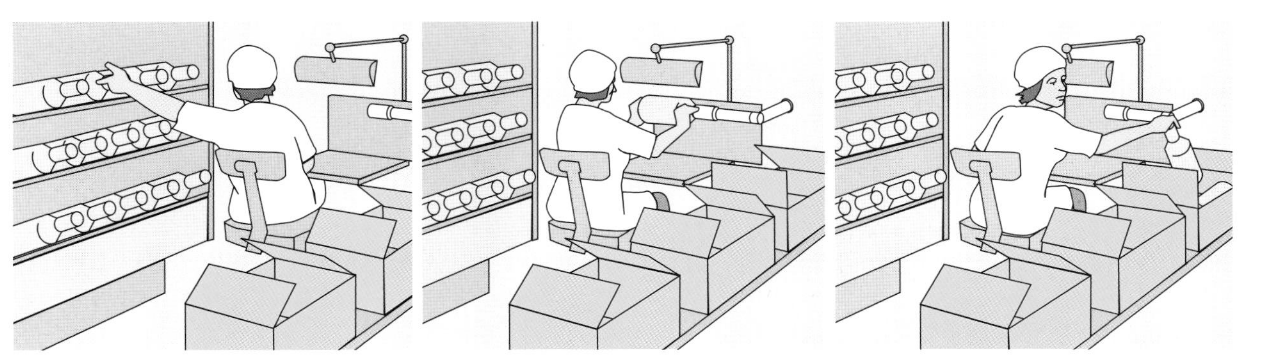

Fig. 4.2 Sedentary worker whose work station is positioned to the side

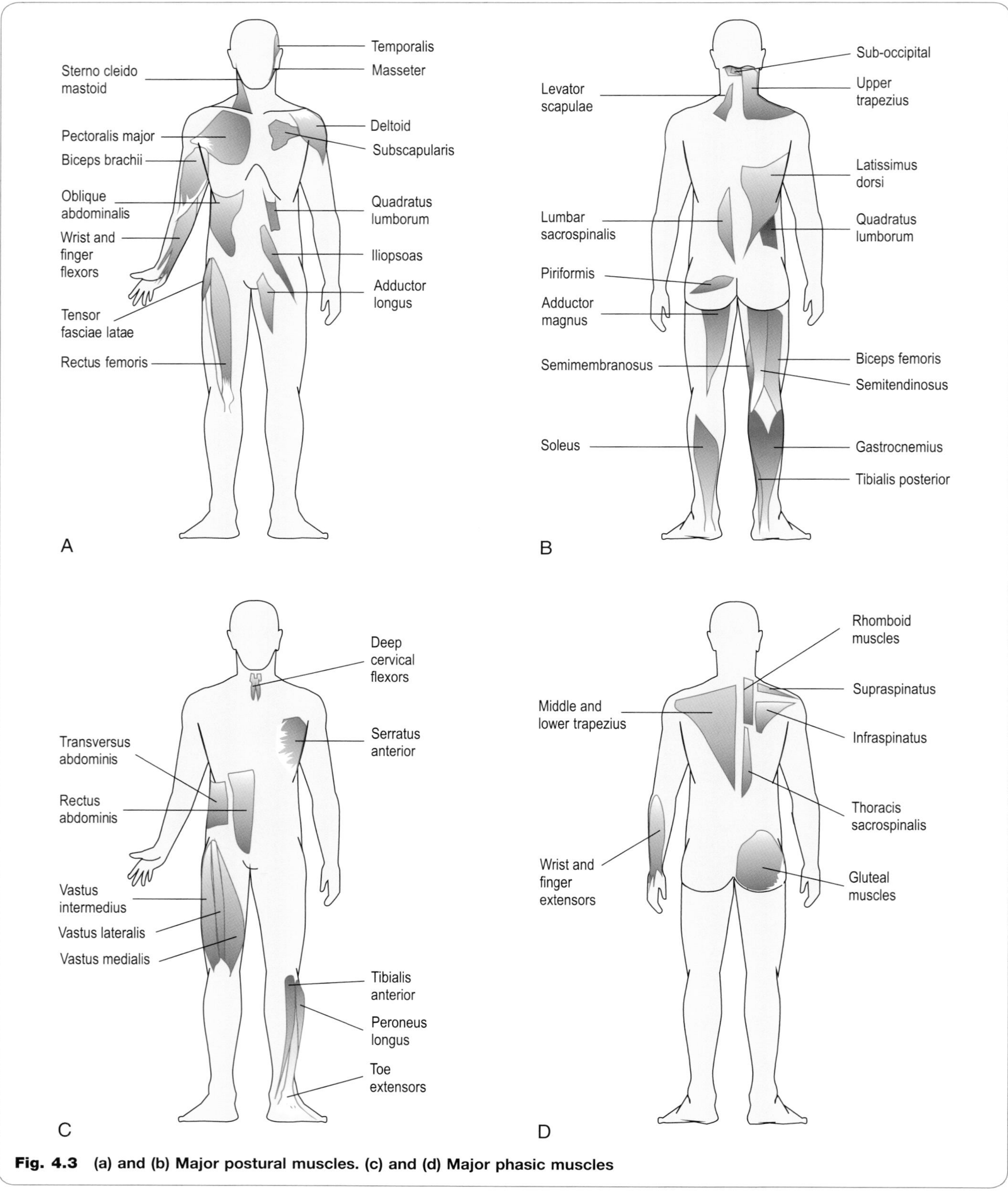

Fig. 4.3 (a) and (b) Major postural muscles. (c) and (d) Major phasic muscles

Case study: The forklift driver (part 2)

If you have looked at the way in which forklifts are driven, you will have noticed that (1) they are not ergonomically designed for individual operators, and (2) the steering wheel is almost horizontal. Operators have to reach forward to steer. Their necks extend so they can raise their eyes. After long periods of driving, an upper crossed syndrome will probably result. The torso is twisted as the driver checks the space behind the forklift while reversing. This position rotates and laterally flexes the spine.

Now, consider the signs and symptoms. Can they be explained in the light of a common postural distortion like upper crossed syndrome? Think about individual muscles or functional groups of muscles which could be affected. See if you can predict which muscles are likely to be locked short and which are likely to be locked long from extended periods of forklift driving. How would you confirm or disprove your predictions?

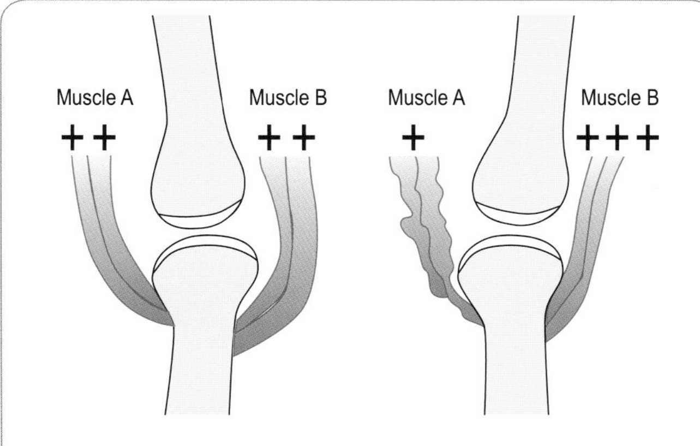

Fig. 4.4 Muscle balance and joint range of motion

There are many instances in which an apparent postural distortion is not directly caused by muscle imbalance. Muscles in the immediate vicinity of injuries and/or painful sites, for example, will often spasm in an effort to immobilise or protect the damaged structure,[15] and in the short term this is not necessarily a problem. An injured person will often adjust their posture to allow continued use of the rest of the body, as in the case of a limp due to an ankle sprain. Posture can also reflect the overall attitude and mood of a person. For example, a depressed person may cast their eyes to the floor, dropping their head and rounding their shoulders. Postural observations should always be interpreted in the light of the client's presenting condition, history and other assessment findings.[10, 15, 18]

TESTING MUSCLES FOR LENGTH

Postural assessment helps identify muscle imbalances. History and questioning provide clues about causes and perpetuating factors[7] and help guide advice and recommendations given to clients. Postural assessment reveals the more visible problem areas and suggests muscles to target. Specific muscle tests help confirm or rule out the involvement of individual muscles.

As mentioned previously, in many cases the muscles which have become hypertonic (locked short) or hypotonic (locked long) are fairly predictable.[5, 15-17] We can now employ techniques which can give valuable information as to the form the treatment might take.

For passive range of motion (PROM) tests, the therapist moves the client's limb with no assistance from contracting muscles.[5, 19] In general, AROM is smaller than PROM because contracting muscles tend to limit bony approximation.[5] There are several things which can limit PROM at any given joint. These include inflammation, instability and changes in any of the structures surrounding or inside the joint itself.[8] Because of this and also because of limitations in reproducibility, PROM measurements are sometimes seen as unreliable and of limited clinical use.[20]

Muscle tissue which is locked short from either spasm or contracture will often restrict the joint by not allowing it to reach its normal range (see Figure 4.4).[5, 7, 21] Spasms in these shortened muscles can be responsible for weakness in their antagonistic groups. Sherrington's Law of Reciprocal Innervation states that when an agonist is contracting, its antagonist will be neurally inhibited in order to allow unopposed joint motion.[5, 22] It is possible that relieving the spasm in the shortened muscle may lead to the withdrawal of the neural inhibition of the locked long muscle with an immediate improvement in function testing results.

Full range of motion depends on both joint range of motion and muscle length. For example, to measure knee flexion joint motion, the client lies supine and the hip is flexed to put rectus femoris in a shortened position so that full joint range of motion can be achieved. To measure the length of rectus femoris, on the other hand, the client lies prone to extend the hip and lengthen the rectus femoris (see Figure 4.5). (See Table 2.7 on page 29, which illustrates length tests of major muscles of the body.)

TESTING MUSCLES FOR STRENGTH

When assessing for muscle imbalance, therapists use strength testing to gauge the ability of a hypotonic muscle to contract. Moreover, a muscle which is locked short, but is actually in contracture (electrically silent) rather than in spasm (electrically active), will usually also test weak during function testing. Hammer[5] suggests that a muscle shortened due to spasm often tests weak due to the number of myosin crossbridges already engaged and because pain associated with muscle spasm may inhibit contractile power.

Whereas injury or pain in inert structures around a joint can often be identified through passive range of motion testing, resisted muscle testing usually elicits pain from dynamic/contractile tissue injuries and can be used to grade these injuries.[5] Acute injuries may involve damage to the fabric of the muscle and/or tendon.[23] Resisted tests for specific muscles are used to ascertain the presence of strains within the musculotendinous unit and also to assess the grades of those particular injuries.[5]

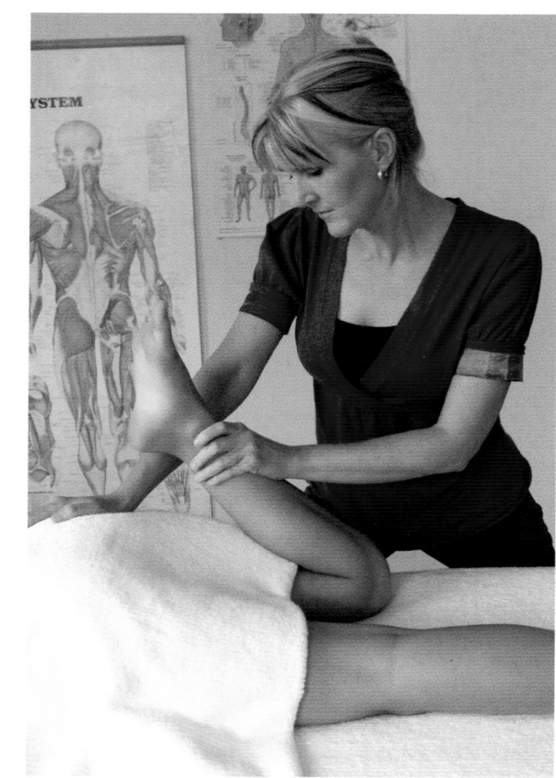

Fig. 4.5 Length test for rectus femoris

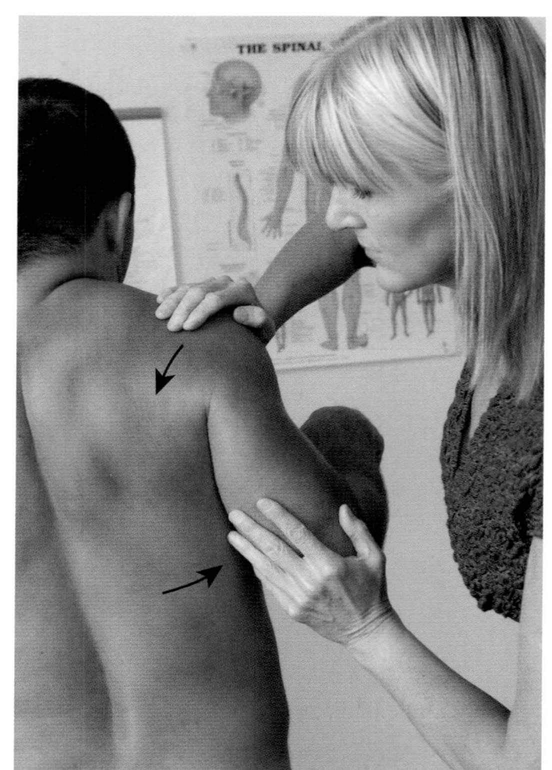

Fig. 4.6 Resisted test for rhomboids

Remedial massage therapists use resisted tests for specific muscles to locate muscle lesions more often than to grade strength (as in break testing[a]).[10] Break testing should be avoided, partly because heavy contraction may damage a compromised muscle, and also because it can be very difficult for the therapist to control accessory movements by the client and accuracy will therefore suffer.[10]

To perform resisted tests for specific muscles the therapist applies resistance as the client contracts the muscle.[5, 10, 12, 19] The amount of resistance matches the client's force so that no movement occurs; that is, an isometric contraction is performed. Contracting a muscle moves its attachment points into closer approximation. To perform a resisted test, the relevant joints and muscles are positioned carefully, proximal regions are stabilised and the client is instructed to perform a movement[12] or to hold the position[10] against resistance. This procedure is carried out initially on the uninjured limb or side wherever possible, to provide a reference for test results on the target muscle. Figure 4.6 shows a resisted muscle test for the rhomboids. Resisted tests for major muscles are described in Chapters 10–20.

Two of the more widely used grading systems for muscle strength are those of Kendall et al[10] and Janda.[12] Differences between the two systems are illustrated in Table 4.1.

Table 4.1 Comparison of muscle strength testing systems of Kendall et al[10] and Janda[12]

Feature	Kendall[10]	Janda[12]
Grading system	12 grades	6 grades
Client positioning	For best fixation and access	For best fixation and access
Stabilisation	Yes	Yes
Therapist resistance	Against line of action, equal and opposite to contraction	Against movement direction, but not overcoming movement
Contraction type	Isometric, against equal resistance	Isotonic, through range
Tests	Muscle, rather than movement	Movement, rather than individual muscle
Tests very weak muscles	Yes	Yes

PALPATION

Although palpation is one of the key assessment procedures used by remedial massage therapists, its findings need to be integrated with others in order to reveal the whole clinical picture.[19, 24] Palpation can be used to locate and identify soft

[a]Break testing refers to resistance applied at the end of a range of motion in the opposite direction to the concentrically contracting muscle.

Table 4.2 Palpatory findings

Condition	Temperature	Pain/tenderness	Hard/soft	Smooth/gritty/crepitation
Acute injury (sprain or strain)	Warm–hot	Yes, on lesion and usually associated with spasm	Palpable defect in Grade 3 injuries, otherwise usually hard (protective spasm)	Normally smooth
Spasm	Varies	Yes, often tender	Hard	Normally smooth
Tendinosis (chronic)	Cool–cold	Not always	Often a thickened area is palpable	May be crepitus on movement Often feels gritty
Fibrosis (muscle)	Cool–cold	Not always	Hard, sometimes stringy/ropey	Often feels gritty
Weakness/ inhibition	Cool–warm	Sometimes (often develop trigger point activity)	If overstretched, may palpate firm; otherwise soft, spongy	Often ropey but may be smooth
Oedema	Hot if acute; variable if chronic	Not always	Spongy, often with some resistance; may retain indent after removal of finger	Usually smooth, but may become gritty over time

tissues lesions, to detect activity (or lack of it) in muscle tissue, and to elicit symptoms, including pain.[5, 10, 18, 19, 25] Massage therapists should be experts in palpation and need to continually refine their skills by practice.[25] Many palpation exercises have been devised to develop fine discrimination and other aspects of palpation skill. The exercise made famous by Gray's *Anatomy*, for example, requires the therapist to develop their skills by palpating a hair through an increasing number of sheets of paper.[25] Researchers are also working on devices, such as a palpation trainer,[26] to enable greater validity and reliability in assessment findings based on palpation.

A good way to begin the development of palpation skills is to palpate normal undamaged muscle which is normally painless to palpation and should feel smooth, soft and resilient when the muscle is relaxed. When the muscle is contracted the therapist can palpate its tension. The muscle will become firmer to the touch. Tendons tend to feel less leathery or resilient than muscles and feel strong and hard when under tension. Bony landmarks may feel the hardest of all, depending upon the tissues which separate them from the skin. The intervening bursae, fat pads, fascia and other tissues will all have their signature quality. After much practice at palpating normal tissues, you will be well equipped to identify damaged or otherwise abnormal tissue.

It is useful to have a wide vocabulary of descriptive terms for palpation findings. These may include terms like *firm*, *tense*, *resistant*, *hard*, *spongy*, *springy*, *warm*, *cold*, *dense*, *ropey*, *cordlike*, *stringy* and *puffy*.[5, 19, 25] Table 4.2 lists some palpatory findings. This table is not exhaustive. Palpatory findings should always be interpreted with caution and correlated with case history and other assessment findings.

REMEDIAL MASSAGE TECHNIQUES

The following section presents some of the most useful and widely used remedial massage techniques for treating muscle injuries and addressing muscle imbalances in the body. These techniques are known by several names. The following terms and abbreviations are used in this book:

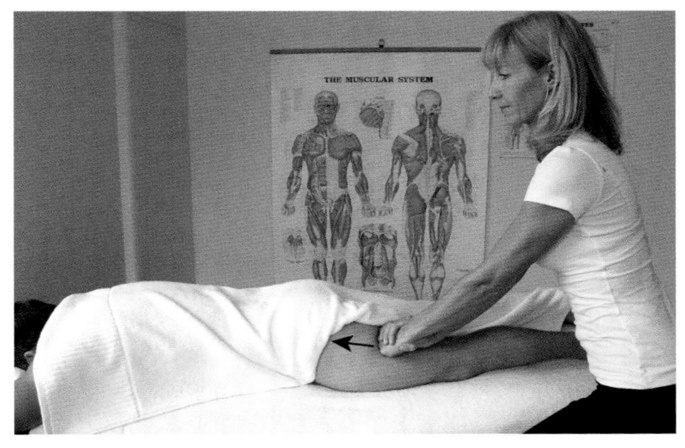

Fig. 4.7 **Deep gliding friction to the hamstring muscle**

- Deep gliding friction (DG)
- Cross-fibre friction (XFF)
- Deep transverse friction (DTF)
- Soft tissue release (STR)

DEEP GLIDING (WITH-FIBRE) FRICTIONS AND CROSS-FIBRE FRICTIONS

The technique referred to here as deep gliding frictions (DG) is also known as *with-fibre frictions*. Cyriax and Russell[27] call it *deep effleurage*, as does Goats.[28] Lowe[29] discusses *deep longitudinal stripping* and *deep tissue massage*. The basic stroke is performed parallel to the muscle fibres in the direction of venous flow. The therapist uses fingers, thumbs, palms, loose fists, forearms or elbows, depending upon the location and the depth required[23, 27, 29] as illustrated in Figure 4.7. Some lubrication is normally used and some measure of discomfort or even pain (always within tolerance, say below 7 out of 10 on a pain scale) is to be expected, but if the client's muscles begin to contract in an attempt to protect the muscle then too much pressure is being used.[29]

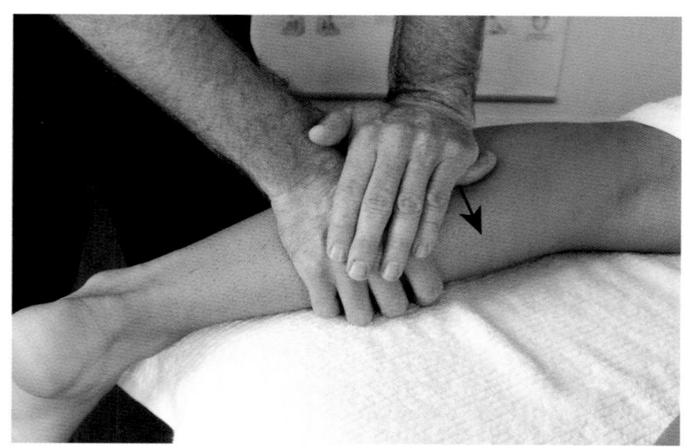

Fig. 4.8 Cross-fibre friction to the gastrocnemius muscle

Claims about the effect of deep gliding frictions include:

- relief of congestion and swelling[23, 27, 28]
- relief of muscle spasm[28, 29]
- acceleration of lymph and blood flow[23, 28]
- localised stretching[28, 29]
- inactivation of trigger points.[29]

Cross fibre friction (XFF), like DG, is a technique that may be performed as part of a Swedish massage routine. As with DG, a lubricant allows the fingers or palms to glide across the skin surface. The difference between the techniques lies in the direction of application: XFF is angled across the muscle fibres, rather than along them (see Figure 4.8). Pressure varies according to the needs of individual clients. The stroke is usually delivered with the fingers together as a unit or the thumb (although therapists should be cautious about overuse of the thumb which can lead to injury and the premature end of a massage career).

The massage literature claims that XFF can:

- separate and broaden muscle fibres[29]
- reduce tension in the muscle[29]
- improve or preserve relative mobility of muscle and connective tissue.[30]

Evidence for the effectiveness of DG and XFF

The scientific literature has few studies specifically addressing the effectiveness of either DG or XFF. There are very few randomised controlled studies which use only these massage techniques as interventions.[31] It seems that many of the claimed effects are extrapolated from physiological phenomena which may or may not be directly related to the application of these specific techniques.

Relevant studies on the effectiveness of DG or XFF include:

- Field et al[32] found that objective measures for stress in adults were reduced by massage strokes of moderate pressure, possibly due to increased vagal activity.
- Lewis and Johnson[33] reviewed 20 studies of massage therapy and muscle pain and found that evidence is inconclusive for any effect. The authors suggested that low-quality studies and small sample sizes may have been partly responsible for the inconclusive findings.
- Best, Hunter, Wilcox et al[34] looked at studies of sports massage (some including friction techniques) and found inconsistent results from case study reports, but moderate evidence from 10 randomised controlled trials.

While it would appear that the evidence does not consistently support claims made for the effects of DG or XFF, we must remember that the paucity of studies and the quality of those studies that do exist may be partly responsible for this. Clearly there is a need for further high-quality research to support or refute claims about the effectiveness of DG and XFF.

CONTRAINDICATIONS

The contraindications for DG and XFF techniques are similar to those for Swedish massage. They include:

- acute injury to tissue, including recent surgery
- active inflammation (redness, pain, swelling, heat, loss of function)
- systemic infection or uncontrolled medical condition
- undiagnosed tumour or swelling
- possibility of thrombosis
- skin infections which may spread (e.g. impetigo)
- osteoporosis.

This list is not exhaustive. Therapists should avoid massage in cases where the pathology involved is either unknown or poorly understood.[35, 36]

DEEP TRANSVERSE FRICTION (DTF)

Deep transverse friction (DTF) has long been held to be one of massage therapy's most powerful tools. Pioneered by James Cyriax, DTF became the technique of choice for the treatment of tendinosis and various other scarring and adhesive conditions in muscles, tendons and ligaments.[5, 27, 29] More recently the technique has been employed to assist in the release of superficial scarring.[30] Two studies suggest that the technique stimulates fibroblast activity and that there is no particular benefit to be gained from applying the technique in a transverse direction.[37, 38] The term *deep transverse friction* is used because of its currency and wide acceptance by the massage profession. A more appropriate term is yet to emerge.

DTF differs from XFF in several ways. First, no lubricant is used. The finger and the skin move together, generating a friction force over the tissues beneath. The stroke is typically applied at 90° to the predominant fibre direction (see Figure 4.9). Care should be taken to ensure sufficient sweep; that is, the stroke should cover the entire lesion although this would normally be less than a centimetre. Pressure usually varies from light to very deep during the specific application.[5, 23, 27-29, 35, 39]

A number of claims have been made about the effectiveness of the technique. Cyriax and Russell list 22 separate disorders which are intractable except by DTF.[27] Some of the apparent effects of DTF are thought to be due to:

- separation of adhesions and broadening of muscle tissue[23, 27, 30]
- analgesia, possibly by activation of the pain gate mechanism[5, 29, 30] or by enhancement of circulation to the area (traumatic hyperaemia)[27]
- stimulation of fibroblastic activity in cases of tendinosis.[5, 29]

Evidence for the effectiveness of DTF

The following research into the effectiveness of DTF found inconclusive support for the technique.

- Stasinopoulos and Johnson[40] found, in a clinical review, that there was no evidence in the literature of any clinical benefit in the treatment of tendinopathy with DTF.
- Pellecchia, Hamel and Behnke[41] compared manual techniques, including DTF, with iontophoresis for infrapatellar tendinitis, and found that iontophoresis was more effective across all measures.
- Gregory, Deane and Mars[42] conducted a histological study and found that a single 10-minute application of DTF to healthy muscle caused cellular damage which mostly healed within 6 days after the treatment. It is unclear whether this effect would be helpful, according to the study.
- A Cochrane review of DTF and tendinitis[43] found inconsistent results across a number of studies and stated that no conclusions could be drawn about the effectiveness of DTF.
- Two studies which are often cited as evidence of increased fibroblastic activity after DTF application used augmented soft tissue mobilisation which involves the use of metal tools to apply friction techniques to the tissue.[37, 38] The studies found that only the deepest ('extreme') pressure produced significant increases in fibroblastic activity. The findings of these studies suggest that the usual application of DTF, involving the use of fingers and thumbs, would not be sufficiently deep to induce such activity.

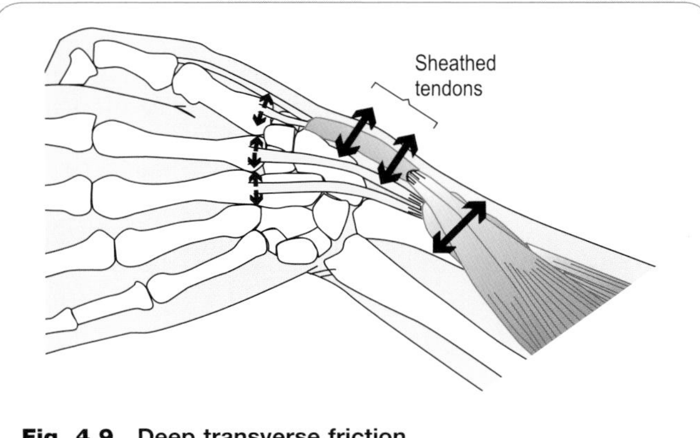

Fig. 4.9 Deep transverse friction

Further research is urgently needed to inform the use of DTF in clinical practice. Some applications of DTF are illustrated in Figure 4.10.

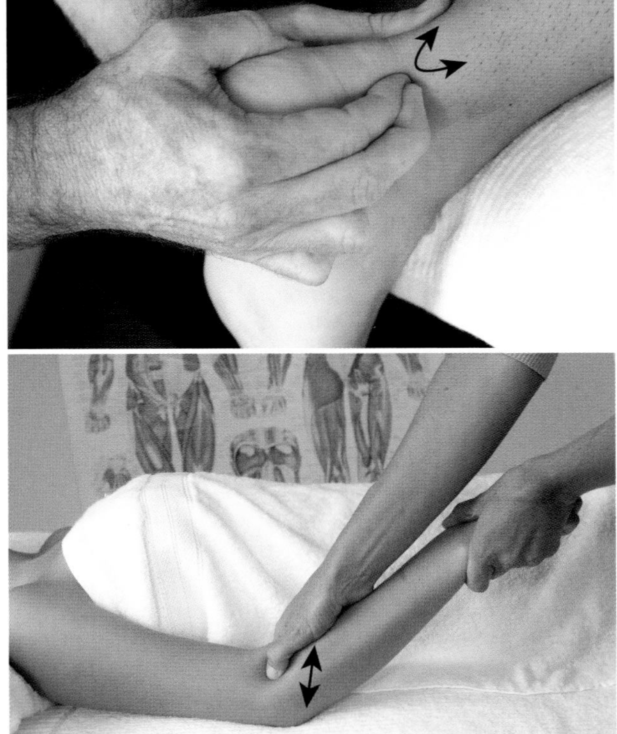

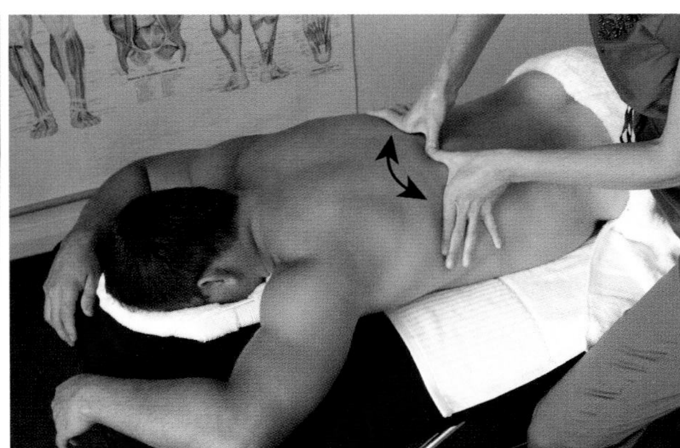

Fig. 4.10 Examples of deep transverse friction in practice

CONTRAINDICATIONS

The literature lists a number of contraindications to DTF application, including:

- active inflammation or infection
- calcification or ossification within tendons, muscles or ligaments
- haematomas
- directly to a peripheral nerve
- rheumatoid arthritis
- bursitis (note that Cyriax and Russell[27] do not recommend DTF for any bursitis. Hammer,[5] on the other hand, states that DTF can be very helpful in chronic cases of hip and subacromial bursitis).

This list is not exhaustive. Avoid DTF in cases where the pathology involved is either unknown or poorly understood.[5, 27]

SOFT TISSUE RELEASE (STR)

Soft tissue release is a group of techniques known by several names and there are small variations in their application. This section describes a myofascial lengthening technique known variously as soft tissue release, directional release, pin and stretch technique[29] or lock and load technique. A patented treatment regimen known as active release technique[44] claims very high success rates with a multitude of soft tissue problems.[44]

Soft tissue release (STR) is applied by fixing specific areas of palpable fibrosis or tension within a muscle and then lengthening the muscle while holding the fixed area still. Two variations within the technique are the passive and active forms. In both of these, the muscle is initially placed in a shortened position and the target area is palpated and pinned or locked by the therapist. This can be done with different parts of the hand, forearm or elbow. The smaller the contact point, the more precise the technique, but the more difficult to maintain control over the tissue.[29, 45]

In the passive variant, move the limb/joint to stretch the target muscle while applying pressure with the other hand (see Figure 4.11). The client can also generate some tension within the target muscle by performing an isometric contraction and maintain this contraction while the therapist pulls the muscle into an eccentric contraction while maintaining the locked tissue.[29] In active STR the client moves the limb/joint through its range of motion while the therapist maintains pressure on the targeted tissue (see Figures 4.12 and 4.13). A good way to think about this technique is to consider that the fixation of the muscle at the selected point creates a false attachment point and the limb/joint movement sets up a new line of stretch, which selectively elongates the desired tissue.[45]

Another variant of this technique involves performing DG frictions or XFF instead of fixing the tissue. This technique is sometimes referred to as *stripping*, especially in sports massage literature.[29, 46] This is a favoured technique when working with athletes as it is considered useful for reaching hard-to-stretch muscles like infraspinatus and the peroneals.[45]

Claims made for the effectiveness of STR include:

- decreasing muscle tension
- stretching contractile and connective aspects of the tissue
- reducing irritation in trigger points.[29, 45]

Evidence for the effectiveness of STR

There is a paucity of research on STR techniques despite its widespread use and acceptance, and much of the evidence underpinning STR appears to be anecdotal. One study looked at the effects of STR on delayed onset muscle soreness (DOMS). The findings suggested that in 20 subjects, the application of STR technique post-exercise actually increased the pain reported due to DOMS and that recovery was not accelerated within the first 48 hours.[47] Clearly, there is a need for more research to support or refute the effectiveness of this technique.

CONTRAINDICATIONS

Contraindications to the technique include those for Swedish massage. In addition,

- easy bruising (stripping, especially, may bruise clients)
- hypermobility in relevant joints.[45]

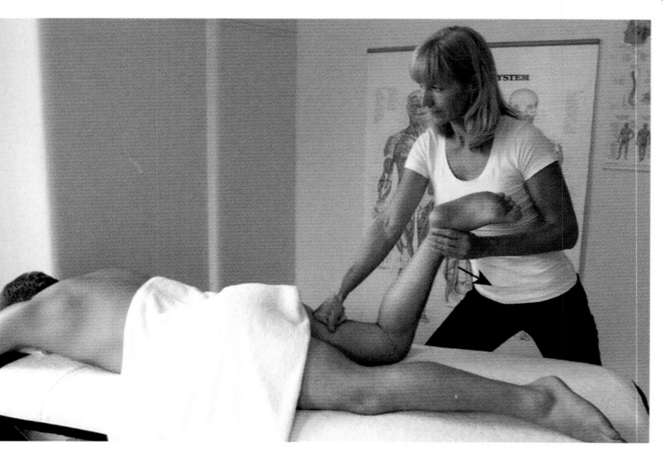

Fig. 4.11 Soft tissue release: passive

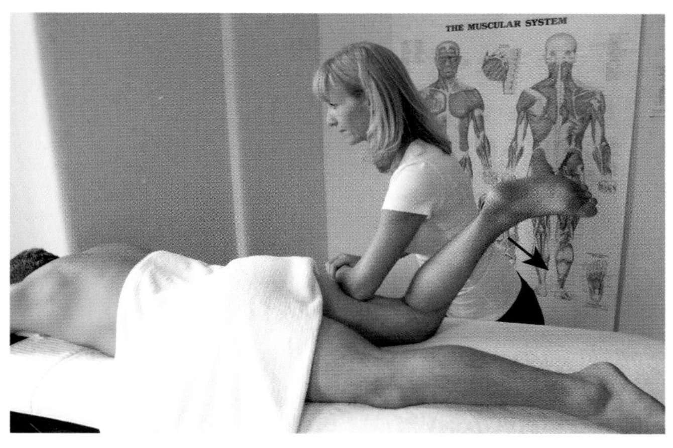

Fig. 4.12 Soft tissue release: active

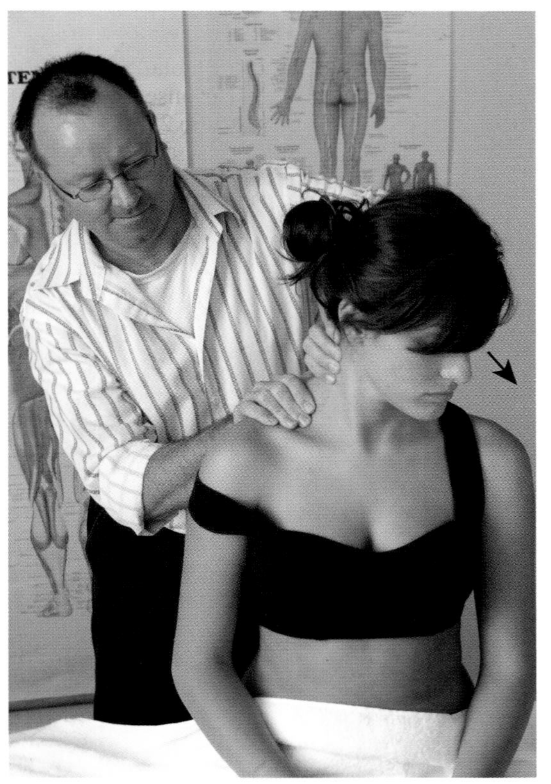

Fig. 4.13 Soft tissue release: active

This list is not exhaustive. Avoid massage in cases where the pathology involved is either unknown or poorly understood.[5, 27]

Table 4.3 summarises the remedial massage techniques for muscles discussed in this chapter. These techniques are perhaps the most widely used by remedial massage therapists. Students and remedial therapists are encouraged to explore further muscle function assessments, like muscle-firing patterns,[47] that are beyond the scope of this book.

KEY MESSAGES

- Remedial massage therapists apply specific techniques to treat muscle injuries and to address muscle imbalances in the body.
- Assessment of muscle injuries and imbalances include case history, postural assessment and functional testing (including functional deficit demonstration and tests for the strength and length of specific muscles).
- Commonly used remedial massage techniques for muscle tissue include deep gliding (DG), cross-fibre frictions (XFF), deep transverse frictions (DTF) and soft tissue release (STR).
- There is insufficient evidence to support or refute the effectiveness of these muscle-specific techniques.

Table 4.3 Major remedial massage techniques for muscles

Technique		Indications	Contraindications
Deep gliding	Deep slow stripping movement along the line of muscle fibres with fingers, knuckles, thumbs, elbows, forearms	Muscle strains, imbalances	As for Swedish massage, including • acute injury • recent surgery • acute inflammation • systemic infection or uncontrolled medical condition • undiagnosed tumour • possible thrombosis • skin infections • osteoporosis
Cross-fibre friction	Deep slow gliding movements perpendicular to the muscle fibres with thumbs, fingers, knuckles, palms, forearms		
Deep transverse friction*	No lubricant Deep friction applied perpendicularly to the line of fibres over the entire lesion (usually <1 cm) with thumbs, fingers, single knuckle, massage tool (e.g. T-bar)	Muscle strains, especially to break down scar tissue/adhesions	As for Swedish massage including • acute inflammation • acute infection • calcification or ossification within tendons, muscles or ligaments • haematomas • peripheral nerves • rheumatoid arthritis • bursitis
Soft tissue release	Practitioner's contacts either static (apply static pressure to lesion with fingers, thumbs, knuckles, elbow) or dynamic (apply deep gliding** with thumbs, fingers, knuckles, forearm) Movement of affected limb either passive (i.e. practitioner moves limb/part) or active (client moves limb/part) 4 variations: i) passive, static ii) passive, dynamic iii) active, static iv) active, dynamic	Muscle strains, imbalances	As for Swedish massage including • easy bruising • joint hypermobility

*DTF may not need not to be restricted to transverse strokes.
**In the dynamic version of STR, deep gliding could be replaced with cross-fibre friction or diagonal gliding.

Review questions

1. Name five procedures that can be used to assess the function of muscles.
2. Give an example of an active functional deficit assessment procedure. Why do some authors prefer active functional deficit assessments to active range of motion assessments in single planes of motion?
3. Why are AROM ranges generally smaller than PROM ranges?
4. What is Sherrington's Law of Reciprocal Innervation? Give an example of how Sherrington's Law could be used in remedial massage practice.
5. How would you test the length of:
   i) latissimus dorsi?
   ii) pectoralis major?
   iii) pectoralis minor?
   iv) quadriceps?
6. What is the difference between the response of postural and phasic muscles to fatigue? How would this fact influence your treatment plan?
7. What do the terms *locked short* and *locked long* mean?
8. What is the difference between a muscle spasm and a contracture? What does this difference mean for treatment of shortened muscle tissue?
9. Joint ranges of motion differ, often markedly, from normative data. This may result from previous conditions or injuries, for instance poorly treated dislocations, or even from training. Name two sports which are associated with either an increased or reduced ROM in specific joints.
10. When assessing a client's right elbow both active and passive ranges of motion appear to be restricted in extension. What can you do to ascertain whether this range is normal for the client?
11. Match column A (condition) with their palpatory characteristics in Column B.

Column A	Column B
Fibrotic tissue	Tender
Oedema	May be crepitus
Acute strain	Hard, sometimes stringy
Chronic tendinosis	Spongy

12. Answer the following questions about deep transverse friction:
    i) What was the technique originally thought to achieve?
    ii) What effects are supported by current research?

REFERENCES

1. Verrall G, Slavotinek J, Barnes P, et al. Clinical risk factors for hamstring muscle strain injury: a prospective study with correlation of injury by magnetic resonance imaging. Br J Sports Med 2001;35:435–40.
2. Orchard J, Seward H. Epidemiology of injuries in the Australian Footbal League, seasons 1997–2000. Br J Sports Med 2002;36:39–45.
3. Orchard J, Best T. The management of muscle strain injuries: an early return versus the risk of recurrence. Clin J Sport Med 2002;12:3–5.
4. Konin JG, Wiksten DL, Isear JA, et al. Special tests for orthopedic examination. New Jersey: Slack; 2006.
5. Hammer WI. editor. Functional soft tissue examination and treatment by manual methods. 2nd edn. Gaithersburg: Aspen; 1999.
6. Chaitow L, Delaney J. Clinical application of neuromuscular techniques – practical case study exercises. Edinburgh: Elsevier; 2005.
7. Travell J, Simons D. Myofascial pain and dysfunction: the trigger point manual. Vol. 1: the upper extremities. Baltimore: Williams and Wilkins; 1983.
8. Cook CE, Hegedus EJ. Orthopedic physical examination tests – an evidence-based approach. New Jersey: Pearson Prentice Hall; 2008.
9. Chaitow L. Soft tissue manipulation. Rochester: Healing Arts Press; 1988.
10. Kendall FP, McCreary EK, Provance PG. Muscles – testing and function. Maryland: Williams and Wilkins; 1993.
11. Chaitow L. Muscle energy techniques. Edinburgh: Churchill Livingstone; 1996.
12. Janda V. Muscle function testing. London: Butterworths; 1983.
13. Vleeming A, Mooney V, Dorman T, et al. Movement, stability and low back pain. New York: Churchill Livingstone; 1997.
14. Myers T. Anatomy trains – myofascial meridians for manual and movement therapists. Edinburgh: Churchill Livingstone; 2002.
15. Chaitow L, Delany JW. Clinical application of neuromuscular techniques. Vol 2: the lower body. Edinburgh: Churchill Livingstone; 2002.
16. Norris C. The muscle debate. J Bodyw Mov Ther 2000;4(4):232–5.
17. Jull G, Janda V. Muscles and motor control in low back pain: assessment and management. In: Twomey L, editor. Physical therapy of the low back. Edinburgh: Churchill Livingstone; 1987.
18. Chaitow L, Delany JW. Clinical application of neuromuscular techniques. Vol. 1: the upper body. Edinburgh: Churchill Livingstone; 2000.
19. Cyriax J. Textbook of orthopedic medicine. Vol. 1: diagnosis of soft tissue lesions. London: Baillière Tindall; 1982.
20. Gracovetsky SA. Range of normality vs range of motion: a functional measure for the prevention and management of low back injury. J Bodyw Mov Ther 2010;14:40–9.
21. Evjenth O, Hamberg J. Muscle stretching in manual therapy – a clinical manual. Alfta: Alfta Rehab Forlag; 1984.
22. Chaitow L. Muscle energy techniques. Edinburgh: Churchill Livingstone; 2001.
23. Brukner P, Khan K. Clinical sports medicine. Sydney: McGraw Hill; 1994.
24. Simmonds MJ, Kumar S. Health care ergonomics, part 1: the fundamental skill of palpation – a review and critique. Int J Ind Ergon 1993;11:135–43.
25. Chaitow L, Chambers G, Frymann V. Palpation and assessment skills. Edinburgh: Churchill Livingstone; 2003.
26. Holsgaard-Larsen A, Myburgh C, Hartvigsen J, et al. Standardized simulated palpation training – development of a palpation trainer and assessment of palpatory skills in experienced and inexperienced clinicians. Man Ther 2010;15:254–60.
27. Cyriax J, Russell G. Textbook of orthopedic medicine. Vol 2: treatment by manipulation, massage and injection. London: Baillière Tindall; 1977.
28. Goats GC. Massage – the scientific basis of an ancient art. Part 1: the techniques. Br J Sp Med 1994;28(3):149–52.
29. Lowe W. Orthopedic massage: theory and technique. 2nd edn. Edinburgh: Mosby Elsevier; 2009.
30. Goats GC. Massage – the scientific basis of an ancient art. Part 2: physiological and therapeutic effects. Br J Sp Med 1994;28(3):153–6.
31. de las Penas CF, Sohrbeck Campo M, et al. Manual therapies in myofascial trigger point treatment: a systematic review. J Bodyw Mov Ther 2005;9: 27–34.
32. Field T, Diego M, Hernandez M. Moderate pressure is essential for massage therapy effects. Int J Neurosci 2010;120(5):381–5.
33. Lewis M, Johnson MI. The clinical effectiveness of therapeutic massage for musculoskeletal pain – a systematic review. Physiotherapy 2006;92(3):146–58.
34. Best TM, Hunter R, Wilcox A, et al. Effectiveness of sports massage for recovery of skeletal muscle from strenuous exercise. Clin J Sport Med 2008;18(5):446–60.
35. Tappan FM. Healing massage techniques – holistic, classic and emerging methods. Norwalk: Appleton and Lange; 1988.
36. Capellini S, Van Welden M. Massage for dummies. 2nd edn. New York: Wiley; 2010.
37. Gehlsen GM, Ganion LR, Helfst R. Fibroblast responses to variation in soft tissue mobilisation pressure. Med Sci Sports Exerc 1999;31(4):531–5.
38. Davidson CJ, Ganion LR, Gehlsen GM, et al. Rat tendon morphologic and functional changes resulting from soft tissue mobilization. Med Sci Sports Exerc 1997;29(3):313–19.
39. Mellion MB. Sports medicine secrets. Philadelphia: Hanley and Belfus; 1993.
40. Stasinopoulos D, Johnson MI. It may be time to modify the Cyriax treatment of lateral epicondylitis. J Bodyw Mov Ther 2007;11:64–7.
41. Pellechia GL, Hamel H, Behnke P. Treatment of infrapatellar tendinitis: a combination of modalities and transverse friction massage versus iontophoresis. J Sport Rehabil 1994;3(2):135–45.
42. Gregory MA, Deane MN, Mars M. Ultrastructural changes in untraumatised rabbit skeletal muscle treated with deep transverse friction. Physiotherapy 2003;89(7):408–16.
43. Brosseau L, Casimiro L, Milne S, et al. Deep transverse friction massage for treating tendinitis. Cochrane Database Syst Rev 2002;(4)CD003528.
44. Leahy M. Active release techniques: logical soft tissue treatment. In: Hammer WI, editor. Functional soft tissue examination and treatment by manual methods. 2nd edn. Gaithersburg: Aspen; 1999.
45. Johnson J. Soft tissue release. Champaign: Human Kinetics; 2009.
46. Walden M, editor. Sports massage tutorials. Accessed: 31 July 2010. Online. Available: http://www.sportsinjuryclinic.net/sports-massage/legs-and-back-sports-massage.php.
47. Micklewright D. The effect of soft tissue release on delayed onset muscle soreness: a pilot study. Phys Ther Sport 2009;10:19–24.

5 Muscle stretching

The content of this chapter relates to the following Units of Competency:
HLTREM503C Plan remedial massage treatment strategy
HLTREM504C Apply remedial massage assessment framework
HLTREM502C Provide remedial massage treatment
HLTREM505C Perform remedial massage health assessment

Health Training Package HLT07

Learning Outcomes

- Assess clients' suitability for muscle stretching.
- Describe the current evidence for the effectiveness of muscle stretching.
- Briefly describe the neurophysiology of muscle reflexes involved in stretching.
- Apply muscle-stretching techniques effectively and safely to a range of clients.
- Advise clients who have been treated with muscle stretching about home exercise.

INTRODUCTION

Therapeutic stretching involves elongating contractile tissue (muscle and associated tendon and connective tissue) within its elastic range of motion. It requires the skilful application of knowledge of anatomy, neuromuscular physiology and biomechanics blended with sound clinical judgment to achieve an optimum predictable outcome. Stretching techniques range from simple stretches of a body part through to re-educating the neuromuscular system of the central nervous system. Although stretching is relatively safe, inappropriate or ill-judged use of stretching techniques can result in injury.[1] When considering the potential benefits of stretching, one should take into account the many functions performed by muscle in vivo. How may stretching assist in the execution of these functions? What criteria do we use to determine a client's suitability for stretching? Should a stretching regimen be part of this client's overall management plan? How can stretching be performed effectively and safely?

FUNCTIONAL ANATOMY

Stretching takes advantage of four properties of muscle:

- Excitability (also called irritability) – the ability to receive and respond to stimuli. The response is contraction of muscle fibres.
- Contractility – muscle can actively shorten its length. This is a unique property of muscle tissue.
- Extensibility – muscle can be stretched beyond its resting length.
- Elasticity – muscle fibre can recoil and resume its resting length after being stretched.

A contractile unit consists of a muscle fibre, tendon and the connective tissue that binds these tissues together. (see Figure 5.1 on p 65)

TISSUE RANGE OF MOTION

All soft tissue of the body has an inherent range of motion. Joints, contractile units and structures that are involved with gross movement are the focus of interest in stretching regimens. However, it is important to consider the influence of a stretching routine on all tissue and the mechanical properties of the affected tissues when developing a routine. For example, a neck-stretching routine must take into account the impact of stretching delicate nerve and vascular tissue within the neck. The type of stretching procedure delivered to the neck must be appropriate for these structures and at the same time must be effective in its primary purpose. Healthy tissue can generally tolerate stretching through a normal range of motion. However, a person suffering vascular disease may be considerably less tolerant of the 'normal' expected range of motion. Give priority to the most at-risk tissue that could be affected by the stretch when planning a stretching routine.

Tissues like bone undergo almost no deformity under tensile loading (stretching) before they fracture. Other tissues are ductile; that is, they undergo plastic (permanent) deformity of shape before they rupture when under load. If stretching allows a ductile tissue (e.g. a ligament) to undergo repeated or prolonged stretch beyond its elastic limit then permanent deformity will ensue. This results in joint hypermobility due to elongation of the ligaments that support the joint and maintain the normal proximity of the congruous articular surfaces. A joint will develop hypermobility only in the directions of excessive stretch. In determining the impact of excessive stretching one must also consider mechanical properties of

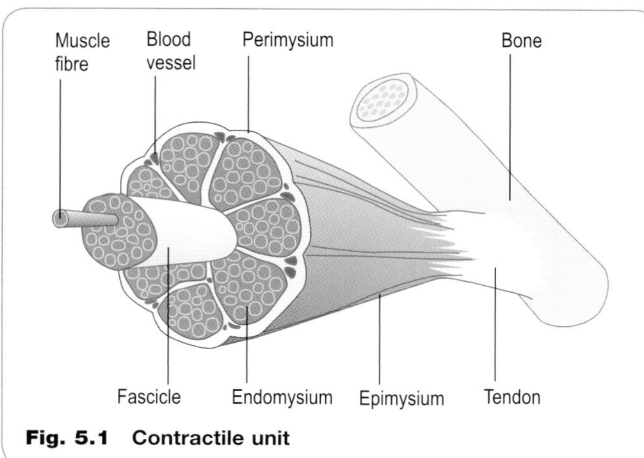

Fig. 5.1 Contractile unit

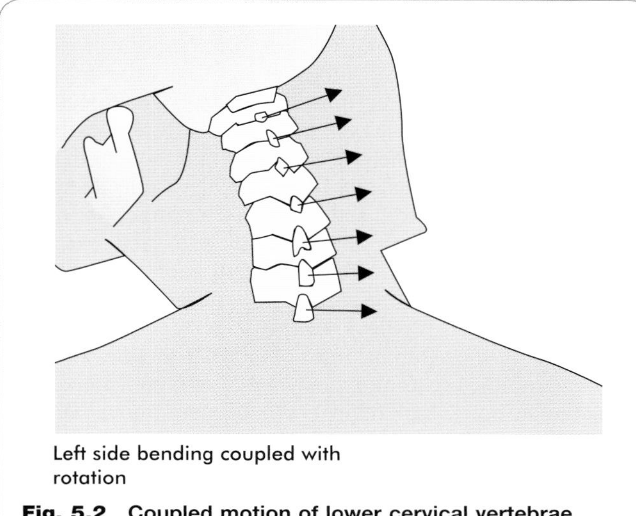

Fig. 5.2 Coupled motion of lower cervical vertebrae

joints including the concept of 'coupled motion' of joints; that is, motion in which translation or rotation about an axis is associated with simultaneous translation or rotation about another axis.[2] Normal cervical movement, for example, involves coupled movement: lateral flexion of the lower cervical spine invokes simultaneous ipsilateral rotation of the vertebrae.[3] (see Figure 5.2)

MUSCLE FUNCTIONS

Muscles produce movement, maintain posture, stabilise joints, generate and maintain body heat, guard orifices and support and protect tissue.

Produce movement

Muscles are responsible for:

- all locomotion of the skeleton and manipulation of the external environment
- movement of fluids via muscle pumping actions. The movement of blood through the body reflects the work of the rhythmically beating cardiac muscle and smooth muscle in the walls of blood vessels. Movement of lymph fluid, urine, bile and faeces results from muscle contractions.

Maintaining posture and position

Adjusting muscles enable us to maintain posture despite external forces acting on the body and the never-ending downward pull of gravity. Righting reflexes are involuntary muscle contractions of the voluntary muscle system that automatically adjust posture and position.

Stabilising joints

Muscles not only pull on bones to create movement, but they also stabilise joints. Muscle tone is a major factor in joint stability.

Generating and maintaining body heat

Muscles generate heat as they contract which is vitally important in maintaining normal body temperature. Involuntary muscles cause the redistribution of heat via the systematic contraction of smooth muscle in blood vessels.

Guard orifices

Sphincter muscles form valves to control passage of substances.

Support and protect soft tissues

Muscle often protects adjacent delicate soft tissue like blood and lymph vessels and peripheral nerves. Strengthening programs are often prescribed to protect hypermobile joints, disc lesions and other tissue injury sites.

TYPES OF MUSCLE CONTRACTIONS

Most body movements are a mixture of both isotonic and isometric contractions.

Isotonic contractions

The tension or tone in a muscle remains the same while the muscle length changes; that is, the muscle shortens while it contracts (e.g. lifting an object overhead, throwing a ball).

- A concentric contraction occurs when the muscle shortens as tension is applied, as in lifting an object or performing a biceps curl.
- In an eccentric contraction the muscle lengthens as it contracts, as when a load is lowered to the ground or running downhill.

Isometric contractions

The muscle length remains the same while the muscle tension increases; that is, a static contraction occurs (e.g. pushing arms against a wall, trying to lift an immovable object).

PHYSICAL CHARACTERISTICS AND NEUROLOGICAL REFLEXES ASSOCIATED WITH STRETCHING

The physical properties of muscle, particularly its limits of shortening and lengthening, are important factors in stretching. The ideal length–stretch relationship within a muscle occurs when a muscle is slightly stretched beyond its normal

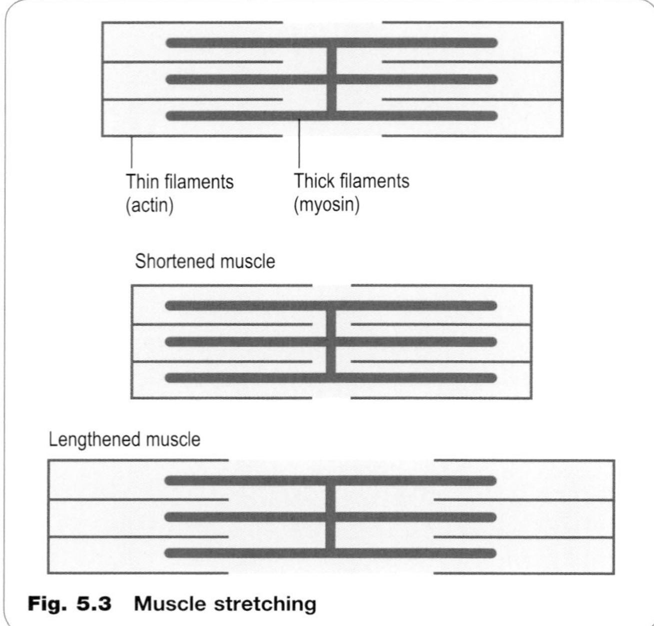

Fig. 5.3 Muscle stretching

resting length. At this length, the actin and myosin filaments within the muscle barely overlap. This permits sliding along the entire length of the filaments. If a muscle is stretched to the extent that the myofilaments do not overlap at all, the muscle cannot generate tension and therefore cannot contract. Conversely, if the muscle is so compressed that the myofilaments are completely overlapping then further shortening is impossible. (see Figure 5.3) Muscles have an optimum operational range of length of 80% to 120% of their normal resting length.[4]

ACTIVE AND PASSIVE INSUFFICIENCY

When multiarticular muscles (i.e. muscles that span more than one joint) contract, they exert force on all the joints they span so that movement can occur at more than one joint simultaneously. Because of limitations in the length of the muscle, these muscles cannot exert enough tension to shorten sufficiently for both joints to achieve full end range movement at the same time. This is called *active insufficiency*. Conversely, it is very difficult for a multiarticular muscle to be stretched enough to allow full end range movement in both joints simultaneously. This is called *passive insufficiency*. These physical properties of muscle should be considered when devising stretching and rehabilitation programs for clients. An example of this principle can be observed in practice when stretching the hamstring muscle. Clients with shortened hamstrings can stretch the muscle by extending the knee with the hip flexed to 90° (i.e. the muscle is stretched across one joint – the knee). For clients with greater hamstring flexibility, flexing at the hip with the knee extended (i.e. stretching the muscle over two joints) may be required to achieve further muscle stretch.

NEUROLOGICAL EVENTS THAT MEDIATE STRETCHING

The neurological events that mediate stretching are briefly reviewed below.

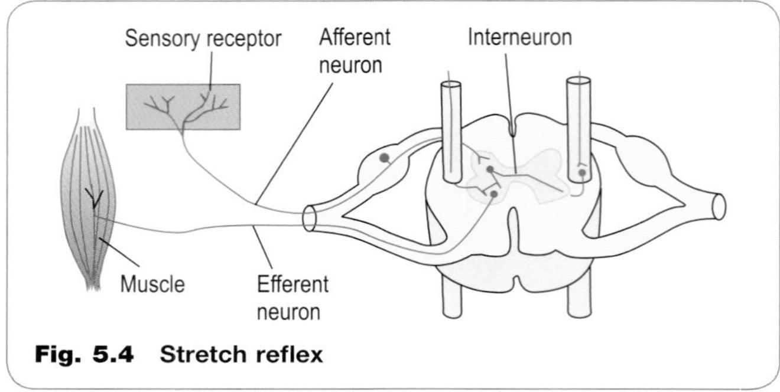

Fig. 5.4 Stretch reflex

Myotatic reflex (stretch reflex)

This is a protective reflex guarding against overstretching muscles. It is mediated within the spinal cord and occurs quickly (1–2 milliseconds). Within all muscles lie nerve endings that respond to the rate and the amount of muscle stretch. Together with the modified muscle fibre to which they attach, they form the muscle spindles. The specialised nerve receptors of these spindles send afferent (sensory) information regarding the rate of stretch and the length of the muscle to the central nervous system. When a muscle spindle is stretched, the stretch reflex causes contraction of the muscle, thereby limiting the muscle's rate and extent of stretch. At the spine the afferent stimuli excite alpha motor neurons which activate the muscle to contract, thus resisting further stretch. (see Figure 5.4)

Branches of the afferent fibres also synapse with interneurons that inhibit the motor neurons of antagonist muscles. Thus, the muscles that oppose the primary movement are stopped from resisting that movement. This is called *reciprocal inhibition*.[4]

Deep tendon reflex

When muscle tension increases during contraction or passive stretching, golgi tendon organ (GTO) receptors within the muscle's tendon are activated. The GTO send afferent impulses to the spinal cord and cerebellum. Motor neurons in the spinal cord that supply the contracting muscle are inhibited and neurons to the antagonist muscles are activated. This process is called *reciprocal activation*.[4] Fine control of muscle coordination is achieved with the help of this system (see Figure 5.5 on p 67).

TYPES OF MUSCLE STRETCHING

Numerous stretching techniques have been developed, including practitioner-assisted stretching and active stretching where the client performs the stretch independently. Some of the major muscle-stretching techniques include:

1. PASSIVE STRETCH

An assistant/practitioner performs a stretch on a client to increase tissue range of motion.

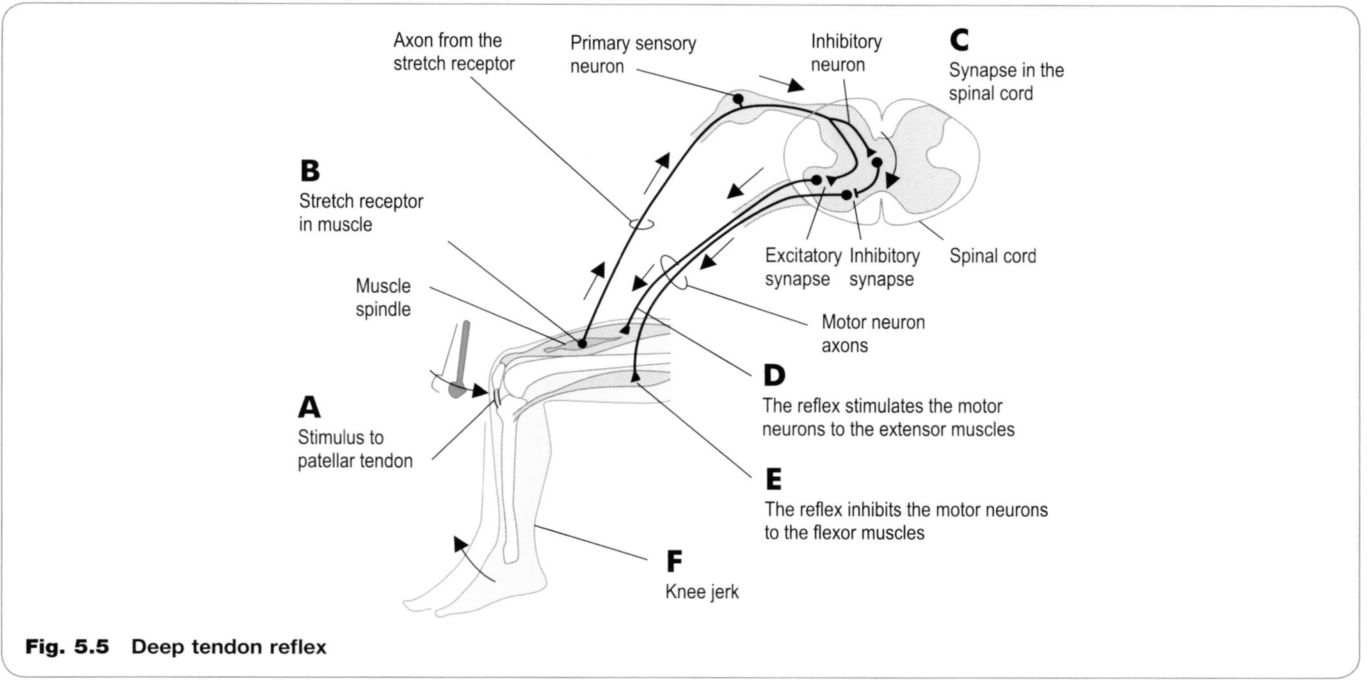

Fig. 5.5 Deep tendon reflex

2. ACTIVE, ACTIVE-ASSISTED STRETCH

Active stretches or self-stretches are inherently safer than passive stretching as the client can judge when the muscle being stretched has reached its comfortable limit.

3. MUSCLE ENERGY TECHNIQUE[5]

Muscle energy technique (MET) involves isometric contraction before stretching. The client uses minimal force during the isometric contraction and this is followed by passive stretching. The main goal of MET is joint mobilisation. The technique uses both reciprocal inhibition and post-isometric relaxation.[5] In post-isometric relaxation the muscle is passively stretched and minimal resistance applied against isometric contraction. When the contraction is released the muscle is taken gently into a further stretch.

4. ACTIVE ISOLATED STRETCH[6]

In this technique, the client actively lengthens the muscle to the point of light irritation and holds for 2 seconds before returning to the starting position. This sequence is repeated 8 to 10 times. The technique is designed to prevent activation of the stretch reflex while activating reciprocal inhibition.

5. BALLISTIC STRETCH

Ballistic stretching involves rapid bouncing performed at the end range of joint motion. It can be an active or passive stretch. Popularised by Beaulieu in 1981[7] ballistic stretching has now fallen out of favour because of the risk of tearing muscle. It produces a strong myotonal reflex, leaving the muscle shorter than before the stretch.[8]

6. DYNAMIC STRETCH

This type of stretching usually occurs in dynamic range of motion warm-up routines. The limbs are moved through their full range of motion slowly in a controlled and comfortable manner. Speed is increased with repetitions.[9]

7. STATIC STRETCH

Bob Anderson, in his book *Stretching*, gives a comprehensive description of static stretching methods for sports, activities of daily living and occupational activities.[10] His method employs slow lengthening of a muscle which is held for 15 to 30 seconds and then repeated, increasing range of motion as the muscle relaxes. Various authors suggest different time intervals for maintaining a static stretch. In one variation, the client holds the position for 30 seconds to two minutes which gradually lengthens a muscle. A study by Ford et al[11] investigated the effect of four different durations (30, 60, 90 and 120 seconds) of static hamstring stretch on passive knee extension range of motion in healthy subjects and found that similar benefits were achieved regardless of the stretch duration. During the holding period or directly afterwards, clients may feel a mild discomfort or warm sensation in the muscles. It is thought that static stretching slightly lessens the sensitivity of muscle spindle receptors which allows the muscle to relax and to be stretched to greater length.

8. PROPRIOCEPTIVE NEUROMUSCULAR FACILITATION

Developed in the 1940s, proprioceptive neuromuscular facilitation (PNF) techniques are the result of the work of Kabat, Knott and Voss.[12–14] They combined their analysis of functional movement with theories from motor development, motor control, motor learning and neurophysiology.[14] PNF can be a valuable part of rehabilitation programs. Most clinicians use PNF to promote muscle stretching and functional movement although it can also be used to develop muscular strength and endurance, improve joint stability or increase neuromuscular control and coordination: 'PNF techniques help develop muscular strength and endurance, joint stability, mobility, neuromuscular control and coordination – all of which are aimed at improving the overall functional ability of patients'.[15] PNF techniques have been used to treat people with neurological and musculoskeletal conditions, most frequently in rehabilitating the knee, shoulder, hip and ankle.[16]

PNF stretching techniques

PNF stretching is regarded by some authors as the most effective of all stretching techniques.[16–18] In PNF stretching neuromuscular inhibition procedures reflexively relax the contractile components of shortened muscles so clients can increase their range of movement. Various techniques are used, among them:

Hold-Relax

This technique is also known as *Contract-Relax.* First, the practitioner lengthens a tight muscle, then the client isometrically contracts it for several seconds. When the contraction is released, the practitioner further lengthens the muscle and holds the stretch at the new end range of motion. Reflexive muscle relaxation occurs as a result of the firing of the golgitendon organ (GTO). Hold-relax technique is easy to perform in clinic and is suitable for home exercises and preventive programs.

It is important to be aware that although activating the GTO can increase flexibility, it may also predispose to injury. PNF stretching applied directly before activity can predispose clients to musculotendinous injury if a sudden stretch occurs during functional activity. PNF stretching techniques have been shown to effectively diminish muscular activity of the biceps femoris, which was apparently due to an inhibition of the myotatic reflex and would therefore permit greater muscle stretching.[19]

Hold (or Contract)-Relax with Agonist Contraction (CRAC)

This technique follows the same procedure as the Hold-Relax technique except that, after the tight muscle is contracted isometrically against the practitioner's resistance, the client concentrically contracts the muscle opposite the tight muscle to actively move the joint through the increased range.[14] A static stretch is then applied at the end of this new range of motion. The process can be repeated several times.

Agonist contraction First, the practitioner passively lengthens the tight muscle (antagonist) to its end range; then the client concentrically contracts the muscle opposite the tight muscle (agonist) to move the joint to a new position in the range of motion.[14] Next, the practitioner applies mild resistance during this contraction, taking care to allow for movement through the available functional range of motion. This technique uses reciprocal inhibition to encourage the tight muscle to lengthen during agonist muscle contraction.

Hold-Relax is one of the most frequently used PNF techniques[16] although over the last decade Hold-Relax with Agonist Contraction has become increasingly popular. Research indicates that sub-maximal contractions that are progressive in intensity over the course of a rehabilitation program increase flexibility.[20] Best outcomes appear to be achieved when practitioners introduce PNF stretching in the early stages of

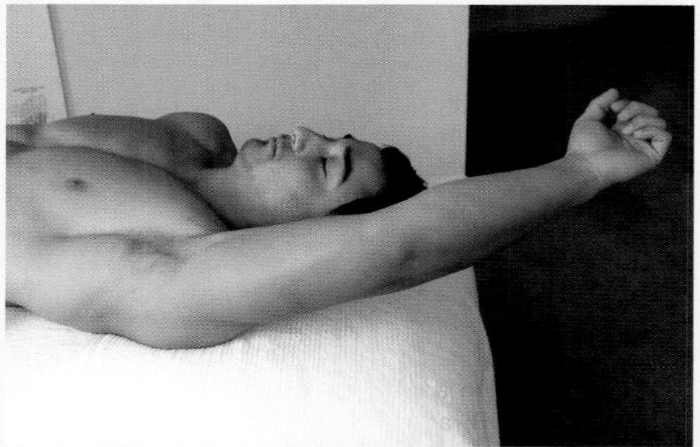

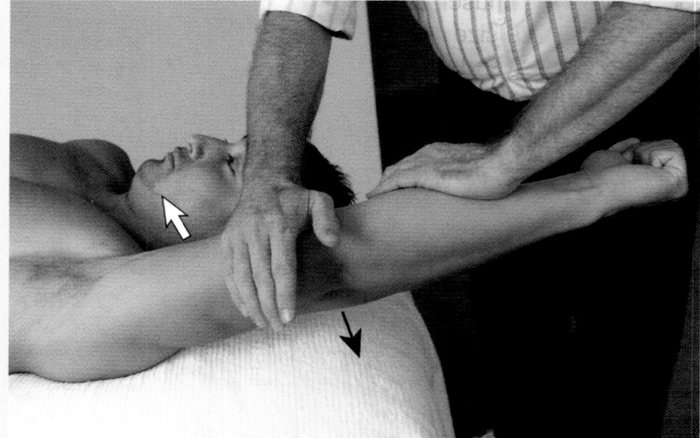

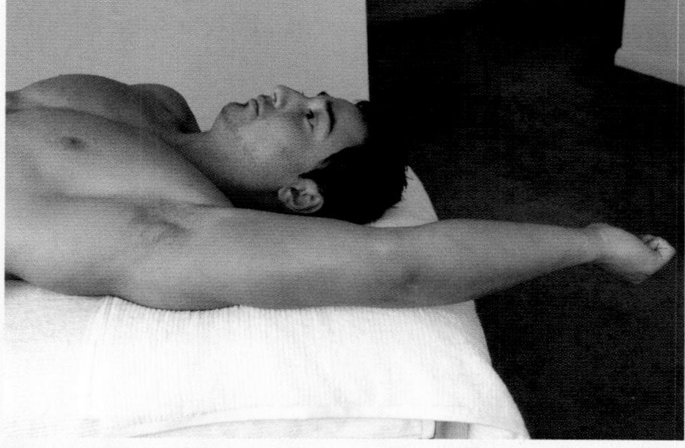

Fig. 5.6 CRAC stretching

[1] Thoughout this book, ➔ represents the direction of the practitioner's pressure; ⇨ represents the direction of the clients' pressure.

Continued

rehabilitation and the intensity of contractions gradually increases throughout rehabilitation.

There is much inconsistency in the use of PNF-related terminology and implementation among practitioners. For example, many practitioners and authors refer to Hold-Relax stretching as Contract-Relax stretching. Some also incorporate a concentric contraction of the tight muscle against minimal resistance before applying a second stretch. This procedure, however, does not allow for maximum gains in flexibility; any firing of GTO is negated by the time the client moves the extremity back to the starting point of the concentric contraction. There are also varying opinions on the duration and number of repetitions. For example, one author recommends performing the PNF technique 3 to 5 times for a given muscle group (resting 20 seconds between each repetition).[21] However, another group suggests that performing 3 to 5 repetitions of a PNF technique for a given muscle group is not necessarily any more effective than performing the technique only once.[22] Walker's[23] PNF stretching method consists of contracting the muscle for 5–6 seconds at a comfortable starting stretch, relaxing the contraction and then further passive stretching for 30 seconds. This is followed by a 30-second recovery period out of the stretch. The sequence is repeated 2–4 times.

Laughlin[24] developed a method of stretching that focuses on injury prevention and rehabilitation. This method uses a contract-relax (C-R) approach. The contract phase involves contracting the muscle for an interval of 2 to 30 seconds depending on its size and location. The intensity of this contraction also depends on the same two variables. The relax phase is composed of two intervals: relaxation of the whole body followed by re-stretch of the muscle in order to exaggerate the stretch. The new stretch is commonly held for a period of 15 to 45 seconds depending on the size and location of the muscle. The C-R stretch can then be repeated. No improvement in range of motion is usually found beyond three repetitions.

PNF strengthening techniques

Spiral-diagonal patterns are observed in normal movements such as swinging the arms across the body during walking. PNF techniques that use spiral-diagonal patterns are designed to restore and enhance coordinately movements through multiple planes and axes of motion.[8] PNF strengthening techniques use spiral-diagonal patterns, often referred to as D1 and D2 patterns. They also apply sensory cues, specifically proprioceptive, cutaneous, visual and auditory feedback, to improve muscular responses.[14] The diagonal movements associated with PNF involve multiple joints moving through various planes of motion. These patterns incorporate rotational movements of the extremities, but also require core stability if patients are to successfully complete the motions.

D1 and D2 patterns can be performed in either flexion or extension.[25] They are referred to as D1 flexion, D1 extension, D2 flexion or D2 extension techniques for the upper or lower extremity.[14] In practitioner-assisted PNF strengthening the practitioner applies manual resistance throughout a range of motion using precise hand positioning while guiding the client through the appropriate range of movement.[14] The practitioner can make minor adjustments as the client's coordination improves or fatigue occurs during the rehabilitation session. In general, the practitioner applies the maximum amount of resistance that allows for smooth, controlled, pain-free movement throughout the range of motion.[25] In addition to manual resistance strengthening, PNF diagonal patterns enhance proper sequencing of muscular contraction, from distal to proximal. This promotes neuromuscular control and coordination.[14]

Variations of PNF technique

To enhance coordination, movement and stability, practitioners use numerous techniques during PNF exercises, among them:

Rhythmic stabilisation

This technique, which incorporates passive movement of the joint through the desired range of motion, is used to re-educate the neuromuscular system to initiate the desired movement. The practitioner passively moves the extremity several times through the movement pattern at appropriate speed. Active assistive and then active movement with resistance are progressively introduced through the same pattern to improve the client's coordination and control.

Slow reversal

This technique involves a dynamic concentric contraction of a strong agonist muscle group, which is immediately followed by a second dynamic concentric contraction of a weak antagonist muscle group.[14] Because rest periods do not occur between contractions this technique promotes the rapid, reciprocal motion that these muscle groups need for coordinated activities.

Slow reversal hold

This technique supplements the technique above with an isometric contraction (hold) at the end range of each muscle group. It is used to enhance dynamic stability of the larger proximal muscle groups (e.g. hip flexors, quadratus lumborum, lower trapezius). This adds a sustained contraction to enhance tone of proximal stabilising muscles.

Alternating isometrics

This technique encourages stability in postural trunk muscles and stabilisers of the hip and shoulder girdle. The practitioner applies manual resistance to the involved limb in a single plane from one side of the body to the other while the client holds the starting position using alternating isometric contractions. This technique can be used to strengthen muscles of the trunk, upper limbs or lower limbs. It can be applied with the limbs in an open kinetic chain (i.e. the hand or foot free to move) or closed kinetic chain position (i.e. the hand or foot fixed).

Alternating rhythmic stabilisation

This technique is an extension of alternating isometrics in which the involved muscle groups co-contract. Rhythmic stabilisation is most commonly performed in a closed kinetic chain position to further enhance muscular co-contraction and joint stability. The practitioner may apply simultaneous manual resistance in a multidirectional pattern, forcing different muscle groups to contract simultaneously to support and stabilise the extremity. This technique is particularly beneficial for isometrically contracting the proximal joint rotators.[14]

STRETCHING TREATMENT GOALS

Using the acronym SMART (Specific, Measurable, Acceptable, Realistic, Time Related), we can develop therapeutic goals that the practitioner and client mutually understand and agree to at the commencement of therapy. This approach facilitates communication and motivates the client to self-assess their needs and re-evaluate any preconceived ideas.

Some defined goals will be almost universal, such as decreasing pain, increasing range of motion, increasing strength and endurance and developing balance between motion and stability. Other goals will be client-specific. Examples are specific performance goals such as walking or running a certain distance in a certain time. Incremental goals established to act as landmarks throughout the course of recovery are particularly helpful.

ASSESSING CLIENTS' SUITABILITY

HISTORY

Clients may complain of muscle aches, pain or stiffness. In some cases clients are not aware of the muscle contractures that have preceded the development of many musculoskeletal complaints, for example headaches from tight upper trapezius and sub-occipital muscles, or knee pain from an overly tight vastus lateralis muscle. Correlating the client's history with other assessment findings helps identify muscle imbalances that may underlie presenting conditions.

POSTURAL ANALYSIS

Postural analysis gives a great deal of information about the way an individual uses their body. It will also give the astute observer insight into aspects of the client's psychological state and how that impacts on their body. Common posture distortions like scoliosis, upper crossed and lower crossed syndrome and hyperlordosis are associated with muscle contractures and weaknesses.

GAIT ANALYSIS

Gait analysis contributes to the functional assessment of the client, enabling identification of appropriate muscles requiring stretching and strengthening. For example, walking on the balls of the feet may indicate shortened gastrocnemius and soleus muscles: abnormal hip rotation in the acceleration phase of gait may indicate weak quadriceps. Assess gait for focal dysfunction and for a global view of the whole kinematic chain affecting the client's gait (see Chapter 2). Reassessing gait at a later date will inform modification to the initial routine as the client's kinematics alter over time.

FUNCTIONAL TESTS

Muscle strains are identified by pain and impaired function which may include decreased strength and impaired ability to lengthen. Muscle length tests help identify muscles requiring stretching. Compare findings to the unaffected side or to population norms (see Chapter 2, Table 2.7).

PALPATION

Palpation is an invaluable tool when assessing muscle tone. Use palpation to confirm findings from postural observation and gait analysis. Assess the perceived level of tension in muscle and tendon. Taut muscle that feels like a stretched fibrous rope suggests chronic hypertonicity. Muscle with a soft, unresponsive, flaccid feel suggests a mechanical dysfunction of the kinematic chain associated with that muscle or neurological deficit.

The WHO's International Classification of Function and Activity and Participation provides a systematic process which is designed to provide and/or maintain the greatest level of functionality available for that individual.[1] It is a useful guide which integrates findings from a range of assessments. At the end of remedial massage assessment the practitioner should be able to describe:

- areas of function
  - pain-free
  - strong
  - able to move and stabilise
  - coordinated and controlled motion
- areas of dysfunction:
  - general functional loss:
    - static – loss of ability to maintain a position.
    - dynamic – loss of ability to move or control motion
- specific deficits:
  - pain
  - weakness
  - decreased ROM due to joint restriction or muscle fatigue or contracture
  - loss of sensation or proprioception
  - deficient sight or hearing
  - deficient motor control
  - lack of endurance.

EVIDENCE FOR EFFECTIVENESS

Many people, both lay and professional, believe that stretching may benefit the user to better prepare the body for activity, reduce the likelihood of injury and post-event muscle soreness, and enhance performance. To date, none of these beliefs can be substantiated by scientific research. Indeed, the clinical effectiveness of stretching remains unclear despite its wide use.[26] Holding, rubbing and stretching affected muscles appears to be a natural response to injury or strenuous activity.

There is a need for rigorous scientific investigation to underpin many stretching techniques commonly used in sports medicine practices. MacAuley and Best[27] point out that much in sport and exercise medicine is not supported by research evidence: 'Stretching is long established as one of the fundamental principles in athletic care … Sport is rife with pseudoscience, and it is difficult to disentangle the evangelical enthusiasm of the locker room from research evidence.' Other unanswered questions about musculoskeletal injury include the value of ice, compression and elevation, as well as the optimal frequency and duration of these treatments. 'Much of sport and exercise medicine and the management of musculoskeletal injury has developed empirically, with little research evidence … Some of the basic principles of caring for acute injuries of the soft tissues have never been questioned, yet there is often little evidence to support common practice.'

Smedes[28] conducted a literature search that examined articles on PNF published between 1990 and 2006 and concluded, 'There is a small amount of support for the PNF concept as an approach for physical rehabilitation. The studies found in this database search vary in subjects and in quality; because of this there is no conclusion over the overall efficacy of the PNF concept. But for specific objectives within the patient management the PNF concept can be beneficial within the physical therapy provided for a wide range of indications.'

According to Herbert and Gabriel,[29] 'Stretching before or after exercising does not confer protection from muscle soreness. Stretching before exercising does not seem to confer a practically useful reduction in the risk of injury, but the generality of this finding needs testing. Insufficient research has been done with which to determine the effects of stretching on sporting performance.' This finding was also confirmed by Barclay[30] who identified five randomised studies in a systematic review of controlled trials. The authors concluded that the effects of muscle stretching were too slight to be effective in preventing delayed onset muscle soreness.

Several studies have demonstrated the effectiveness of PNF exercises for a range of client populations. Klein et al[31] found that using PNF techniques for older adults improved range of motion, isometric strength and selected physical function tasks. Additional studies have shown that PNF stretching is superior to static stretching in improving hamstring flexibility in people 45 to 75 years of age.[32] One study compared PNF stretching to static stretching in active seniors. While static stretching and PNF stretching yielded gains in hamstring flexibility, PNF stretching was most beneficial in participants younger than 65.[33] Another study demonstrated the value of PNF stretching versus static stretching when comparing the techniques in Special Olympic athletes.[34]

A number of studies found that joints spanned by muscles undergoing pre-event PNF stretching demonstrated an increased range of motion but at the same time the mean power of the stretched muscles was reduced.[35, 36] This effect may leave the joint prone to overstretch and injury. This possible effect should be taken into consideration when performing pre-event PNF stretching.

CONTRAINDICATIONS AND PRECAUTIONS

Contraindications and precautions for muscle stretching include:

- joint instability
- pain in the region of treatment
- pre-existing injury in muscle or tendon being treated
- active local inflammation of tissues
- geriatric clients – connective tissue begins losing elasticity from around the age of 30 years
- children – according to Appleton,[21] PNF stretching is not recommended when bones are still growing
- post surgery
- pre-event and post-event athletics
- recent or unresolved haematoma
- advanced osteoporosis and conditions that weaken bone such as osseous tumour and osteomalacia
- muscle fatigue or weakness.

APPLYING MUSCLE STRETCHING IN REMEDIAL MASSAGE

Muscle stretching is a common component of remedial massage, not only for treating specific muscle strains but also for releasing muscle contractures associated with chronic conditions like degenerative joint disease and postural deviations like upper and lower crossed syndrome. Swedish massage or heat application to the area usually precedes muscle stretching and other remedial techniques. Stretches performed during the consultation are often supplemented by a stretching program performed by the client at home.

ADAPTING STRETCHES FOR INDIVIDUAL CLIENTS

Stretches can be performed in a number of ways. Consider, for example, hamstring stretches which can be performed in various positions including sitting with legs straight and touching toes, lying and raising a straight leg or standing and bending forward towards the toes. Characteristics of individual clients, including age, fitness and history of previous injury need to be taken into account when performing or recommending stretches. Use the See-Move-Touch principle described in Chapter 2: passive techniques are performed after observing the client move the muscle/joint through its active range of motion. This principle alerts you to the client's functional range of motion and helps ensure that further assessments and treatments are performed safely.

THERAPIST'S POSITION

When applying stretching in remedial massage, consider your position as the therapist relative to the client, to the equipment and to gravity. You must ensure at all times that your own position is strong, supported and able to transmit force from your body to the client's body in the most efficient manner possible. This will minimise the load on your body and the energy expenditure required to perform the technique while maintaining the client's confidence and comfort.

A stretching routine should form part of a health promotion program for massage therapists, who may be prone to repetition strain injury, particularly of the lower back, upper back, wrist and hand.[37, 38] Using a variety of techniques and a variety of contacts (in particular substituting forearms and elbows for thumbs) and maintaining correct posture and table height are imperative. Stretches for the pectoral muscles, shoulder internal rotators, elbow flexors and wrist extensors are advisable and may be accompanied by strengthening exercises for the middle trapezius, rhomboids, serratus anterior as well as lumbar exercises tailored to the needs of individual practitioners.

RECOMMENDATIONS

Recent research suggests that passive treatments like remedial massage (including passive stretching) are most beneficial in the first 4 to 6 weeks after injury.[39] From about 6 weeks post injury, clients have been shown to have better outcomes if they take an increasingly active part in their rehabilitation. Home exercise programs to support remedial massage treatment are recommended. Muscle stretching is usually prescribed to achieve competent joint motion before strengthening programs are introduced. Some forms of yoga are considered to be stretching routines for the whole body and are recommended by some practitioners.

Guidelines for active stretching:

1. Always warm up before stretching.
2. Stretch before and after exercise.
3. Stretch all major muscle groups and their antagonists.
4. Stretch slowly and gently.
5. Stretch only to the point of tension (not pain).
6. Use breathing awareness and control during the stretching procedures.

MUSCLE STRETCHING IN PRACTICE

The choice of specific technique depends on the functional requirements and personal characteristics of individual clients (e.g. age and agility). The range of stretching techniques includes simple active stretches performed by clients, passive stretches which are designed to elongate the contractile unit and soft tissue around the joint so as to increase joint mobility and connective tissue flexibility, and facilitated neuromuscular coordination techniques such as CRAC variations to induce proximal muscle stability. When recommending home exercises you should demonstrate or carefully explain them and observe clients performing them correctly before they leave the clinic. The following examples have been selected to demonstrate the wide range of stretching techniques in the clinical setting.

Scalene group

Hypertonicity is common in the scalene muscles. This can result in functional impairment of their ability to spontaneously respond to mechanical vectors and loading; for example, for maintaining efficient head carriage. An appropriate stretching technique in this case could be CRAC which involves neurological co-ordination.

For the posterior and medial fibres, place the client's head in approximately a third of their available range of lateral flexion (i.e. close to neutral). Your hand is placed on the side of the head to isolate the involved muscle. The client tries to further laterally flex their neck against your resistance (i.e. the muscle is isometrically contracted). Passively move the client's head to stretch the involved muscle as far as possible within its comfortable range and hold the stretch for 10 seconds. The procedure is repeated but this time starting at two-thirds of the client's available range of lateral flexion. A final repetition starts at the fully stretched position. (see Figure 5.7)

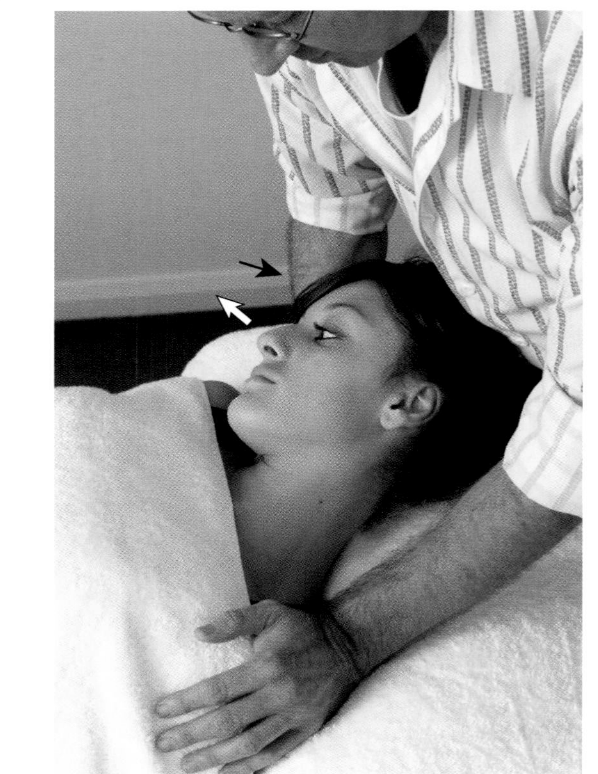

Fig. 5.7 **Scalene stretch**

Upper trapezius

A number of practitioner-assisted stretches of the upper trapezius can be performed. In one example, a practitioner-assisted stretch may be performed with the client supine. Stand at the head of the table. Place your ipsilateral hand medial to the acromioclavicular joint over the top of the shoulder; the contralateral hand supports the occiput. Slowly move the client's neck into contralateral lateral flexion and slight ipsilateral rotation. Your ipsilateral forearm can be used as a pivot against the head to assist lateral flex.

For an active stretch for the upper trapezius the client sits on a chair and holds the seat of the chair with the ipsilateral hand. The client's contralateral hand reaches over their head and contacts the side of the head around the temple. The client uses their contralateral hand to laterally flex their neck and simultaneously lift their head (see Figure 5.8 on p 73). Further lateral flexion can be obtained by leaning the body contralaterally against the resistance of the hand holding the chair.

Pectoral muscles

Chronic shortening of the pectoral muscles is associated with protraction of scapulae in upper crossed syndrome (see Chapter 12). An active stretch for the pectoral muscle group is the doorway stretch. The client stands side-on in a doorway and places the arm in the stop sign position with the forearm against the doorframe. The body is turned away from the doorframe until a comfortable stretch is felt across the front of the shoulder. The position is held for 20 seconds. (see Figure 5.9 on p 73)

This stretch can be enhanced by introducing PNF. The starting position is similar to the position described above except that the client's arm position is more anterior. The client pushes the forearm against the doorframe to isometrically contract the pectoral muscles. This is held for 5 seconds

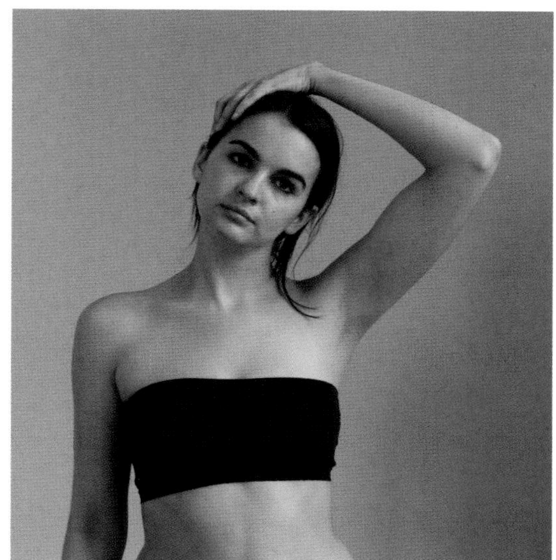

Fig. 5.8 **Upper trapezius stretch**

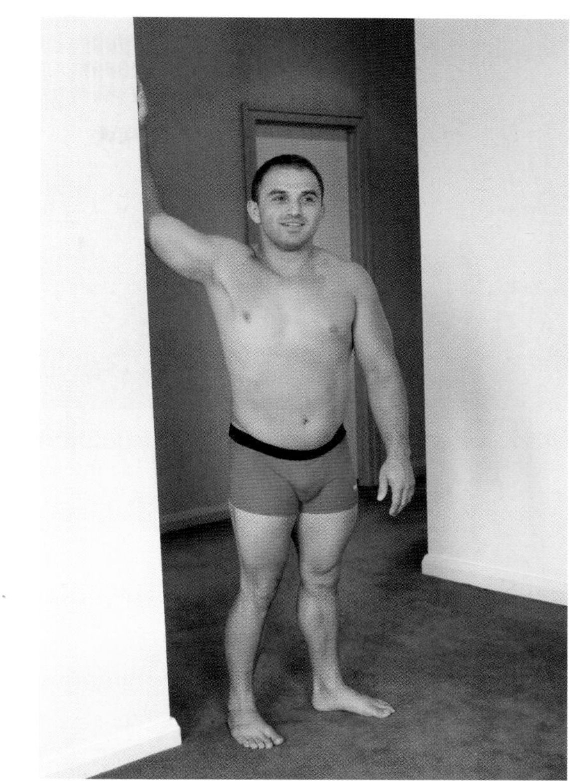

Fig. 5.9 **Pectoralis major stretch: Doorway stretch**

before relaxing. The muscle is stretched to its new comfortable limit by progressively turning the body away from the doorframe after each contraction is released. The procedure should be repeated three times.

Levator scapulae

This stretch is similar to the active upper trapezius stretch. With the ipsilateral hand holding under the seat of the chair, the client leans their body diagonally forward. The contralateral hand reaches over the top of the head and holds the lateral aspect of the occiput behind the ear. The client simultaneously flexes and laterally flexes the neck so that the stretch can be localised to the scapula insertion of the muscle. Hold for 10 seconds. (see Figure 5.10)

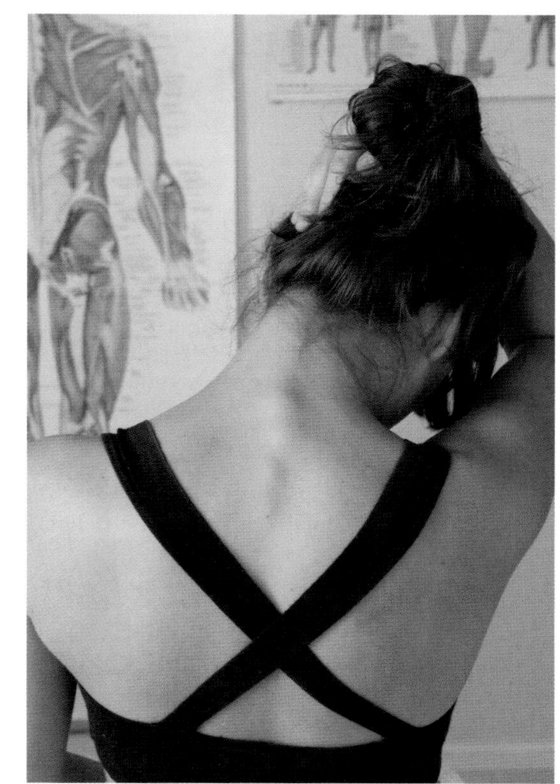

Fig. 5.10 **Levator scapulae stretch**

Wrist flexors/extensors

Actively stretching the wrist flexor and extensor muscles stretches fibrous repair tissue along lines of pull which contributes to normal fibre orientation.

To perform a PNF stretch to the wrist extensors, the client's elbow is extended. The wrist is flexed by the client's other hand holding the dorsum of the hand on the side to be stretched. The client pulls the wrist to exaggerate wrist flexion. The stretch is held for 15 seconds before releasing. The stretch can be repeated in several positions by rotating the forearm around an arc to find the position that maximally stretches the lesion. Each stretch is held for 15 seconds, released for a minimum of 5 seconds and repeated. Note: stretching is always performed within the client's pain tolerance.

A similar procedure is used to stretch the wrist flexors except that the wrist is extended to stretch the flexor muscles. Active stretches for the wrist extensor and floxor muscles are demonstrated in Figures 5.11 and 5.12 respectively on p 74.

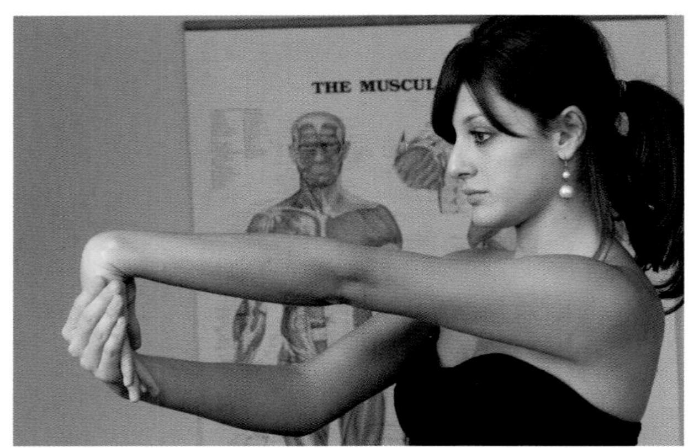

Fig. 5.11 Wrist extensor stretch

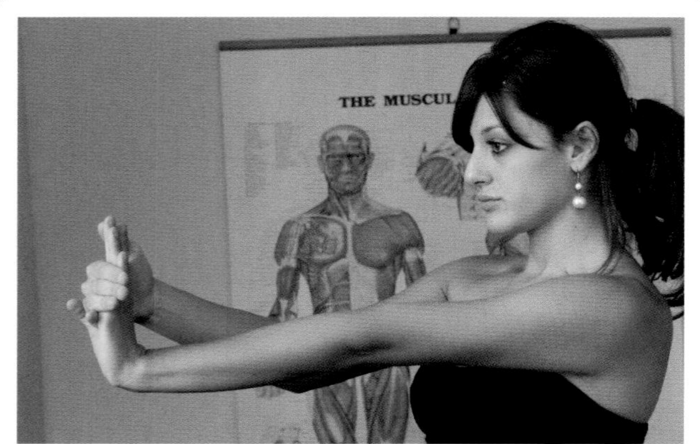

Fig. 5.12 Wrist flexor stretch

Piriformis

When trigger points are present in the muscle or if the client has piriformis syndrome (see Chapter 10) stretching is appropriate treatment. Passive stretching is commonly used in clinical practice and active stretches are prescribed for home.

For a practitioner-assisted stretch, the client is supine with their knee flexed and foot placed over the opposite leg just below the knee. Guide the client's flexed knee to the opposite side (laterally) with one hand stabilising the pelvis on the involved side by holding the ipsilateral anterior superior iliac spine. Hold the stretch for 20 to 40 seconds. Repeat the stretch three or four times. (see Figure 5.13)

Do not use PNF if the client has piriformis syndrome to avoid irritation of the sciatic nerve. However, in chronic cases, PNF can be used to enhance the muscle's range of motion. Stretch the muscle to mid range and perform a resisted submaximal contraction against your resistance for 15 seconds. The client relaxes and you passively stretch the muscle to its full range. Release the stretch slightly and repeat resistance and stretch.

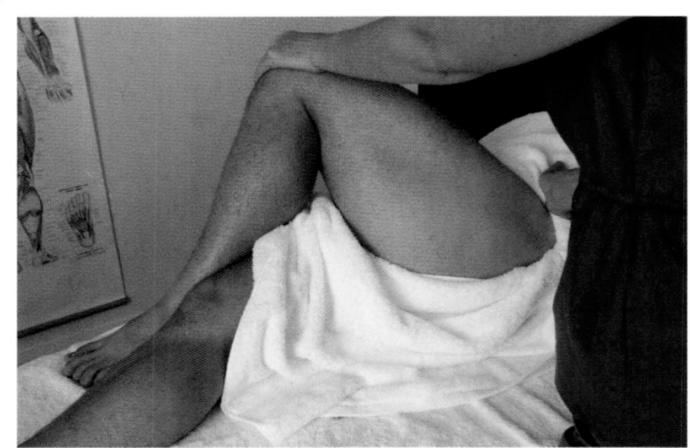

Fig. 5.13 Piriformis stretch

Psoas

Psoas is commonly treated to induce symmetry in length and strength of the muscle in order to maintain lumbar and pelvic biomechanical balance. An active stretch is performed by the client in a lunge position. The client adopts a fencer's stance with one foot in front of the other, feet pointing forward. The feet should be shoulder width apart. The pelvis should face the front; the low back straight. Body weight is transferred to the front foot and the psoas stretch should be felt in the groin region on the back leg. The stretch should be held for 10 seconds, then repeated four times on each leg. (see Fig 5.14 on p 75)

Quadriceps

HIP FLEXOR STRETCH (RECTUS FEMORIS AND ILIOPSOAS)

For a practitioner-assisted stretch, the client lies prone, knee flexed to 90°. Hold the distal thigh with the caudal hand. With the other hand, contact the posterior aspect of the hip to stabilise the pelvis. The client's knee should be maintained at 90°. Raise the thigh until the client feels a comfortable stretch of rectus femoris. Hold the stretch for 20 seconds. (see Figure 5.15a)

HIP FLEXORS, VASTUS LATERALIS, VASTUS INTERMEDIALIS AND VASTUS MEDIALIS

Alternatively, with the client prone, a pillow can be placed under the distal thigh to extend the hip. Move the client's heel towards their buttock until they feel a comfortable stretch. (see Figure 5.15b on p 75)

Hamstrings

For a PNF stretch, the client lies supine and flexes their hip and knee to 90°. Support the anterior aspect of the knee with the cephalad hand; the other hand holds the Achilles region. Extend the knee to comfortably stretch the hamstrings. Hold the stretch for 20 seconds. Maintaining this position, the client contracts the hamstrings against your resistance for 5 seconds and then releases. Passively extend the knee to the

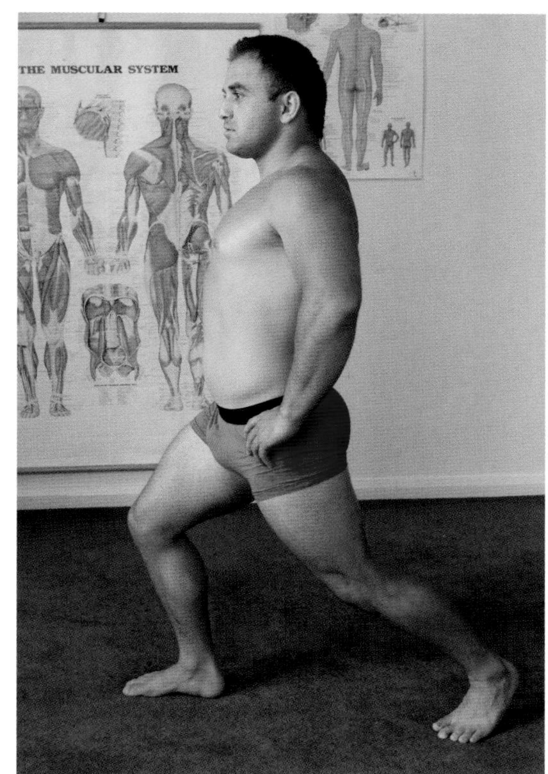

Fig. 5.14 Psoas stretch

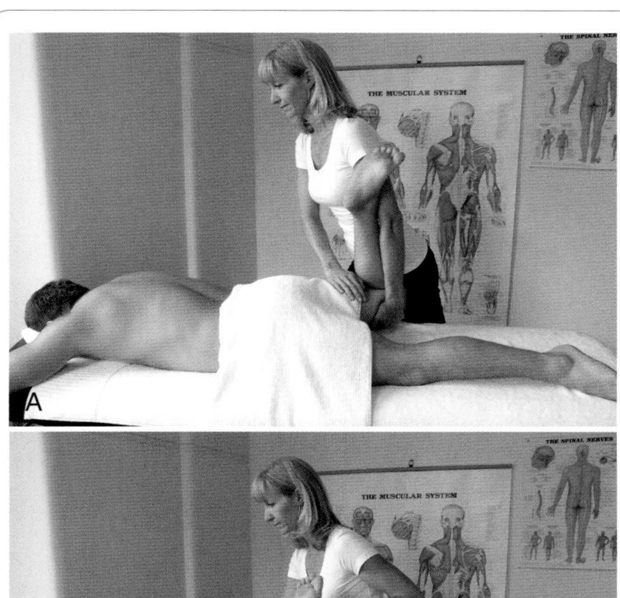

Fig. 5.15 (a) Hip flexor stretch, (b) hip flexor and quadriceps stretch

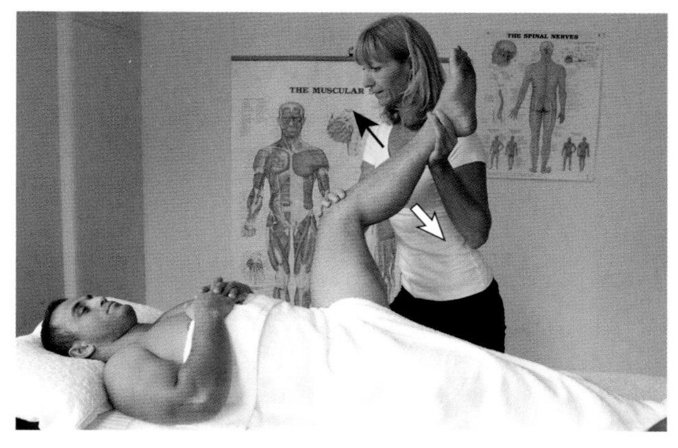

Fig. 5.16 Hamstring stretch

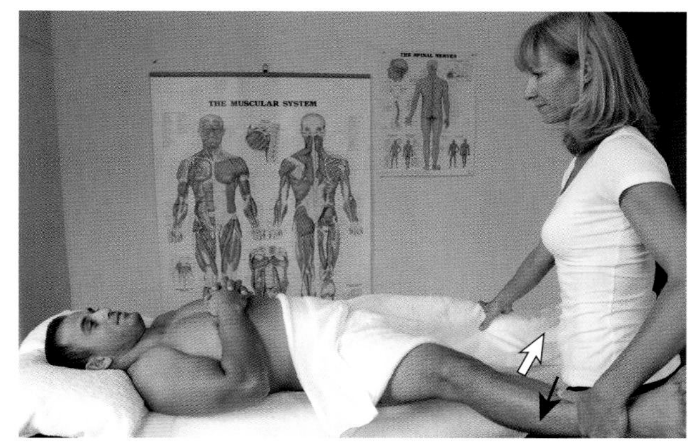

Fig. 5.17 Hip adductor stretch – draping

new point of comfortable stretch. Repeat this procedure three times. (see Figure 5.16 on p 75)

Adductors

For a PNF stretch, the client lies supine. Abduct the client's leg and stand between it and the table distal to client's knee. Hold the ankle of the uninvolved leg to prevent any movement. The client tries to bring the abducted leg back to the midline against resistance by your thigh or other hand. The client releases the contraction after 5 seconds and then you abduct the client's leg further. When a comfortable maximum stretch is achieved the client adducts their leg again. Release after 5 seconds and abduct the leg further to the new comfortable maximum stretch. (see Figure 5.17)

Gastrocnemius

For an active home stretch the client rolls a towel to make a rope and loops it around the ball of the foot. Holding the ends of the towel in each hand the client pulls the towel towards their head to stretch the gastrocnemius. The stretch is held for 20 seconds, released for 5 seconds and repeated six times. (see Figure 5.18 on p 76)

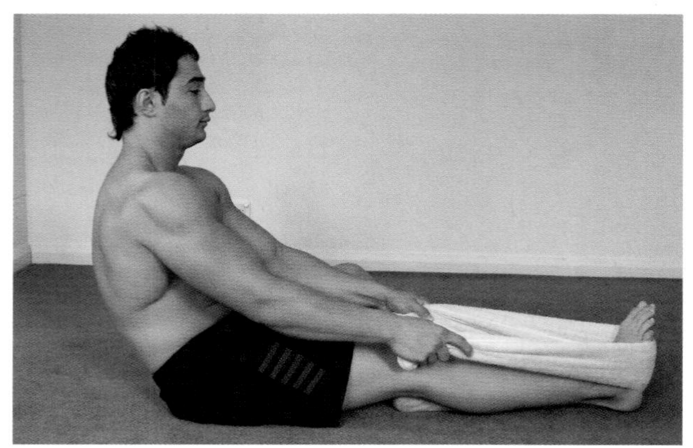
Fig. 5.18 Gastrocnemius stretch

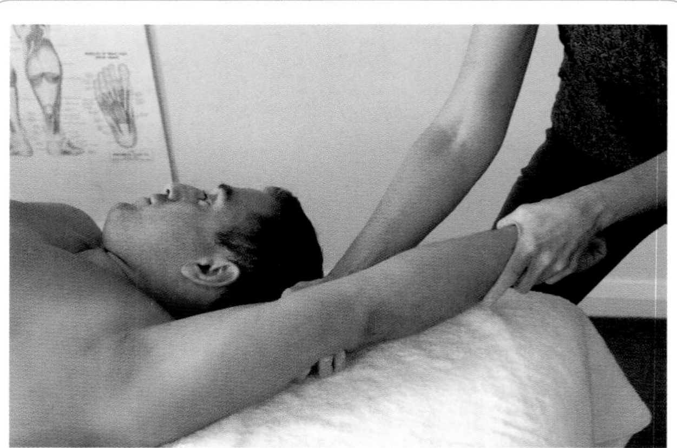
Fig. 5.20 Latissimus dorsi stretch

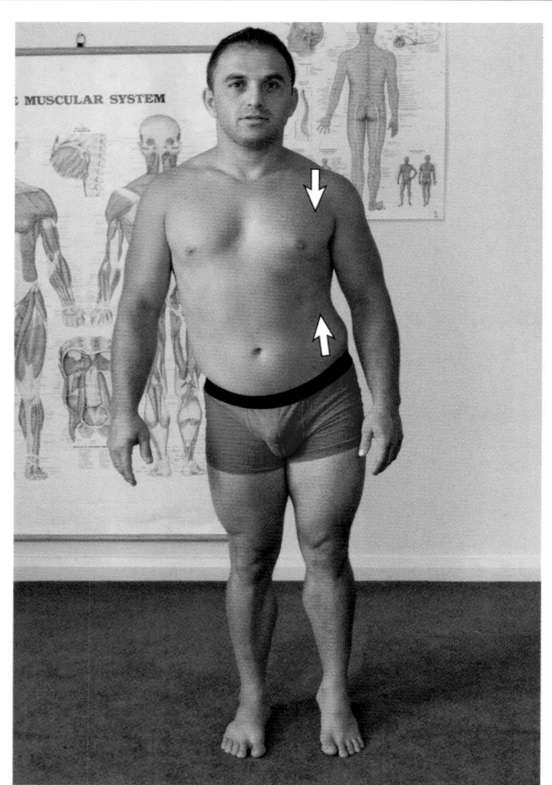

Fig. 5.19 Quadratus lumborum stretch

Quadratus lumborum

Quadratus lumborum may be recruited to assist splinting of low back lesions. This technique involves mobilisation of the lumbar spine through alternating contractions of the quadratus lumborum and muscles of the abdominal wall.

The client stands upright with knees extended throughout the procedure. The client raises one heel while simultaneously lowering the shoulder on the same side. Instruct the client to maintain their spine in a vertical line. Imagine the shoulder and hip getting closer together while the back remains straight. Lower the heel and level the shoulders and repeat on the other side. This is a repetitive action (do not hold position). Repeat for up to 2 minutes. Stop the exercise if the client experiences any discomfort. (see Figure 5.19)

Latissimus dorsi

Latissimus dorsi is an important muscle to consider when treating shoulder problems. Imbalance of latissimus dorsi is commonly involved in rounded shoulder posture involving scapula protraction and internal rotation of the upper limb. When chronically contracted, it inhibits shoulder abduction and external rotation. Latissimus dorsi is also often involved in lumbar and pelvic problems because of its attachments to the lumbosacral fascia and innominate bones. To passively stretch latissimus dorsi, the client lies supine. Abduct and externally rotate the involved arm and laterally flex the trunk contralaterally. The stretch is held for 5 to 40 seconds. (see Figure 5.20)

Review questions

1. What are the four properties of muscle?
2. What is the difference between post-isometric relaxation stretching and CRAC stretching?
3. Name four contraindications to stretching.
4. What palpatory findings suggest tissue that will benefit from stretching?

Continued

Review questions—cont'd

5. Match items in Column A with their function in Column B.

A	B
Hold-relax	muscle stretching
Rhythmic stabilisation	stability in postural trunk muscles and hip and shoulder stabilisers
Muscle energy technique	muscle stretching
CRAC	joint mobilisation
Alternating isometrics	motor coordination and control

6. How would you integrate stretching into your remedial massage plan?
7. How would you modify your recommended home stretch for the hamstring muscles for:
   a) an athlete?
   b) a 35 year old who plays football once a week, does no other exercise and has a sedentary job?
   c) a 70 year old?
8. When running downhill the gastrocnemius and soleus contract:
   a) Concentrically
   b) Eccentrically
   c) Isometrically
9. When a muscle spindle is stretched an impulse is immediately sent to the spinal cord and a response to contract the muscle is received. This is known as:
   a) Post-isometric relaxation
   b) Reciprocal inhibition
   c) Stretch reflex
10. Afferent fibres from muscle spindles send information about the length of a muscle and rate of stretch to the spinal cord. Branches of the afferent fibres synapse with interneurons that inhibit the motor neurons of the antagonist muscle. This is known as:
    a) Post-isometric relaxation
    b) Reciprocal inhibition
    c) Stretch reflex
11. Which form of stretching is generally regarded as the most dangerous?
    a) Static
    b) PNF
    c) Ballistic
    d) Passive
12. Which form of stretching is generally regarded as the most beneficial?
    a) Dynamic
    b) Passive
    c) PNF
    d) Ballistic

REFERENCES

1. Adler S, Beckers D, Buck M. PNF in practice: an illustrated guide. 3rd edn. Heidelberg: Springer Medizin Verlag; 2008.
2. Eriksen K. Upper cervical subluxation: a review of the chiropractic and medical literature. Baltimore, MD: Lippincott Williams and Wilkins; 2004.
3. Kapandji I. The physiology of the joints. 6th edn. Oxford: Churchill Livingstone; 2008.
4. Marieb E. Essentials of human anatomy and physiology. 9th edn. San Francisco, CA: Benjamin Cummings; 2008.
5. Chaitow L. Muscle energy techniques. 2nd edn. Edinburgh: Churchill Livingstone; 2001.
6. Mattes A. Active isolated stretching: the Mattes method. Sarasota, FL: A. Mattes Therapy; 2000.
7. Beaulieu J. Developing a stretching program. Phys Sportsmed 1981;9(11):59–69.
8. McAtee R, Charland J. Facilitated stretching. 3rd edn. Champaign, IL: Human Kinetics; 2007.
9. Murphy D. Dynamic range of motion training: an alternative to static stretching. Chiropractic Sports Med 1994;8:59–66.
10. Anderson B. Stretching: 20th Anniversary. Bolinas, CA: Shelter; 2000.
11. Ford G, Mazzone M, Taylor K. The effect of 4 different durations of static hamstring stretching on passive knee-extension range of motion in healthy subjects. J Sport Rehabil 2005;14(2):95–107.
12. Knott M, Voss D. Proprioceptive neuromuscular facilitation. Philadelphia PA: Harper and Row; 1968.
13. Morris S, Sharpe M. PNF revisited. Physiother 1993;9(1):43–51.
14. Kisner C, Colby L. Therapeutic exercise: foundations and techniques. Philadelphia PA: FA Davis; 2002.
15. Scifers J. Therapeutic exercise: foundations and techniques. Advance Newsmagazines [serial on the Internet] 2004;13(10). Online. Available: http://physical-therapy.advanceweb.com/
16. Surburg P, Schrader J. Proprioceptive neuromuscular facilitation in sports medicine: a reassessment. J Athlet Train 1997;11(4):34–9.
17. Spernoga S, Uhl T, Arnold B, et al. Duration of maintained hamstring flexibility after a one-time, modified hold-relax stretching protocol. J Athl Train 2001;36(1):44–8.
18. Funk D, Swank A, Mikla B, et al. Impact of prior exercise on hamstring flexibility: a comparison of proprioceptive neuromuscular facilitation and static stretching. J Strength Cond Res 2003;17(3):479–92.
19. Carter A, Kinzey S, Chitwood L, et al. Proprioceptive neuromuscular facilitation decreases muscle activity during the stretch reflex in selected posterior thigh muscles. J Sport Rehabil 2000;9(4):269–78.
20. Schmitt G, Pelham T, Holt L. A comparison of selected protocols during proprioceptive facilitation stretching. Clin Kinesiol 1999;53(1):16–21.
21. Appleton B. Stretching and flexibility: everything you wanted to know. Cited: 6 Aug 2010. Online. Available: www.crossroads.com/bradapp/docs/rec/stretching/stretching_5.html; 1994.
22. Shields A, editor. The health for life training advisor. Los Angeles: Health for Life; 1990.
23. Walker B. The stretching handbook. Robina, Qld: Walkerbout Health; 2011.
24. Laughlin K. Stretching and flexibility. Sydney: Simon and Schuster; 2000.
25. Prentice W. Rehabilitation techniques in sports medicine. 3rd edn. Boston: McGraw-Hill; 1999.
26. Freiwald J, Engelharadt M. Stretching: possibilities and limits. Ther Umsch 1998;55(4):267–72.
27. MacAuley D, Best T. Evidence-based sports medicine. Malden, MA: Blackwell, 2007.
28. Smedes F. Is there support for the PNF-concept? a literature search on electronic databases. Online. Available: www.ipnfa.org/download/FredSmedes2006.pdf; 2006.
29. Herbert RD, Gabriel M. Effects of stretching before and after excerise on muscle soreness and risk of injury: systematic review. BMJ 2002;325(7362):468–70.
30. Barclay L. Reading the risk of injury due to exercise: stretching before exercise does not help. BMJ 2002;325(7362):451–2.
31. Klein D, Stone W, Phillips W, et al. PNF training and physical function in assisted-living older adults. J Aging Phys Act 2002;10(4):476–88.
32. Ferber R, Gravelle D, Osternig L. Effect of proprioceptive neuromuscular facilitation stretch techniques on trained and untrained older adults. J Aging Phys Act 2002;10(2):132–42.
33. Feland J, Myrer J, Merrill R. Acute changes in hamstring flexibility: proprioceptive neuromuscular facilitation versus static stretching senior athletes. Phys Ther Sport 2001;2(4):186–93.

34. Stopka C, Morley K, Siders R, et al. Stretching techniques to improve flexibility in Special Olympic athletes and their coaches. J Sport Rehabil 2002; 11(1):22–34.
35. Nelson A, Driscoll N, Landin D, et al. Acute effects of passive muscle stretching on sprint performance. J Sports Sci 2005;23(5): 449–54.
36. Marek S, Cranmer J, Fincher A, et al. Acute effects of static and PNF stretching on muscle strength and power output. J Athlet Train 2005;40(2):94–103.
37. Holder N, Clark H, Di Blasio J, et al. Cause, prevalence, and response to occupational musculoskeletal injuries reported by physical therapists and physical therapy assistants. Phys Ther 1999;79(7):642–52.
38. Albert W, Currie-Jackson N, Duncan C. A survey of musculoskeletal injuries amongst Canadian massage therapists. J Bodyw Mov Ther 2008; 12(1):86–93.
39. WorkCover NSW. Management of soft tissue injuries using work related activity. Gosford, NSW: WorkCover NSW; 2006.

Myofascial trigger points

6

The content of this chapter relates to the following Units of Competency:

HLTREM503C Plan remedial massage treatment strategy
HLTREM504C Apply remedial massage assessment framework
HLTREM502C Provide remedial massage treatment
HLTREM505C Perform remedial massage health assessment

Health Training Package HLT07

Learning Outcomes

- Assess clients for the presence of myofascial trigger points.
- Describe current theories posited to explain the pathogenesis of trigger points.
- Apply myofascial trigger point therapy effectively and safely to a range of clients, adapting the therapy to suit individual client needs.
- Advise and resource clients who have been assessed and treated for myofascial trigger points.

INTRODUCTION

Myofascial trigger points were first described in 1952 by Janet Travell and Seymour Rinzler in an article entitled *The Myofascial Genesis of Pain.*[1] During her long and productive career Travell helped develop new techniques for treating muscle pain using procaine injections and vapocoolant sprays. Today myofascial trigger point therapy is widely used by many physical therapists, including chiropractors, physiotherapists, osteopaths and remedial massage therapists. This chapter presents a brief overview of the identification and treatment of common myofascial trigger points. Remedial massage therapists who plan to use trigger point therapy in their practices should consult the original texts, *Myofascial Pain and Dysfunction: The Trigger Point Manual (Volume 1: The upper half of body* (Simons, Travell and Simons)*; Volume 2: The lower extremities* (Travell and Simons)).[2, 3] Travell's books contain very practical information on postural corrections and rehabilitation exercises to accompany manual trigger point therapy. Trigger point charts displayed on the wall of treatment rooms are another useful way to become familiar with trigger points.

WHAT IS A TRIGGER POINT?

A trigger point is a focus of hyperirritability in a tissue that is locally tender when compressed and if sufficiently tender refers pain in a particular pattern that is similar in all clients. It is thought that pain is initiated when the trigger point area is stimulated by stressors like cold, postural distortions and emotional stress which set up a self-perpetuating pain cycle that long outlasts the initiating stimulus. Trigger points are commonly misdiagnosed as muscular rheumatism, myalgic spots and fibrositis.[2, 4] There is also much interest in the relationship between acupuncture points and trigger points, a number of studies reporting considerable overlap.[5, 6] According to Peng[6] 95% of trigger points (235 out of 255) corresponded to acupuncture points in anatomical location and clinical indications.

LOCATING TRIGGER POINTS

Trigger points can be found in skeletal muscles and tendons, joint capsules, ligaments, fascia, periosteum and skin (usually in scar tissue). They tend to develop more readily in postural muscles (e.g. upper trapezius, levator scapulae, quadratus lumborum, iliopsoas, piriformis and tensor fasciae latae) than in phasic muscles,[7] and in high-demand muscles more than in low-demand muscles. Trigger points in skeletal muscles usually develop at the origins and insertions (attachment trigger points), and bellies of muscles, particularly at the neuromuscular junction (central trigger points). According to Fritz,[8] trigger points tend to be found near origins and insertions in long eccentrically contracted muscles, and in muscle bellies in short concentrically contracted muscles. Areas of muscles that are prone to mechanical strain, impaired circulation and muscular or fascial adhesions are also common sites.

CLASSIFYING TRIGGER POINTS

ACTIVE AND LATENT TRIGGER POINTS

The main difference between active and latent trigger points is the presence of pain. Active trigger points are always painful and refer pain at rest and/or when the specific muscle containing the trigger point is moved. Active trigger points prevent full lengthening of muscles and weaken the muscle. They can mediate a local twitch response (i.e. a brisk contraction of a taut band of skeletal muscle fibres elicited by snapping palpation of a trigger point[9]) and often produce autonomic phenomena such as local sweating and vasomotor activity, generally in the pain reference zone. Active trigger points are likely to be found in postural muscles of the neck, shoulder and pelvic girdle and the muscles of mastication.

Latent trigger points do not refer pain until pressed but are tender on palpation. They may become active through physical or emotional events such as sleeping position, chilling or viral disease. Latent trigger points are often found incidentally during routine massage.

Satellite and secondary trigger points

Simons et al[2] also described associated trigger points, which can be either:

i. Satellite trigger points which are activated because the muscle in which they are located is in the referral zone of another muscle; or
ii. Secondary trigger points which are activated because the muscle is a synergist or an antagonist of the muscle with the primary trigger point and becomes overloaded.

Key trigger points

Key trigger points have also been identified. It appears that by treating key trigger points, satellite trigger points can also be reduced or eliminated.[10, 11] Key trigger points are listed in Table 6.1.[12]

Table 6.1 Key trigger points

Key trigger point	Associated satellite trigger point
sternocleidomastoid	temporalis, masseter
upper trapezius	temporalis, masseter
scalene	deltoid, extensor carpi radialis, extensor digitorum communis
splenius capitis	temporalis
supraspinatus	deltoid, extensor carpi radialis
infraspinatus	biceps brachii
pectoralis minor	flexor carpi radialis, flexor carpi ulnaris
latissimus dorsi	triceps brachii, flexor carpi ulnaris
serratus posterior superior	triceps brachii, extensor digitorum communis, extensor carpi ulnaris
quadratus lumborum	gluteus maximus, piriformis
piriformis	hamstrings
hamstrings	gastrocnemius, soleus

WHAT CAUSES TRIGGER POINTS?

A number of theories have been proposed to explain possible causes of myofascial trigger points. However the pathogenesis of myofascial pain syndrome remains unclear. Simons et al[2] posited the following theory:

> *An acute or chronic muscle strain leads to cellular disruption of the muscle fibre sarcoplasmic reticulum and the release of stored calcium ions. Increased calcium ions then cause a sustained muscle fibre contraction (taut palpable band) which eventually leads to muscle fatigue. Damage due to trauma may also affect small blood vessels of the area and cause the release of proinflammatory substances like serotonin and histamines which further sensitise pain receptors in the region. The resultant muscle contraction will cause further release of histamines and the depletion of local adenosine triphosphate so the fibres will remain in a state of permanent contraction. Sustained contractions decrease the blood flow to the area, which limits the removal of local metabolites and further sensitises pain receptors.*

The pain cycle may be initiated by any stimulus that acts directly or indirectly on the area containing the trigger point (e.g. direct trauma, strain, fatigue, heat, cold, nerve root irritation, visceral dysfunction, emotional factors, chronic conditions or overuse). The *injury pool theory*[2] suggests that trigger points are activated when these trigger events combine with other predisposing factors (see below).

Perpetuating factors of trigger points

- Mechanical stresses (e.g. skeletal asymmetry, poor lifting techniques, poor posture, prolonged immobility)
- Nutritional inadequacies (low level of vitamins B_1, B_6, B_{12}, and C, folic acid, calcium, potassium, iron)
- Metabolic and endocrine inadequacies (thyroid underactivity, hyperuricaemia, hypoglycaemia) or any impairment to muscle metabolism (anaemia, hypoxia)
- Psychological factors
- Chronic infection
- Allergy, impaired sleep, radiculopathy, chronic visceral disease

(adapted from Fritz et al[8])

There have been a number of studies demonstrating abnormal spontaneous electrical activity, spike activity and local twitch responses at trigger point sites.[13–16] Hong[17, 18] postulated that many small sensitive loci are distributed throughout affected muscles but they concentrate in trigger point referral zones. Sensitive loci are probably sensitised nociceptors which are widely distributed through the muscle but concentrated in the endplate zone. Motor (active) loci are also present. These are probably dysfunctional endplates since they exhibit spontaneous electrical activity similar to endplate noise recorded in abnormal endplates. Trigger points develop when sensory loci and motor (active) loci coincide. Referred pain and local twitch responses are mediated through spinal cord mechanisms. 'The pathogenesis of myofascial trigger points appears to be related to the integration in the spinal cord (formation of myofascial trigger point circuits) in response to the disturbance of the nerve endings and abnormal contractile mechanism of multiple dysfunctional endplates.'[17] Several studies suggest that referred pain and local twitch responses are related to nerve degeneration and disintegration of motor and sensory nerves in the spinal cord. A study by Chang et al[19] found evidence of neuroaxonal degeneration and neuromuscular transmission disorders in trigger point muscles of 23 myofascial pain syndrome patients.

Hypothesis: A trigger point is formed when a sensitive locus (nociceptor) and an active locus (abnormal motor endplate) coincide. Referred pain patterns, local twitch responses and autonomic phenomena are related to interneuronal integration in the spinal cord.[17]

IDENTIFYING TRIGGER POINTS

Likely trigger points are often identified during history (e.g. by descriptions of the nature of pain, location of pain in referral pattern, onset) and confirmed by physical examination. Reliability of physical examination for the presence of trigger points is as yet unconfirmed because of the lack of high-quality studies.[20]

CHARACTERISTICS OF TRIGGER POINTS

Symptoms

- Deep, dull aching pain
- Pain referred in a specific pattern that is characteristic of each trigger point
- Activated directly by acute overload, overwork, fatigue, trauma, chilling
- Activated indirectly by disease, arthritic joints, emotional stress
- Vary in irritability from hour to hour and day to day
- Symptoms long outlast the precipitating event
- Occasionally autonomic reactions (e.g. sweating, local vasoconstriction, lacrimation, coryza, salivation, pilomotor activity) and proprioceptive disturbances (e.g. dizziness and tinnitus)
- Affected muscles are shortened and weakened

Signs

- Flat or pincer palpation identifies trigger points (circumscribed spots of exquisite tenderness in taut bands of muscle)
- Pressure on an active trigger point usually elicits a jump sign (i.e. the client quickly pulls away when the trigger point is palpated)
- Snapping palpation (rapid movement across the muscle so that fibres snap back) frequently evokes a local twitch response
- Skin sometimes evinces dermographia (elevations or wheals caused by scratching the skin) or panniculosis (sensitive thickenings or nodules in the subcutaneous tissue) in the area overlying trigger points

Strategies to identify trigger points are summarised in Table 6.2.

TREATING TRIGGER POINTS

The most important consideration in the treatment of trigger points is eliminating or reducing causative or aggravating factors.[22] If the aetiology is not addressed, the trigger point may be temporarily deactivated but is likely to recur. When trigger points were first described, Travell and Simons recommended two options for reducing trigger points: (1) injecting trigger points with local anaesthetics, followed by muscle stretching, or (2) spraying the skin overlying the trigger point referral pattern with a vapocoolant spray (see Simons et al[2] and Travell and Simons[3] for directions for spraying specific muscles). Most treatment options that have been developed for trigger points since the 1950s still maintain the original two-phase procedure: (1) hyperstimulation analgesia and counter-irritation to break the pain cycle and (2) stretching the affected muscle to realign the muscle fibres. The following treatment methods are used in a range of practices including physiotherapy, chiropractic, osteopathy, acupuncture, general practice and remedial massage:

1. Injection and stretch. Injection with local anaesthetic, corticosteroids, botulinum A toxin, sterile water and sterile saline followed by stretching of the affected muscle.
2. Vapocoolant spray (e.g. ethyl chloride) and stretch. Spray from the trigger point towards the pain referral zone in a slow sweep (up to 6 seconds) covering the full length of the zone, then stretch the affected muscle. Spray in slow sweeps over the entire width of the muscle, maintaining the passive stretch. Repeat this until the full range of motion of the muscle group is reached, re-warming the area with moist heat at least every three repetitions. Avoid prolonged exposure to the spray and overstretching. This technique was considered by Simons et al[2] to be the most effective non-invasive method to deactivate trigger points.
3. Ice/ice massage (see Chapter 3).
4. Acupuncture. Chou et al[23] studied the effect of acupuncture on pain referred from trigger points and recorded reductions in both subjective reports of pain intensity and changes in endplate noise amplitude in the trigger point region of the upper trapezius during and after acupuncture treatment.
5. Electrical stimulation (e.g. transcutaneous electrical were stimulation (TENS) electrodes are placed at the trigger point site or along the referred pain zone).
6. Muscle energy and other remedial massage techniques. Remedial massage therapists sometimes use muscle energy techniques, positional release and direct muscle manipulation methods such as cross-fibre frictions (see Chapter 4) and a variety of muscle-stretching techniques. Such techniques are particularly useful for trigger points which are not easily accessible (e.g. trigger points in iliopsoas and subscapularis).

Table 6.2 Identifying trigger points

History	History of onset usually related to trauma or overload of affected muscle.	Patients are rarely aware of the existence of trigger points. They experience pain and/or other symptoms.
	Nature of pain ■ deep, steady, aching ■ varies from hour to hour and day to day ■ outlasts initial event.	Active trigger points produce steady, deep, aching pain. The pain is rarely felt as a burning pain. Occasionally it is described as sharp, lancing pain. (Compare prickling pain, numbness or paraesthesia of peripheral nerve entrapment/ nerve root irritation; throbbing pain of vascular origin.)
	Location of pain. Characteristic pain referral pattern.	Referred pain differentiates trigger point pain from fibromyalgia and other tender points. Referred pain does not coincide with dermatological or neuronal distributions. Pain usually accompanies muscle function change.
	Muscle function. Restricted range of motion. Affected muscle feels tight or weak.	
Physical examination	Palpation Focus of exquisite tenderness in taut band identified by flat or pincer palpation (Figure 6.1). Trigger points tend to be located centrally in the bellies of muscles or at the attachments of muscles.	Trigger points are always in hypertonic muscle fibres. They are common in the neck, shoulder and lower back muscles. Palpation of taut bands requires practice. Less experienced practitioners may need to rely on clients' identification of exquisite pain sites and pain referral patterns until they develop their palpation skills.
	Digital pressure on the trigger point reproduces the client's symptoms.	
	Jump sign.	The client flinches and pulls away from pain; the reaction is out of proportion to the pressure applied.
	Local twitch response when the taut band is snapped near the site of the trigger point.	Brisk contraction of muscle fibres in and around the taut band.
	There can be autonomic signs.	For example, increased vasomotor activity, changes in skin temperature, erythema of overlying skin, lacrimation, coryza, sweating, goose bumps.[21]
	Resisted and length tests for affected muscles.	Affected muscles may have altered length and strength.

7. Dry needling. In this technique an acupuncture needle is inserted into a trigger point. The trigger point is needled many times to elicit a local twitch response and reproduce the patient's symptoms. The needle can remain inserted for 2 minutes.[24] Dr Ma's technique involves inserting a one-inch 32-gauge acupuncture needle perpendicularly through subcutaneous tissue until a density change is encountered. The needle is 'bounced on the muscle' at a rate of 1–3 times per second until the tissues soften.[25] Recent studies suggest that dry needling a primary trigger point may inhibit activity in satellite trigger points situated in the zones of pain referral.[10, 11]
8. Direct manual ischaemic compression. Pressure is applied to the trigger point with increasing intensity and maintained until the patient reports a significant reduction in pain or the practitioner palpates a release of the taut band of muscle. After the digital pressure is released, the muscle is stretched.

MANUAL TECHNIQUES

Since the identification of central and attachment trigger points[2] it has become apparent that each requires a different treatment approach. The traditional manual techniques that were previously used to treat all trigger points are now recommended for central trigger points only. Such deep techniques may inflame or irritate tissues near attachment trigger points and cold applications are now recommended for attachment trigger points. A treatment protocol including currently recommended trigger point treatments is presented in Table 6.3. Trigger point therapy should be integrated into a short-term treatment plan that may focus on relieving symptoms and a long-term treatment plan that tries to address the underlying causes.

Typically, Swedish massage is applied to the area before specific trigger points are treated. Remedial massage therapists have commonly used direct ischaemic pressure on the trigger point followed by specific muscle stretching. Steady pressure is applied using the thumb, fingers, elbow or knuckle to the trigger point to within the client's pain tolerance (between 4 and 7 on a pain scale of 1 to 10) for up to 60 seconds. Chaitow[26] recommends gradually increasing the pressure until the client reports a 7 or 8 out of 10 on the pain scale, maintaining pressure until the client reports a reduction to 3 or 4 and then increasing the pressure again up to 7 or 8. This process is repeated up to three times or until the therapist feels a tissue change in the trigger point area. Using variable pressure prevents further irritation to the trigger point. The trigger point is pressed onto the underlying bone, or if there is no underlying bone (e.g. sternocleidomastoid muscle), the trigger point can be squeezed using a pincer grip[a]. The aim is to cause mechanical disruption of sensory nerve endings that contribute to trigger point activity. Other authors suggest that pressure need only be sufficient to release contracted sarcomeres and that heavy ischaemic pressure is not required.[2]

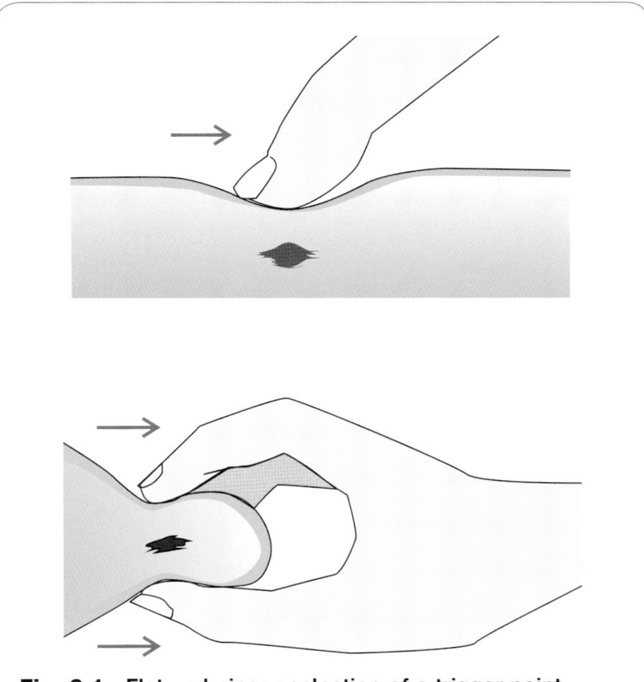

Fig. 6.1 Flat and pincer palpation of a trigger point. *adapted from Simons, Travell and Simons.[2]*

After pressure has been applied to the trigger points in a muscle group, the muscles are gradually stretched to their full range of motion.[7] Most sources describe passive stretching following the hyperstimulation phase of treatment. As discussed in Chapter 2, use active stretching wherever possible before passive stretching. An overview of a remedial massage treatment that incorporates myofascial trigger point therapy is presented in Table 6.3.

Save your body

A lot of strain can be placed on therapists' joints and muscles during sustained ischaemic compression. McMahon et al[27] found that 65% of physiotherapists who responded to a survey had experienced thumb problems at some stage during their working lives. Trigger point therapy was reported as one of the factors that were significantly associated with thumb problems. Vary the contact (use your thumbs sometimes, knuckles and elbows at other times) and avoid flexion and extension, especially of metacarpophalangeal joints or interphalangeal joints when applying pressure (see Figure 6.2). Some therapists use a T-bar made of wood, plastic or metal, and often rubber capped, to save their hands. Another study compared muscle load to the shoulder using three different trigger point

[a]Special caution is required when treating trigger points in the sternocleidomastoid muscle because of the proximity of the carotid artery, jugular vein, cervical and brachial plexuses, and cervical lymph nodes.

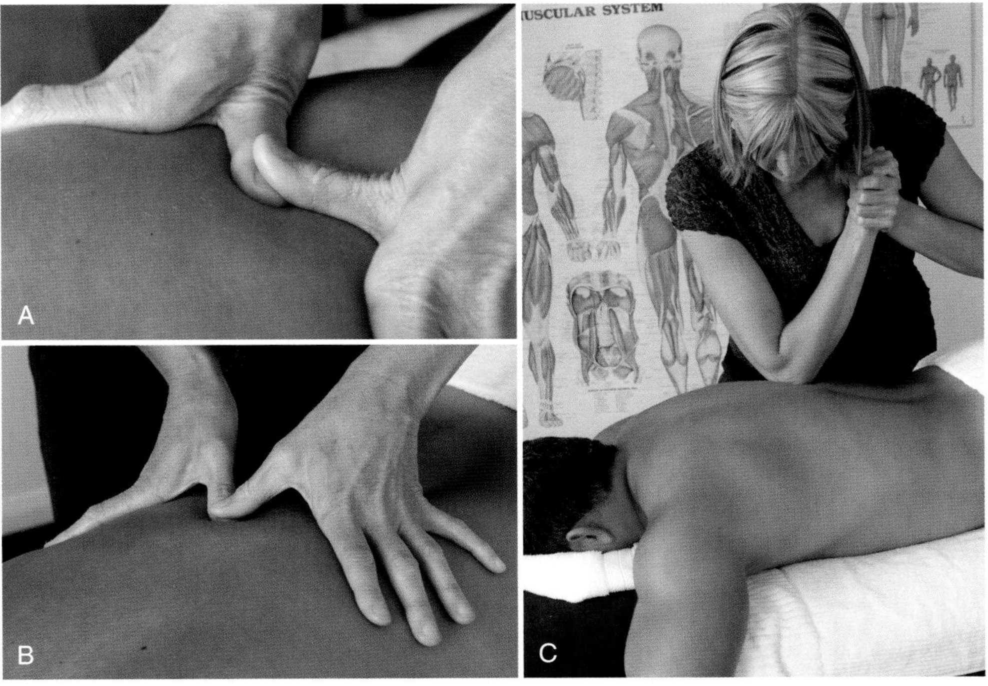

Fig. 6.2 (a) incorrect, and (b) and (c) correct ergonomics for intermittent, (c) digital pressure

Table 6.3 Remedial massage treatment of myofascial trigger points

1. Swedish massage	Massage the whole muscle, muscle group or region.	Improves circulation (increased oxygenation, removal of waste products); increases awareness of the body's adaptations to external and internal stressors, locates taut bands in muscles, relaxes the client.
2. Apply a range of remedial massage techniques		
i) *Trigger point techniques* Treat key trigger points first	Usually only two or three and not more than five trigger points are treated at any one time. Treat the most painful, the most medial and the most proximal trigger points first. Key trigger points are closest to the head and to the midline.[7]	Deactivating key trigger points may also deactivate or reduce satellite and attachment trigger points.
Treat central trigger points before attachment trigger points.	A range of massage techniques can be used to treat central trigger points including: *Intermittent digital pressure*	Apply gradually increasing pressure to 7 or 8 out of 10 on the pain scale, maintain the pressure until the client reports 3 or 4 out of 10, then gradually increase the pressure to 7 or 8 again. Repeat the process up to three times. Note: There is no need for heavy ischaemic pressure (only sufficient pressure to release contracted sarcomeres).[2]
	Gliding massage techniques from the muscle belly out towards the muscle attachments.	To lengthen shortened sarcomeres in the belly of the muscle and reduce tension on muscle attachments.
	Mild stretching	Full range of motion stretches could irritate attachment trigger points. Newly activated trigger points can be deactivated by slow passive stretching.[2, 29]
	Thermotherapy	Heat packs to the affected muscles.
	Deep stroking or stripping massage over the trigger point area.[2]	Deep gliding along the line of the fibres and then cross-fibre frictions,[24] 6–12 strokes per trigger point.[30] Thought to be the most effective direct manual treatment.[2]
	Other techniques including joint mobilisation, friction massage, myofascial release, lymphatic drainage massage.	Fernandez-de-las-Penas[31] recommended joint mobilisation in the management of trigger points based on indicators that muscle sensitivity reduced after spinal manipulation. Avoid deep pressure or friction as it could aggravate surrounding tissues.
Treat attachment trigger points.	Ice massage Short 20–30 second cold applications.[7]	
Return muscle to its normal resting length.	Regardless of the method used to deactivate the trigger point, restoring the normal resting length of the muscle is recommended.[7]	Gradual, gentle, pain-free stretching (especially muscle energy techniques and myofascial release).
ii) *Apply a range of remedial massage techniques to eliminate perpetuating factors where possible.*	Techniques to correct or reduce mechanical factors predisposing to trigger points: (e.g. postural distortion, muscle imbalance, joint dysfunction).	Trigger points are a culmination of a number of events. Find and correct the cause if possible. Trigger point treatment techniques can permanently eliminate pain cycles. However, if the cause is remote, such as a visceral or emotional cause, a new stream of noxious stimuli can reactivate the trigger.
3. Client education	Action to eliminate perpetuating factors. Advise clients about causes including mechanical stress (e.g. prolonged immobilisation, inadequate training for sport) and systemic factors (e.g. metabolic and endocrine dysfunction, chronic infection, dietary insufficiencies especially vitamin B_{12}, folic acid, vitamin C and iron[2], psychological stress).	For example, if psychological stress is a perpetuating factor then the client might benefit from referral to a counsellor, yoga teacher or for a course of relaxation massage.
	Home exercise program.	Exercises to stretch and strengthen the affected muscle(s) as required.

therapy techniques: digital ischaemic pressure using a single hand contact, a double hand contact and a treatment tool. The authors found that using the treatment tool decreased the muscle load to the shoulder of the contact arm although they were unable to comment on where the load was redistributed.[28]

Some key trigger points and their associated muscle stretches are illustrated in Appendix 6.1.

EVIDENCE-BASE OF TREATMENTS FOR TRIGGER POINTS

Vernon and Schneider[32] conducted a literature search and summarised the evidence for myofascial trigger point therapy as follows:

- Manipulation and ischaemic pressure for immediate pain relief at trigger points is supported by moderately strong evidence. Long-term pain relief is supported by limited evidence.
- The use of laser therapy for treating myofascial trigger points and myofascial pain syndrome has strong support in the literature.
- Moderate evidence supports the use of electrical nerve stimulation, acupuncture and magnet therapy for treating myofascial trigger points and myofascial pain syndrome.
- The use of electrical muscle stimulation, high-voltage galvanic stimulation, interferential current and frequency-modulated neural stimulation for treating myofascial trigger points and myofascial pain syndrome is supported by limited evidence.
- The use of ultrasound therapy for treating myofascial trigger points and myofascial pain syndrome is supported by weak evidence.

Delaney et al[33] found that healthy subjects had increased parasympathetic activity and improved measures of relaxation after a 20-minute treatment which combined massage strokes, pressure and circular friction to trigger points of the head, neck and shoulders.

A systematic review conducted in 2001 concluded that direct needling of myofascial trigger points appeared to be an effective treatment but the hypothesis that needling therapies have efficacy beyond placebo is neither supported nor refuted by the evidence.[34] A more recent systematic review and meta-analysis of seven randomised controlled trials on acupuncture and dry needling in the management of myofascial trigger points found limited evidence from one study that deep needling directly into trigger points has an overall treatment effect when compared to standardised treatment.[35]

CONTRAINDICATIONS AND PRECAUTIONS

As well as the usual contraindications of massage therapy (e.g. acute inflammation, moles, varicose veins, breast tissue, pregnancy, rheumatoid arthritis), the following special considerations apply when using trigger point therapy:

- The heaviness of digital ischaemic pressure makes it unsuitable for clients with osteoporosis. The technique must be adapted to the size, age and level of fitness of the client.
- Resistance stretching techniques (see Chapter 5) are unsuitable for hypertensive clients.
- Potentially painful massage (including trigger point therapy) has been associated with increased blood pressure and should be avoided in hypertensive clients.[36]
- Muscle stretches, including home exercise programs, must make allowance for age and levels of fitness.
- Where a trigger point is maintaining joint stability in a hypermobile client, a strengthening program may need to be introduced before deactivation of the trigger point.[7]

KEY MESSAGES

- Trigger point therapy is widely used in the treatment of myofascial pain. One current hypothesis about the pathogenesis of trigger points suggests that a pain cycle may be set up by a stimulus that acts directly or indirectly on muscles, joint capsules or ligaments including direct trauma, strain, fatigue, heat, cold, nerve root irritation, visceral dysfunction, emotional factors or overuse. It appears that a trigger point forms when a sensitive locus (nociceptor) coincides with an active locus (abnormal motor endplate). Nerve degeneration and disintegration of motor and sensory nerves in the spinal cord may be responsible for pain referral, local twitch responses and autonomic phenomena associated with trigger points.
- Trigger points are identified by client history (e.g. deep dull aching pain, pain referral pattern, variability of symptoms) and physical assessment including muscle function tests, palpation (e.g. a hyperirritable and very painful spot in a taut band of muscle) and by eliciting the jump sign and local twitch response.
- Treatment techniques for trigger points include spray and stretch, dry needling, and a range of manual techniques. Treat central trigger points with intermittent digital pressure (or deep gliding, cross-fibre friction, thermotherapy, etc). Attachment trigger points require 20–30-second cold applications. Follow the deactivation of trigger points with gentle pain-free stretching.
- Eliminating key trigger points may also deactivate their associated satellite trigger points. Treat key trigger points first.
- Treat the most painful, the most medial and the most proximal trigger points first.
- Address predisposing or contributing factors to prevent re-activation of trigger points.
- Intermittent digital pressure is suitable for most clients; digital ischaemic pressure is contraindicated in osteoporotic and hypertensive clients.

Review questions

1. What is the difference between an active trigger point and a tender point in a tight band of muscle? List five distinguishing features.
2. What is the difference between an active trigger point and a latent trigger point?
3. List five perpetuating factors of trigger points. Discuss the impact of perpetuating factors on treatment.
4. Draw an X on the following diagrams to indicate the locations of trigger point(s) in each of the following muscles.

i) Levator scapulae

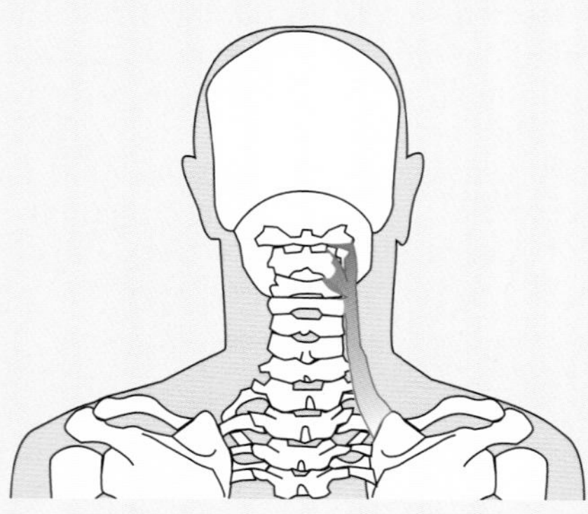

ii) Upper trapezius

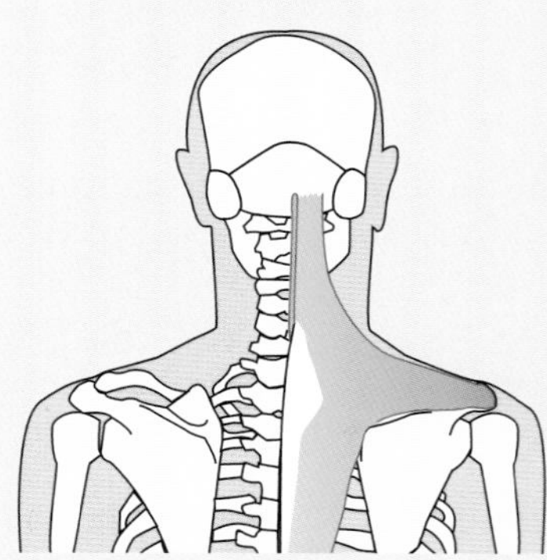

iii) Iliopsoas

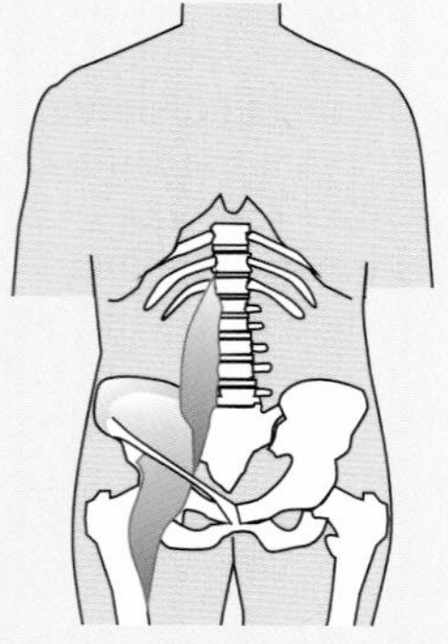

iv) Piriformis

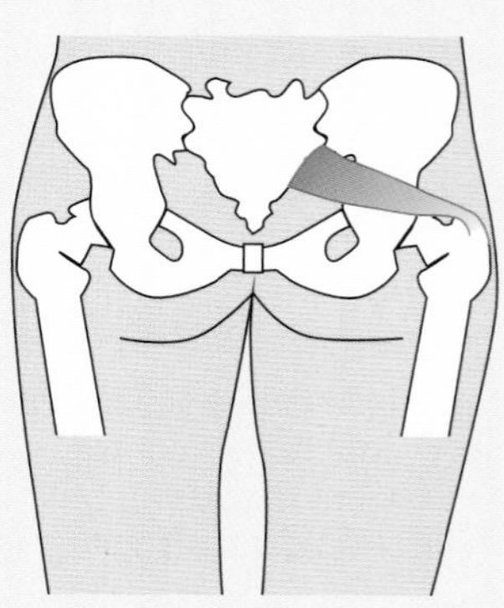

Review questions—cont'd

5. On the following diagrams, draw in the pain referral patterns for the trigger points indicated.

i) Quadratus lumborum

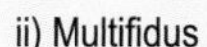

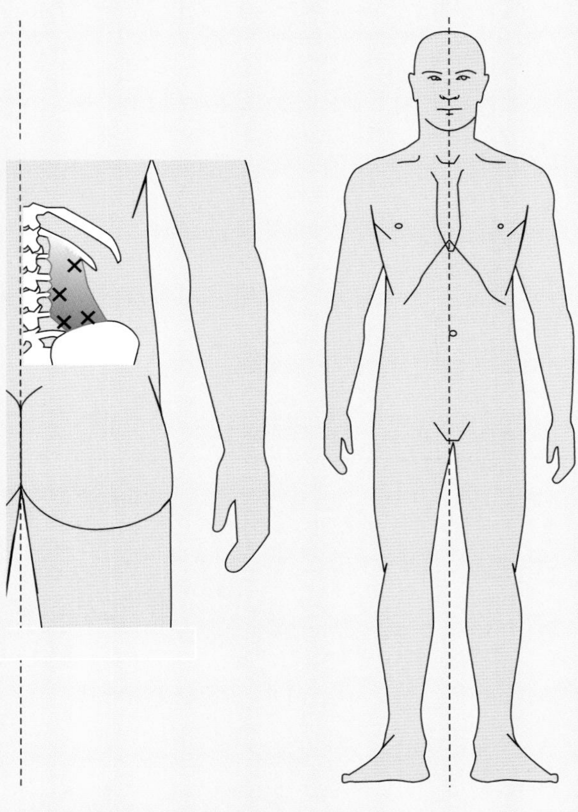

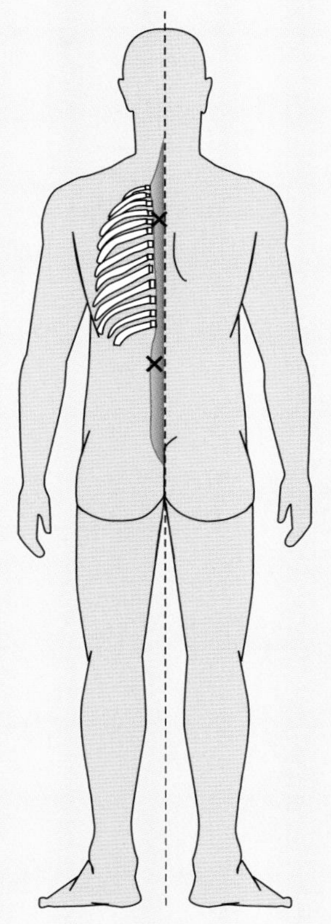

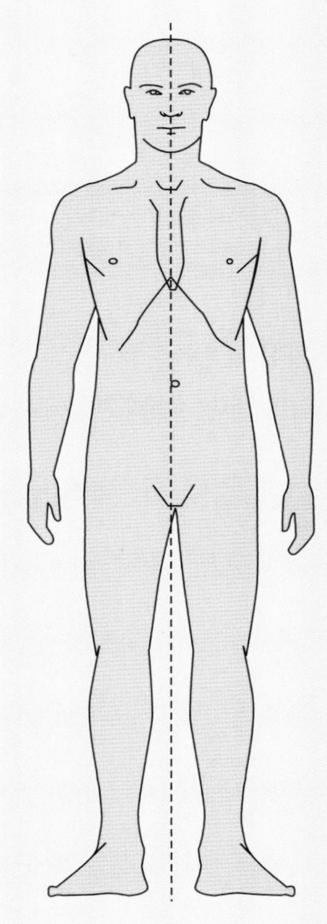

iii) Rhomboids

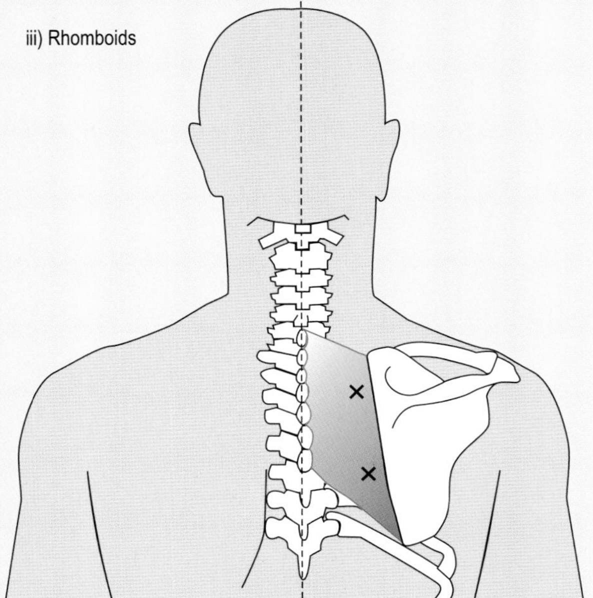

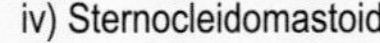

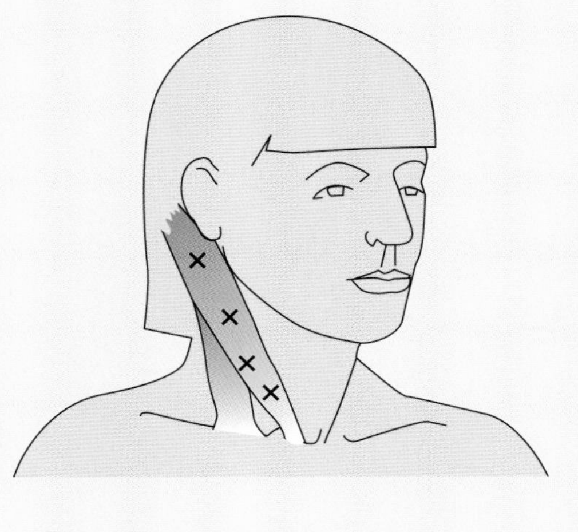

Review questions—cont'd

6. Draw a stretch of (or otherwise describe a stretch for) the following muscles:
   i) Erector spinae muscles
   ii) Upper trapezius muscle
   iii) Piriformis
7. What effect does the presence of a trigger point have on the function of a muscle?
8. What is the difference between digital ischaemic pressure and intermittent digital pressure?
9. How is a twitch response elicited?
10. Give two examples of autonomic signs associated with the presence of a trigger point.
11. What is a key trigger point? Give an example of a key trigger point and its associated satellite trigger points.
12. A client is found to have trigger points in the right piriformis, gastrocnemius and hamstring muscles. If all three trigger points are described as equally painful, in what order would you treat these trigger points?
13. Briefly describe your treatment for:
    a) a central trigger point in the upper trapezius
    b) an attachment trigger point in the hamstring muscles.

APPENDIX 6.1
Some key trigger points

Muscle	Trigger point	Stretch
Sternocleidomastoid	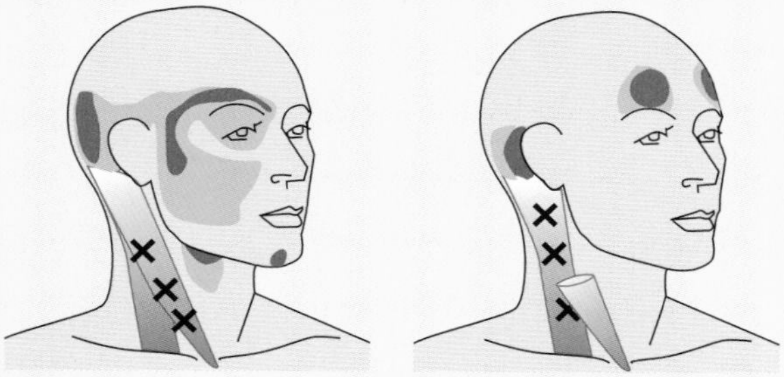	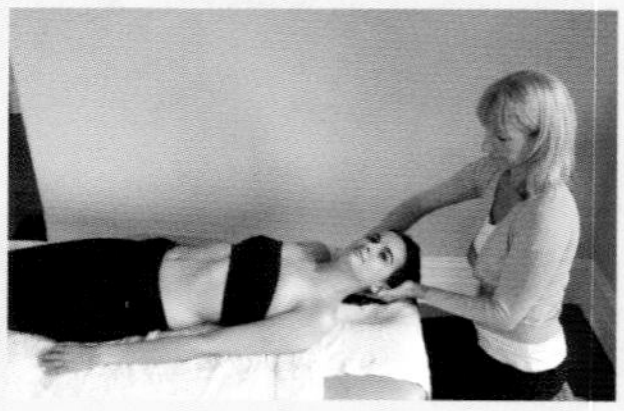
Upper trapezius	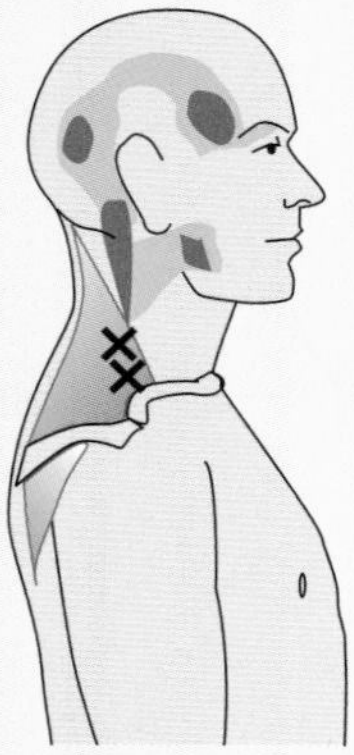	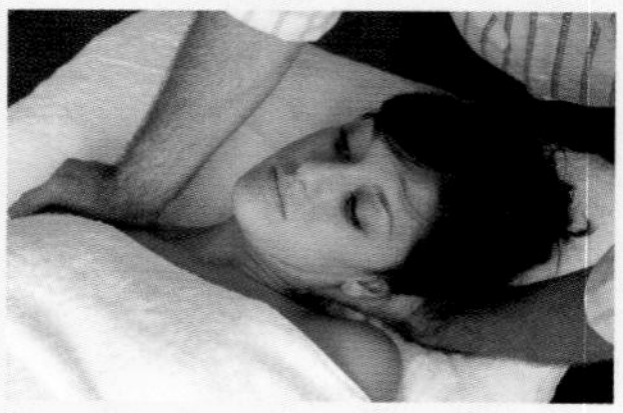

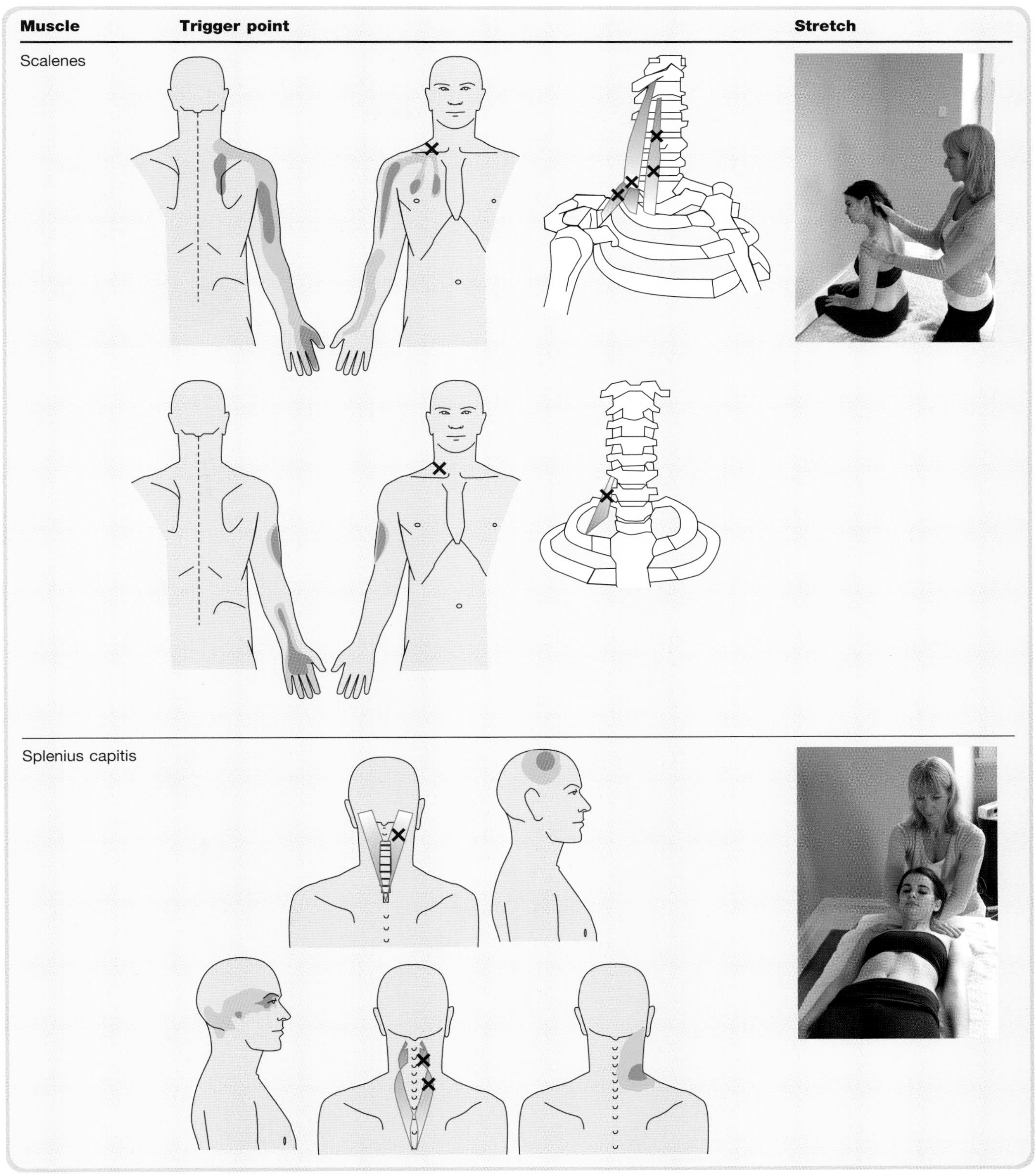

Continued

Muscle	Trigger point	Stretch
Supraspinatus	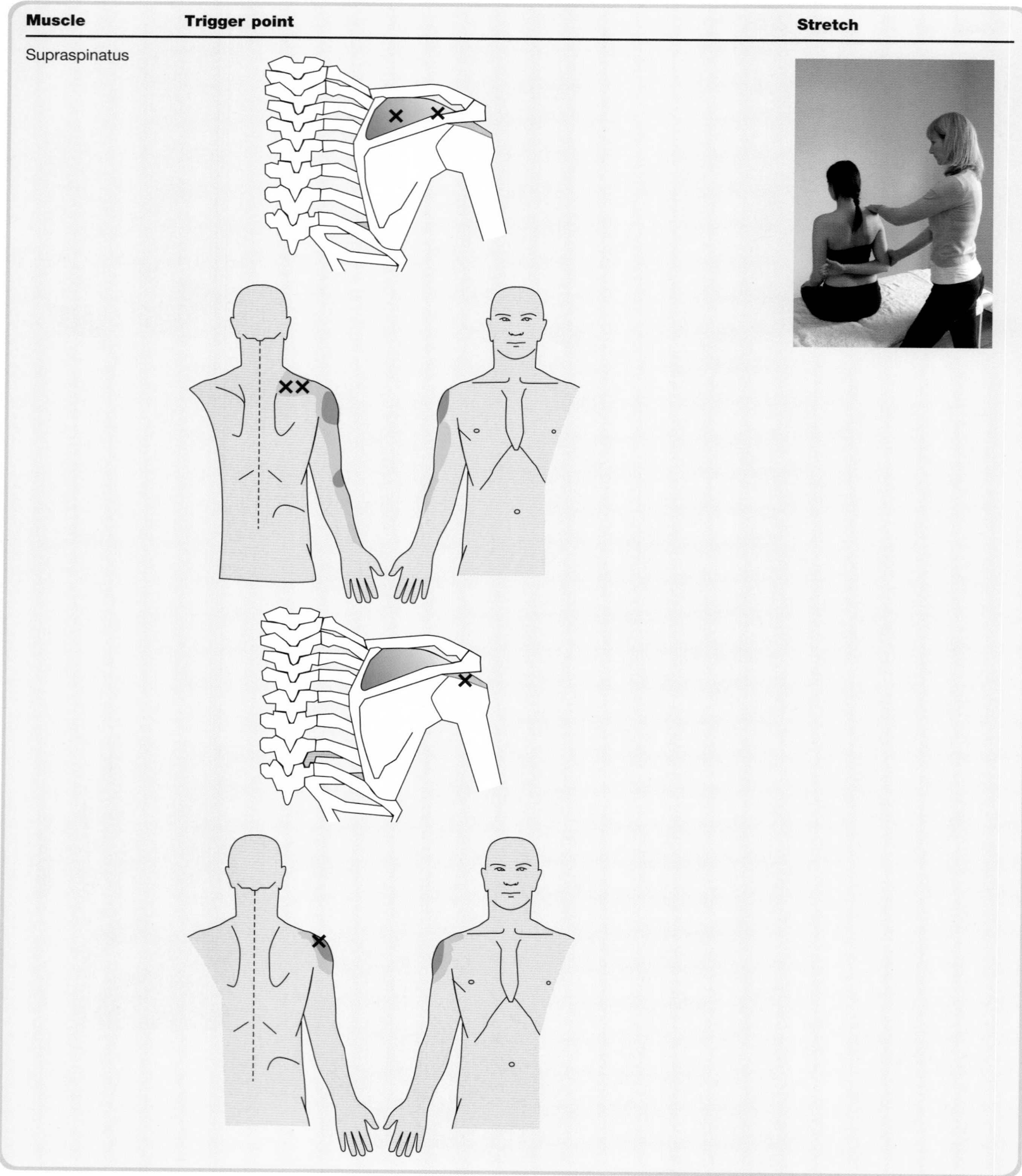	

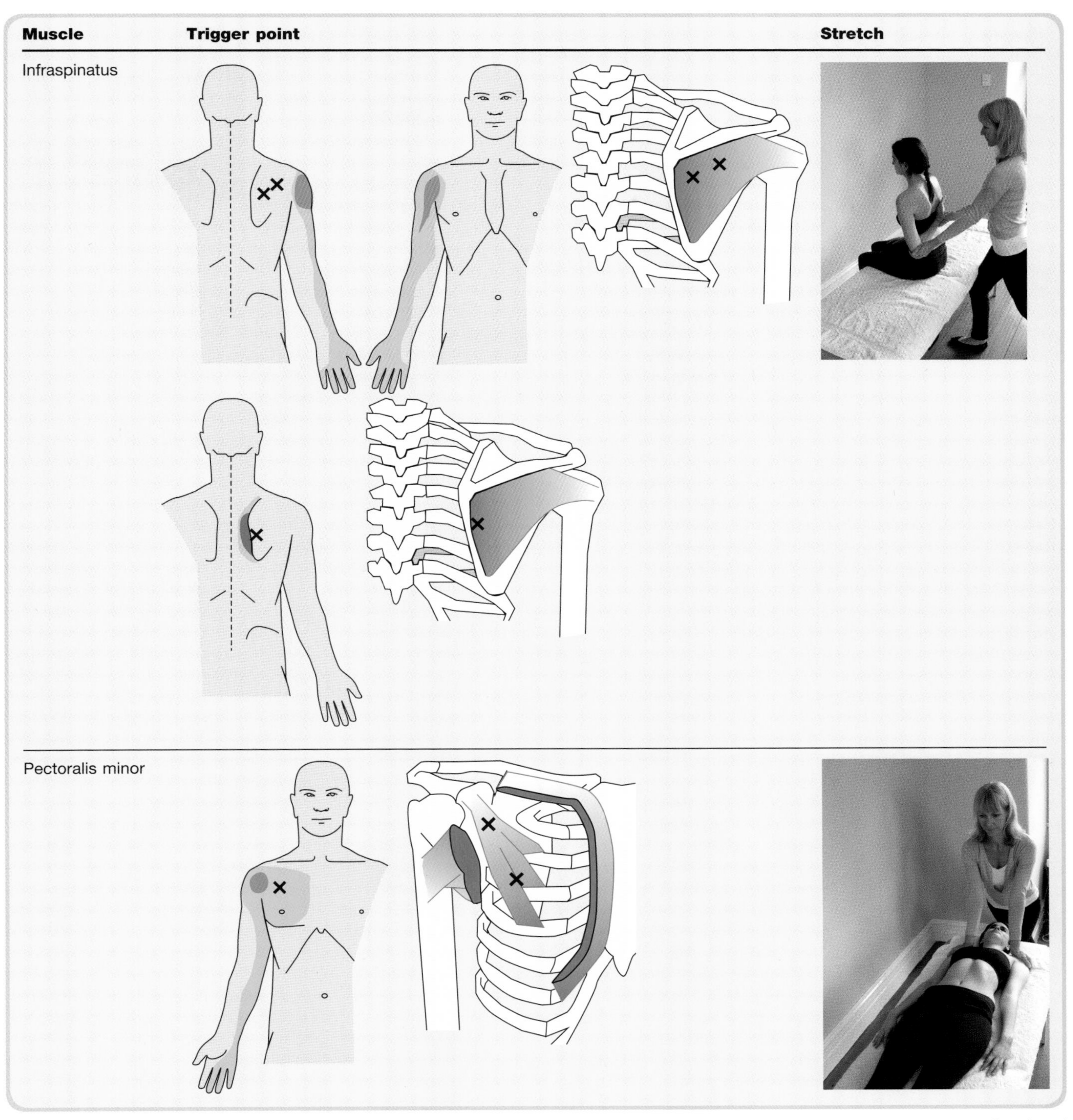
Muscle
Trigger point
Stretch
Infraspinatus
Pectoralis minor

Continued

Muscle	Trigger point	Stretch
Latissimus dorsi	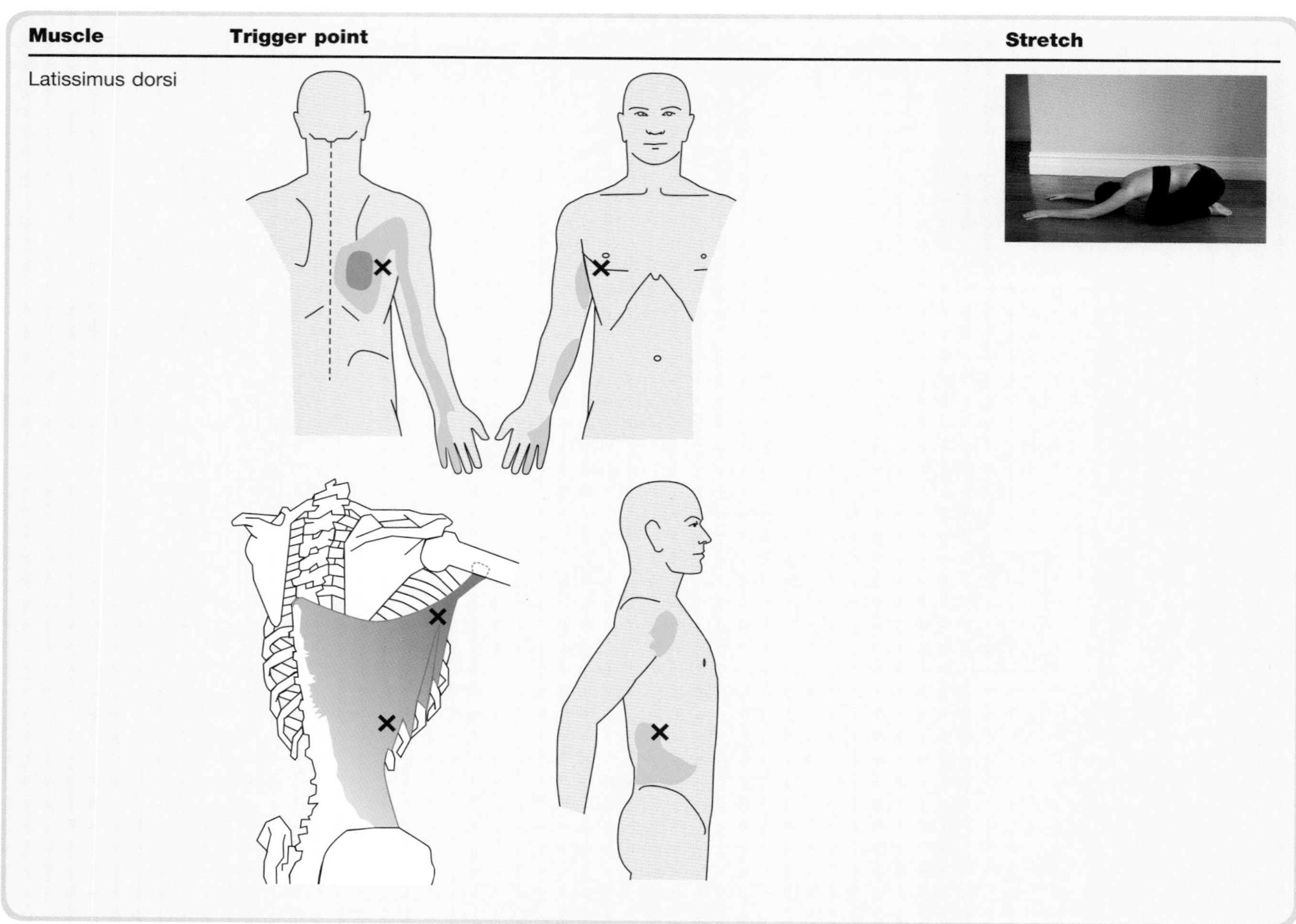	

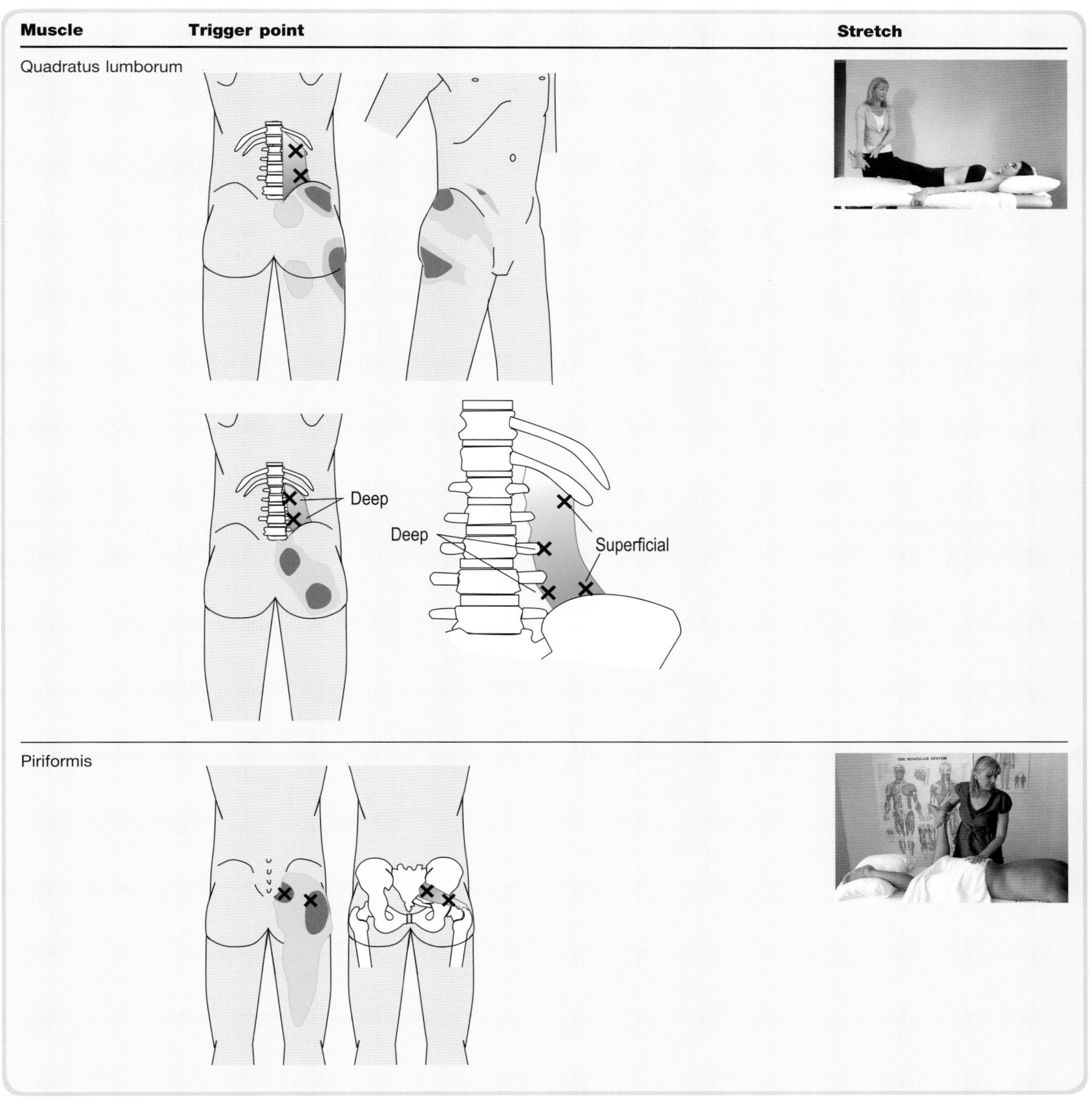
Muscle
Trigger point
Stretch
Quadratus lumborum
Deep
Deep
Superficial
Piriformis

Continued

Muscle	Trigger point	Stretch
Hamstrings	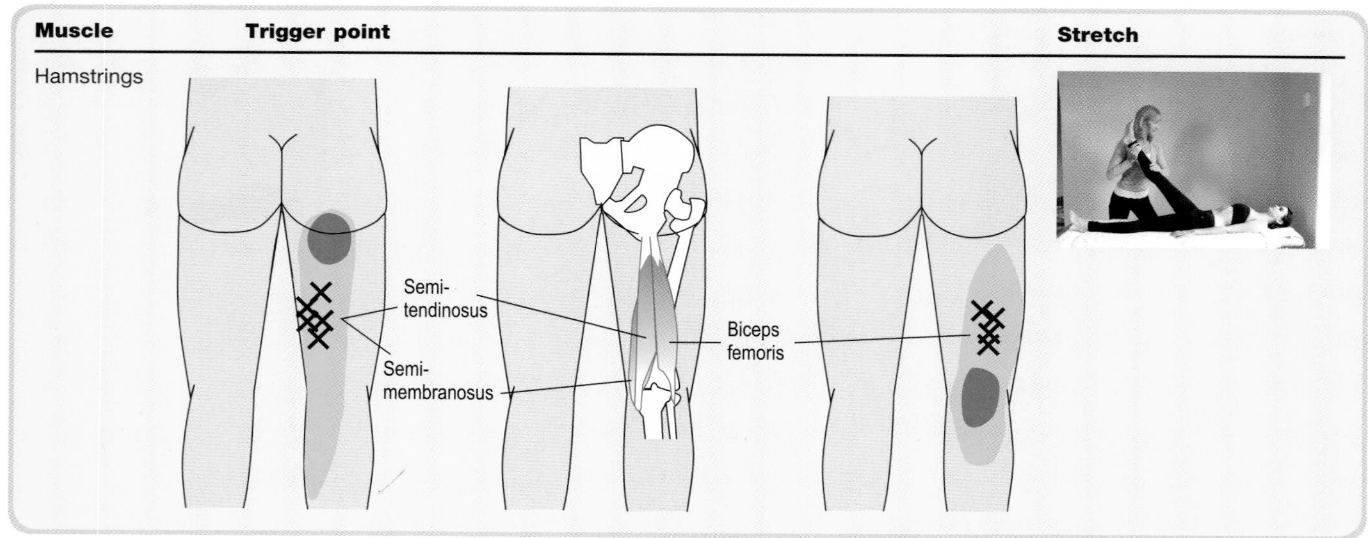	

REFERENCES

1. Travell J, Rinzler S. The myofascial genesis of pain. Postgrad Med 1952;11(5):424–34.
2. Simons D, Travell J, Simons L. Myofascial pain and dysfunction: The trigger point manual. Vol 1: Upper half of body. 2nd edn. Philadelphia: Williams and Wilkins; 1999.
3. Travell J, Simons D. Myofascial pain and dysfunction: The trigger point manual. Philadelphia: Lippincott Williams and Wilkins; 1993.
4. Offenbacher M, Stucki G. Physical therapy in the treatment of fibromyalgia. Scand J Rheumatol Suppl [Review] 2000;113:78–85.
5. Dorsher PT, Dorsher PT. Myofascial referred-pain data provide physiologic evidence of acupuncture meridians. J Pain 2009;10(7):723–31.
6. Peng ZF. Comparison between western trigger point of acupuncture and traditional acupoints. Zhongguo zhenjiu. [Comparative Study English Abstract] 2008; 28(5):349–52.
7. Chaitow L, Fritz S. A massage therapist's guide to understanding, locating and treating myofascial trigger points. Edinburgh: Churchill Livingstone, 2006.
8. Fritz S, Chaitow L, Hymel GM. Clinical massage in the healthcare setting. St Louis, MI: Mosby Elsevier; 2008.
9. Hong CZ. Persistence of local twitch response with loss of conduction to and from the spinal cord. Arch Phys Med Rehabil 1994;75(1):12–16.
10. Tsai C, Hsieh L, Kuan T, Kao M, et al. Remote effects of dry needling on the irritability of the myofascial trigger point in the upper trapezius muscle. Am J Phys Med Rehabil 2010;89(2):133–40.
11. Hsieh Y, Kao M, Kuan T, et al. Dry needling to a key myofascial trigger point may reduce the irritability of satellite MTrPs. Am J Phys Med Rehabil 2007;86(5):397–403.
12. Hong C, Simons D. Remote inactivation of myofascial trigger points by injection of trigger points in another muscle. Scand J Rheumatol 1992; 21(s94):25.
13. Hubbard D, Berkoff G. Myofascial trigger points show spontaneous needle EMG activity. Spine 1993; 18:1803–7.
14. Simons D, Hong CZ, Simons L. Endplate potentials are common to midfiber myofascial trigger points. Am J Phys Med Rehabil 2002;81:212–22.
15. Chung J, Ohrbach R, McCall W. Characteristics of electrical activity in trapezius muscles with myofascial pain. Neurophysiol Clinic 2006; 117:2459-66.
16. Kuan T, Hsieh Y, Chen S, et al. The myofascial trigger point region: Correlation between the degree of irritability and the prevalence of endplate noise. Am J Phys Med Rehabil 2007;86:183–9.
17. Hong CZ. Myofascial trigger points: Pathophysiology and correlation with acupunture points. Acupunct Med 2000;18(1):41–7.
18. Hong CZ, Hong C-Z. New trends in myofascial pain syndrome. Chung Hua I Hsueh Tsa Chih Zhonghua Yi Xue Za Zhi (Taipei) [Review] 2002;65(11): 501–12.
19. Chang CW, Chen YR, Chang KF, et al. Evidence of neuroaxonal degeneration in myofascial pain syndrome: a study of neuromuscular jitter by axonal microstimulation. Eur J Pain 2008;12(8):1026–30.
20. Lucas N, Macaskill P, Irwig L, et al. Reliability of physical examination for diagnosis of myofascial trigger points: a systematic review of the literature. Clin J Pain 2009;25(1):80–9.
21. Lavelle ED, Lavelle W, Smith HS, et al. Myofascial trigger points. Anesthesiol Clin [Review] 2007; 25(4):841–51.
22. Hong CZ. Myofascial pain therapy. In: Pongatz D, Mense S, Spaeth M, editors. Soft tissue pain syndromes: Clinical diagnosis and pathogenesis. New York: Hawthorn Medical Press; 2004. pp. 37–43.
23. Chou LW, Hsieh YL, Kao MJ, et al. Remote influences of acupuncture on the pain intensity and the amplitude changes of endplate noise in the myofascial trigger point of the upper trapezius muscle. Arch Phys Med Rehabil [Randomized Controlled Trial] 2009;90(6):905–12.
24. Niel-Asher S. Concise book of trigger points. Berkeley, CA: North Atlantic; 2005.
25. Ma Y-t. Biomedical acupuncture for sports and trauma rehabilitation: Dry needling technique. St Louis, MI: Elsevier; 2010.
26. Chaitow L. Osteopathic self-treatment. London: Thorsons; 1990.
27. McMahon M, Stiller K, Trott P, et al. The prevalence of thumb problems in Australian physiotherapists is high: an observational study. Aust J Physiother 2006;52(4):287–92.
28. Smith EK, Magarey M, Argue S, et al. Muscular load to the therapist's shoulder during three alternative techniques for trigger point therapy. J Bodywork Mov Ther [Clinical Trial] 2009; 13(2):171–81.
29. Lewitt K. Manipulation in rehabilitation of the motor system. 3rd edn. London: Butterworths; 1999.
30. Davies C. The trigger point therapy workbook. 2nd edn. Oakland, CA: New Harbinger Publications; 2004.
31. Fernandez-de-Las-Penas C, Alonso-Blanco C, Cuadrado ML, et al. Are manual therapies effective in reducing pain from tension-type headache?: a systematic review. Clin J Pain 2006;22(3): 278–85.
32. Vernon H, Schneider M. Chiropractic management of myofascial trigger points and myofascial pain syndrome: A systematic review of the literature. J Manipulative Physiol Ther 2009;Jan 32(1):14–24.
33. Delaney JP, Leong KS, Watkins A, et al. The short-term effects of myofascial trigger point massage therapy on cardiac autonomic tone in healthy subjects. J Adv Nurs 2002;37(4):364–71.
34. Cummings T, White A. Needling therapies in the management of myofascial trigger point pain: a systematic review. Arch Phys Med Rehabil 2001; 82(7):986–92.
35. Tough EA, White AR, Cummings TM, et al. Acupuncture and dry needling in the management of myofascial trigger point pain: a systematic review and meta-analysis of randomised controlled trials. Eur J Pain 2009;13(1):3–10.
36. Cambron JA, Dexheimer J, Coe P. Changes in blood pressure after various forms of therapeutic massage: a preliminary study. J Altern Complement Med 2006;12(1):65–70.

Joint articulation

7

The content of this chapter relates to the following Units of Competency:
HLTREM503C Plan remedial massage treatment strategy
HLTREM504C Apply remedial massage assessment framework
HLTREM502C Provide remedial massage treatment
HLTREM505C Perform remedial massage health assessment

Health Training Package HLT07

Learning Outcomes

- Describe the benefits of joint articulation for remedial massage clients.
- Assess clients for treatment with joint articulation.
- Describe the current evidence for the effectiveness of joint articulation.
- Apply joint articulation techniques effectively and safely to a range of clients.
- Advise and resource clients who have been treated with joint articulation.

INTRODUCTION

As part of a remedial massage program, articulations of joints are designed to improve range of motion and to reduce pain or other symptoms generated from joint dysfunction. Passive joint articulations move joints beyond their active range of motion until an elastic barrier is reached (see Figure 7.1 on p 96).[1] Such manoeuvres are distinct from manipulative techniques which overcome the elastic barrier but remain within the limit of anatomical integrity. As with all remedial massage techniques there are some clients for whom joint articulation is not suitable and it is important to assess the particular joint for indications and contraindications before performing the technique. Joint articulation and mobilisation techniques are widely used among manual therapists to treat mobility restrictions and pain.[2]

WHAT IS JOINT ARTICULATION?

Joint articulation involves the practitioner moving a joint through its ranges of motion without active participation on the client's part. Joint movement is described as:

- Physiological; that is, movements that clients can perform themselves. The ranges of motion that are possible for physiological movements are determined by concentric or eccentric muscle contractions.
- Accessory; that is, movements within the joints that are necessary for normal activities but that cannot be performed actively by the client. Accessory movements represent the movement permitted by the articulating surfaces, ligaments and joint capsule. Accessory movements include component movements (e.g. rotation of the scapula and clavicle when the shoulder joint is flexed) and joint play (determined by the laxity of the joint capsule).

Joint articulation uses accessory movements to improve range of motion and decrease pain. They are specific for each joint. The joint surfaces are slowly moved through an increased range of motion by gentle traction or by slow pressure. The movement can be stopped by the client at any stage. The practitioner attempts to restore normal movement within the joint and normal balance to muscles which have been sustained in a shortened or lengthened position.

EVIDENCE FOR THE EFFECTIVENESS OF JOINT ARTICULATION AND MOBILISATION

Although joint articulation is an integral part of most manual therapy treatments much research is required to determine its application and integration with other manual therapies for optimal client outcomes. Massage and mobilisation of the feet and ankles made a significant improvement in the balance of 28 elderly adults compared with a placebo.[3] It appears that intensive passive mobilisation techniques in end-range positions are more effective in improving glenohumeral joint mobility and reducing disability than passive mobilisations performed within the pain-free range for clients with adhesive capsulitis.[4]

The literature reports several case studies or trials using a single patient. For example, one case report described clinically meaningful improvements in passive range of motion measures and functional activities during a course of care of

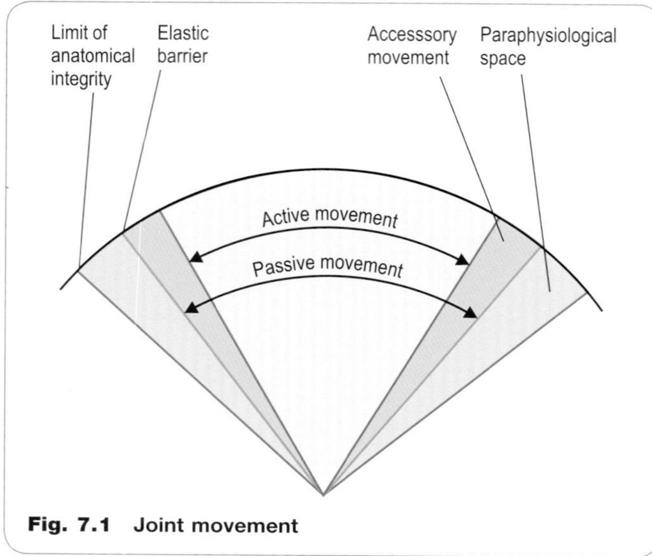

Fig. 7.1 Joint movement

a client with severely restricted hip motion following bilateral hip resurfacing arthroplasty. Treatment was multimodal with an emphasis on joint mobilisation.[5]

Several studies compared the effectiveness of joint articulation over other manual techniques and exercise programs. For example, Cleland et al[6] compared short-term effects of thrust versus non-thrust mobilisation of the thoracic spine in clients with neck pain and found significantly greater short-term reductions in pain and disability in the thrust group. Another study into the effectiveness of passive mobilisation following distal radius fractures found that routine passive mobilisation did not appear to have any additional benefit over advice and a home exercise program for clients.[7] Van der Wees et al[8] conducted a systematic review of the effectiveness of exercise therapy and manual mobilisation in ankle sprain. The authors concluded that manual mobilisation has an initial effect on dorsiflexion range of motion but the clinical relevance of these findings for physiotherapy practice may be limited. Tal-Akabi and Rushton[9] compared the effectiveness of carpal bone mobilisation and median nerve mobilisation in 21 clients diagnosed with carpal tunnel syndrome and could find no statistically significant difference in effectiveness between the two treatment methods.

Several mechanisms have been proposed for the effects of manual therapy including the gate-control mechanism[a].[10] A systematic review conducted by Schmid et al[11] found evidence for concurrent activation of both pain modulatory and sympathetic nervous system effects suggesting that key brain region areas are involved in coordinating these responses. The authors support a neurophysiological model based on stimulation of areas within the central nervous system to explain the effectiveness of passive joint mobilisation.

[a]The gate-control theory of pain postulated that pain perception is modulated by intrinsic neurons and controls from the brain.[10]

ASSESSING CLIENTS FOR TREATMENT

A number of assessment procedures are used to determine the suitability of clients for remedial massage, the types of tissue(s) to be treated, and the application of specific techniques (see Chapter 2). Assessing clients' suitability for treatment with joint articulation includes history, passive range of motion (PROM) testing and palpation. Findings from all assessments should be integrated and used to guide the treatment plan.

HISTORY

Case history enables practitioners to identify red flags of potentially serious medical conditions requiring referral including:

- Fractures (history of trauma, history of minor trauma if over 50 years or osteoporotic or taking corticosteroid medication, excessive pain, obvious deformity)
- Tumour (past history of malignancy, age over 50 years, failure to improve with treatment, unexplained weight loss, pain at multiple sites, pain at rest)
- Infections (fever, malaise, risk factors for infection including underlying disease process or immunosuppression)[12]

Ask questions to determine whether the pain is mechanical (e.g. pain aggravated by activity, relieved by rest, associated with morning stiffness). Be vigilant for systemic conditions that may present with joint pain including:

- Ankylosing spondylitis: A chronic inflammatory disorder that mainly affects the sacroiliac joints and spine and leads to ankylosis. It usually begins between 15 and 35 years of age and is four times more common in men than women. Symptoms are worse after periods of inactivity. Night pain may be present.
- Fibromyalgia: A chronic pain condition characterised by generalised pain and muscle stiffness. Clients with fibromyalgia often complain of extreme fatigue and difficulty sleeping. The whole body becomes hypersensitive to pain. It is thought to be related to biochemical changes in the central nervous system, abnormal central processing of nociceptive pain or central sensitisation. It is sometimes confused with polymyalgia rheumatica, a type of arthritis with associated muscle symptoms.
- Gout: A group of metabolic conditions associated with urate crystal deposits leading to acute arthritis. The client is usually between 30 and 60 years; the ratio of males to females is 20 to 1. The most common presentation is an acutely inflamed joint, usually the first metatarsophalangeal joint.
- Psoriatic arthritis: An autoimmune disease associated with psoriasis and polyarthritis. The usual age of onset is 35 to 55 years. It is slightly more common in females than males. Digits of the hands and feet may be affected first. Between 2% and 10% of people with psoriasis develop psoriatic arthritis.
- Reiter's syndrome: A polyarthropathy with three main symptoms: conjunctivitis, urethritis and polyarthritis. The age of onset is 20 to 60 years, often following venereal acquired infection. The ratio of males to females is 15 to 1.

- Rheumatoid arthritis: This chronic autoimmune inflammatory disease usually begins in the proximal interphalangeal and metacarpophalangeal joints bilaterally and is characterised by symmetrical joint pain and swelling. Women are three times as likely to have rheumatoid arthritis than men and the usual age of onset is between 20 and 40 years of age.
- Systemic lupus erythematosus: A chronic autoimmune inflammatory disease that can affect every organ system of the body. The ratio of females to males is 20 to 1. It can occur at any age but most commonly between 30 and 50 years. It is associated with pleurisy, pericarditis, oral ulcers, arthritis, blood disorders, seizures and a malar (butterfly) rash over the cheeks and nose.[13]

Joint articulation is commonly used to manage joint pain and improve restricted range of motion in the subacute or chronic phases of the above conditions.

FUNCTIONAL TESTS

Passive range of motion testing is the most important functional test for assessing joint function. Passive range of motion testing should always follow active range of motion testing which provides information about the client's functional movement and level of impairment (the See-Move-Touch principle described in Chapter 2). Ranges of motion are determined by the anatomical structure of the joint. When a joint becomes injured certain ranges of motion may become limited. If the joint capsule is tightened the limitation of movement is often referred to as a capsular pattern (see Table 7.1). Capsular patterns are thought to indicate joint degeneration and may be associated with hard and leathery end-feels, although recent research has questioned the validity of capsular patterns for the diagnosis of degenerative joint disease.[14, 15]

Table 7.1 Capsular patterns of major joints of the body

Joint	Capsular pattern of limitation of joint range of motion
Cervical spine	lateral flexion = rotation, extension
Lumbar spine	lateral flexion = rotation, extension
Shoulder joint	external rotation > abduction > flexion > internal rotation
Elbow joint	flexion > extension; pronation = supination
Wrist joint	flexion = extension
Metacarpophalangeal and interphalangeal joints	flexion > extension
Hip joint	flexion > internal rotation > abduction (order varies)
Knee joint	flexion > extension
Ankle joint (talotibial joint)	dorsiflexion = plantarflexion
Subtalar joint	inversion > eversion
Metatarsophalangeal joints (2nd–5th)	flexion > extension
Metatarsophalangeal joint (1st)	extension > flexion

PALPATION

Palpation is used to identify different types of end-feel including:

Hard end-feel

Hard end-feel describes the practitioner's palpatory sensation when a joint is stopped within its normal range by bony approximation, such as a foreign object inside the joint. This could be a piece of floating bone or cartilage or bony block which can occur with osteoarthritic changes in the joint.

Soft end-feel

Soft end-feel is palpated when joint range of motion is limited by inflammation, pain, excessive muscle mass or even a soft tissue tumour.

Leathery end-feel

This is felt when joint range of motion is limited by ligament tightness or shortening.

Sometimes crackling sounds (crepitus) are associated with joint movement. It may be audible or felt as a grating sensation. It indicates degeneration in the joint and often occurs in osteoarthritis. It can also be caused by loose particles or debris (e.g. small pieces of cartilage) in the joint. Crepitus may be a signal to discontinue the technique. Discontinue if pain is elicited as the techniques are performed.

TREATING CLIENTS

Relaxing the muscles around the joint is essential before performing joint articulations. As an introductory procedure apply a general massage around the joint and related areas. Alternatively, the area may be warmed with a heat pack in preparation for joint articulation.

GUIDELINES[16, 17]

- Place the joint in mid-range. In general, mid-range positions are loose-packed, that is the articulating surfaces are maximally separated and the joint has the greatest amount of free play. For example, the resting (loose-packed) position of the glenohumeral joint is 55° to 70° abduction and 30° horizontal adduction.
- Stabilise the body part.
- Your hands should be as close to the joint as possible.
- Usually the proximal bone is stabilised and the distal bone is mobilised.
- Work with gravity where possible.
- Work within the client's pain tolerance.

After treatment advise clients to avoid all aggravating conditions. Wearing shoes with good shock absorption and controlling body weight is advisable, especially for clients with low back or lower limb complaints. Range of motion exercises within pain tolerance should be encouraged and heat therapy may provide pain relief. A program of muscle stretching and strengthening can be introduced to address specific muscle imbalances around the joints. Refer clients for osseous manipulation, acupuncture and/or herbal/nutritional support as required.

If joint articulation is carried out after adequate warm-up and within the pain-tolerance then adverse effects are unlikely. If joint inflammation does occur after treatment, advise the client to use ice and rest the joint for a day or two. If symptoms persist, refer clients for further investigation.

TECHNIQUES

The following terms are used to describe the practitioner's position with respect to the client.

- Cephalad: Towards the head
- Caudal: Towards the feet
- Ipsilateral: On the same side as the body part
- Contralateral: On the opposite side to the body part
- Primary Contact: The hand used to move a bone
- Secondary Contact: The hand used to stabilise a bone

1. Cervical spine

Articulation of the cervical vertebrae requires particular caution. It should only be performed after a full assessment of the cervical spine has been carried out (See-Move-Touch principle). Perform all articulations slowly and gently and stop immediately if the client experiences symptoms.

CERVICAL LATERAL FLEXION

This technique is contraindicated if active cervical lateral flexion produces symptoms or if there is a history of disc lesions or neurological symptoms.

With the client supine, stand at the head of the table. Place one hand on the client's shoulder; the other hand is placed horizontally under the occiput. Apply gentle pressure to anchor the shoulder and slowly laterally flex the client's neck towards the opposite shoulder. This is best achieved if you lunge to the opposite side and keep knuckles in contact with the table to avoid cervical flexion. Hold for 5 seconds and repeat on the other side. (see Figure 7.2)

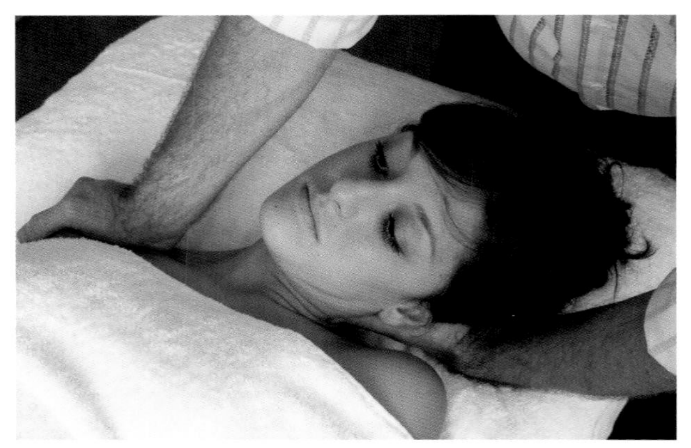

Fig. 7.2 **Cervical lateral flexion**

CERVICAL ROTATION

This technique is contraindicated if active cervical rotation produces symptoms or if there is a history of disc lesions or neurological symptoms.

With the client supine, stand or sit at the head of the table. Hold the side of the client's head with one hand and slowly and gently rotate the head and neck as far as the client can move comfortably to one side. Hold the rotation for 5 seconds and then repeat on the other side. (Fig 7.3)

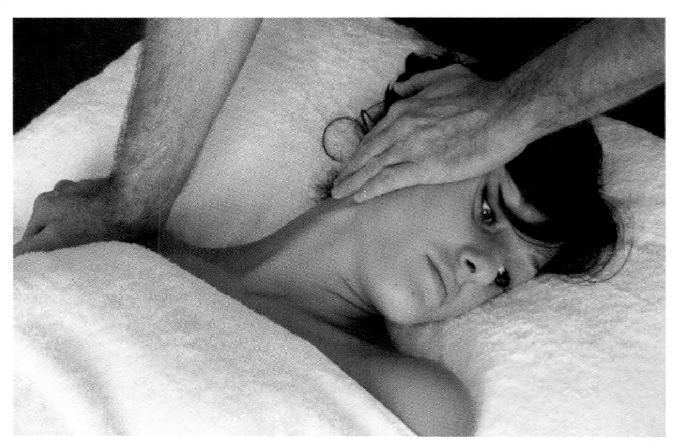

Fig. 7.3 **Cervical rotation**

CERVICAL EXTENSION

The client is supine. Sit at the head of the table. Begin at the lower cervical spine. Using index fingers of both hands placed either side of the spinous processes, gently and slowly lift fingers anteriorly so that the head and neck extend over the practitioner's contact. Hold for 3 to 5 seconds and release. Move the fingers to the next cervical vertebra and repeat the technique. Continue moving the fingers up the cervical spine and extending the cervical spine at each level up to the occiput (see Figure 7.4).

When this technique is applied at the occiput/C1 articulation it is sometimes referred to as the occipital release or cranial base release. Some practitioners prefer to use fingertips spread across the base of the occiput. Extension of the suboccipital area is then achieved by extending the interphalangeal joints and sometimes also the metacarpophalangeal joints.

CERVICAL HORIZONTAL TRACTION

This technique is contraindicated if cervical distraction causes symptoms. Sit at the head of the table or stand with one foot forward and the other back to maintain balance. Cup one hand horizontally under the occiput and place the other under the client's chin. Ask the client to hold onto the sides of the table to anchor their shoulders. Gently and slowly apply horizontal traction with the hand contacting the occiput. Hold for 5 seconds and slowly release. No pressure is applied to the contact under the client's chin. Be careful not to apply pressure to the client's throat. (see Figure 7.5)

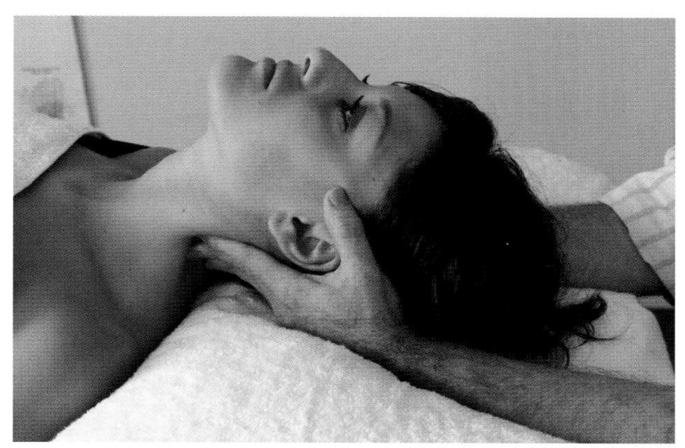

Fig. 7.4 **Cervical extension**

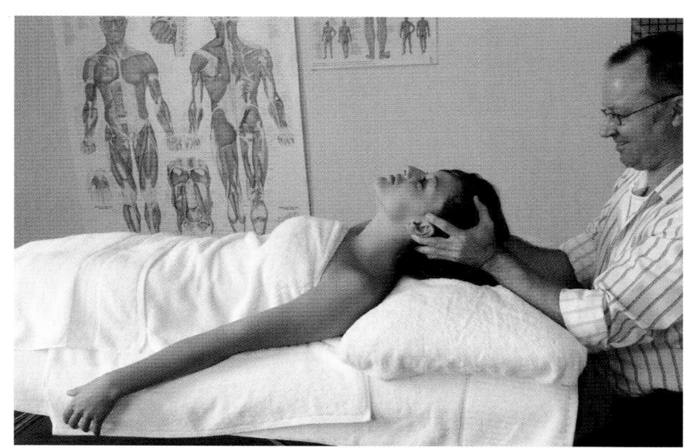

Fig. 7.6 **Cervical stair-step manoeuvre**

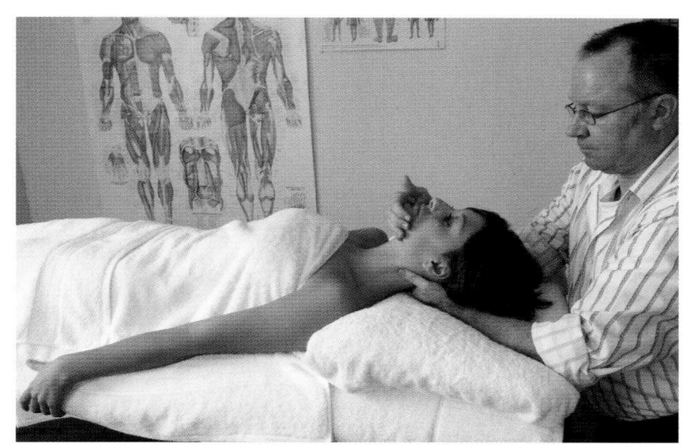

Fig. 7.5 **Cervical horizontal traction**

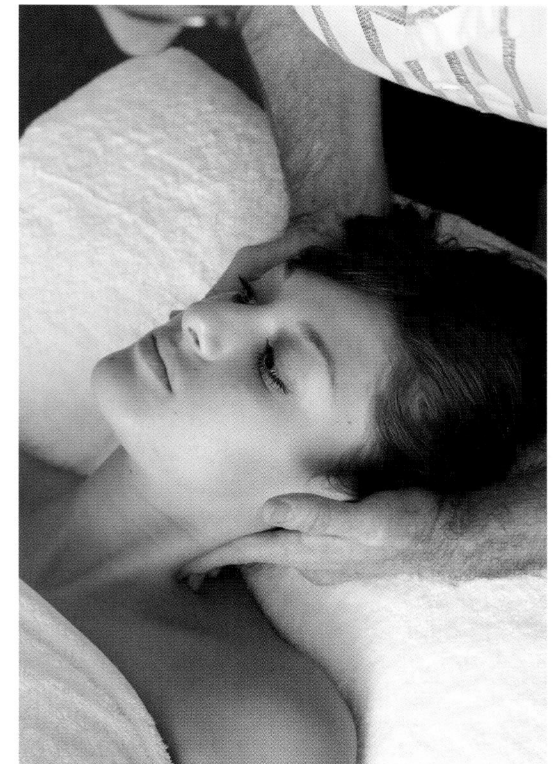

Fig. 7.7 **Cervical facet rotation**

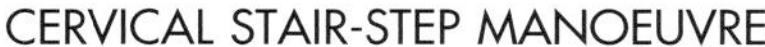

CERVICAL STAIR-STEP MANOEUVRE

This technique is contraindicated if the client's symptoms increase with cervical compression or if the client has a history of cervical disc lesion or neurological symptoms.

With the client lying supine, sit at the head of the table. Slowly and gently apply pressure with both palms over the client's parietal bones in inferoanterior direction. Feel for the *steps* as the head moves downward and forward. Rock the head forward and backward over segments that feel restricted or if the head jolts forward too quickly. Consider each cervical segment in turn. (see Figure 7.6)

CERVICAL FACET ARTICULATION

Cervical facet articulations are contraindicated if active range of motion produces symptoms or if the client has a history of cervical disc lesion or neurological symptoms. For both facet rotation and lateral flexion the client lies supine and the practitioner is seated at the head of the table.

i. Rotation

Place the palms of the hands over the client's ears. The fingers contact the facet joints and laminae of C6 or C7. Gently and slowly rotate the head in small movements (< 10°) about the point of contact in the facet joints. After several rotations to each side, move the fingers up the spine and repeat the small rotations at C5 or C4. When restrictions are located, continue gently rocking and rotating the facet joints several times to improve their range of motion. Continue moving up the cervical spine, repeating the small rotations at each level. (see Figure 7.7)

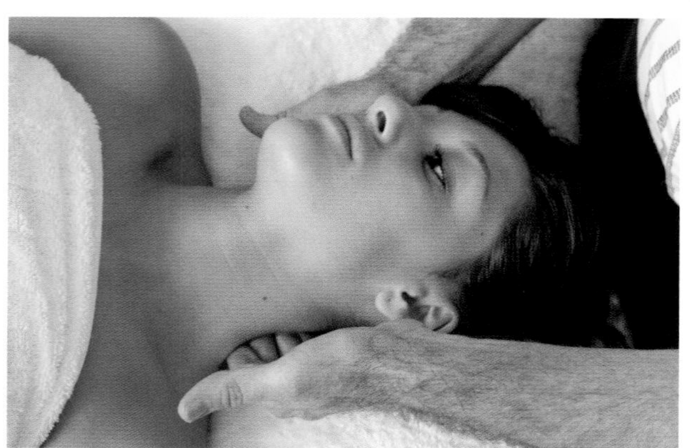

Fig. 7.8 **Cervical facet lateral flexion**

ii. Lateral flexion

Place the hands in the same position as above but this time move the fingertips more laterally. Gently rock the client's head in small movements from side to side at the level of the point of contact on the facet joints. If restrictions in the movement are palpated, continue gently rocking the facet joints several times to improve their range of motion. Move up the cervical spine, laterally flexing the facets at each level. (see Figure 7.8)

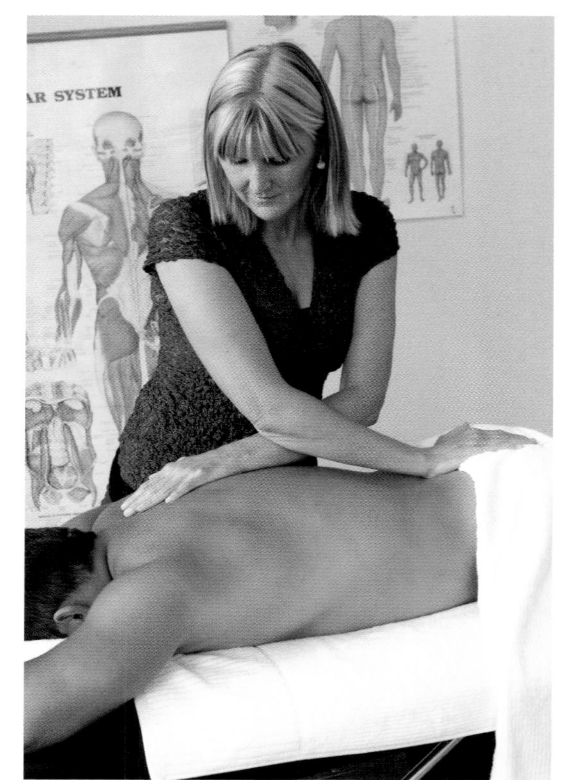

Fig. 7.9 **Thoracic longitudinal mobilisation**

2. Thoracic spine and rib cage

The following mobilisations are designed to reduce thoracic hypomobility. All thoracic and rib cage techniques are contraindicated if the client is osteoporotic.

THORACIC LONGITUDINAL MOBILISATION

The client is prone. If the client is covered with a towel, extra folds of towel are placed in the lumbar area so that the movement is not restricted. Hook the heel of one hand over the sacral base, fingers pointing towards the feet. The heel of the other hand contacts the spinous process of one of the lower thoracic vertebrae. Your arms are crossed. As the client exhales, apply pressure on the body contacts and slowly separate your hands. Hold for 5 seconds and release the stretch slowly. Move the thoracic hand to a new position contacting a spinous process in the mid thoracic spine and repeat the stretch as the client exhales. Repeat again with the thoracic hand contacting the spinous process of one of the upper thoracic vertebrae. (see Figure 7.9)

THORACIC DIAGONAL MOBILISATION

Similar to the longitudinal mobilisation above, except that the heel of one hand contacts the iliac crest and the heel of the other hand contacts the rib angles in the lower thoracic area on the opposite side. As the client exhales, your hands are moved apart to create a diagonal stretch of the lower thoracic region. Hold for 5 seconds. Repeat the technique on the middle and upper rib angles and on the other side. (see Figure 7.10)

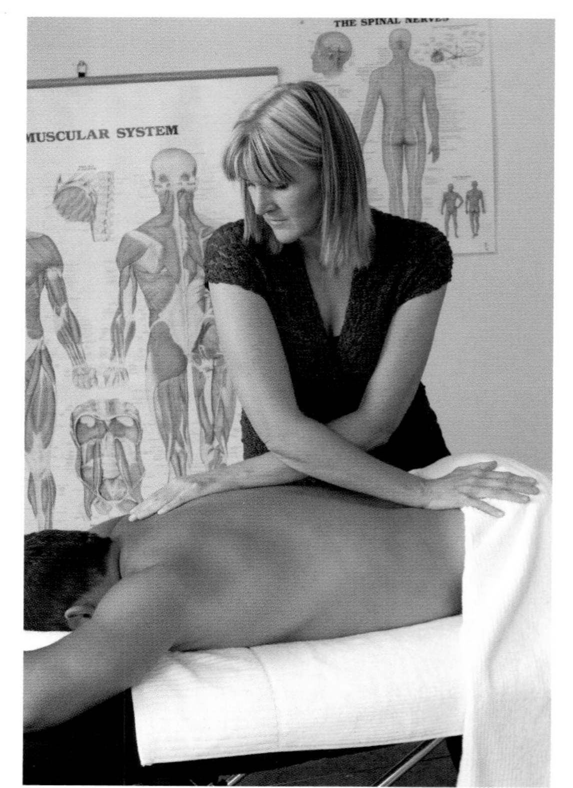

Fig. 7.10 **Thoracic diagonal mobilisation**

THORACIC ROCKING

The client is prone. Stand facing across the client. Using the heels of both hands in unison, contact the contralateral rib angles and gently push laterally in a rhythmical fashion to create a rocking motion through the rib cage. The rib cage recoils passively between lateral pushes. Contacts move up and down the rib angles. Repeat on the other side. (see Figure 7.11)

ARM OVERHEAD RIB MOBILISATION

The client lies supine.

i. Upper ribs. (The technique is described here for the client's left upper ribs. Reverse the contacts for the right upper ribs.) Stand at the head of the table. The client's arm is abducted as far as possible. Hold the client's left arm at the elbow with your left hand. Your right palm contacts the client's upper pectoral area lateral to the sternum, fingers pointed laterally. In this position rib mobilisation is achieved by gentle pressure on the upper ribs as the client exhales. Repeat three times maintaining some pressure between exhalations.
ii. Lower ribs. Stand at the side of the table between the client's arm and the table. Hold the client's left arm at the elbow with your right hand, abduct the arm as far as possible and face towards the client's feet. Use a lunge position to stand low. With your left hand, contact the client's lower ribs in the mid-axillary line. Stretch is achieved by gentle pressure inferiomedially as the client exhales. Repeat three times, maintaining some pressure between exhalations. Repeat on the other side. (see Figure 7.12)

Fig. 7.11 Thoracic rocking

RIB ROTATION

This technique is contraindicated if the client experiences symptoms on thoracic and/or lumbar rotation or during the technique.

The client is seated and places their interlocked fingers behind their neck. Stand behind the client and place one hand through the loop of one elbow from anterior to posterior and place it on top of the client's hands. The heel of the other hand contacts the lower rib angles on the opposite side. As the client exhales, use both hands to rotate the client away from the rib contact hand. Hold the stretch for 5 seconds then repeat to the other side. (see Figure 7.13 on p 102)

3. Lumbar spine and pelvis

The following mobilisation may be beneficial for clients with lumbar facet syndrome. Lumbar mobilisations are contraindicated if the client is osteoporotic or has a history of disc lesion or neurological symptoms.

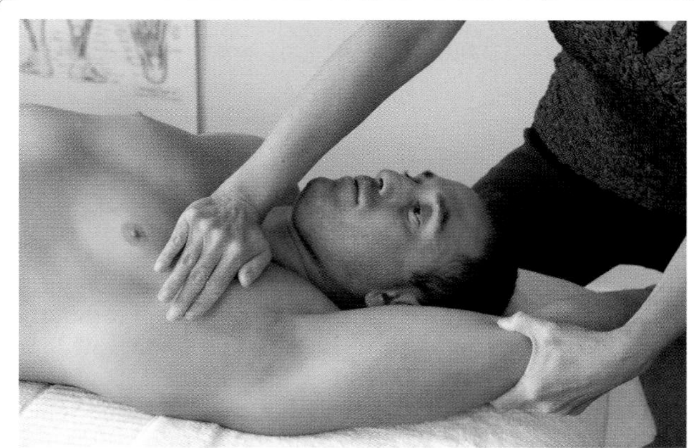

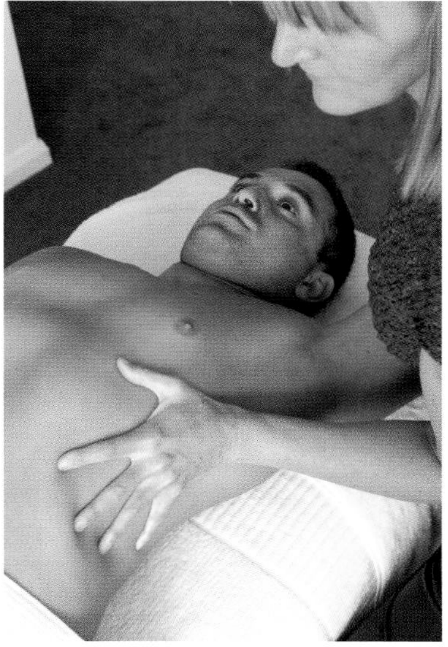

Fig. 7.12 Arm overhead upper and lower rib mobilisation

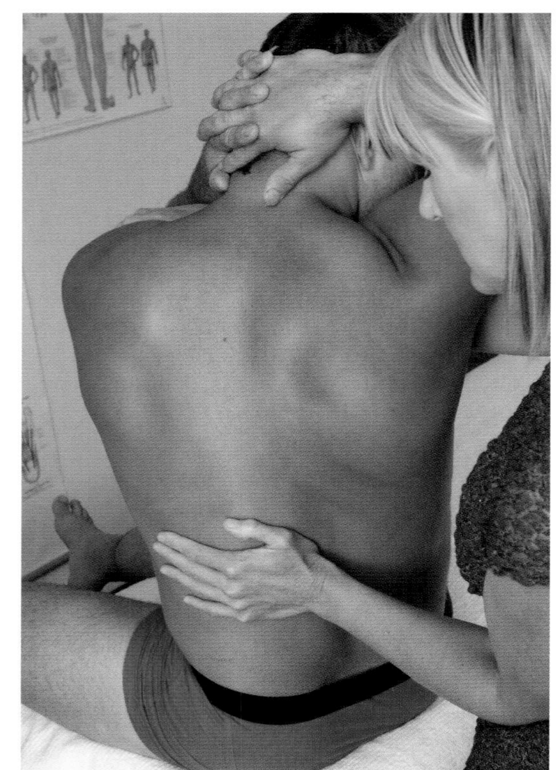

Fig. 7.13 Sitting rib rotation

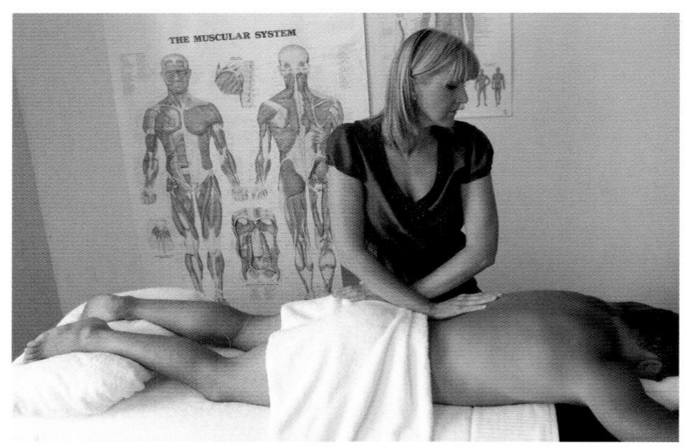

Fig. 7.14 Lumbar longitudinal mobilisation

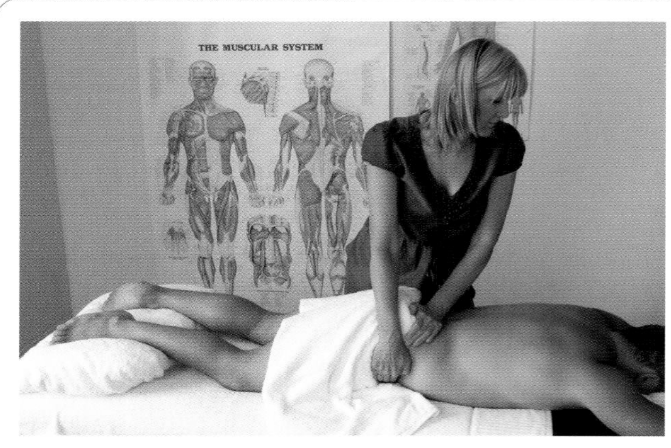

Fig. 7.15 Lumbar rotational mobilisation

LUMBAR LONGITUDINAL MOBILISATION

The client is prone. If the client is covered with a towel, extra folds of towel are made in the lumbar area so that the towel does not restrict movement. Stand at the side of the table facing across the client. Hook the heel of the cephalad hand on the sacral base. The heel of the caudal hand contacts the spinous process of one of the lower lumbar vertebrae, fingers pointing superiorly. Your arms are crossed. As the client exhales, apply pressure to the bony contacts and slowly separate your hands. Hold the stretch for 5 seconds before releasing slowly. Repeat with the cephalad hand contacting the spinous processes of an upper lumbar vertebra. (see Figure 7.14)

LUMBAR ROTATIONAL MOBILISATION

This technique may be helpful for restricted sidebend coupling of the facet joints. It is contraindicated for clients with hyperlordosis, spondylolisthesis or pain on lumbar rotation.

The client lies prone. Stand facing across the patient. Fold a towel in quarters and drape it across the client's pelvis. Place the heel of the cephalad hand along the contralateral paravertebral muscles in the lumbar area. The caudal hand is placed over the towel and under the contralateral anterior superior iliac spine. As the client exhales, gently apply pressure towards the floor to the lumbar paravertebral muscles. Maintain the pressure and gently lift the pelvis with the caudal hand. This creates a slight rotation of the lumbar spine. Hold for 5 seconds. Release gently. Repeat on the other side. (see Figure 7.15)

SI JOINT MOBILISATION

This technique is contraindicated if sacroiliac ligaments are sprained. The client lies prone, covered with a towel. Stand level with the pelvis facing across the client. Place your caudal hand over the client's sacrum, fingers pointing superiorly. The cephalad hand contacts the gluteal area on one side, fingers pointing inferiorly. Your arms are crossed. Apply gentle pressure inferiorly with the caudal hand and superiorly with the cephalad hand and hold for 5 seconds. Repeat on the other side. This technique applies a slight rotational force through the sacroiliac joint. (Note: the inferior pressure on the ilium makes the leg on that side appear to lengthen during this technique.) Repeat with hands reversed. (see Figure 7.16 on p 103)

4. Shoulder joint

SHOULDER ROTATION

With the client supine, lying close to the side of the table, stand at the side of the table in lunge position facing towards the client's head. Hold the client's elbow with the lateral hand, and place your other hand over the shoulder. Using both hands in unison, rotate the glenohumeral joint. Use your body weight by alternately bending and straightening your knees to perform the shoulder rotation. You can also slowly abduct the client's

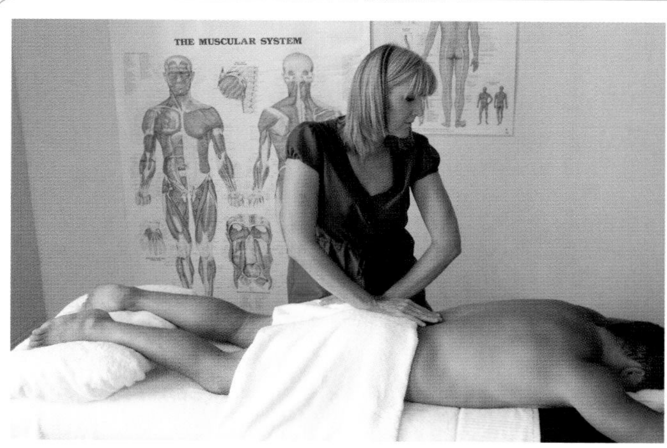

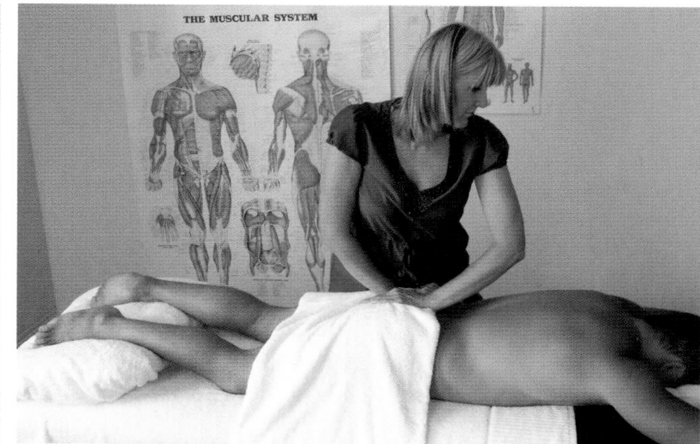

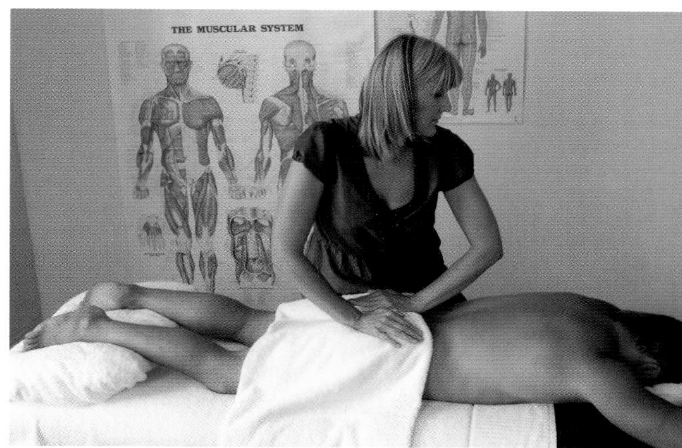

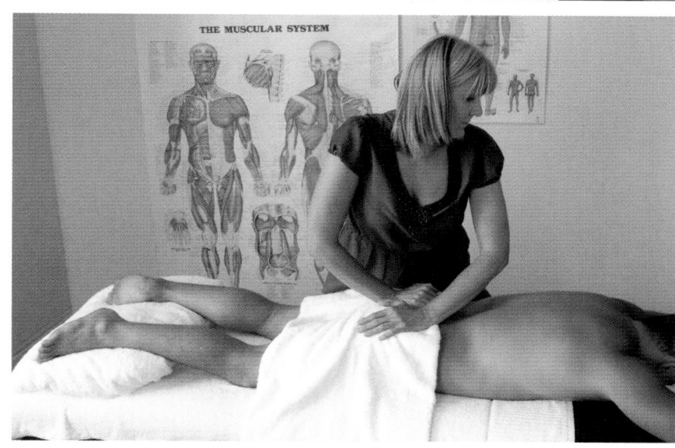

Fig. 7.16 **SI joint mobilisation**

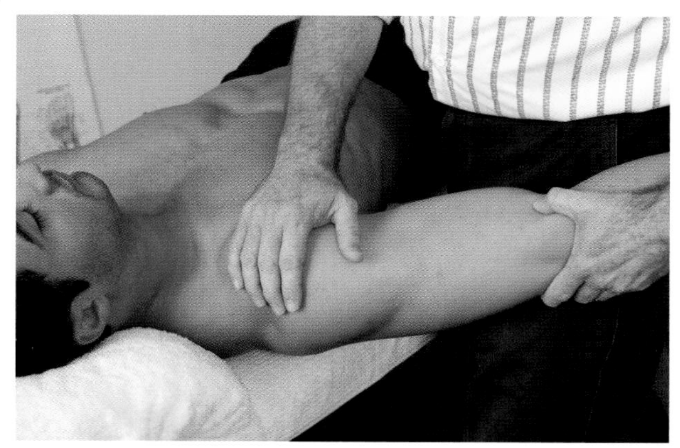

Fig. 7.17 **Shoulder rotation**

arm while continuing to rotate the shoulder joint. Care must be taken if abduction is painful (as is the case in many shoulder conditions). (see Figure 7.17)

SHOULDER TRACTIONS

The glenohumeral joint is gently tractioned in five ranges of motion. The client is supine.

i. Inferior traction. Face the client's head and stand in lunge position. Hold the upper limb with both hands (e.g. one proximal to the wrist and the other proximal to the elbow). Gently traction the client's glenohumeral joint in an inferior direction by transferring weight from the front foot to the back foot.
ii. Anterior traction. Hold the upper limb with both hands (e.g. one proximal to the wrist and the other proximal to the elbow). Raise the client's arm to 90° flexion and gently traction the client's arm towards the ceiling.
iii. Superior traction. Stand at the head of the table. Hold the upper limb with both hands, one proximal to the wrist and the other proximal to the elbow. The client's arm is raised overhead to its comfortable limit. (Note that full flexion may be limited in many clients with shoulder problems.) Gently traction the client's glenohumeral joint in a superior direction within the client's pain-free range.
iv. Lateral traction. Stand facing across the client. The client's arm is abducted to 90° (or to its comfortable limit). Hold the upper limb with both hands, one proximal to the wrist and the other proximal to the elbow. Traction the client's glenohumeral joint in a lateral direction.
v. Medial traction. Stand on the contralateral side. Place the client's arm into adduction by moving the arm

across the chest with the elbow flexed. Apply gentle traction to the arm across the body. (see Figure 7.18)

SHOULDER PROGRESSIVE CYLINDRICAL ARTICULATION

This technique is designed to circumduct the humeral head at the glenohumeral joint. The client lies supine close to the side of the table. Stand on the ipsilateral side of the client between the client's arm and the table and face cephalad. Place the palm of the medial hand just distal to the shoulder joint. The palm of the other hand holds the client's elbow and stabilises the arm close to your side.

Use both contacts in unison to transcribe a cylinder with the humerus emphasising the posterior pressure. While this motion is maintained, slowly abduct the arm by gradually moving cephalad. The degree of abduction is limited by the client's mobility but rarely needs to reach more than 120°. (see Figure 7.19 on p 105)

SHOULDER PROGRESSIVE HUMERAL EXTERNAL ROTATION

The purpose of this technique is to externally rotate the humeral head at the glenohumeral joint. The client lies supine close to the side of the table, forearm supinated, elbow flexed to approximately 90° and arm abducted to 45°. Stand on the ipsilateral side of the client facing cephalad and hold the client's wrist with the lateral palm on the anterior aspect of the wrist, and the medial hand holding under the client's elbow.

Repeatedly lift and lower the client's elbow with the medial hand while the other hand passively maintains elbow flexion. This repetitive action with the elbow causes the humerus to

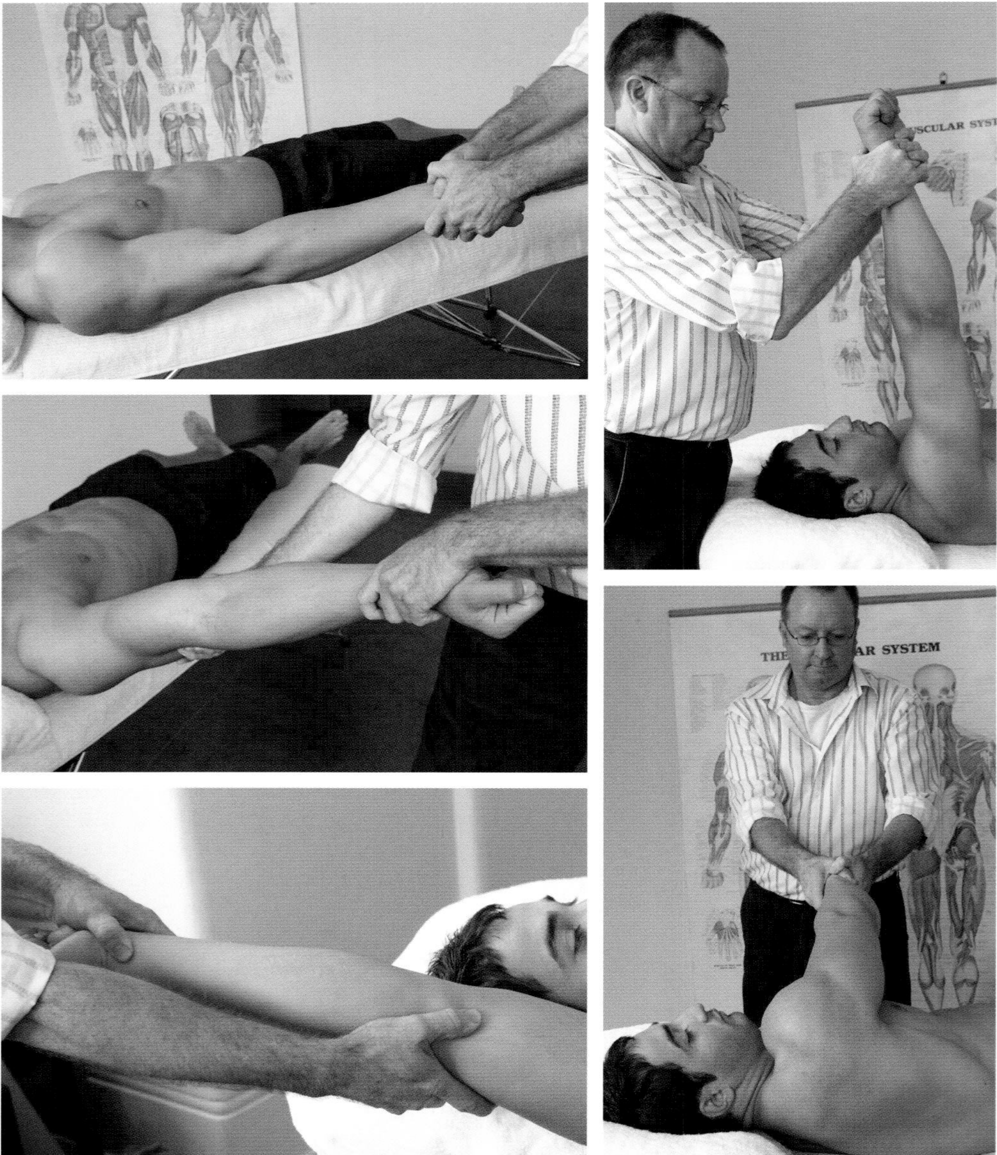

Fig. 7.18 Shoulder tractions

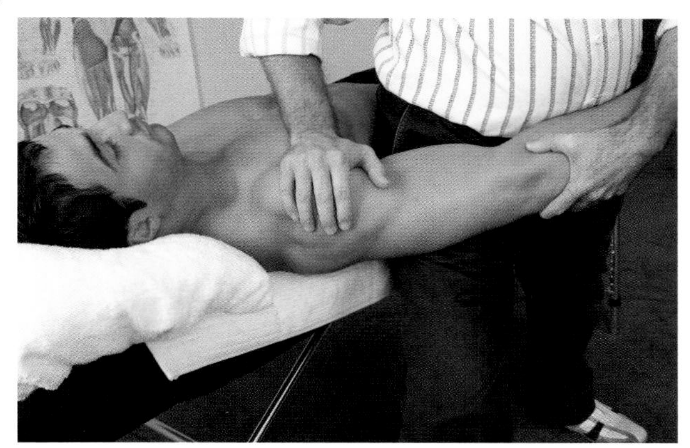

Fig. 7.19 Shoulder progressive cylindrical articulation

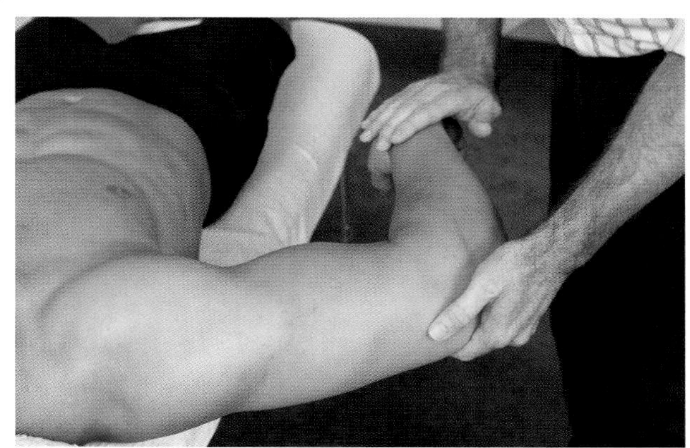

Fig. 7.21 Shoulder progressive humeral internal rotation

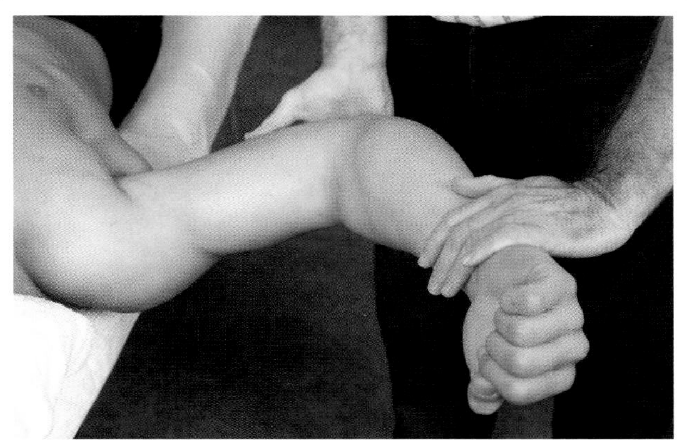

Fig. 7.20 Shoulder progressive humeral external rotation

externally rotate. Continue repetitions of shoulder external rotation as the humerus is slowly abducted to approximately 120°. (see Figure 7.20)

SHOULDER PROGRESSIVE HUMERAL INTERNAL ROTATION

This technique is similar to progressive humeral external rotation except that the humerus is internally rotated at the glenohumeral joint. The client's pronated arm is abducted to 45° with the elbow flexed to 90°. Face across the client and hold under the client's elbow with the cephalad hand and over the top of the client's wrist with the caudal hand. Progressively lift and lower the client's elbow with the caudal hand while the other hand passively maintains elbow flexion. This repeated lifting and lowering of the client's elbow causes the humerus to internally rotate. Continue repetitions of shoulder internal rotation while taking small steps backwards to abduct the humerus to approximately 120°. (see Figure 7.21)

SHOULDER FIGURE-8

The client is supine, clasping their elbows with their hands. Stand at the head of the table, hold under the client's forearms distal to the elbows and flex the client's shoulders to 90°. Apply slight traction to the shoulders by gently raising the client's arms towards the ceiling. Create a figure-8 movement by slowly making circles first with one elbow and then the other. (see Figure 7.22 on p 106)

5. *Elbow joint*

ELBOW ARTICULATION

The client is supine lying near the side of the table with their extended arm raised vertically with the palm facing medially. Stand on the ipsilateral side of the client facing across them. Place the palm of your caudal hand on the dorsal aspect of the elbow. Wrap your fingers around the medial aspect of the elbow. Hold the client's wrist with the cephalad hand. Your caudal hand moves the client's elbow in a small anticlockwise circle for the left elbow, or clockwise circle for the right elbow. (see Figure 7.23 on p 106)

ELBOW JOINT CAPSULE STRETCH

The client is supine. Hold the client's arm either side of the elbow. Traction is applied in both directions to gently stretch the joint capsule. Hold for 5 seconds. (see Figure 7.24 on p 106)

6. *Wrist and hand*

WRIST PRONATED LONGITUDINAL THENAR KNEADING

This technique is designed to articulate the carpal bones in a sagittal plane. The client lies supine with the arm pronated and elbow extended. Stand on the ipsilateral side of the couch and face cephalad. Place the thenar eminences of both hands together on the dorsum of the client's hand over the proximal metacarpal heads. Point your thumbs superiorly along the client's forearm. With the second, third and fourth fingers, apply counterpressure to the palm of the client's hand. The client's arm may be raised to a comfortable position off the table. While maintaining pressure, move your hands alternately up and down in a sagittal plane causing carpal shearing. Repeat several times before moving the contacts proximally by about 1 cm. Repeat the process. The contacts move progressively proximal until they reach the proximal carpal row. (see Figure 7.25 on p 106)

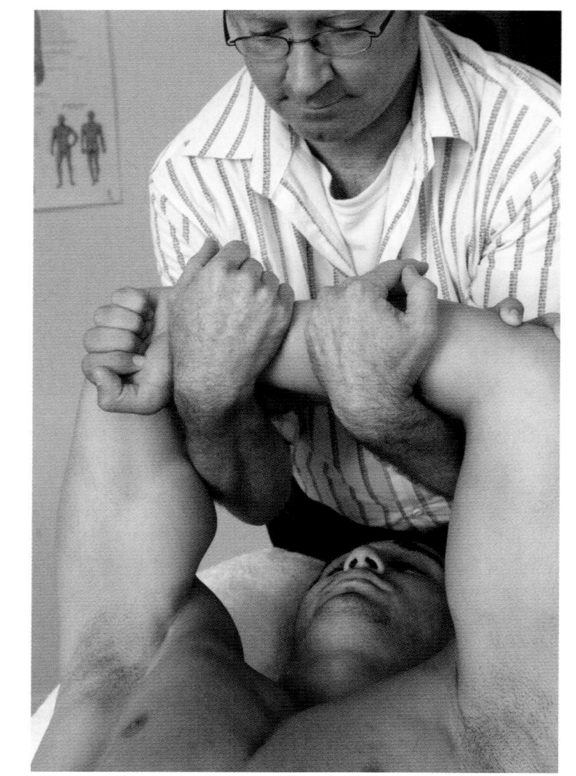

Fig. 7.22 Shoulder figure-8

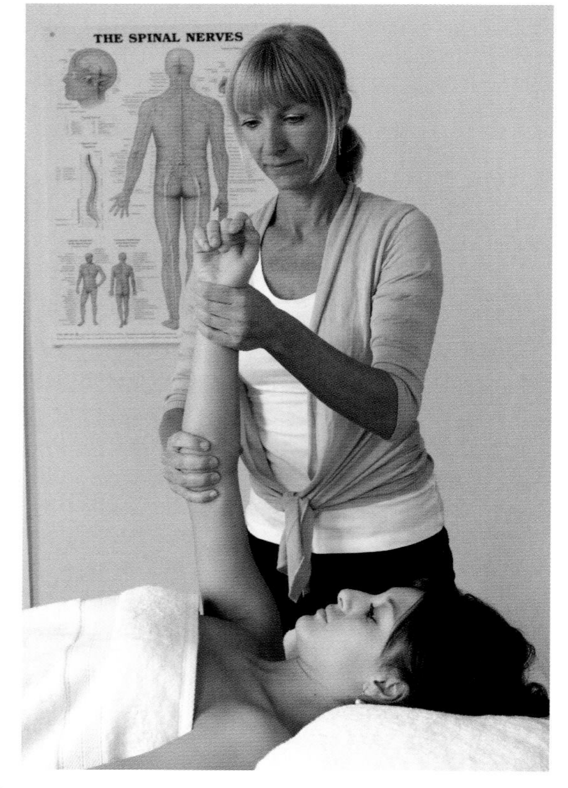

Fig. 7.23 Elbow articulation

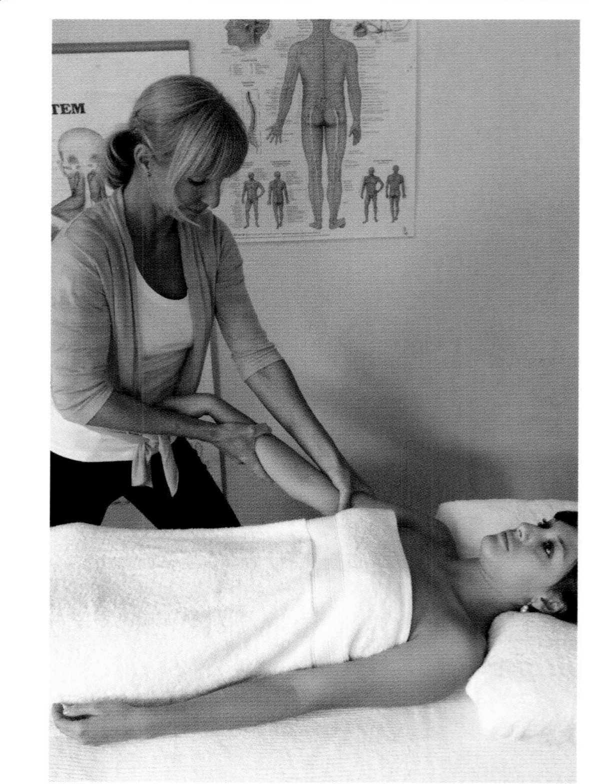

Fig. 7.24 Elbow capsule stretch

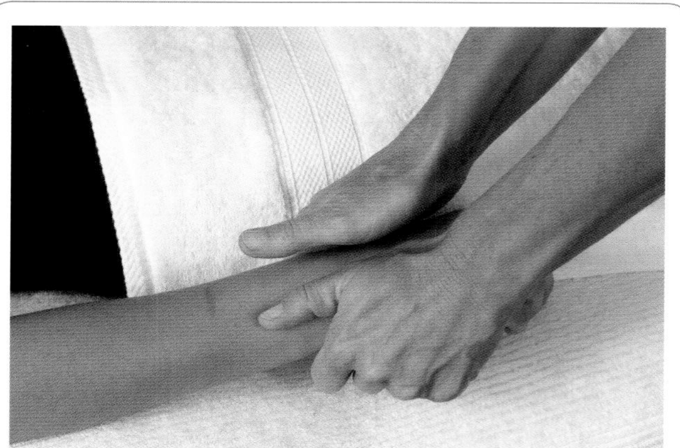

Fig. 7.25 Wrist pronated longitudinal thenar kneading

WRIST PRONATED TRACTION AND CIRCUMDUCTION

This technique is designed to articulate the carpal bones under traction. The client is supine with the arm raised to about 20–30° and the forearm pronated. Stand on the ipsilateral side and face cephalad. Place the thenar eminences of both hands together on the dorsum of the client's hand over the wrist. Place your fingertips under the client's wrist either side of the carpal tunnel. Gently traction and circumduct the client's arm keeping the client's hand pronated. (see Figure 7.26 on p 107)

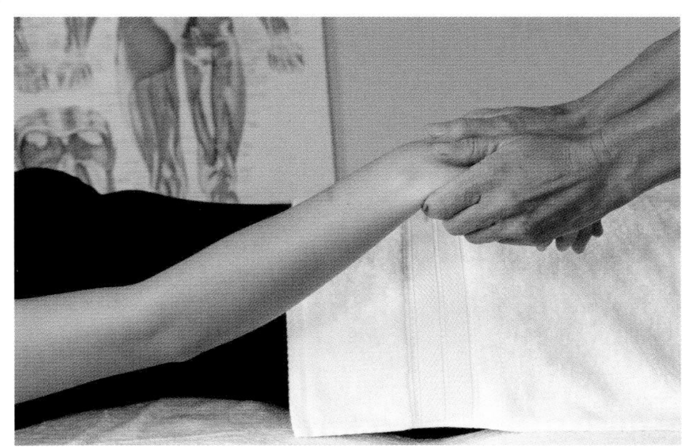

Fig. 7.26 Wrist pronated traction and circumduction

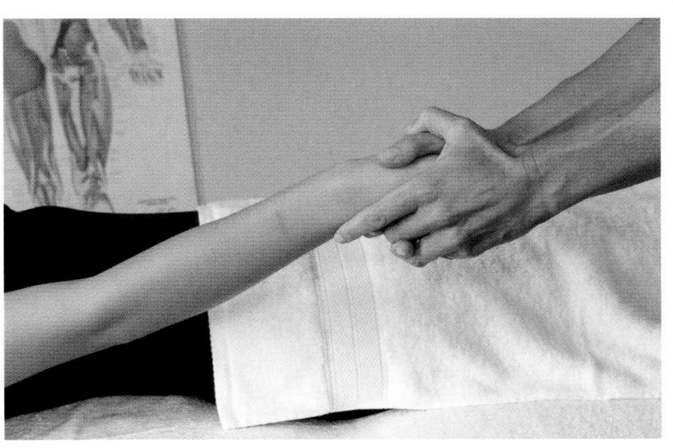

Fig. 7.27 Wrist semi-supinated traction and circumduction

WRIST SEMI-SUPINATED TRACTION AND CIRCUMDUCTION

This technique is similar to the pronated traction and circumduction technique except that the client's hand is semi-supinated. (i.e. thumb points towards the ceiling) This technique articulates the carpal bones under traction with emphasis on the radiocarpal and ulnacarpal articulations. Place the thenar eminences of both hands together on the radial side of the client's wrist with thumbs crossed. The fingertips are placed under the wrist. Maintaining pressure with the hands, slowly circumduct the arm, keeping the client's hand semi-supinated. (see Figure 7.27)

WRIST OVERHEAD TRACTION AND CIRCUMDUCTION

The client lies supine with the extended arm raised overhead with palms facing the ceiling. Stand ipsilaterally at the level of the client's shoulders and face cephalad. Place the webs of both hands just proximal to the client's trapezium and pisiform. Lunge superiorly to traction the client's carpal bones. With traction maintained, the client's hand is slowly circumducted in both directions. (see Figure 7.28)

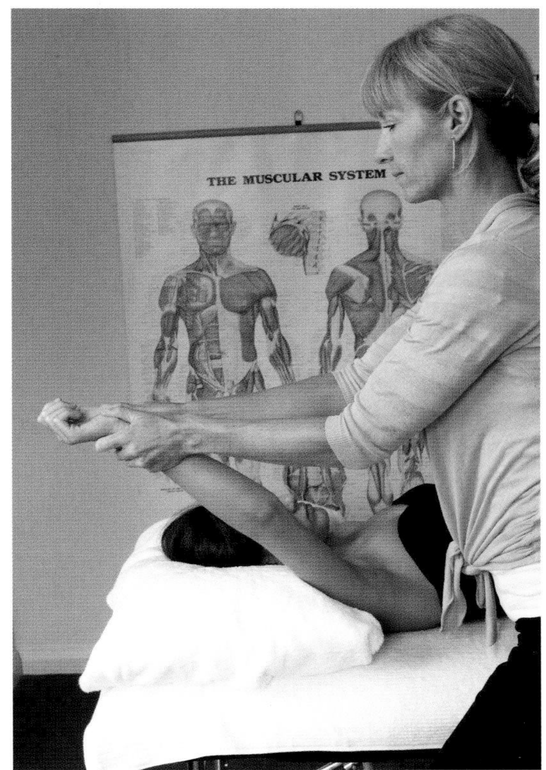

Fig. 7.28 Wrist overhead traction and circumduction

METACARPOPHALANGEAL AND INTERPHALANGEAL MOBILISATION

The client is seated or lies supine with their arm raised to about 20° flexion. Stand on the ipsilateral side and face towards the client's head. Isolate the joint to be mobilised by placing thumb or finger contacts either side of the joint and close to the joint. A number of mobilisations can be performed including flexion/extension, rotation and traction. (see Figure 7.29 on p 108)

METACARPAL SHEARING

The client is supine or seated, forearm pronated. Contact the dorsum of the client's hand with your thenar eminence and your fingers wrapped around the client's palm. Shear each metacarpal individually in an anterior–posterior direction. (see Figure 7.30 on p 108)

7. Hip joint

HIP ROTATION

The purpose of this technique is to mobilise the femoral head in the acetabulum. It is useful for stretching the acetabular capsule. The client lies supine near the side of the table with the hip and knee flexed. Stand on the ipsilateral side of the client in lunge position and face towards the client's head. Place your clasped hands over the client's knee. Lie your caudal forearm along the medial aspect of the client's tibia. By transferring weight alternately between your front foot and back foot, make small circles with the client's knee. (Note the

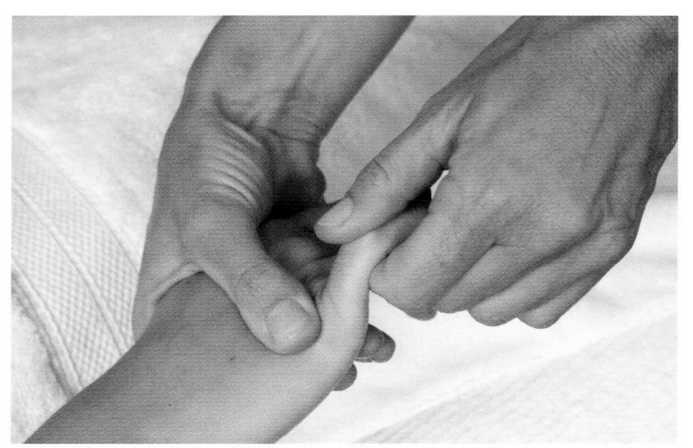

Fig. 7.29 Metacarpophalangeal and interphalangeal mobilisation

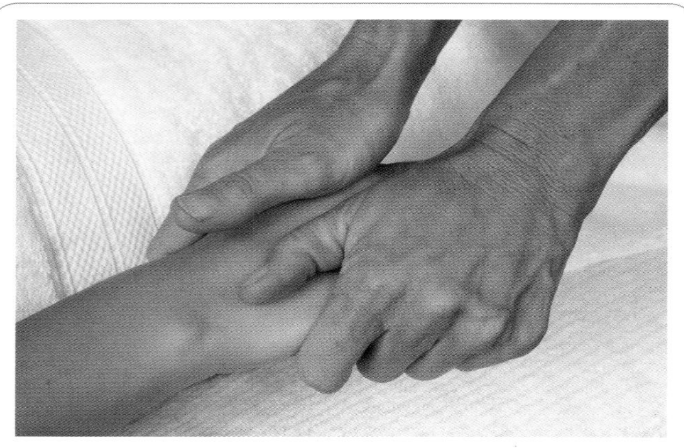

Fig. 7.30 Metacarpal shearing

comparatively restricted end-feel of the medial arc of hip rotation.) (see Figure 7.31)

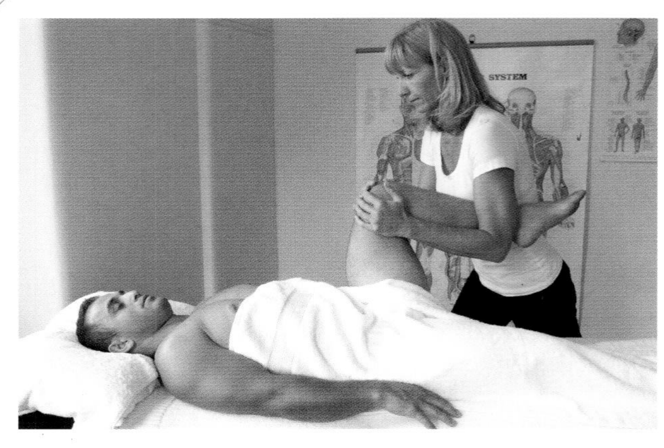

Fig. 7.31 Hip rotation

HIP FIGURE-8

The client lies supine with hip and knee flexed to 90°. Face across the client and place one hand over the knee joint and the other under the Achilles tendon. Maintaining the lower leg parallel to the table, alternately trace small circles with the knee and with the foot which creates a figure-8 of the hip joint. (see Figure 7.32)

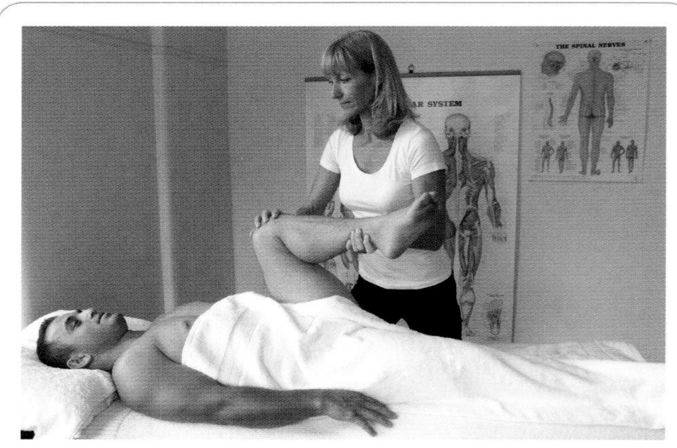

Fig. 7.32 Hip figure-8

HIP TRACTION

The client is supine and holds the top of the table with both hands overhead. A towel folded into a strap is placed on the posterior aspect of the lower leg under the Achilles tendon. The ends of the towel are crossed over the dorsum of the foot and wrapped under the plantar aspect of the foot. Next the lateral end of the towel is twisted over the medial end. This has the effect of internally rotating the leg. Firmly grip the twisted ends of the towel, further internally rotate the leg and raise it 20° off the table. Slow and gentle traction is applied to the leg. Hold for 5 seconds and slowly release. (see Figure 7.33)

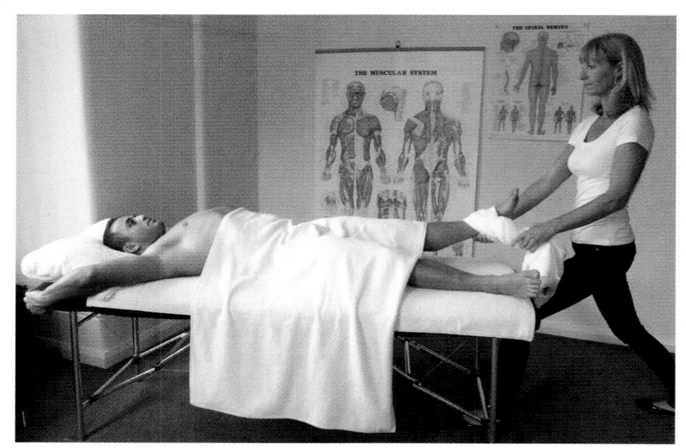

Fig. 7.33 Hip traction

HIP ROTATION SIDELYING

This technique aims to mobilise the femoral head anteromedially at the acetabular joint. The client lies on the uninvolved side close to the edge of the table and slightly bends the hip and knee of the lower leg. Stand behind the client facing across the client. The upper leg is straight. The client holds

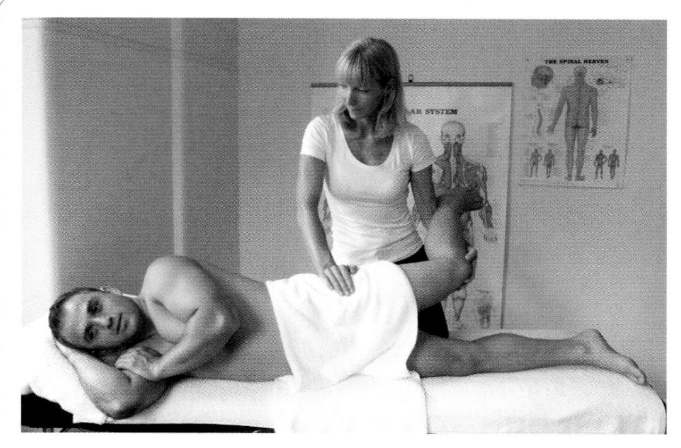

Fig. 7.34 Hip rotation sidelying

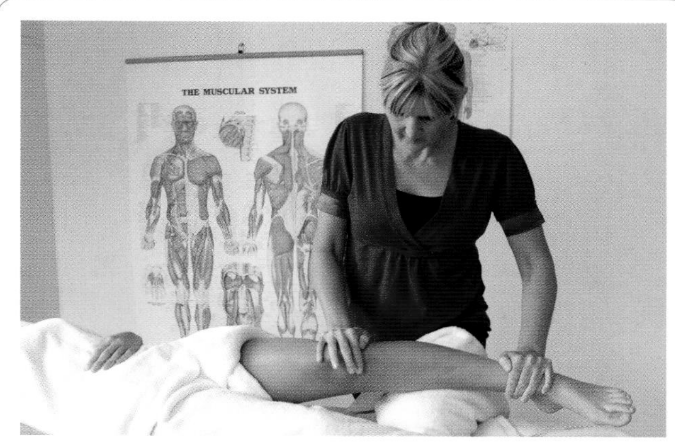

Fig. 7.36 Knee articulation (lateral approach)

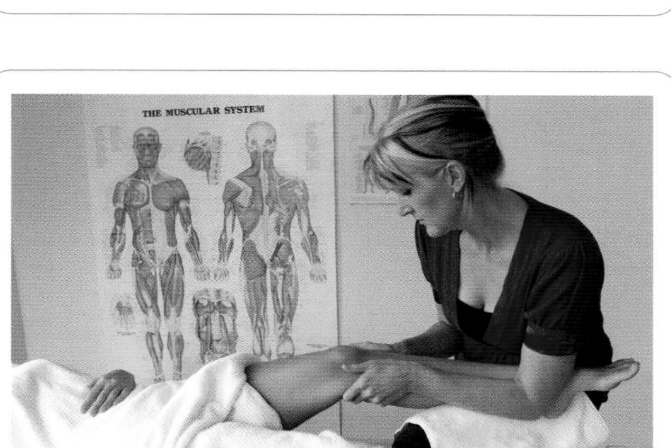

Fig. 7.35 Knee rotation (inferior approach)

the edge of the table in front to prevent rolling forward. Rest your caudal knee on the edge of the table for balance. Place your cephalad palm over the lateral aspect of the client's greater trochanter, fingers and thumb pointing anteriorly. With your other palm, reach under the ipsilateral leg and hold the femur just proximal to the knee. The upper leg is extended, abducted and internally rotated and then slowly circumducted while anteromedial pressure is maintained on the greater trochanter with your cephalad hand. (see Figure 7.34)

8. Knee joint

KNEE ARTICULATION (INFERIOR APPROACH)

The client lies supine, near the side of the table. Stand on the ipsilateral side of the client just inferior to the knee, and face cephalad. Rest your medial tibia on the table with your flexed knee pointing superomedially. Rest the client's mid calf over your knee. Place your lateral palm over the lateral aspect of the knee joint and the medial palm over the medial aspect of the knee joint. Wrap the fingers of both hands around the sides of the knee, point the thumbs superiorly and contact the sides of the patella. Lie your caudal forearm along the medial edge of the tibia to stabilise the leg. Slowly rotate the client's knee, keeping the lower leg still with your medial forearm. (see Figure 7.35)

KNEE ARTICULATION (LATERAL APPROACH)

This technique is contraindicated in clients with medial collateral ligament sprains. The client is supine. Face across the client and place your caudal knee on the table. Place the client's mid calf across your thigh. Place the palm of your cephalad hand over the knee, and your caudal palm over the front of the ankle. In this position, slightly internally rotate the client's leg. Using your hands, alternately make small circles with the knee and ankle in a bicycle-pedalling motion. (see Figure 7.36)

9. Ankle and foot

ANKLE PRONE CIRCUMDUCTION

The client lies prone near the side of the table with the knee flexed to 90°. Stand on the ipsilateral side and face across the client. Lie the palm of your cephalad hand over the plantar aspect of the calcaneus. Hold the dorsal aspect of the metatarsophalangeal joints with the palmar aspect of your caudal hand. Circumduct the talotibial joint and its adjacent articulations in both directions. (see Figure 7.37 on p 110)

CALCANEUS PRONE ARTICULATION

The client is prone with feet overhanging the end of the table. The client's knee is flexed to 90° or less. Stand at the foot of the table facing cephalad. Place your palms on the lateral and medial aspects of the calcaneus with your fingers interlocked, and take a firm grip on the calcaneus. Articulate the calcaneus in all directions. (see Figure 7.38 on p 110)

TARSALS PRONE PLANTARFLEXION

The client lies prone close to the side of the table with the knee flexed to 90°. Stand on the ipsilateral side and face inferomedially. Place the palm of the caudal hand on the dorsum of the foot. With your other hand, hold the plantar surface of the foot just distal to the calcaneus, fingers running transversely across the mid-plantar area. The client's foot is fully plantar flexed and inverted. From this position, *fold* the client's forefoot towards the calcaneus to mobilise the tarsal joints. (see Figure 7.39 on p 110)

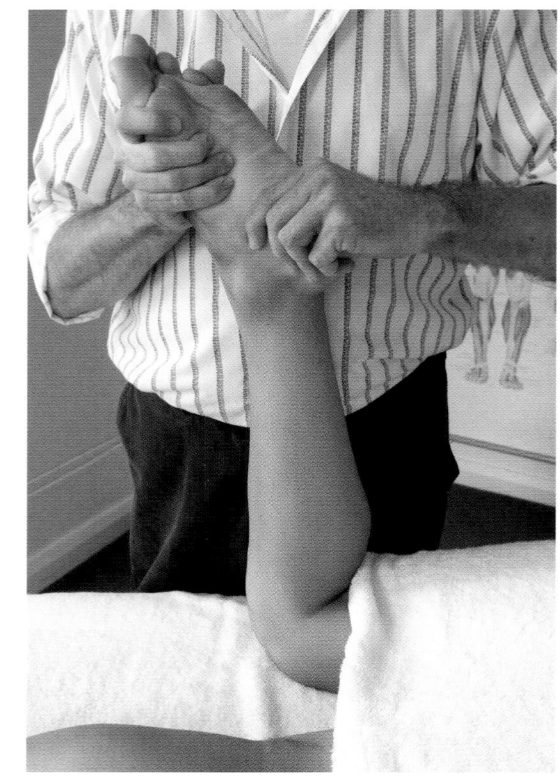

Fig. 7.37 Ankle prone circumduction

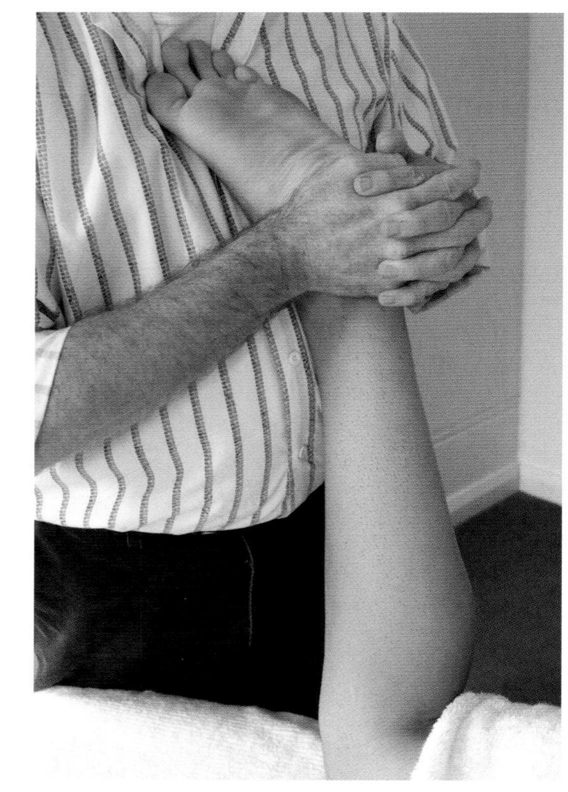

Fig. 7.38 Calcaneus prone articulation

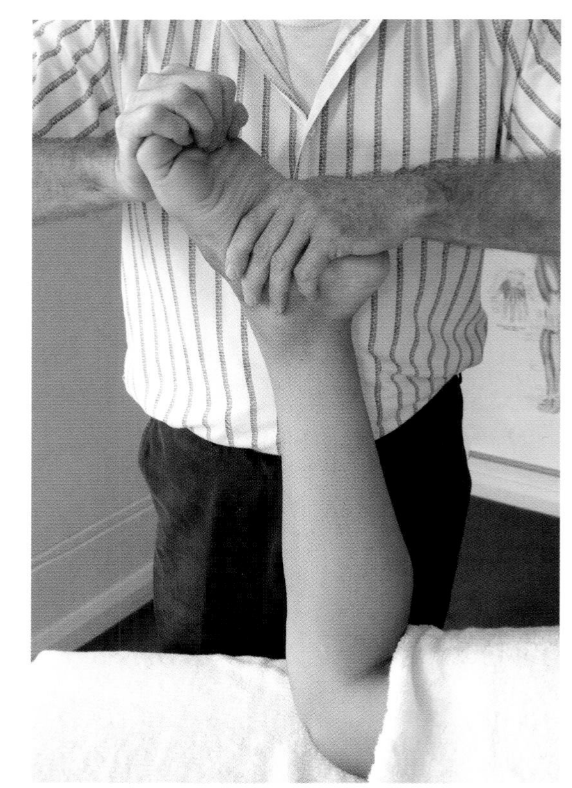

Fig. 7.39 Tarsals prone plantarflexion

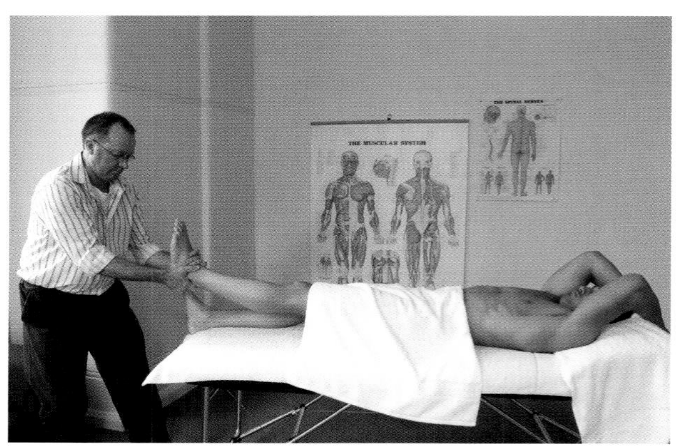

Fig. 7.40 Ankle traction

ANKLE TRACTION

The client is supine and holds the head of the table with both hands. Stand at the foot of the table facing cephalad. Place your medial hand on the client's medial arch, thumb under the sole and fingers wrapping over the dorsum of the foot. Hold the ankle with your lateral hand, the thumb across the front of the ankle and the fingers wrapping around the Achilles tendon. Apply gentle traction in an inferior direction to the client's slightly dorsiflexed foot. Hold the traction for 5 seconds, and slowly release. (see Figure 7.40)

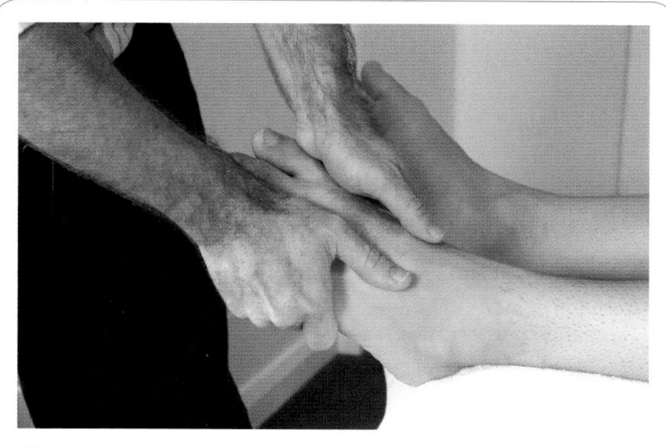

Fig. 7.41 Metatarsal shearing

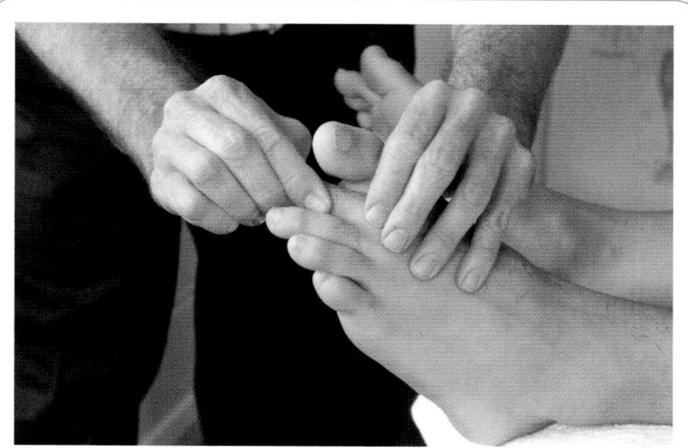

Fig. 7.42 Phalanges mobilisation

METATARSAL SHEARING

The client is supine. Stand at the foot of the table facing cephalad. Place thenar pads of both hands over the dorsal surface of the metatarsal heads, fingers wrapping around to the plantar surface. Slowly shear each metatarsal several times in an anterior–posterior direction. (see Figure 7.41)

PHALANGES MOBILISATION

The client is supine. Stand or sit at the foot of the table. Contact either side of the metatarsophalangeal or interphalangeal joint to be mobilised using thumb and index finger contacts. The proximal contact stabilises the joint. Perform a slow rotation in both directions and apply gentle traction. (see Figure 7.42)

CONTRAINDICATIONS

Contraindications include all those for Swedish massage as well as contraindications that apply specifically to joint articulation:[18]

- acutely inflamed joints
- recent fracture
- osteoporosis
- malignancy
- joint instability
- rheumatoid collagen necrosis
- joint ankylosis
- vertebrobasilar insufficiency (for cervical articulation)
- infections
- joint replacement
- severe degenerative joint disease
- history of disc lesions or radiculopathy.

Caution is required for:

- pregnancy
- hypermobility
- neurological signs
- spondylolisthesis.

KEY MESSAGES

- Passive joint articulation is an important treatment tool for joint pain and stiffness.
- Assessing clients for joint articulation includes history, functional tests and palpation.
- Capsular pattern refers to limitations of specific ranges of motion that develop when the joint capsule tightens. The concept has not been supported by recent research findings.
- A leathery or hard end-feel may indicate joint degeneration.
- Crepitus is sometimes heard when joints move. It suggests joint degeneration.
- Joint articulations are performed when the surrounding muscles are relaxed and warm. Joints are usually placed in mid-range. Generally the practitioner stabilises the proximal bone and articulates the distal one.
- Joint articulations are performed within the limits of accessory movements of joints and within the client's pain tolerance.
- The usual contraindications of Swedish massage apply to joint articulation as well as joint instability or ankylosis, joint replacement, severe rheumatoid arthritis or degenerative joint disease, vertebrobasilar insufficiency (cervical articulation) and history of disc lesions or radiculopathy.

Review questions

1. What is the difference between joint articulation/mobilisation and joint manipulation?
2. Circle true or false:
   a) Physiological movements can be actively performed by clients. True/False
   b) Component movements are determined by the laxity of the joint capsule. True/False
   c) Joint articulation uses physiological and accessory movement. True/False
   d) Component movements can be actively performed by clients. True/False
3. What does the term loose-pack joint position mean?
4. What is the capsular pattern for:
   a) cervical spine?
   b) shoulder?
   c) hip?
   d) knee?
5. List four contraindications for joint articulation.
6. How would you integrate joint articulation into a remedial massage treatment for a 60-year-old male with degenerative joint disease of the right hip?
7. What recommendations would you give a client after treatment with joint articulation?
8. What assessments would you carry out to determine the client's suitability for joint articulation?
9. Name three conditions of the shoulder joint that would benefit from joint articulation.
10. A 31-year-old male presents with chronic pain and inflammation that began in the sacroiliac joints four years ago and has spread to the low back, shoulders and hips. He reports pain that wakes him at night and recent night sweats. His pain seems to get worse after periods of inactivity. This history could suggest:
    a) Reiter's syndrome
    b) Anklyosing spondylitis
    c) Fibromyalgia
    d) Psoriatic arthritis

REFERENCES

1. Esposito S, Phillipson S. Spinal adjusting technique: the chiropractic art. Sydney, Australia: Well Adjusted Publishing; 2005.
2. Maitland G, Hengeveld E, Banks K, et al. Maitland's vertebral manipulation. 7th edn. London: Elsevier; 2005.
3. Vaillant J, Rouland A, Martigne P, et al. Massage and mobilization of the feet and ankles in elderly adults: effect on clinical balance performance. Man Ther 2009;14:661–4.
4. Vermeulen HM, Rozing PM, Obermann WR, et al. Comparison of high-grade and low-grade mobilization techniques in the management of adhesive capsulitis of the shoulder: randomized controlled trial. Phys Ther 2006;86(3):355–68.
5. Crow J, Gelfand B, Su E. Use of joint mobilization in a patient with severely restricted hip motion following bilateral hip resurfacing arthroplasty. Phys Ther 2008;88(12):1591–600.
6. Cleland JA, Glynn P, Whitman JM, et al. Short-term effects of thrust versus nonthrust mobilization/manipulation, directed at the thoracic spine in patients with neck pain: a randomized clinical trial. Phys Ther 2007;87(4):431–40.
7. Kay S, Haensel N, Stiller K. The effect of passive mobilisation following fractures involving the distal radius: a randomised study. Aust J Physiother 2000;46(2):93–101.
8. van der Wees PJ, Lenssen AF, Hendriks EJ, et al. Effectiveness of exercise therapy and manual mobilisation in ankle sprain and functional instability: a systematic review. Aust J Physiother 2006;52(1):27–37.
9. Tal-Akabi A, Rushton A. An investigation to compare the effectiveness of carpal bone mobilisation and neurodynamic mobilisation as methods of treatment for carpal tunnel syndrome. Manual Ther 2000;5(4):214–22.
10. Melzack R, Wall P. Pain mechanisms: a new theory. Science 1965;150(699):971–9.
11. Schmid A, Brunner F, Wright A, et al. Paradigm shift in manual therapy? Evidence for a central nervous system component in the response to passive cervical joint mobilisation. Manual Ther 2008;13:387–96.
12. Australian Acute Musculoskeletal Pain Guidelines Group. Evidence-based management of acute musculoskeletal pain. a guide for clinicians. Bowen Hills, Qld: Australian Academic Press; 2004.
13. Carnes M, Vizniak N. Quick reference evidence-based conditions manual. 3rd edn. Burnaby, BC: Professional Health Systems; 2009.
14. Klassbo M, Harms-Ringdahl K, Larsson G, et al. Examination of passive ROM and capsular patterns in the hip. Physiother Res Int 2003;8(1):1–12.
15. Bijl D, Dekker J, van Baar ME, et al. Validity of Cyriax's concept capsular pattern for the diagnosis of osteoarthritis of hip and/or knee. Scand J Rheumatol 1998;27(5):347–51.
16. Tomberlin J, Saunders D. Evaluation, treatment and prevention of musculoskeletal disorders: extremities. 3rd edn. Chaska, MN: Educational Opportunities; 1995.
17. Hertling D, Kessler R. Management of common musculoskeletal disorders. 3rd edn. Philadelphia: Lippincott; 1996.
18. Lepak V. Principles of joint mobilizations. Online. Available: http://moon.ouhsc.edu/llepak/7223/lecture/Joint%20mobilization.pdf.

8 Myofascial release

The content of this chapter relates to the following Units of Competency:

HLTREM503C Plan remedial massage treatment strategy
HLTREM504C Apply remedial massage assessment framework
HLTREM502C Provide remedial massage treatment
HLTREM505C Perform remedial massage health assessment

Health Training Package HLT07

Learning Outcomes

- Describe the properties and function of fascia and the causes and consequence of myofascial restrictions.
- Assess clients for myofascial restrictions.
- Describe the current evidence for the effectiveness of myofascial releasing techniques.
- Apply myofascial releasing techniques effectively and safely to a range of clients.
- Advise and resource clients who have been assessed and treated with myofascial releasing techniques.

INTRODUCTION

Myofascial release has been used in one form or another for a very long time. Andrew Taylor Still, the father of osteopathy, practised gentle release methods for connective tissue restrictions in the nineteenth century to assist in bringing about three-dimensional functional symmetry to his clients. The term *myofascial release* was coined in 1981 when it was first used to describe courses taught at Michigan State University. Other pioneers working with fascia include Janet Travell, Ida Rolf, Milton Traeger and John Barnes, each of whom developed their own approaches to assessing and treating clients with fascial restrictions.

Myofascial techniques are generally classified as direct (deep) or indirect (gentle). Direct techniques work on deep fascial restrictions. Ida Rolf's work, developed in the 1950s, involved direct myofascial techniques and movement education. Many contemporary myofascial techniques like structural integration, postural integration and deep tissue massage techniques have been developed from Rolf's original work. Indirect techniques, on the other hand, use gentle tractions to generate heat and increase blood flow, thereby releasing fascial restrictions.

John Barnes first developed his myofascial techniques to alleviate long-standing post-operative pain from spinal fusion in a client who had not responded to other techniques. Pain relief is one of the main uses of myofascial release today, including treatment and management of post-operative pain and sporting and other injuries. It is a very efficient technique for managing clients with either physical or emotional trauma. The gentle myofascial techniques in particular are welcomed by physical therapists who acknowledge the benefits for clients suffering chronic pain who can be treated without adding further mechanical stress to their already traumatised systems. The gentleness of indirect myofascial technique is also well suited to treating children, older clients and clients suffering from stress and anxiety-related conditions.

FUNCTIONAL ANATOMY REVIEW

The body is made up of different types of connective tissue including bone, adipose tissue, lymph, blood and fascia that support and protect most structures in the body. Fascia is a three-dimensional web of tough connective tissue that spreads throughout the body as a single structure. It gives the body its form and scaffolding and connects all structures of the body.[1] The analogy that is commonly used to describe fascia is that of a knitted sweater: just as pulling one sleeve affects the whole sweater, fascial distortions or restrictions in any area can affect the whole body.[2]

The main functions of fascia are:

- maintaining normal shape
- maintaining vital organs in their correct position
- resisting mechanical stress (strength, support, elasticity and cushioning)
- nutritive: loose connective tissue contains fluid that serves as a transport medium for cellular elements of other tissues, blood and lymph
- providing an additional surface area for muscle attachments (deep fascia)
- conserving body heat in fat stores (superficial fascia)
- fighting bacterial infection: histiocytes offer defence when infectious substances pass through planes in connective tissue

- healing: fascia deposits collagen fibres (scar tissue) to assist in healing injuries.

Connective tissue is characterised by few cells dispersed in a large extracellular matrix. The extracellular matrix contains a fibrous component made up of elastin and collagen and a non-fibrous component called ground substance. Ground substance contains proteins that attract and bind water. Different structures of the body require collagen and elastin in different proportions depending on their function.[3, 4]

Fascia is a colloid, which means that it is composed of particles of solid matter suspended in fluid.

- The fluid (ground substance) contains glycosaminoglycans (predominantly hyaluronan), proteoglycans, glycoproteins and water. Ground substance is highly viscous. It is hydrophilic (water-loving) which aids lubrication and resists compression like a shock absorber.
- The solid matter (fibrous component) is made up of fibroblasts, chondrocytes, collagen and elastin. Collagen provides strength and elastin fibres allow structures to return to their original shape after stretching. The fibres align along lines of stress to absorb tensile forces.

Superficial and deep fascia are dense irregular connective tissue containing thick bundles of collagen arranged irregularly to resist tension applied in many directions. Deep fascia is a coarse sheet of connective tissue that surrounds and infuses with muscles, bones, nerves, blood vessels and organs. It includes fascia surrounding a group of muscles, epimysium surrounding individual muscles, and perimysium surrounding fascicles within muscles (see Figure 8.1). The deepest fascia is the dura of the craniosacral system. Superficial fascia (hypodermis) lies directly below the skin. It contains fat, muscle tissue, cutaneous blood vessels and nerves.

Myers[2] describes the fascial system as conveying mechanical information through its response to pushes and pulls. He described a number of myofascial meridians or common pathways for this mechanical communication including (see Figure 8.2 on p 115):

- Superficial back line
- Superficial front line
- Spiral line
- Arm lines
- Functional lines
- Deep front line

Most changes in connective tissue are degenerative.[4] Fascia can also become restricted as a result of physical strain, which has been shown to increase collagen and fascial myofibroblasts, which can cause fascial contraction.[5] Overuse, trauma, infectious agents, poor posture, inactivity and psychological states can result in pain, muscle tension and diminished blood flow. If fascia is immobilised for any reason the ground substance gradually solidifies making it difficult for collagen fibres to slide over each other. Eventually adhesions form and connective tissue thickens (becomes fibrotic) which in turn can lead to further pain and irritation. Myofascial releasing techniques aim to break this cycle.[6]

WHAT IS MYOFASCIAL RELEASE?

Myofascial release is an interactive hands-on technique for evaluating and treating the whole body via its fascial network. The body's connective tissue network responds to mechanical pressure. The aim of myofascial release is to return the body as closely as possible to balanced structural alignment so as to allow greater flexibility and ease of movement. In particular, myofascial release aims to:

- lengthen contracted tissue
- reduce fascial adhesions
- increase range of motion
- decrease compartment pressure
- restore elasticity.

Because of its viscous nature, fascia resists compression forces. Its resistance increases in proportion to the pressure

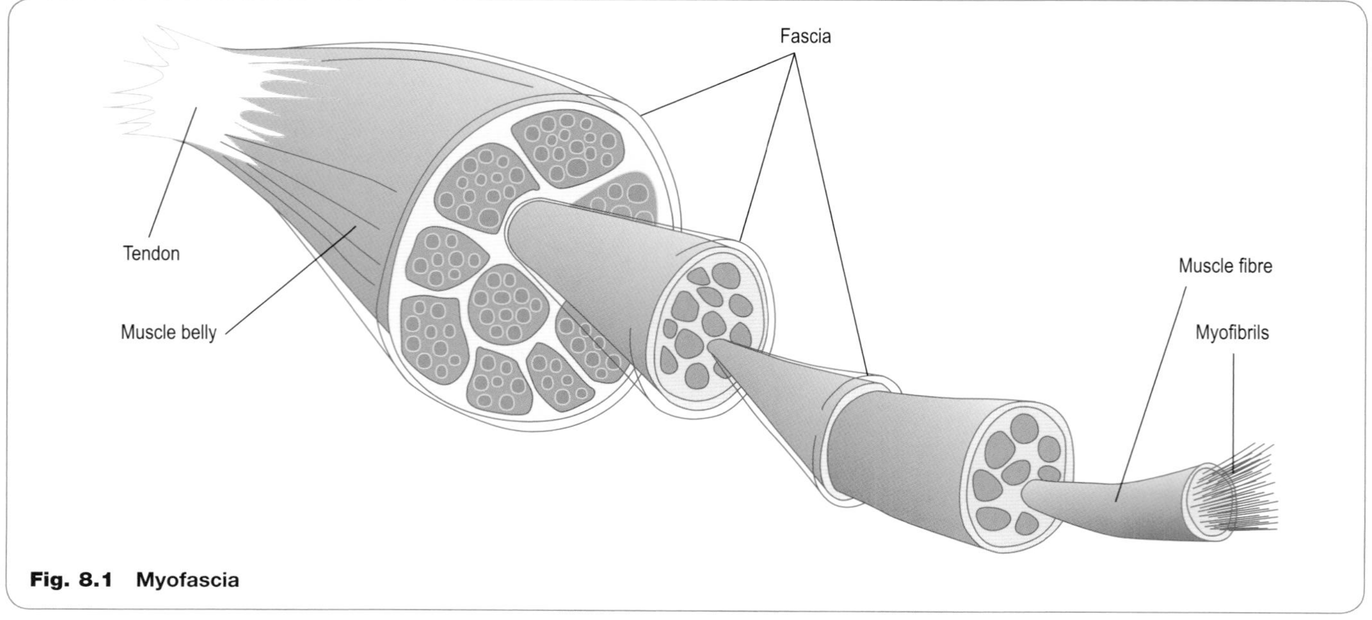

Fig. 8.1 Myofascia

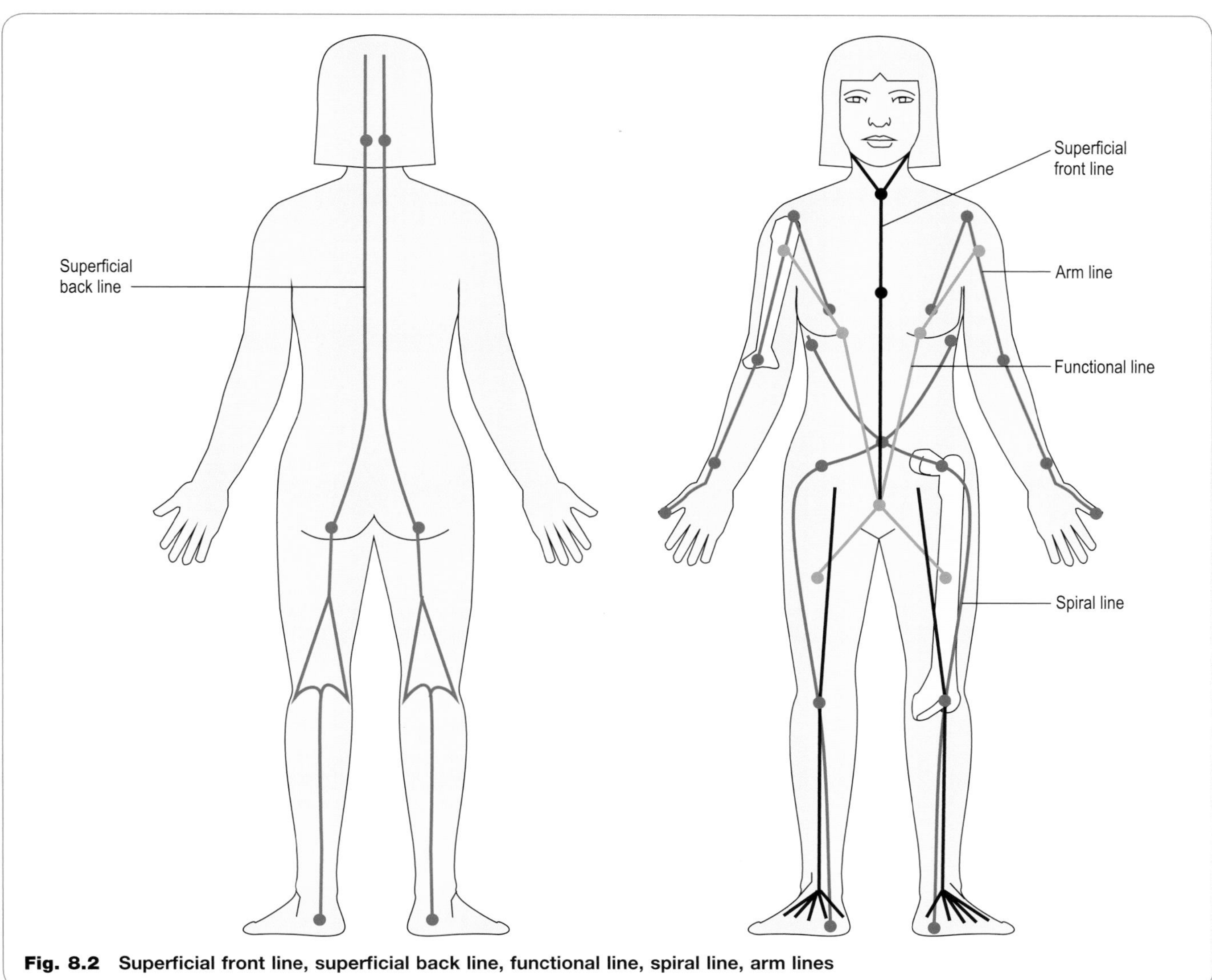

Fig. 8.2 Superficial front line, superficial back line, functional line, spiral line, arm lines

applied to it. This means that gentle sustained pressure is required to affect fascia. Colloids also respond to heat by changing from a gel-like consistency to a more watery state.

Deep myofascial releasing techniques (including rolfing, postural integration, deep connective tissue massage) have evolved to include the integration of controlled breathing techniques and specific body positioning so that practitioners can reach deep myofascial layers within the client's pain tolerance. Deep myofascial release works by breaking adhesions, elongating and stretching fascia. The deeper forms of myofascial release are often associated with a psychological or emotional response. Rolf proposed that releasing muscle tension also released associated emotional trauma.[7] However, even gentle applications of myofascial release can arouse an emotional response in susceptible clients. Refer clients to a psychologist, counsellor or medical practitioner when dealing with emotional responses that are beyond the scope of remedial massage therapy.

ASSESSING CLIENTS

Assessment procedures for all remedial massage clients includes case history, postural analysis, functional testing and palpation. For myofascial release, palpatory findings are particularly informative.

HISTORY

Myofascial restrictions do not produce referred pain in the same way as trigger points. The site of the original injury gradually spreads and tightens in many directions producing pain and discomfort. The progression of such symptoms as aching pain, headaches, discomfort, limited range of motion and impaired respiration suggests myofascial restrictions. Clients are often not aware of an original event (e.g. trauma, overuse, jaw clenching, surgery) that may be the cause of their present pain especially if symptoms are felt at a site that is distant from the original injury site. As with all case histories, it is important to identify the presence of red or yellow flags and to refer clients where appropriate (see Chapter 2).

POSTURAL ANALYSIS

Myofascial restrictions influence the way the body moves and performs adaptive responses and may be evident in postural analysis. For example, internal or external hip rotation, pelvic imbalance, leg length discrepancy, forward head carriage, shoulder protraction, hyperkyphosis and hyperlordosis may be associated with myofascial restrictions. The fascial lines of the body are observed and compared (e.g. left lateral line compared to the right, left spiral line compared to the right). Figure 8.3 shows two examples of postural analysis using fascial lines. Treatment plans can then be developed for stretching restricted fascial lines.[2]

FUNCTIONAL TESTS

Clients with myofascial restrictions usually have muscle imbalances that can be observed during functional testing (active, passive and resisted range of motion) (see Chapter 2). Findings from functional testing direct practitioners to target tissues.

PALPATION

Palpatory assessments provide further information including temperature, dryness and tissue adhesions. Fascial restrictions often palpate as cold and dry and with reduced fascial glide. Practitioners need to be mindful that they are palpating myofascial restrictions, not specific muscles. Fascia tend to run in straight lines.[2, 8] The superficial back line, for example, runs from the plantar fascia to the gastrocnemius, hamstrings, sacrotuberous ligament, erector spinae and then to the fascia of the scalp. Fascial lines also run at a consistent depth. They are tied to underlying tissues at muscle and ligament attachments.

Some practitioners describe a myofascial end-feel, the practitioner's perception of barriers to movement. Myofascial end-feel is described as soft and rubbery.

TREATING CLIENTS

Myofascial release techniques are interactive in that the practitioner monitors feedback from the client's body which determines the direction, force and duration of the techniques. The direction of the movement does not depend on the direction of specific muscles. Fascia is an extensive three-dimensional network and treatments applied to one area can affect the entire network. A leg traction, for instance, can facilitate a fascial release in the neck.

Myofascial release is performed in a step-by-step progression as each restriction responds to treatment. As the release occurs the practitioner usually palpates a relaxation and elongation of tissues and may observe other involuntary physiological reactions like tonic muscular activity and eye movements.[9] The client may report a sensation of heat, cold or tingling. Changes to the client's posture do not normally happen quickly. The central nervous system takes time to be re-educated to maintain more energy-efficient postures.

Through the combined effect of the client's responses to myofascial release and the therapist's ability to *listen with their hands*, normal functioning may be restored to tissues.

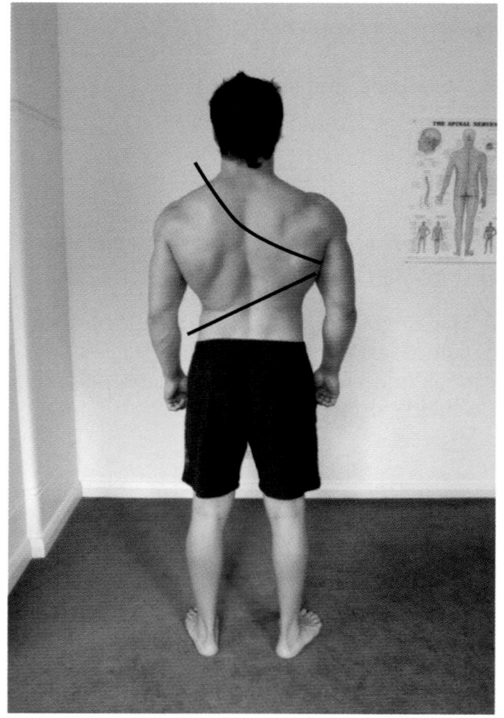

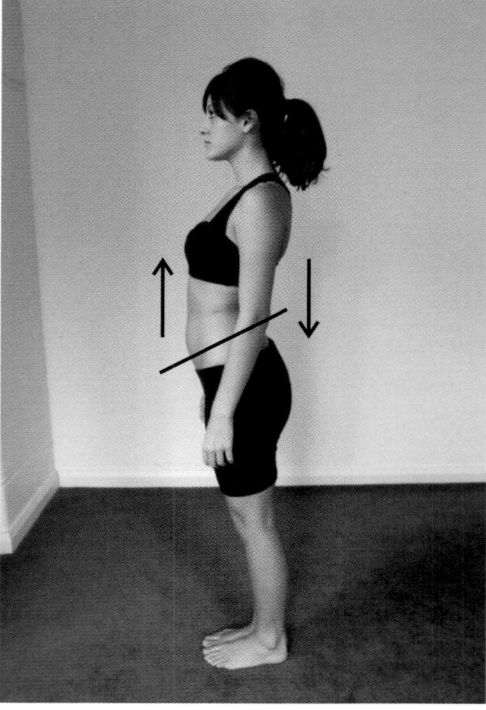

Fig. 8.3 Postural analysis using fascial lines

This is achieved by removing pressure from nerves, blood vessels, organs and joints and promoting re-alignment and improved range of motion to the structures of the body.

EVIDENCE FOR THE EFFECTIVENESS OF FASCIAL RELEASING TECHNIQUES

Several studies investigating the effectiveness of myofascial release have found promising results. For example:

- Meltzer et al[10] conducted an in vitro study to potentially explain the immediate clinical outcomes associated with myofascial release. The authors concluded that treating with myofascial release following modelled repetitive motion strain resulted in normalisation in apoptic (cell death) rate and cell morphology. This could reflect tissue texture changes and increased myofascial elasticity.
- Martin[11] performed 20 sessions of myofascial release on one client with diffuse systemic sclerosis and found remodelling of the connective tissue affected by diffuse systemic sclerosis. The client was found to have increased range of motion in joints, reduced effects of Raynaud's phenomenon and reduced pain.
- Barnes et al[12] investigated the efficacy of myofascial release on pelvic symmetry using 10 subjects with unilateral anterior rotation of the innominate of more than 10 mm and perceived low back and/or sacroiliac symptoms. The authors concluded that myofascial release has the potential to be effective in facilitating a change in pelvic position towards symmetry.
- Arroyo-Morales et al[13] studied 62 healthy individuals for the usefulness of massage as a recovery method after high-intensity exercise and concluded that myofascial release favours the recovery of heart ventilation and diastolic BP after high-intensity exercise.

As with all research, caution is required when interpreting results of studies of low methodological quality.

APPLYING THE TECHNIQUES

Myofascial release can be used as a modality in its own right or in combination with other manual therapies including other remedial massage techniques, sports massage and craniosacral therapy. Myofascial techniques are usually performed without oil or lubricant so as to prevent sliding over the tissues.

Good ergonomics are required, whether applying deep or gentle techniques, to minimise stress on the practitioner. Massage therapists are prone to musculoskeletal injuries, especially of the low back, wrists and thumbs.[14, 15] All massage techniques should be based on sound biomechanical principles and adapted to suit the needs of individual therapists. Correct table height and stance are fundamental. Awkward and prolonged techniques, particularly those using thumbs or extended wrists, should be replaced by the correct use of forearms, knuckles and fists.[16]

MFR techniques

1. DEEP TECHNIQUES

Deep connective tissue release focuses on the deeper tissue structures of the muscle and fascia to provide physiological release of tension or adhesions in tissues and psychological release from stored emotional memories.[17] Deep myofascial release involves the use of slow, deep pressure applied with fingers, knuckles, fists, forearms or elbows. (see Figure 8.4 on p118)

Technique

- Lower the table height so that body weight can be used efficiently.
- Do not use oil so that the superficial layers of skin and fascia are moved. (Note: a small quantity of cream or lotion may be used if the client has very dry or fragile skin.)
- Warm up the area using compressions or other dry warm-up techniques.
- Use body supports (e.g. thoracic roll) and body positioning to stretch tissues before applying the techniques.
- Work with the client's breathing. Work through superficial tissues to locate deep layers and advance the contact as the client exhales.
- Work within the client's pain range and ask for regular feedback.
- Apply slow short strokes over small areas.
- Always maintain correct posture and use body weight to reduce pressure on joints (e.g. transferring weight from the back leg to the front) and use a variety of body parts including knuckles, fist, forearm and elbow. For good biomechanics hyperextending thumbs and wrists should be avoided. Elbows should be kept straight but not locked. Riggs suggests internally rotating the arm to keep the wrist in a neutral position.[16]
- Use larger contacts (e.g. forearms) before smaller contacts (e.g. thumb and fingers).
- After applying the technique, stretch the muscle and/or take the joint slowly through its full range of motion.
- Instruct the client to drink plenty of water.

Techniques can be applied to specific regions of the body or along fascial lines. For example, techniques applied to the superficial back line could include:

- knuckles to plantar fascia
- knuckles around lateral malleoli
- thumb frictions across the lateral ligaments
- knuckles around calcaneus
- knuckles/forearm to gastrocnemius
- thumbs or fingertips to separate gastrocnemius and soleus
- forearms and fists to hamstrings
- knuckles around ischial tuberosity (flex and externally rotate the hip for better access)
- fists to gluteals (face across the client and glide from sacrum inferolaterally)
- thumb/knuckles to sacrotuberous ligament
- forearms/knuckles along erector spinae
- fists/knuckles to posterior cervical muscles
- fingers to scalp fascia.

2. GENTLE TECHNIQUES

The style of myofascial release described in this section is based on the work of John Barnes.[17] This style uses gentle open-handed touch to maximise the contact area (except for small children where finger contact may be more appropriate). The technique is progressively applied to one area and after a softening and elongation of affected tissues has been

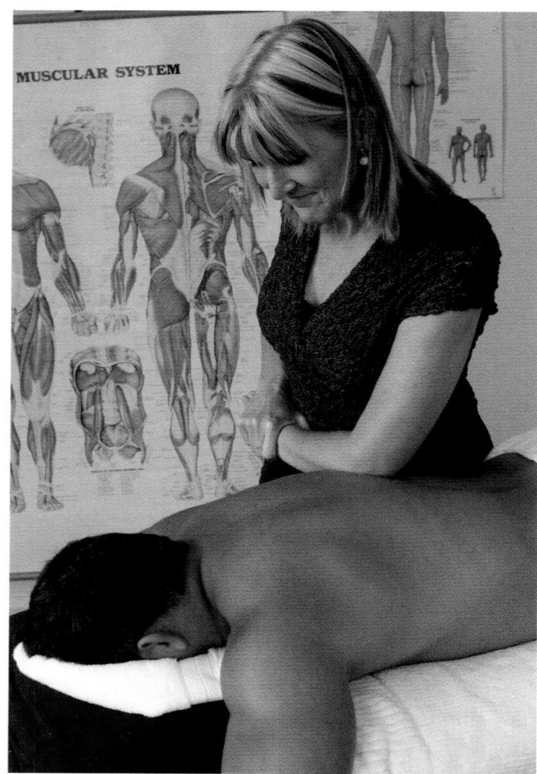

Fig. 8.4 Deep myofascial release

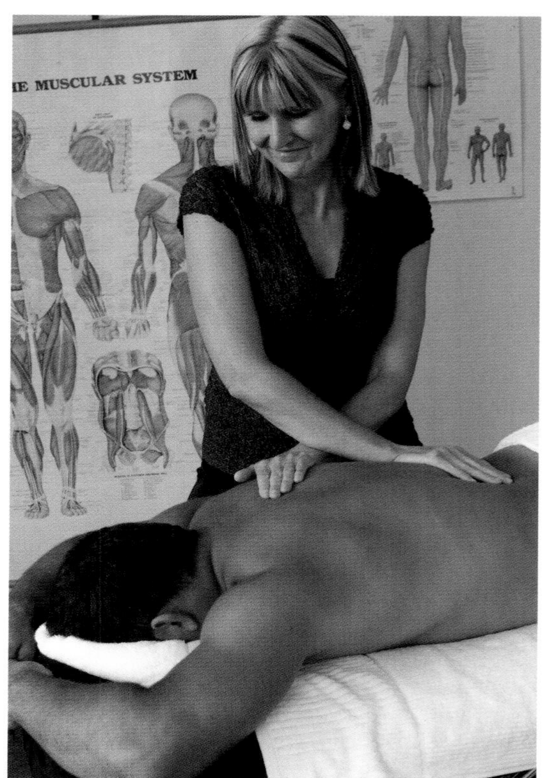

Fig. 8.5 Cross-hand technique

achieved, then to another restricted area. Myofascial release is a very safe technique. Appropriate monitoring of clients' responses prevents inadvertently overstretching the soft tissues of the body.

Key features of gentle myofascial releasing techniques are:

- Light
- Sustained
- Interactive
- Progressive.

Applying gentle techniques involves:

- locating the restriction (e.g. palpate for cold, dry, tight tissue)
- applying gentle pressure to engage the elastic component of the myofascia which has a springy feel (if your hands are not allowed to sink into the first barrier before proceeding, the client may experience a burning sensation as the skin is overstretched)
- gently stretching target tissue between your contacts until a resistance to further stretch is felt – this stretch realigns the elastin and collagen fibres, and is maintained until the hands stop at a firmer (collagen) barrier
- holding until the soft tissues relax or elongate ('calm sensation of relaxation'[6]) for usually 3–5 minutes. After the initial release, further releases may occur without any change in contact (Bertolucci[9] described a 'singular springy sensation that causes the force of the practitioner to rebound', and then further suggested that this 'sense of firmness' is a hallmark of MFR and should increase in intensity as the technique is applied)
- from this new (elongated) position, further stretching the tissues between your hands to take up the tissue slack until another barrier is felt[17]
- repeating the process until the tissues are fully elongated.

Gentle pressure is required to overcome barriers because of the viscous nature of fascia. A low load applied slowly and gently facilitates more flow in a viscous medium than a high load applied quickly or with heavy pressure. Thermotherapy may also be beneficial.

Techniques

1. Cross-hand technique

One commonly used technique, the cross-handed technique, can be applied all over the body on areas of fascial restriction. The hands are placed lightly onto an area of fascial restriction and allowed to sink into the tissues until a barrier is perceived. This is sometimes called the depth barrier. Next, the hands separate slowly until another barrier is felt. This is called the elastic and muscular barrier. Your hands now follow the tissues in whatever direction they move until a release or softening and elongation of the tissue is achieved. This usually takes from 3 to 5 minutes. Fascial release may be felt between 90 and 120 seconds but it may be premature to release the technique at this point. Maintaining the technique for 3–5 minutes may achieve longer-lasting results (see Figure 8.5).[18]

To minimise stress on your own body, place your hands on the area being treated and lean forward so that depth is achieved with your own body weight. The arms are kept flexed at the elbows, ensuring that you follow the tissues as they release rather than pushing through them.

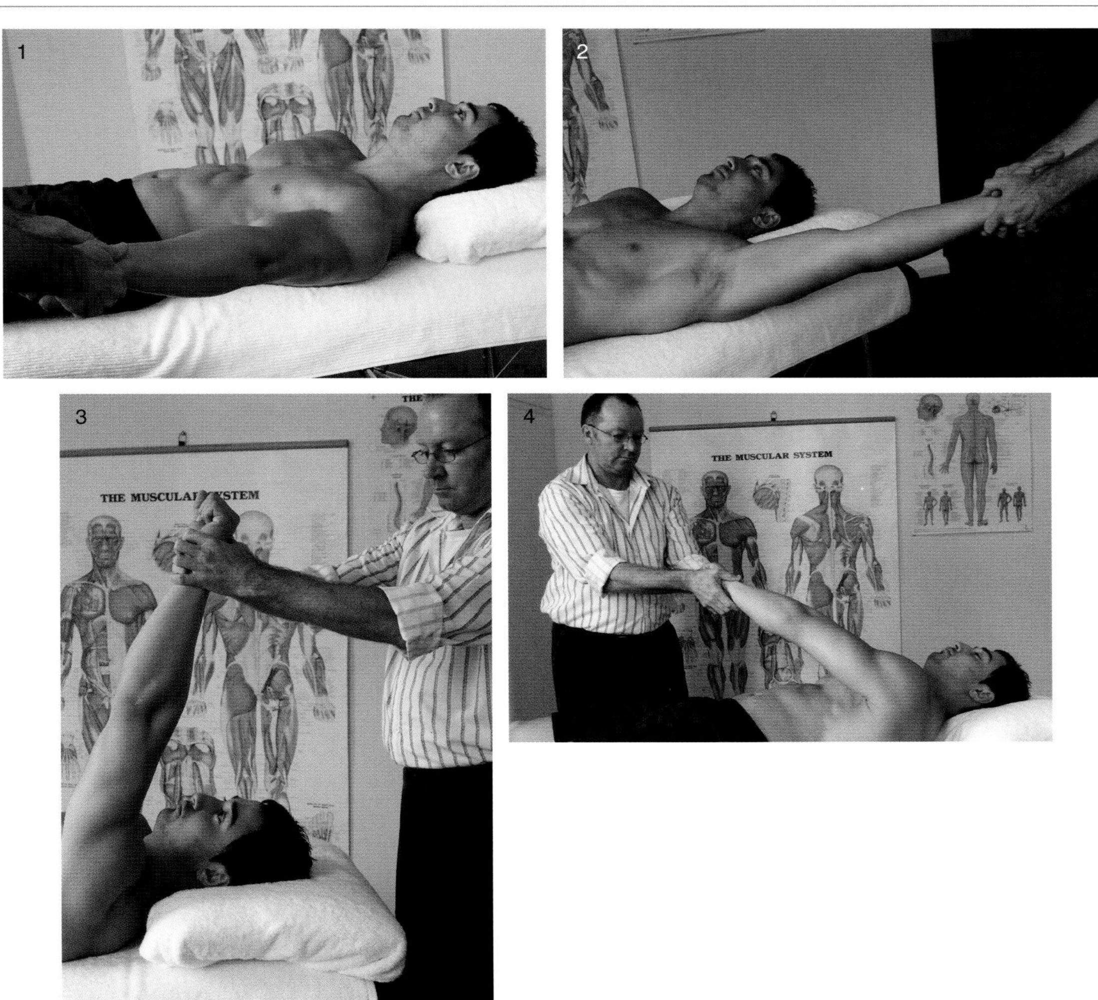

Fig. 8.6 Arm pull

2. Traction techniques

When performing traction techniques (i.e. leg and arm pulls, (see Figures 8.6 and 8.7 on page 119–120) both the client and the practitioner sense the elongation in the treated limb. Apply a gentle, slow, sustained traction to the whole limb, holding at each restriction before moving onto the next. The limbs move through an arc into abduction and then across the body into adduction. When a myofascial release has taken place the limb feels heavy and loose.[6] Traction techniques can increase the range of motion of the extremity. These techniques take time. Rushing the movements will not provide any long-lasting changes. The results of waiting and working with the tissues are worth the effort.

Try to keep your upper trapezius muscles relaxed and your knees flexed while performing this technique. Contacts for the arm pull are usually two hands around the wrist, or one hand at the wrist and the other at the elbow. For the leg pull, the contacts are either two hands at the ankle, or one hand at the knee and one at the ankle. Be careful not to hold the limb too tightly. Change hand contacts as often as is required for the client's comfort and to minimise the stress on you.

3. Transverse holds

Fascia in the body is predominantly vertically oriented. However, there are very important transverse planes. These can be found at the areas of transitional spinal curves (i.e. C7–T1, T12–L1 and L5–S1) and at each joint. The hyoid bone and cranial base can also be regarded as a transverse plane. These areas are quite often places of major dysfunction as they can be subject to large amounts of stress.

Myofascial release for the thoracic inlet and the respiratory and pelvic diaphragms are usually performed with clients in the supine position. (However, if the client is unable to lie supine, the techniques can be performed with the client prone or in a sidelying position.) Sit or stand at the side of the table level with the transverse structure being treated. Place the cephalad hand under the client's back, and the caudal hand on the anterior aspect of the body at the level of the transverse plane. Light anteroposterior pressure is applied with the caudal hand until a barrier is felt. After 90 to 120 seconds you may feel a movement in the tissues. Follow this movement with your caudal hand until an end-feel has been perceived. Remove both hands slowly.

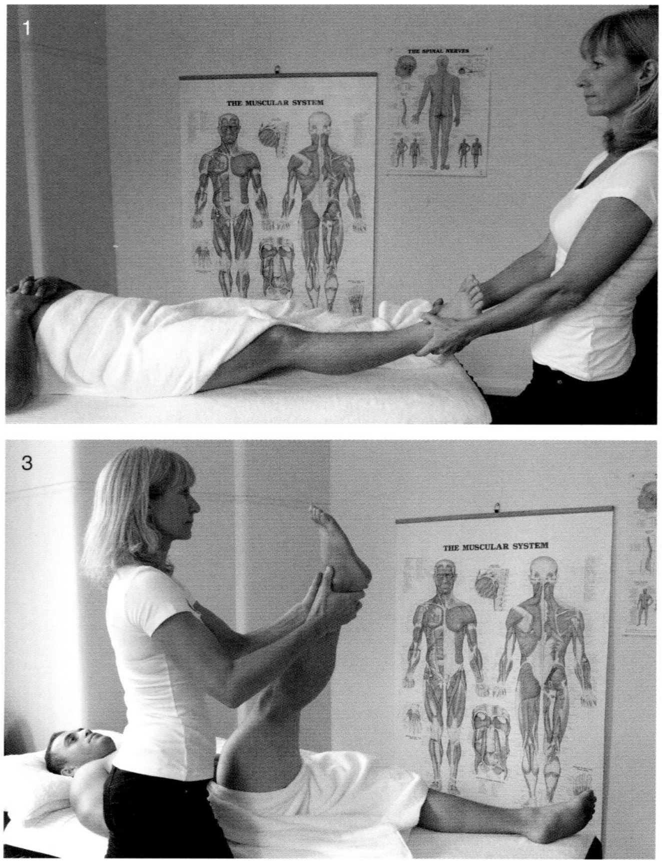

Fig. 8.7 Leg pull

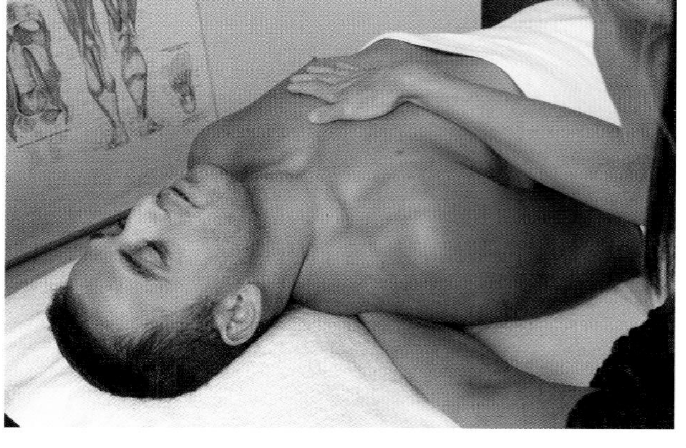

Fig. 8.8 Thoracic inlet release

C7–T1 Thoracic inlet/anterior chest wall For the thoracic inlet the anterior hand is placed just under the clavicles at the sternoclavicular joint. The thoracic inlet release is often used before myofascial releasing techniques for the neck, shoulder or cranium. It is beneficial for clients with breathing problems, musculoskeletal problems of the neck, shoulder and upper limb, and to promote lymph drainage. (see Figure 8.8)

T12–L1 Respiratory diaphragm release For the respiratory diaphragm release, the anterior hand is placed over the xiphoid process and on the upper part of the abdomen. This technique is useful for low back pain because iliopsoas and quadratus lumborum muscles communicate with this diaphragm. The quadratus lumborum is also involved in breathing. The respiratory diaphragm and thoracic inlet release can be used to open the chest for more efficient breathing. (see Figure 8.9 on p 121)

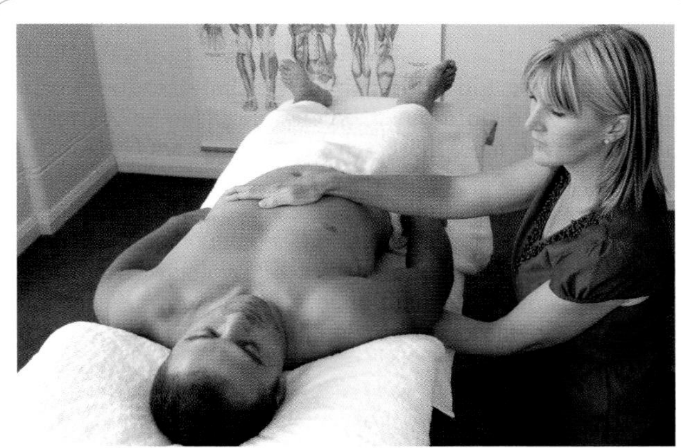
Fig. 8.9 Respiratory diaphragm release

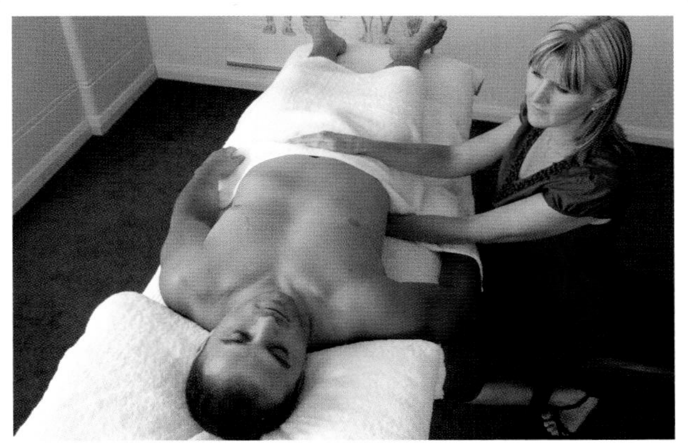
Fig. 8.10 Pelvic diaphragm release

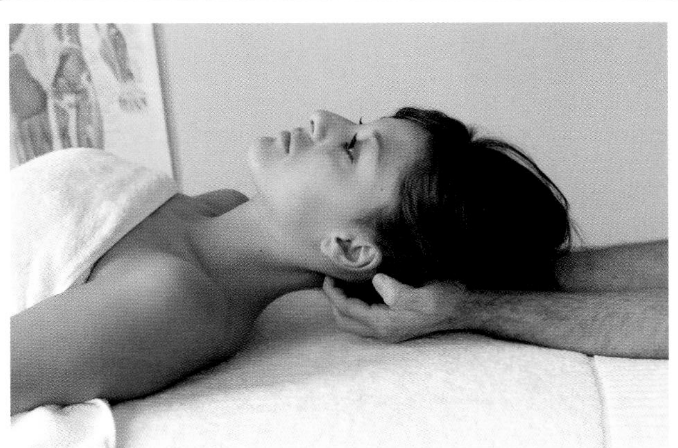
Fig. 8.11 Cranial base release

L5–S1 Pelvic diaphragm release For the pelvic diaphragm release, the anterior hand is placed on the abdomen with the hypothenar eminence at the superior border of the pubic ramus and the rest of the hand over the suprapubic region. The pelvic diaphragm release may be beneficial for low back pain, sacral pain and lower abdominal discomfort. (see Figure 8.9)

4. Cranial base release

Sit at the head of the table with the client lying supine. Cup the client's occiput in both hands and let your hands rest on the table. Spreading fingers of both hands, place your fingertips under the occiput and appy slow gentle pressure with the fingertips in an anterior direction. As the tissues relax and elongate, the client's head extends over your fingertips. This is a very useful technique for the treatment of neck pain, stress and headache. (see Figure 8.11)

INTEGRATING MYOFASCIAL RELEASING TECHNIQUES WITH REMEDIAL MASSAGE

Myofascial techniques are often used at the beginning of a remedial massage before oil has been applied, or at the end of the treatment after the oil has been removed. The use of myofascial release before any other remedial techniques may enhance the efficacy of the entire treatment and may also reduce your workload. Table 8.1 presents some of the key considerations associated with the integration of myofascial release into a remedial massage treatment.

CONTRAINDICATIONS AND PRECAUTIONS

Contraindications for myofascial release are similar to those for other forms of manual therapies including:

- any red flag (indication of serious underlying medical condition)
- acute inflammation
- lumps and tissue changes
- rashes and hyperaemia
- obstructive oedema
- mood alterations (e.g. depression, anxiety)
- contagious or infectious disease that may be spread by the upper respiratory tract or by direct contact with the skin
- fever
- cellulitis
- osteoporosis (for deep myofascial release)
- the client being unable to give informed consent
- the client being under the influence of alcohol or other substance.

Perform myofascial release with caution when the following conditions are present:

- Hypotension. Myofascial release may lower blood pressure. Instruct the client to lie quietly for a few minutes after treatment and to get up slowly as they may feel light headed.
- Haematoma, open wounds, recent surgery, healing fracture. Work away from the involved area.
- Osteoporosis and advanced degenerative changes. Work gently and focus on uninvolved areas.

Table 8.1 Integrating myofascial release (MFR) into remedial massage treatment

1. MFR initially, augmented by remedial massage techniques	The aim of the first session is to eliminate the client's initial symptoms. ■ Treat the area of the main presenting condition first. ■ Monitor for signs that may arise in an area distant to the tissues being treated. Signs could include heat, cold, tingling or pain sensations (vasomotor responses) indicating a further area in need of treatment. ■ Treat with transverse plane releases, cross-hand technique or leg or arm pull techniques. In subsequent sessions search for the cause of the problem. This may involve areas of discomfort which may be distant from the site of initial symptoms (*treat the pain, look elsewhere for the cause*). ■ Eliminate causative and perpetuating factors where possible. ■ Mechanical stresses cause myofascial restriction. Restrictions occur at the injury site and because of fascia's extensive network, pain and restrictions may migrate in many directions. ■ Work systematically through the body with MFR to release the symptoms and the cause for long-term relief. Work in the correcting direction according to postural analysis (e.g. moving the superior frontal line superiorly and the superficial back line inferiorly). Work superficial layers before deep ones then work on places where fascial meridians cross, especially spiral and functional lines.[2] ■ Use a range of remedial techniques (e.g. trigger point therapy, muscle stretching, soft tissue releasing techniques, deep transverse friction) to eliminate mechanical factors such as chronic inefficient postural adaptations, inefficient movement patterns. Use Swedish massage or other relaxation techniques to eliminate systemic factors such as emotional stress.
2. Other remedial techniques initially, augmented by MFR	MFR aims to improve circulation, relieve pressure on pain-sensitive structures, allow for greater cellular nutrition, respiration and elimination, improve range of motion. ■ Upper body treatment using remedial techniques. Include respiratory diaphragm and thoracic inlet release. ■ Lower body treatment with remedial technique. Include respiratory diaphragm and the pelvic diaphragm. ■ Use cross-hand technique on affected areas.
3. Client education	■ Advise the client to drink plenty of water after treatment. ■ Educate the client in ways to minimise mechanical stresses. ■ Eliminate causative factors (e.g. chronic inefficient postural habits) where possible. ■ Encourage the client to be aware of the effects of poor postures and to adopt good postural habits.[8] ■ Heat packs may be beneficial. ■ Suggest exercises such as Pilates, yoga, walking. If stress of any sort is a factor, meditation, tai-chi or Qigong may be beneficial.

- Anti-coagulant therapy. Be aware that the client may bruise easily.

KEY MESSAGES

- Myofascial release is an interactive hands-on technique for assessing and treating conditions such as musculoskeletal pain, tight muscles, limited range of motion and poor posture.
- Myofascial release techniques fall into two main categories: direct (deep) myofascial release and indirect (gentle) myofascial release.
- Assessment of clients for myofascial release includes history, postural analysis, functional assessment and palpation.
- Myofascial postural analysis involves observing distortions in posture in relation to myofascial meridians.
- Fascial restrictions often palpate as tight, cold and dry.
- Fascia responds to mechanical approaches that influence its viscous and plastic properties. Deep myofascial release involves working through superficial layers, slowly applying pressure to a deep myofascial layer, working in time with the client's breathing and using a pain scale; gentle myofascial release involves gentle sustained pressure (3–5 minutes).
- Treatment involves beginning in one area of myofascial restriction, and waiting for release (elongation) of tissues before moving to another area.
- Treatment can be applied locally or throughout the whole body, usually along myofascial meridians. When working myofascial meridians, begin with superficial lines before deep lines.
- Myofascial release is associated with release of stored emotional memory.
- The gentle nature of indirect myofascial release makes it a popular and safe technique.

Review questions

1. Fascia is a colloid, which means it is made up of:
   a) loose and dense connective tissue
   b) solid matter suspended in a fluid
   c) regular, irregular and elastic connective tissue
   d) areolar and reticular connective tissue
2. The solid matter of fascia includes:
   a) glycosaminoglycans and water
   b) glycosaminoglycans and fibroblasts
   c) fibroblasts and chondrocytes
   d) water and collagen
3. One of the aims of deep myofascial release is to:
   a) loosen adhesions between connective tissue layers
   b) excite nerve endings
   c) sedate nerve endings
   d) facilitate fibroblast production
4. Fascial restrictions are usually palpated as:
   a) red, hot and swollen
   b) cold, moist and tight
   c) cold, moist and painful
   d) cold, dry and tight
5. What influence does temperature have on fascia?
   a) the lower the temperature, the more liquid the ground substance
   b) the higher the temperature, the more solid the ground substance
   c) the lower the temperature, the more solid the ground substance
   d) temperature has no influence on fascia
6. The resistance of a colloid increases in proportion to the pressure applied to it. True / False
7. Thoracic inlet release is useful for clients with breathing problems. True / False
8. Myofascial release is performed progressively towards the heart. True / False
9. Gentle myofascial release is suitable for most clients. True / False
10. When fascia is immobilised the ground substance gradually liquefies. True / False
11. List five functions of fascia.
12. Some clients experience an emotional release during myofascial release. How would you manage such a response in a client?
13. Fascia is hydrophilic. How does this property influence the application of techniques?
14. List three ways in which the application of deep myofascial release techniques differs from the application of other remedial massage techniques.
15. How can myofascial release be integrated with other remedial techniques?
16. Describe the tissue feel when fascia reaches its maximum release.
17. How does palpation for myofascial restriction differ from palpation for trigger points?

REFERENCES

1. Clay J, Pounds D. Basic clinical massage therapy: integrating anatomy and treatment. Philadelphia: Wolters Kluwer/Lippincott Williams and Wilkins; 2008.
2. Myers T. Anatomy trains. Edinburgh: Churchill Livingstone; 2001.
3. Marieb E. Essentials of human anatomy and physiology. 9th edn. San Francisco, CA: Benjamin Cummings; 2008.
4. Fritz S, Grosenbach M. Mosby's essential sciences for therapeutic massage. 3rd edn. St Louis, MO: Mosby Elsevier; 2009.
5. Schliep R, Zorn A, Els M, et al. The European fascia research project. Online. Available: http://www.somatics.de/FasciaResearch/ReportIASIyearbook06.htm; 2006.
6. Manheim C. The myofascial release manual. 4th edn. Thorofare, NJ: Slack; 2008.
7. Rolf I. Rolfing: the integration of human structures. Michigan: The University of Michigan; 1977.
8. Schultz R, Feitis R. The endless web: fascial anatomy and physical reality. Berkeley, CA: North Atlantic Books; 1996.
9. Bertolucci L. Muscle repositioning: a new verifiable approach to neuro-myofascial release? J Bodyw Mov Ther 2008;12(3):213–24.
10. Meltzer K, Cao T, Schad J, et al. In vitro modeling of repetitive motion injury and myofascial release. J Bodyw Mov Ther 2010;14(2):162–71.
11. Martin M. Effects of the myofascial release in diffuse systemic sclerosis. J Bodyw Mov Ther 2009;13(4):320–7.
12. Barnes M, Gronlund R, Little M, et al. Efficacy study of the effect of a myofascial release treatment technique on obtaining pelvic symmetry. J Bodyw Mov Ther 1997;1(5):289–96.
13. Arroyo-Morales M, Olea N, Martinez M, et al. Psychophysiological effects of massage-myofascial release after exercise: a randomized sham-control study. J Altern Complement Med 2008;14(10):1223–9.
14. Albert W, Currie-Jackson N, Duncan C. A survey of musculoskeletal injuries amongst Canadian massage therapists. J Bodyw Mov Ther 2008;12(1):86–93.
15. Holder N, Clark H, Di Blasio J, et al. Cause, prevalence, and response to occupational musculoskeletal injuries reported by physical therapists and physical therapy assistants. Phys Ther 1999;79(7):642–52.
16. Riggs A. Deep tissue massage: Part 1 – the tools. Massage and bodywork 2005;38–46.
17. Barnes JF. Myofascial release: the search for excellence. Padi, Pennsylvania; 1990.
18. Wolfe-Dixon M. Myofascial massage. Maryland: Lippincott Williams and Wilkins; 2007.

9 Lymphatic drainage massage

The content of this chapter relates to the following Units of Competency:

HLTREM503C Plan remedial massage treatment strategy
HLTREM504C Apply remedial massage assessment framework
HLTREM502C Provide remedial massage treatment
HLTREM505C Perform remedial massage health assessment

Health Training Package HLT07

Learning Outcomes

- Describe the reported benefits of lymphatic drainage massage.
- Assess clients' suitability for lymphatic drainage massage.
- Describe the current evidence for the effectiveness of lymphatic drainage massage.
- Apply basic lymphatic drainage massage effectively and safely to a range of clients.
- Advise and resource clients who have been assessed and treated with lymphatic drainage massage.

INTRODUCTION

Lymphatic drainage massage is a gentle, light-touch, non-invasive technique which can be used to treat specific conditions, complement existing healthcare protocols or as a relaxing massage treatment. It is a style of bodywork which is designed to promote the free flow of lymph throughout the body. Lymphatic drainage massage is distinctly different from other types of massage which generally use strokes that manipulate the soft tissues of the body (muscles, tendons, ligaments, fascia, joints or connective tissue) in that it is mainly concerned with the flow of lymph in the superficial lymph vessels just below the surface of the skin. 'Lymphatic drainage is a specialised massage technique designed to activate and cleanse the human fluid system. Because the lymphatic system itself is responsible for optimum functioning of fluid circulation and immune system, lymphatic drainage is a key to maximising our ability to rejuvenate and to establish resistance to stress and disease.'[1]

Manual Lymphatic Drainage (MLD) was developed in France by Emil Vodder in the 1930s. Over the years many scientists, doctors and therapists have contributed to Dr Vodder's techniques which has enabled MLD to gain worldwide acceptance and recognition in medicine and physiotherapy. MLD and other forms of lymphatic drainage massage have become popular in contemporary massage therapy, particularly to relieve post-traumatic oedema. Its reported benefits, which arise from mechanical stimulation of the flow of lymph,[2] include:[3–8]

- reducing or preventing lymphoedema
- alleviating fluid congestion (e.g. swollen ankles, puffy eyes)
- stimulating the immune system to reduce frequency of recurring infections (e.g. colds, flu, ear or chest infections)
- promoting healing (e.g. wounds, acute injuries, burns). After traumatic injury lymphatic drainage massage is performed proximal to the injury and not directly over it
- inducing relaxation and restful sleep
- reducing pain (e.g. in arthritic conditions)
- relaxing hypertonic muscles
- reducing cellulite
- stimulating bowel and bladder movements
- promoting hormone balance (some menstrual conditions and menopause)
- removing metabolic wastes, excess water, toxins, bacteria, large protein molecules and foreign substances from the tissues
- promoting general health and wellbeing
- improving many chronic conditions (e.g. sinusitis, scleroderma, acne and other skin conditions, chronic fatigue)
- assisting in conditions arising from venous insufficiency
- scar treatment (lymphatic drainage massage may soften and improve elasticity of scar tissue)
- assisting treatment of some neurological disorders (e.g. multiple sclerosis, migraine, Parkinson's disease, trigeminal neuralgia).

EVIDENCE FOR THE EFFECTIVENESS OF LYMPHATIC DRAINAGE MASSAGE

There have been a number of studies investigating the effects of lymphatic drainage massage which have promising results. For example, a number of studies found that the application of pressure and gliding movements enhanced movement of fluid out of tissues[9, 10] and that lymph drainage massage was effective in reducing oedema.[1, 11, 12] A study published in 2009 compared the effects of manual lymph drainage and connective tissue massage in women with primary fibromyalgia. The findings suggested that both techniques yield improvements in pain, health status and health-related quality of life. Manual lymph drainage was found to be more effective than connective tissue massage for morning tiredness and anxiety.[13] Schillinger et al[14] found that manual lymph drainage after treadmill exercise was associated with a faster decrease in serum levels of muscle enzymes. According to the authors, this may indicate improved regenerative processes related to structural damage of muscle cell integrity.

However, much research in this area has been criticised for its low methodological quality. A Cochrane review on the use of physical therapies for reducing and controlling lymphoedema of the limbs reviewed three trials and found that all three trials had methodological limitations. The authors concluded that there is a need for well-designed randomised trials of the whole range of physical therapies.[15]

FUNCTIONAL ANATOMY REVIEW[7]

The term *lymph* comes from the Latin *lympha*, which means water. Lymph is a colourless or slightly yellowish fluid, whose composition is similar to blood plasma except that the protein and cholesterol content of lymph are a little lower. Body tissues are bathed in intracellular fluid (i.e. fluid which lies inside the cells and makes up about two-thirds or approximately 25 litres of the body's water) and interstitial fluid (i.e. the remaining one-third of the body's water or approximately 10–12 litres which is located between the cells).

Blood carries oxygen and nutrients to the cells and carries away carbon dioxide and other wastes. Fluid leaks out of the blood capillaries and is reabsorbed again through diffusion. The rate at which fluid leaks from the capillaries is determined by pressures on either side of the capillary walls. These pressures (*Starling forces*) are exerted by fluid and protein on either side of the capillary wall. All body cells are bathed in interstitial fluid. In order to keep the volume of fluid in the interstitial compartment constant, excess interstitial fluid (about 10% or approximately 2 litres) and large proteins must be returned to the bloodstream. This process is carried out almost entirely by the lymphatic system, which forms an elaborate system of drainage vessels. (see Figure 9.1)

Excess interstitial fluid first drains into small, thin walled lymphatics (initial lymphatics) and then into larger lymphatics. Larger lymphatics contain valves to ensure that lymph flow is one-way and have muscular walls which can pump the interstitial fluid (now termed *lymph*) towards lymph nodes. Lymphocytes within lymph nodes police all fluid which passes through them and an immune response may be initiated if a foreign body is encountered (this is why our lymph nodes swell when we are unwell).

From the lymph capillaries the fluid passes to pre-collectors, then to collectors and finally to lymphatic trunks, which return the fluid back to the bloodstream at the junction of the venous angle in the neck. The thoracic duct is the largest of the lymphatic vessels and drains lymph from the lower limbs and many internal organs. It opens into the left venous angle, the junction of the subclavian and internal jugular veins. The much smaller right lymphatic duct drains part of the heart, lungs, right arm, right side of the face, head and neck emptying into the right venous angle. (see Figure 9.2 on p 126)

Lymph nodes (sometimes called lymph glands) are found throughout the body and are generally located in adipose tissue. These nodes consist of lymphoid tissue, which contains specialised cells that can help fight infection and other diseases such as cancer. Lymph nodes vary greatly in size, some being as small as a pinhead and others up to 3 cm long. There are about 500–700 lymph nodes in the body. The number of nodes varies from person to person and in different parts of the body. (see Figure 9.3 on p 126) The branched sinus system in the nodes slows the lymph flow allowing macrophages to phagocytose toxins, cell debris, bacteria, infectious organisms or cancer cells. Lymph nodes have more lymph vessels entering them (afferent vessels) than leaving them (efferent vessels). Seventy per cent of the fluid that enters a lymph node is absorbed into the veins of the node. (see Figure 9.4 on p 126)

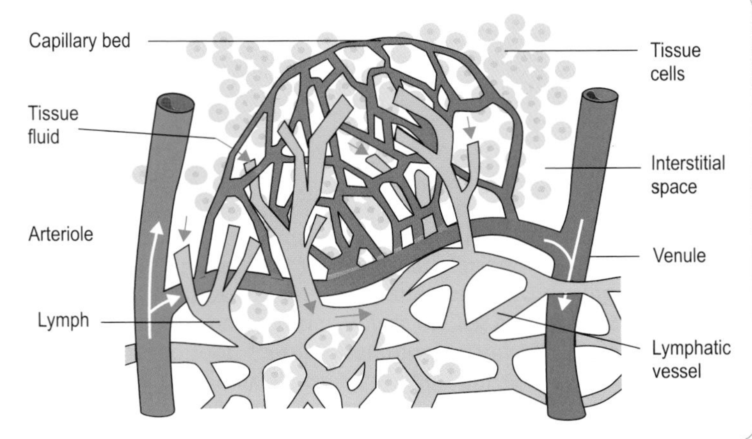

Fig. 9.1 Relationship between a blood capillary and lymphatic capillaries

FUNCTION OF THE LYMPHATIC SYSTEM

One of the major functions of the lymphatic system is to remove protein from interstitial fluid. Other functions include the production of small lymphocytes which play a key role in cellular immunity, and the production of large lymphocytes which are capable of synthesising antibodies. It also acts as a drainage system to return interstitial fluid containing dead cells, proteins, bacteria, foreign bodies, pathogenic agents and fats back to the cardiovascular system to be flushed out of the body. Lymph nodes act as filters for debris and infective agents that have gained access to the lymphatic system. In the gut the lymphatic system carries absorbed fats to the blood via the thoracic duct so that metabolism of the fats can commence.

The major function of the lymphatic system that concerns massage therapists is the movement of interstitial fluid and protein via the lymph vessels back to the bloodstream. If this protein-rich fluid accumulates, oedema prevents normal tissue function and metabolism.

OEDEMA

Oedema is a condition where excessive tissue fluid accumulates in the body. Oedema is the result of an imbalance between incoming and outgoing fluid which causes an abnormal amount of water to collect in the tissues. It should never be considered a diagnosis but rather a symptom of an underlying disorder. There are many possible causes of oedema including:

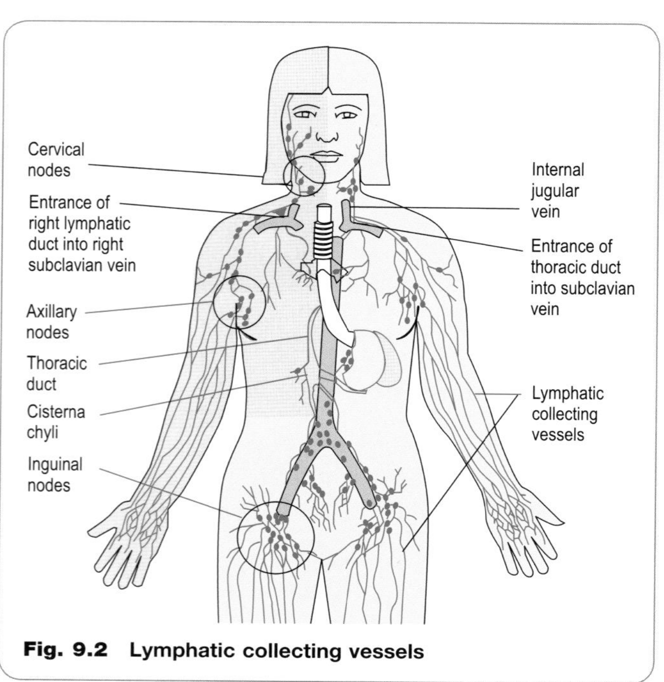

Fig. 9.2 Lymphatic collecting vessels

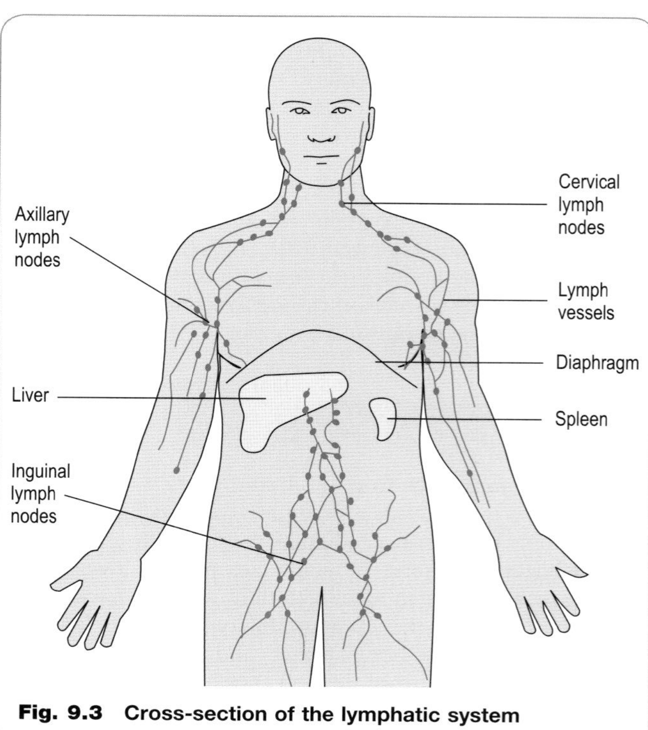

Fig. 9.3 Cross-section of the lymphatic system

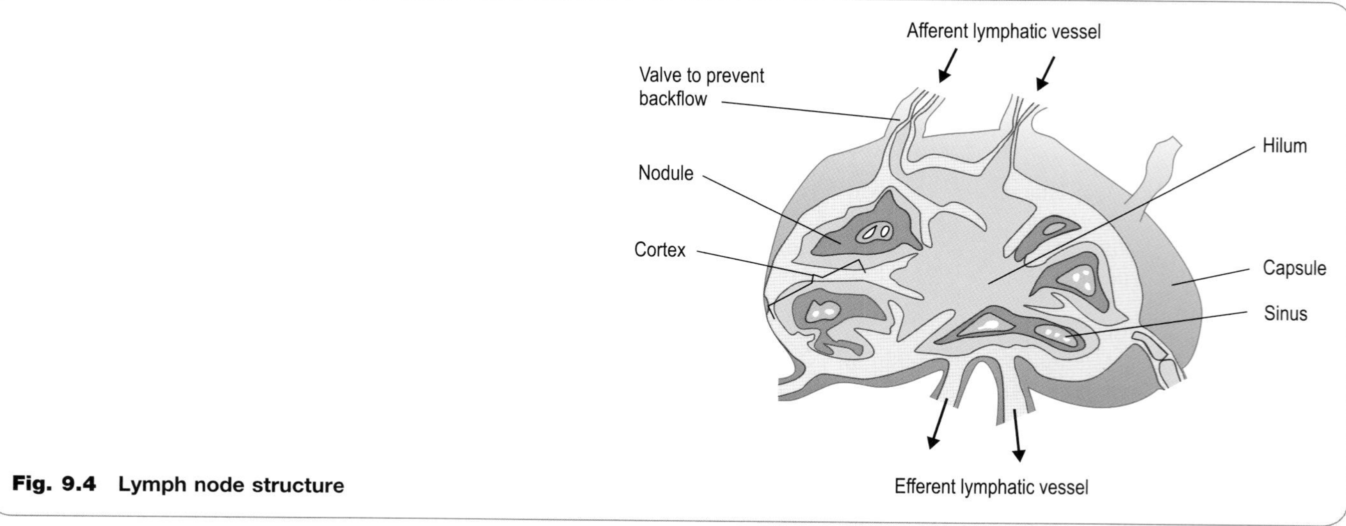

Fig. 9.4 Lymph node structure

- acute nephritic syndrome
- heart failure
- Hodgkin's disease or non-Hodgkin's lymphoma
- deep vein thrombosis
- pregnancy
- pulmonary oedema
- acute injury or allergic reaction – the hormones histamine and bradykinin act by raising the permeability of the capillary wall which leads to greater filtration of proteins and fluids in the tissues
- sodium excess – oedema can result from excessive table salt which causes water retention and increased protein excretion in the urine (renal oedema – the first visible signs of renal oedema are swelling of the eyelids and oedema in both lower legs)
- reduced protein uptake or impaired protein processing – lower blood protein level reduces the colloid osmotic pressure in the plasma (e.g. from malnutrition, malabsorption or protein loss due to gastrointestinal disease)
- hydrodynamic congestion due to local impediment to blood flow such as thrombosis or fibrosis.

The primary consequence of oedema is mechanical impairment of organ function. Oedema may have been present for some time before it is noticeable in areas of the body. The longer an oedema is present in tissue, the greater the chance that fibrosis can occur. Fibroblasts in the connective tissue are activated by free proteins that produce granulation tissue. This tissue is soft at first but gradually hardens and becomes sclerotic as further collagenous fibre is produced.

Lymphoedema

Lymphoedema refers to localised oedema due to lymphatic obstruction. According to the International Society of Lymphology,[16] 'In its purest form the central disturbance is a low output failure of the lymphvascular system, that is, overall lymphatic transport is reduced … lymphatic transport has fallen below the capacity needed to handle the presented load of microvascular filtrate including plasma protein and cells that normally leak from the bloodstream into the interstitium. Swelling is produced by accumulation in the extracellular space of excess water, filtered/diffused plasma proteins, extravascular blood cells and parenchymal/stromal cell products.' One of the main reasons for the prevalence of lymphoedema is surgical intervention and lymph node dissections as can occur in mastectomy to prevent the spread of breast cancer. It is estimated that 20% of patients treated for melanoma, breast, gynaecological or prostate cancer will experience secondary lymphoedema.[17] Other reasons for lymphoedema are trauma to lymph vessels, deep vein thrombosis, venous insufficiency, filariasis,[a] impaired venous circulation, dysplasia of lymphatic vessels and radiation therapy.

Lymphoedema is classified as primary or secondary.

PRIMARY LYMPHOEDEMA

Primary lymphoedema is not common. It almost exclusively affects the lower extremity and there is usually no family history. Primary lymphoedema originates from a developmental abnormality that is present but not always clinically evident at birth. It may become visible months after birth or many years later in life. A trauma or a simple event such as an insect bite can trigger a lymphoedema to occur. In primary lymphoedema the person may have had defective lymphatic drainage for many years before problems occur. If the lymphoedema is only mild, it may disappear within a few days or may stay and continue to worsen.

SECONDARY LYMPHOEDEMA

Secondary lymphoedema can occur in any part of the body (limbs, joints or viscera) and usually develops as a result of surgery, radiation, chronic venous insufficiency, trauma, paralysis of a limb or parasites. Damage to lymph vessels or nodes always entails the risk of developing lymphoedema which may occur immediately or weeks, months or even years later. It may also occur after an infection, insect bite, aircraft travel or sunburn.

STAGES OF LYMPHOEDEMA

Any lymphoedema left untreated gradually worsens and will progress through the following stages:

Latency stage

- Subclinical stage of lymphoedema
- Transport capacity reduced
- No visible or palpable oedema
- Complaints of discomfort or heaviness

Stage 1

- Visible signs of oedema
- Pitting on pressure
- Reduces on elevation or overnight, returns gradually during the day
- Smooth texture of skin and softness of tissue

Stage 2

- Accumulation of protein-rich oedema
- No longer pits easily
- Connective tissue proliferation causing fibrosis
- Oedema does not reduce overnight or on elevation
- Prone to developing infections

Stage 3

- The third stage is known as lymphostatic elephantiasis
- Extreme increase in volume
- The extremity is column-shaped, resembling the limb of an elephant
- Natural skin folds are extremely deepened, the dermal tissues progressively harden and the back of the hand or foot is massively swollen
- Non-pitting
- Skin changes (e.g. papillomas, hyperkeratosis)
- Fibrosis and sclerosis

ASSESSING CLIENTS

All potential lymphatic drainage clients need to be screened for red flags for serious conditions and to determine their suitability for the technique. Case history, observation and

[a]Filariasis is an infectious tropical disease caused by roundworms.

palpation are particularly useful assessment tools for lymphatic drainage massage clients.

HISTORY

A thorough case history should be taken before commencing lymphatic drainage massage. It is necessary to know about medication, past illness, surgery and any current illness. As lymphatic drainage massage is not appropriate for all conditions, the case history enables you to determine the suitability of the client for treatment. A referral may be necessary to rule out contraindications before treatment can begin.

Indications of increased interstitial fluid volume include increased physical activity followed by 24–48 hours of inactivity or insufficient recovery time, increased salt or decreased fluid intake, or increased water intake without electrolyte balance.[18] Clients may complain of delayed onset muscle soreness, stiffness or sluggishness.

Clients with lymphoedema may have a history of surgery or radiation therapy. Signs or symptoms of lymphoedema may include:

- sensation of heaviness and tightness in the limb
- pins and needles in the limb
- rings, watches or clothing becoming tight
- pain, which may be shooting, or tenderness in the affected limb.

RED FLAG CONDITIONS FOR OEDEMA[19]

- Sudden onset
- Significant pain
- Shortness of breath
- History of a heart disorder or an abnormal cardiac examination
- Haemoptysis, dyspnoea, or pleural friction rub
- Hepatomegaly, jaundice, ascites, splenomegaly or haematemesis
- Unilateral leg swelling with tenderness

Chronic heart, kidney or liver disorder are suggested by generalised oedema that develops slowly.

POSTURAL ANALYSIS

Postural observation should note the presence of any of the following:

- loss of muscle definition
- swollen appearance (e.g. puffy face, hands, feet and legs)
- swollen joints.

FUNCTIONAL TESTS

- Decreased joint range of motion may result from fluid accumulation.

PALPATION[18]

Palpation can show oedema to be boggy, spongy or soggy and may elicit tenderness. The overlying skin and superficial fascia feel taut. Determining the nature of the oedema (e.g. pitting or non-pitting) helps identify its cause. Pitting refers to the persistence of the indentation after digital pressure has been released. Pitting oedema can occur when any pressure is applied to the limb (e.g. wearing tight socks). In non-pitting oedema the indentation does not persist after the pressure is released. Non-pitting oedema occurs in conditions like lymphoedema and hyperthyroidism.

DIFFERENTIAL DIAGNOSIS

- Small lymph nodes are often detected in the axilla and groin of healthy individuals.
- Localised lymphadenopathy is common and usually the result of local infection.
- In Hodgkin's disease the lymph nodes palpate as rubbery; in tuberculosis they may feel matted; in metastatic carcinoma they feel craggy.
- Tender nodes usually indicate acute infection.
- Nodes which are fixed to deep structures or skin are usually malignant.[20]
- Peripheral causes of oedema include orthostatic oedema, lymphoedema, lipoedema or chronic venous insufficiency (see Table 9.1).

Table 9.1 Peripheral causes of oedema[21]

Type of oedema	Process	Nature of oedema	Skin thickening	Ulceration	Pigmentation	Foot involvement	Bilateral
Orthostatic	Prolonged standing or sitting	Soft pitting	–	–	–	Yes	Always
Lymphoedema	Lymphatic obstruction	Soft early, later hard and non-pitting	Marked	Rare	–	Yes	Often
Lipoedema	Fatty deposits in legs	Minimal	–	–	–	–	Always
Chronic venous insufficiency	Deep venous obstruction or valvular incompetence	Soft, pitting; later brawny	Occasional	Common	Common	Yes	Occasionally

TREATING CLIENTS

It is important to remember that lymphatic drainage massage is a specialist treatment and should be provided by practitioners who are trained in this technique. Practitioners must not provide healthcare of a type that is outside the scope of their training and experience.

Due to the success of lymphatic drainage massage in treating lymphoedema many hospitals and medical centres to employ lymph drainage therapists to participate in treatment.

BASIC PRINCIPLES

1. Clear the major lymph nodes in the area first. Proximal areas are treated before distal areas and the direction of massage follows lymph flow. The massage sequence is designed to clear an area before directing lymph into it. For example, the upper arm is massaged before the forearm; the thigh before the lower leg; and the abdomen before the legs.
2. Pressure is light. Contact is superficial; that is, only to skin depth, not muscle depth. Firm pressure is used only when fibrosis or hard oedema is present. Lymphatic drainage massage should not cause pain.
3. The massage movements should be done at a moderate pace. This is important as lymphatic drainage massage causes mechanical emptying and filling of the lymphatic vessels. If the massage movements are too fast the vessels are not given the opportunity to fill completely before the next movement is applied, rendering the massage inefficient.
4. Movements should be smooth, rhythmic and repetitious. The object is to stimulate a peristaltic wave-like action within the lymph vessels so as to stimulate the lymphangions, the functional units of lymph vessels. Smooth muscles in the walls of the lymphatic vessels cause the lymphangions to contract sequentially to aid the flow of lymph.
5. Movements are predominantly circular and performed in a wave-like rhythm which also promotes general relaxation.
6. Movements have a pressure or working phase which promotes the movement of fluid in the desired direction, followed by a relaxation phase to allow lymph capillaries to refill.
7. Each movement should be repeated 5–7 times to stimulate the lymph collectors.

LENGTH OF TREATMENT

General lymphatic drainage massage takes about 60 minutes but treatment time should not be fixed. Shorter treatment times (e.g. 20 minutes) may also be of value to many clients. The treatment time will depend on the age and health of the client and the purpose of treatment. Lymphatic drainage massage is an effective and powerful therapy. If treatment time is too long the client may develop side effects like mild headache, nausea or fatigue.

EXPLANATION OF TREATMENT

Always explain lymphatic drainage massage to your clients, including the reason for lightness of pressure, the duration of the treatment, recommended treatment frequency and areas to be massaged. Also discuss what to expect from the treatment including how clients may feel after treatment and how they may assist treatment. Recommendations for the immediate period after treatment could include drinking plenty of water, doing only light exercises and refraining from eating a heavy meal. Other recommendations include epsom salts baths and a diet that is rich in diuretic foods like pineapple, papaya, berries, cucumbers, radishes, celery, aloe vera juice and watermelon.[18]

Pressure

To be most effective the pressure of lymphatic drainage massage needs to be light to avoid compression of the superficial lymph vessels and lymph collectors which would prevent or considerably hamper the flow of lymph during massage. Correct pressure is achieved when the top layer of skin moves against the level immediately beneath, not against muscle which would indicate pressure that is too heavy. A reddening of the skin may also indicate that the pressure is too heavy. Lymphatic drainage massage should not be painful. Firm pressure may be indicated when treating chronic lymphoedema which has become fibrotic. Note that fibrosis occurs in the connective tissue not in the muscle. Pressure should always be applied within the client's pain-free range. Overworking an area or using too much pressure may cause bruising or inflammation.

Strokes

There is a small number of specific strokes used in lymphatic drainage.

1. STATIONARY CIRCLES

These strokes are used more frequently than all other strokes. As the name implies the stroke is stationary – it does not generally glide or slide over the skin. The movements may be small or large stationary circles, clockwise or anti-clockwise, using flat fingers or the whole of the palm. The strokes stretch the skin numerous times in the one area before moving to the next area (see Figure 9.5 on p 130).

2. PUMP TECHNIQUE

Pumping is performed with the palm of the hand and fingers. It is an exaggerated movement of the wrist using a hinge action to carry the hand forward over the area being treated (see Figure 9.6 on p 130).

3. SCOOP TECHNIQUE

The scoop technique involves turning the palms out from the body by rotating the wrists in a corkscrew motion (see Figure 9.7 on p 130).

4. ROTARY TECHNIQUE

This movement uses the palm of the hand and thumb to create sweeping circular movements in the direction of lymph flow. The writs are used to increase and decrease the pressure of the stroke (see Figure 9.8 on p 130).

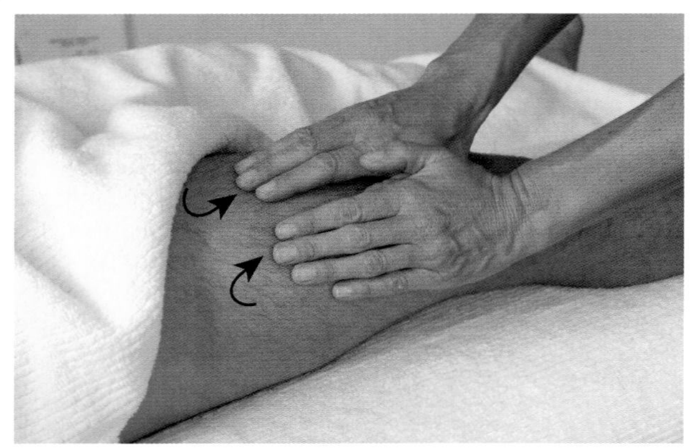

Fig. 9.5 **Lymphatic drainage strokes: stationary circles**

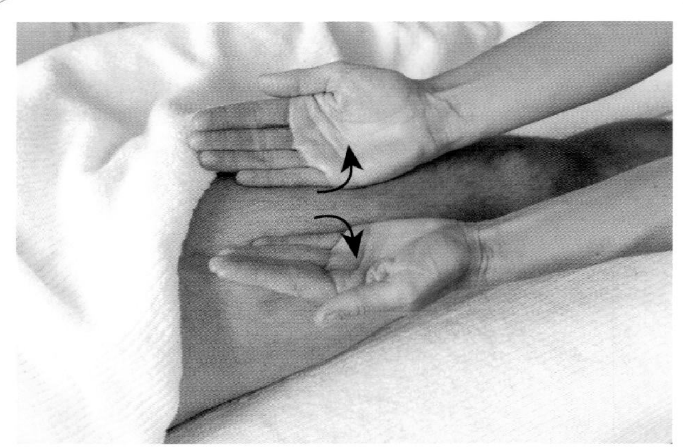

Fig. 9.7 **Lymphatic drainage strokes: scoop technique**

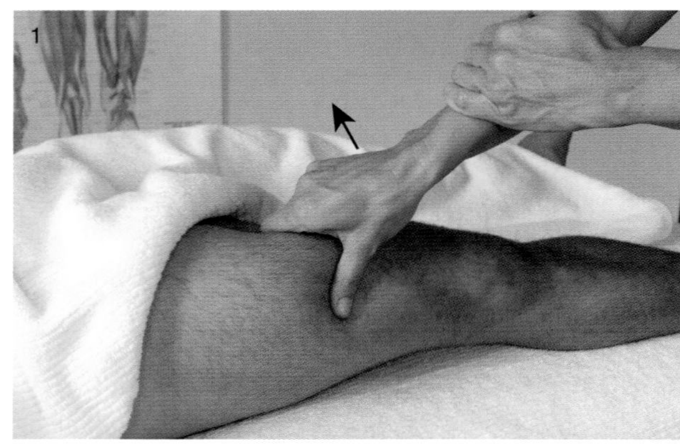

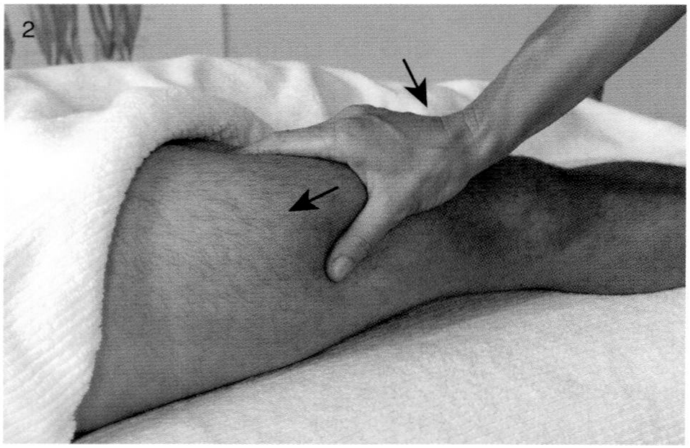

Fig. 9.6 **Lymphatic drainage strokes: pump technique**

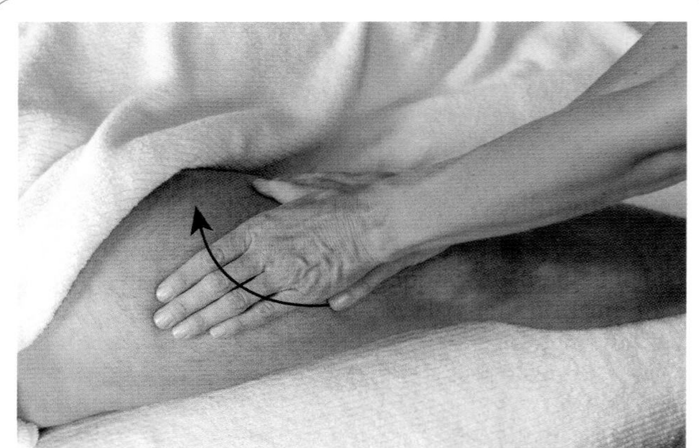

Fig. 9.8 **Lymphatic drainage strokes: rotary technique**

These four movements are combined to produce pressure-on/pressure-off kneading movements that can be circular, oval, deep, shallow, large or small.

Summary

- Massage slowly. Lymph is thicker than blood and moves more slowly. Flow rates of lymph in the skin vary from one area of the body to another (e.g. lymph from the head and neck moves more slowly than lymph in the legs). Strokes should be rhythmical and performed at the rate of one stroke per second but this may vary depending on the individual treatment.
- Use gentle pressure to increase lymph production and lymph flow through stimulation of lymph capillaries and lymph collectors. Heavy pressure may hamper the flow of lymph or cause the delicate lymph vessels to spasm.
- Drain in the correct direction. Knowing the direction of lymph flow is required for effective lymphatic drainage massage.
- Apply pressure smoothly during the working phase and release pressure during the resting phase of each stroke. This allows for filling or refilling of lymph vessels and the stimulation of the lymph collectors during the massage (see Figure 9.9 on p 131).
- The area closest to the terminus (the triangular area just above the clavicle where lymph returns to the subclavian veins) is treated first so that the peripheral areas can be drained. On the extremities, regional lymph nodes are treated first, then the massage begins proximally and continues distally.

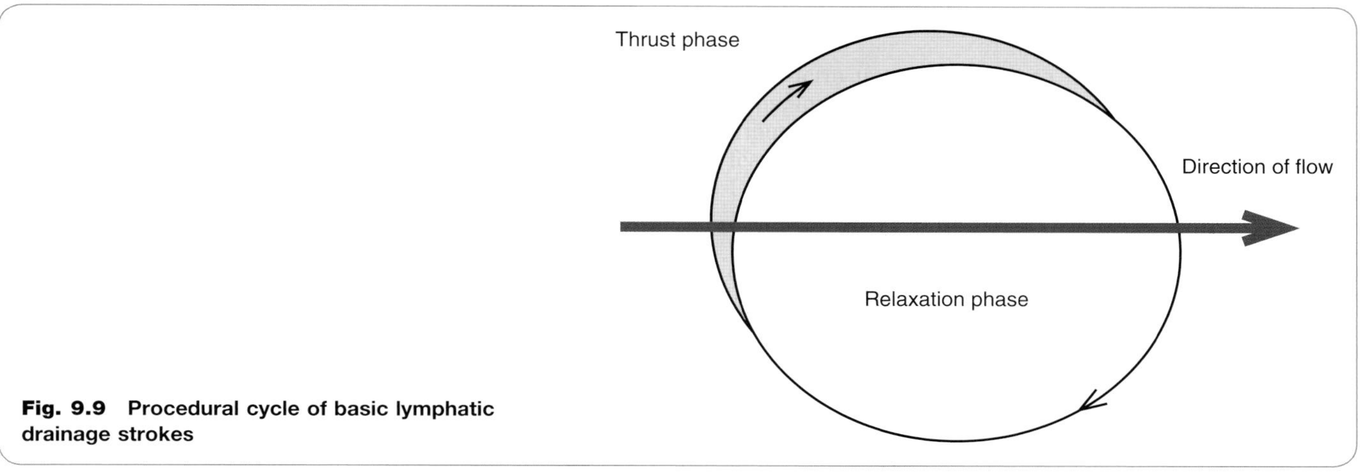

Fig. 9.9 Procedural cycle of basic lymphatic drainage strokes

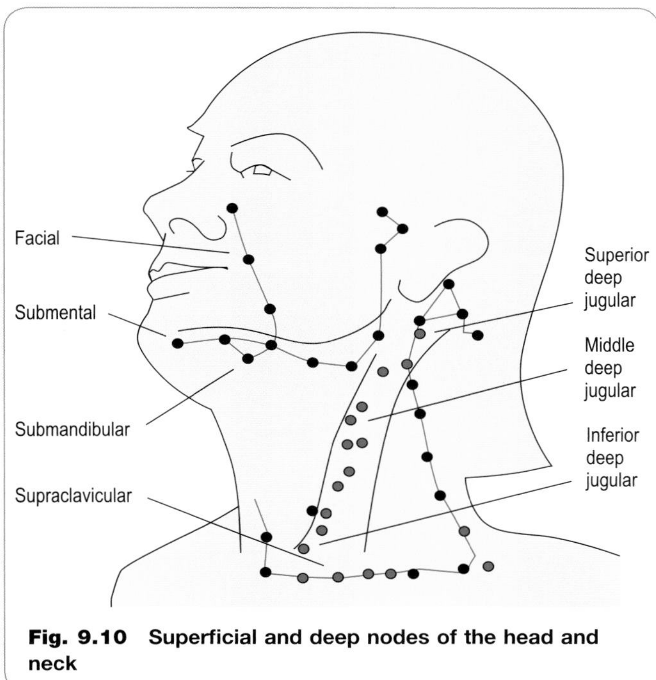

Fig. 9.10 Superficial and deep nodes of the head and neck

REGIONAL LYMPHATIC DRAINAGE MASSAGE

The following section presents an overview of lymph anatomy, direction of lymph flow and indications for lymph drainage massage for specific regions of the body: the head and neck, upper torso, upper limb, lower torso, lower limb and thorax.

The head and neck

The lymphatics of the neck are arranged in deep and superficial chains (see Figure 9.10):

- The deep jugular chain extends from the base of the skull to the clavicle and consists of superior, middle and inferior groups of lymph nodes. The *superior deep jugular nodes* receive primary drainage from oral cavity tonsils, the larynx, pharynx, pyriform sinus and above the vocal folds. This group of lymph nodes also receives lymph from more superficial nodes in the upper head and neck (retropharyngeal, spinal accessory, parotid, superficial cervical and submandibular nodes).

  The *middle deep jugular nodes* receive primary drainage from the larynx above the vocal folds, lower pyriform sinus (located on each side of the laryngeal orifice) and posterior cricoid. They receive secondary drainage from the deep jugular nodes above them and the lower retropharyngeal nodes. The *inferior deep jugular nodes* receive primary drainage from the thyroid, trachea and cervical oesophagus. They receive secondary drainage from the deep jugular nodes above them and the paratracheal nodes. The retropharyngeal and paratracheal nodes lie posteriorly around the midline viscera. They receive drainage from these viscera and from the deep structures in the midline of the head; that is, the nasopharynx, posterior nasal cavity, paranasal sinuses and posterior oropharynx. They drain towards the deep jugular chain. The superficial nodes tend to drain secondarily, as mentioned, to the deep nodes (see Figure 9.11 on p 132).
- The superficial nodes are the submental, superficial cervical, submandibular, spinal accessory and anterior scalene. The *submental nodes* drain the chin, the middle of the lower lip, tip of the tongue and anterior mouth. These nodes in turn drain to the submandibular nodes. The submandibular nodes drain the upper lip, lateral lower lip, lower nasal cavity, anterior mouth and the skin of the cheek. The *submandibular nodes* in turn drain to the superior deep jugular nodes (see Figure 9.12 on p 132). The *superficial cervical nodes* located along the external jugular vein receive drainage from the cutaneous lymphatics of the face, especially from around the parotid gland, behind the ear, parotid and occipital nodes.

  The superficial cervical nodes then drain into the superior deep jugular nodes. The nodes in the posterior triangle lie along the spinal accessory nerve. These nodes drain the parietal and occipital regions of the scalp. The upper nodes drain to the superior deep jugular nodes while the lower nodes drain down to the supraclavicular nodes. The anterior scalene (Virchow's) nodes receive drainage from the thoracic duct and are located at the junction of the thoracic duct and left subclavian vein. The supraclavicular nodes receive drainage from the spinal accessory nodes and from infraclavicular sources. All of these lymphatics eventually drain into the venous system either through or together with the thoracic duct on the left, or the right lymphatic duct (see Figure 9.13).

Indications for lymphatic drainage of the head and neck include:

- acne vulgaris or rosacea
- facial muscle contractures
- puffy eyes
- after root canal surgery and tooth extraction
- sinusitis
- nasal congestion
- syringitis (inflammation of the eustachian tube)
- Bell's palsy

The upper torso

All lymph vessels of the upper torso drain into the axilla (see Figure 9.14 on p 133). The superficial nodes begin in lymphatic plexuses in the skin and end at the axillary lymph nodes. The deep vessels follow the principal vascular and neurovascular bundles and end in the lateral axillary lymph nodes.

Axillary lymph nodes are the regional group for the whole of the upper extremity. There can be 20 to 30 large nodes in this area.

- The lateral group lies medial to and behind the axillary vein. This group receives lymph from the whole upper arm except for the lymph vessels that accompany the cephalic vein.
- The anterior (pectoral) group lies along the lower border of the pectoralis minor. Vessels from the skin and muscles of the anterior and lateral walls of the trunk above the

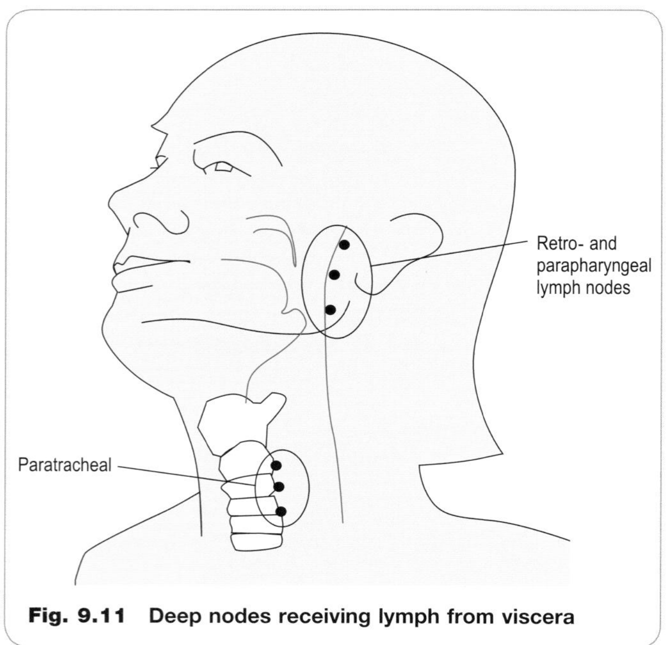

Fig. 9.11 Deep nodes receiving lymph from viscera

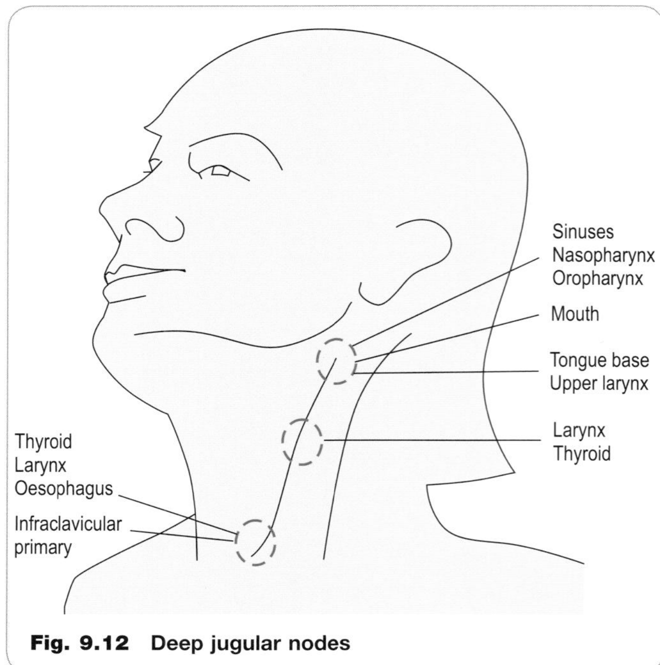

Fig. 9.12 Deep jugular nodes

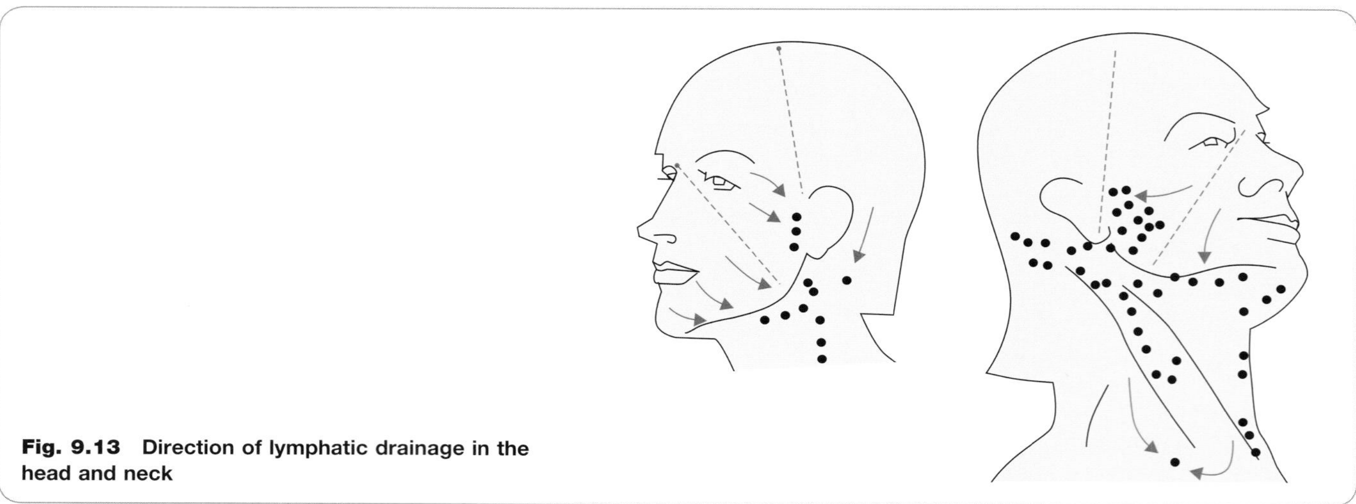

Fig. 9.13 Direction of lymphatic drainage in the head and neck

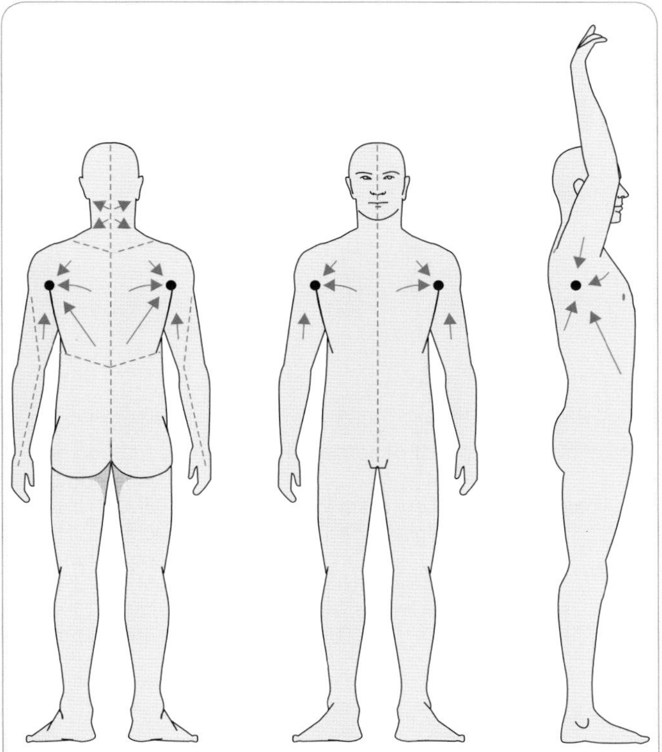

Fig. 9.14 **Direction of lymphatic drainage of the upper torso**

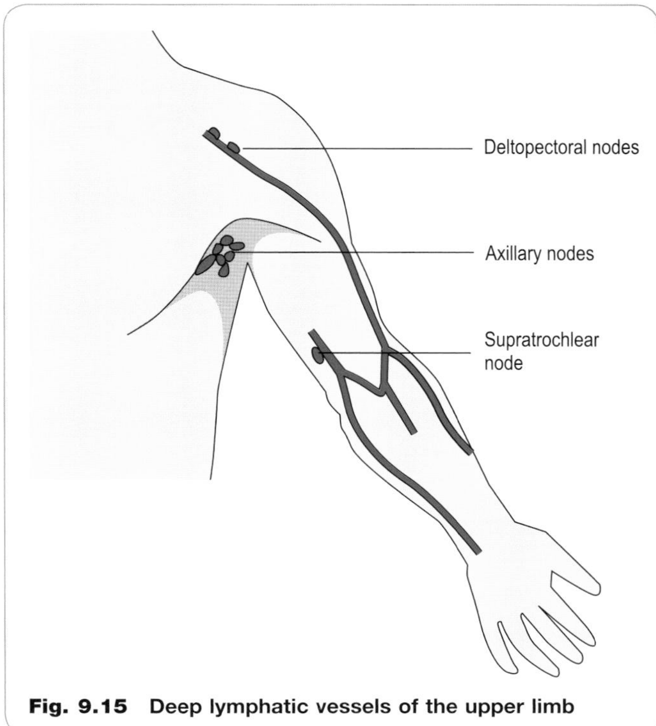

Fig. 9.15 **Deep lymphatic vessels of the upper limb**

umbilicus and the central and lateral areas of the breast drain into these nodes.

- The posterior (subscapular) group lies along the lower margin of the posterior wall of the axilla. Vessels from the skin and muscles of the lower part of the back of the neck and the dorsal aspect of the trunk drain into these nodes.
- The central group is embedded in the fat of the axilla and receives lymph from all the preceding groups of axillary lymph nodes.
- The apical group is situated posterior to the upper border of the pectoralis minor, above its lower border and extends to the apex of the axilla. Lymph vessels that accompany the cephalic vein drain into these nodes as do lymph vessels from part of the breast and all other axillary nodes. The efferent vessels of this group unite to form the subclavian trunk which opens either into the internal jugular and subclavian vein or into the jugular lymphatic trunk. On the left side it may end in the thoracic duct.

Superficial vessels on the anterior surface begin in the palm of the hand, draining the fingers towards the wrist. The vessels on the front of the wrist pass into the forearm following the median vein up to the cubital region. From there they follow the medial border of the biceps to pierce the deep fascia at the axillary fold to end at the lateral axillary nodes. On the dorsal surface most of the vessels run parallel upwards finally passing around the borders of the limb to join the vessels on the anterior aspect. Some of the lateral vessels reach the level of the deltoid where they mostly incline medially to join the anterior vessels; a few continue with the cephalic vein and end in the infraclavicular nodes. Collecting vessels from the front and back of the deltoid pass around to the anterior and posterior axillary fold to end in the axillary nodes.

Deep vessels are less numerous than the superficial ones with which they have some communication at intervals along their course. They follow the main neurovascular bundles, the radial, ulnar, interosseous and brachial and end in the lateral axillary nodes. A few lymph nodes occur along the course of these vessels (see Figure 9.15).

Indications for lymphatic drainage massage of the upper limb include:

- lymphoedema
- acute and chronic conditions of the upper limb (e.g. adhesive capsulitis, tendinitis, lateral epicondylitis, osteoarthritis, repetition strain injury).

The lower torso

Most of the lymph from the lower torso drains into the inguinal lymph nodes located in the groin (see Figure 9.16 on p 134).

The superficial inguinal lymph nodes are arranged in two groups:

- An upper group situated below the inguinal ligament. This group receives lymph from the abdominal wall below the umbilicus, gluteal region and part of the lateral region of the upper thigh. The inferior nodes of the upper group receive vessels from external genitalia, part of the anal canal, the perianal region and uterine lymph vessels.
- A lower group situated along the terminal end of the great saphenous vein. Vessels from the entire lower torso (superficial) except for the back and lateral aspects of the calf drain into these nodes.

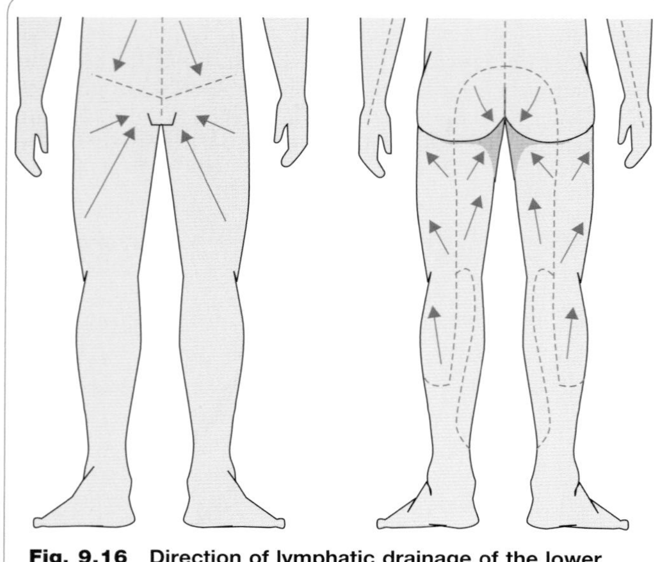

Fig. 9.16 Direction of lymphatic drainage of the lower torso and lower limb

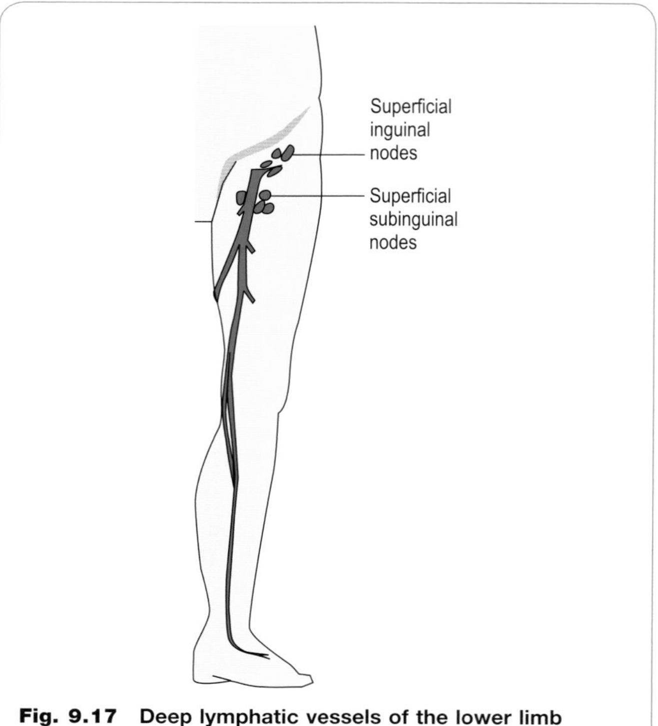

Fig. 9.17 Deep lymphatic vessels of the lower limb

The few deep inguinal nodes are located on the medial side of the femoral vein. These nodes receive the lymph vessels that accompany the femoral vessels, vessels from the external genitalia and a few vessels from the superficial nodes. Vessels from the superficial and deep nodes pass through the femoral canal to the external iliac lymph nodes.

The popliteal lymph nodes are embedded in the fat of the popliteal fossa. There are approximately five to seven small lymph nodes which receive vessels from the back and lateral aspects of the calf. The efferent vessels from these nodes ascend with the femoral blood vessels to the deep inguinal nodes.

Superficial vessels begin in the foot: a median set follow the great saphenous vein and a lateral set follow the small saphenous vein. The vessels of the medial group begin on the dorsum of the foot (tibial side), ascend in front of or behind the malleolus and accompany the great saphenous vein to the groin. They end in the lower group of the superficial inguinal nodes. The vessels from the lateral set begin on the dorsum of the foot (fibular side). Some join the medial group; the others accompany the small saphenous vein and end in the popliteal lymph nodes.

The deep vessels accompany the main blood vessels (anterior tibial, peroneal, popliteal and femoral groups) to pass directly to the deep inguinal nodes except where some vessels from the lower leg end at the popliteal nodes. (see Figure 9.17)

Indications for lymphatic drainage massage of the lower limb include:

- lymphoedema
- chronic venous conditions
- acute injuries
- chronic injuries and conditions (e.g. arthritis)
- leg ulcers
- restless leg syndrome
- heavy, tired legs
- fluid retention.

The thorax

The groups of vessels and nodes in the thorax are known as the intercostal, diaphragmatic, internal mammary, innominate and tracheo-bronchial, the first three of which are discussed here.

- Intercostal lymph nodes are located near the vertebral end of each intercostal space and receive vessels from the parietal pleura of the posterior abdominal wall. The vessels that accompany the intercostal arteries come from the costovertebral and intervertebral joints and also drain into these nodes. The efferents of the nodes of the upper 6–7 intercostals on both sides run independently of the thoracic duct to empty into the subclavian vein. The lower five join on each side to form a descending intercostal trunk, which passes through the aortic opening to enter the cisterna chyli.
- The diaphragmatic lymph nodes make up three groups: the posterior, anterior and middle. The *posterior* group is situated at the lower part of the oesophagus and receives vessels from the oesophagus, back of the pericardium and diaphragm. Efferents from these nodes empty directly into the thoracic duct or the descending intercostal lymph trunks. The *anterior* group is large and situated on the sternal and costal origins of the diaphragm behind the xiphoid process and the seventh costal cartilages. They receive vessels from the front of the pericardium, anterior intercostal lymph nodes and anterior part of the diaphragm and from the anterior and upper surface of the liver. The *middle* group of vessels from the lateral part of the diaphragm and their efferents pass to the anterior or posterior groups.

- Internal mammary lymph nodes are situated in the upper four intercostal spaces close to the sternum, where they receive vessels from the anterior (diaphragmatic) nodes and the vessels which accompany the intercostal and branches of the internal mammary arteries. The anterior intercostal afferent vessels of the internal mammary chain drain the parietal pleura almost as far back as the angles of the ribs. Vessels also drain the skin of the breast and the medial part of the stroma. (see Figure 9.18)

Superficial lymph drainage of the trunk and back covers the cutaneous area of the trunk extending from the level of the umbilicus to the clavicle in front to halfway up the neck on the back. These vessels originate in the fascia and converge on the axillary lymph nodes. On the back the vessels run downwards from the lower part of the neck, horizontally from the area of the scapula and upward from the iliac crest to converge round the posterior fold of the axilla. The cutaneous vessels on the front, from the level of the umbilicus to below the breast, run diagonally upward, horizontally over the pectoral area and downward from the clavicle, again to converge on the axillary nodes (see Figure 9.19 on p 136).

Indications for lymphatic drainage massage for the thoracic and lumbar areas include:

- after surgery (mastectomy, lumpectomy)
- painful or swollen breasts
- lower back and neck pain
- chronic conditions (e.g. osteoarthritis, chronic bronchitis, emphysema).

CONTRAINDICATIONS AND PRECAUTIONS

The new levels of acceptance and high public use of manual lymph drainage calls for high levels of responsibility on the part of practitioners to apply techniques safely and

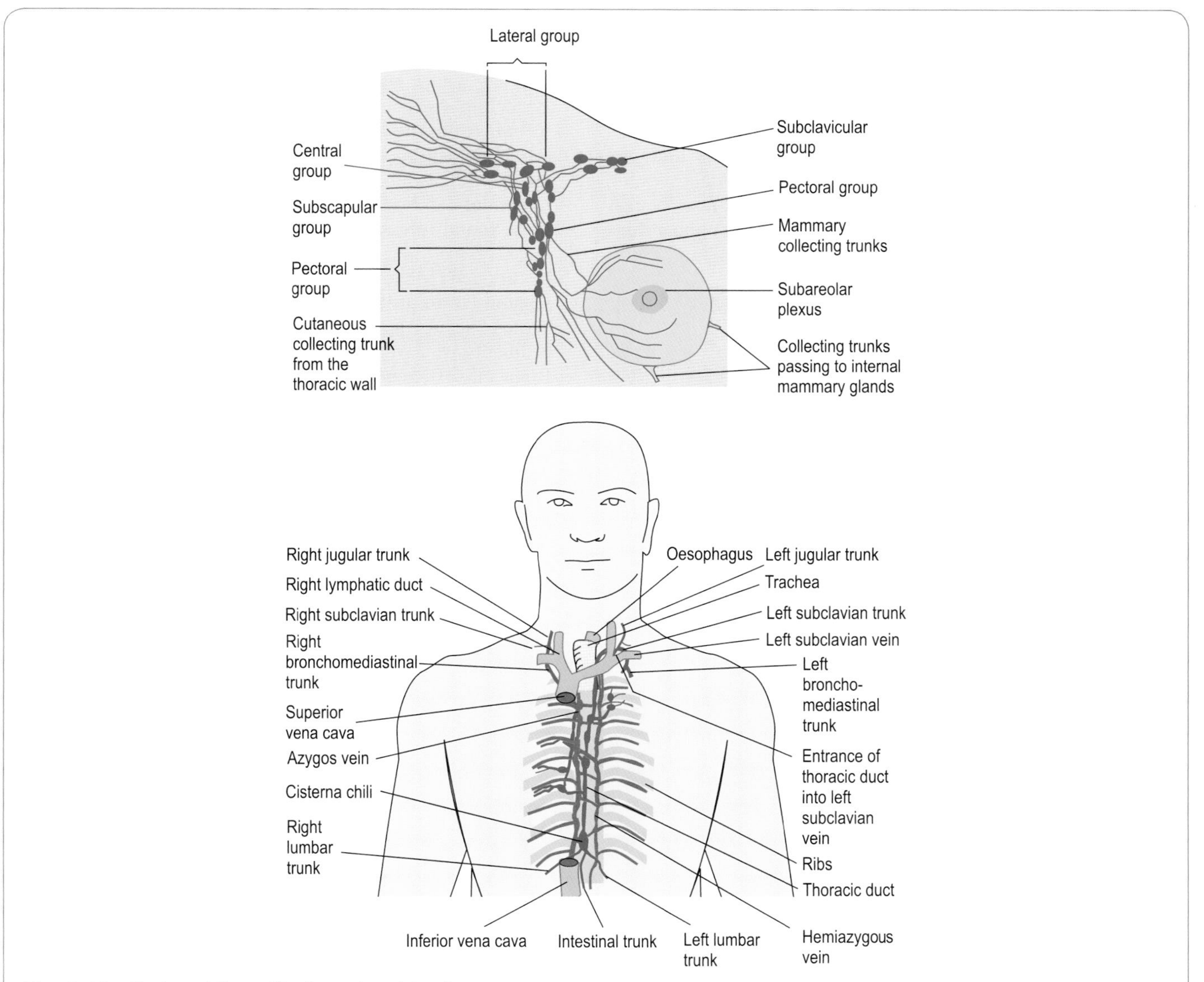

Fig. 9.18 Nodes of the axilla, breast and trunk

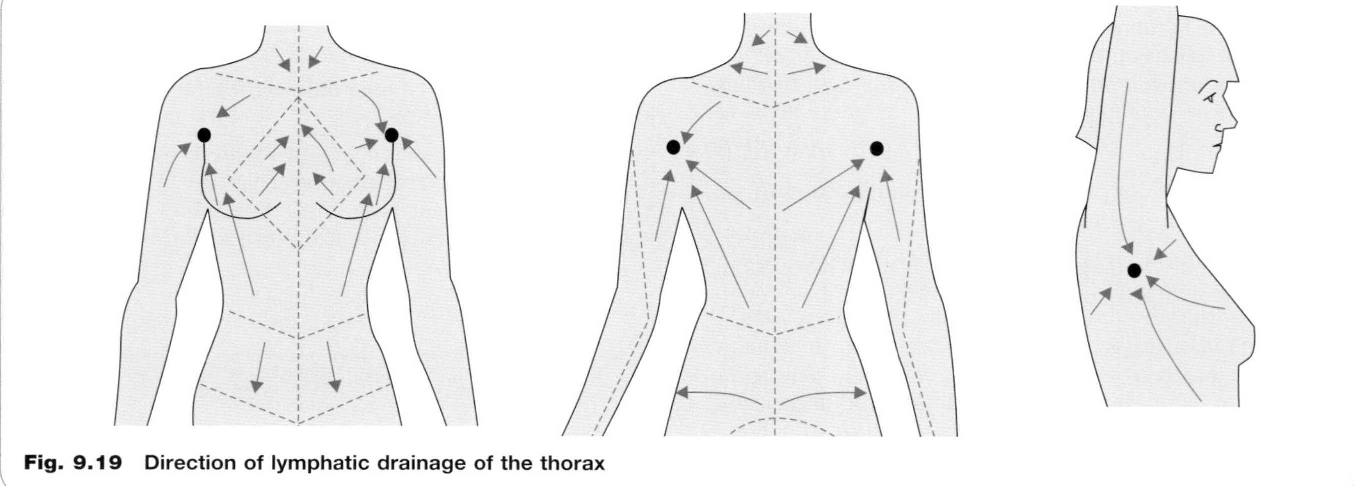

Fig. 9.19 Direction of lymphatic drainage of the thorax

competently. There are only a few absolute contraindications to lymph drainage massage (see below). There are also conditions for which it is advisable to seek clearance from the client's doctor before commencing treatment. Practitioners who feel uncertain about working with a client should refer them to a more experienced practitioner. Lymph drainage massage is often recommended as a complementary therapy for cancer treatment. Previous thinking that massage could cause the spread of cancer from the primary tumour is being challenged as no evidence has been produced to support this claim. Furthermore the scientific literature cites numerous positive benefits of massage for cancer.[22]

Contraindications for lymphatic drainage massage can be classified as absolute, relative and local.[7]

ABSOLUTE CONTRAINDICATIONS

- Chronic congestive heart failure, untreated heart failure or cardiac oedema, acute renal insufficiency. A load is placed on the venous system when there is an increase in the volume of lymph arriving at the subclavian veins. Significantly increasing the load could place strain on the heart and kidneys.[2]
- Acute infections and fever.
- Acute deep vein thrombosis (known or suspected).
- Unexplained pain.
- After recent surgery.
- After recent trauma (e.g. whiplash, fractures, sprains or dislocations, or when the extent of the injury is not known).
- Severe unstable hypertension (i.e. elevated blood pressure above the normal range for a prolonged period of time).
- Systemic illness (e.g. fever, diarrhoea, vomiting, unexplained oedema).
- Oedema that contributes to joint stability.[18]

RELATIVE CONTRAINDICATIONS

- Malignancies. Advise clients who have active cancer or who are recovering from cancer to get clearance from their doctor before commencing lymphatic drainage massage.
- Recent thrombosis. Older clients, clients with veins in poor condition and past history of thrombosis may be a contraindication.
- Varicose veins. Massage above the involved area.
- Bronchial asthma. Treat clients when the condition is receding, omitting sternum and chest massage. Never treat bronchial asthma in an acute phase. Care should always be taken with asthmatics to keep treatments short as over-treatment can bring on a mild attack of asthma.[4]
- Low blood pressure. A full body lymphatic drainage massage may lower blood pressure. Treatment time should be reduced for the first session and increased in subsequent sessions if no problems occur.[4]
- Moles, beauty spots, burns, fresh scars, bruises or skin problems.
- Renal insufficiency or clients receiving haemodialysis. Care should be taken to keep treatments short as such clients tire and bruise easily.
- Gynaecological cysts and other conditions of the uterus. Avoid deep abdominal massage.

LOCAL CONTRAINDICATIONS

- Varicose veins, thrombosis after inflammation has subsided.
- Local inflammation without fever (e.g. open wound, sprains).
- Sports injuries with oedema or inflammation.

Neck

- Hypersensitivity of the carotid sinus.
- Hyperthyroidism.

Abdomen

- Pregnancy.
- During menstruation.
- After recent abdominal surgery.
- Radiation fibrosis.
- After pelvic deep venous thrombosis.
- Crohn's disease.
- Diverticulosis.

Review questions

1. Name three functions of the lymphatic system.
2. Complete the following:
   a) Lymph is filtered as it passes through ______________ as it travels through the body.
   b) Contractions of the smooth muscle in the walls of the ________________ (the functional units of lymphatic vessels) stimulates the flow of lymph towards the thorax.
   c) There are approximately ___________ lymph nodes in the body.
3. Lymph from the right upper quadrant empties into the
   a) thoracic duct
   b) bright lymphatic duct
   c) left lymphatic duct
   d) cisterna chyli
4. What is the primary consequence of oedema?
5. How does lymphoedema differ from oedema?
6. What is the main cause of lymphoedema?
7. Complete the following table:

Primary lymphoedema	Secondary lymphoedema
Mainly affects __________	Occurs in any part of the body
Developmental abnormality. Can be triggered by ______	Usually develops after ___________________

8. Name three contraindications for lymphatic drainage massage.
9. Select the most correct answer. Orthostatic oedema:
   a) is associated with skin pigmentation, ulceration and pits on pressure
   b) is occasionally bilateral and is sometimes associated with skin thickening
   c) is always bilateral and pits on pressure
   d) is always bilateral and does not usually involve the feet
10. Complete the following guidelines for lymphatic drainage massage.
    a) The pressure of lymphatic drainage massage is ___________
    b) The rate of lymphatic drainage is ___________
    c) Begin lymphatic drainage massage at the __________________________
    d) Lymphatic drainage massage is always performed in the direction of _______________________
    e) In lymphatic drainage massage each stroke is performed _________ times.
    f) Strokes are predominantly circular and __________________
    g) Each stroke has a working phase and a resting phase to create a variation in _____________________
11. Which of the following is *not* an indication for lymphatic drainage massage?
    a) chronic pain
    b) sub-acute inflammation
    c) shortness of breath
    d) slowly developing generalised oedema
    e) lymphoedema
    f) acne vulgaris
    g) severe pain

REFERENCES

1. Chikly B. Silent waves: theory and practice of lymphatic drainage therapy. Scotsdale, AZ: LHH Publishing; 2002.
2. Fritz S, Grosenbach M. Mosby's essential sciences for therapeutic massage. 3rd edn. St. Louis, MO: Mosby Elsevier; 2009.
3. Cash M. Sport and remedial massage therapy. London: Edbury Press; 1996.
4. Wittlinger G, Wittlinger H. Introduction to Dr Vodder's manual lymphatic drainage. Rev edn. Heidelberg: Karl V. Haug: Verlag; 1990.
5. Yates J. A physician's guide to therapeutic massage: its physiological effects and their application to treatment. Vancouver: Massage Therapists' Association of British Columbia; 1990.
6. DelLisa J, Gans B. Rehabilitation medicine: principles and practice. 2nd edn. Philadelphia: Lippincott; 1993.
7. Foldi M, Foldi E, editors. Foldi's textbook of lymphology for physicians and lymphedema therapists. 2nd edn. Munich: Elsevier GmbH; 2006.
8. Piller N, O'Connor M. The lymphoedema handbook: causes, effects and management. Melbourne: Hill of Content; 2002.
9. Kriederman B, Myloyde T, Bernas M, et al. Limb volume reduction after physical treatment by compressions and/or massage in a rodent model of peripheral lymphedema. Lymphology 2002;35(1): 23–7.
10. Leduc O, Leduc A, Boureois P, et al. The physical treatment of upper limb edema. Cancer 1998;83 (12 Suppl American):2835–9.
11. Haren K, Backman C, Wiberg M. Effect of manual lymph drainage as described by Vodder on oedema of the hand after fracture of the distal radius: a prospective clinical study. Scand J Plast Reconstr Surg Hand Surg 2000;34(4):367–72.
12. Johansson K, Albertsson M, Ingvar C, et al. Effects of compressive bandaging with or without manual lymph drainage treatment in patients with postoperative arm lymphedema. Lymphology 1999;32(3):103–10.
13. Ekici G, Bakar Y, Akbayrak T, et al. Comparison of manual lymph drainage therapy and connective tissue massage in women with fibromyalgia: a randomised controlled trial. J Manipulative Physiol Ther 2009;32(2):127–33.
14. Schillinger A, Koenig D, Haefele C, et al. Effect of manual lymph drainage on the course of serum levels of muscle enzymes after treadmill exercise. Am J Phys Med Rehabil 2006;85(6): 516–20.
15. Preston N, Seers K, Mortimer P. Physical therapies for reducing and controlling lymphoedema of the limbs. Cochrane Database Syst Rev 2004;(4) CD003141.
16. International Society of Lymphology. The diagnosis and treatment of peripheral lymphedema: 2009 Consensus document of the International Society of Lymphology. Online. Available: www.u.arizona.edu./~witte/ISL.htm; 2009.
17. National Breast and Ovarian Cancer Centre. Lymphoedema – what you need to know. Online. Available: www.nbocc.org.au; 2008.
18. Fritz S, Chaitow L, Hymel GM. Clinical massage in the healthcare setting. St. Louis, MI: Mosby Elsevier; 2008.
19. Beers M, Porter R. The Merck manual of diagnosis and therapy. 17th edn. West Point, PA: Merck; 1999.
20. Munro J, Campbell I, editors. Macleod's clinical examination. Edinburgh: Churchill Livingstone; 2000.
21. Bickley L, Szilagyi P, editors. Bates' guide to physical examination and history taking. 10th edn. Philadelphia: Lippincott-Raven; 2009.
22. Russell N, Sumier S, Beinhorn C, et al. Role of massage in cancer care. J Altern Complement Med 2008;14(2):209–14.

10 The low back and pelvis

The content of this chapter relates to the following Units of Competency:

HLTREM503C Plan remedial massage treatment strategy
HLTREM504C Apply remedial massage assessment framework
HLTREM502C Provide remedial massage treatment
HLTREM510B Provide specialised remedial massage treatment

Health Training Package HLT07

Learning Outcomes

- Assess clients with conditions of the low back and pelvis for remedial massage, including identification of red and yellow flags.
- Assess clients for signs and symptoms associated with common conditions of the low back and pelvis and treat and/or manage these conditions with appropriate remedial massage therapy.
- Develop treatment plans for clients with conditions of the low back and pelvis, taking into account assessment findings, duration and severity of the condition, likely tissue types, the best available evidence and client preferences.
- Develop short- and long-term treatment plans to address presenting symptoms, underlying conditions and predisposing factors, and to progressively increase the self-help component of therapy.
- Adapt remedial massage therapy to suit the needs of individual clients based on duration and severity of injury, the client's age and gender, the presence of underlying conditions and co-morbidities, and other considerations for special population groups.

INTRODUCTION

It is estimated that 70–85% of the populations in developed countries are likely to experience low back pain at some time in their lives.[1, 2] In the period 2004–2005, 15% of the total population of Australia reported having back problems.[3] Clients with non-specific low back pain (i.e. pain that cannot be given a precise pathoanatomical diagnosis) account for 85–95% of clients[4, 5] and many such clients consult remedial massage therapists. Serious medical causes of low back pain are rare but it is vital that remedial massage therapists can identify red flags and other conditions that require specific precautions for safe practice. In most cases of acute low back pain, X-rays and blood tests are not required.

FUNCTIONAL ANATOMY REVIEW

The lumbar spine is designed for both stability and mobility. Five large vertebrae and discs bear the weight of the upper body. Between pairs of vertebral bodies are intervertebral discs which are composed of an annulus fibrosus (concentric rings of fibrocartilage) and a nucleus pulposus (a central mass of pulpy tissue). The discs act as shock absorbers and give the spine its flexibility. When the vertebral column is flexed, extended or bent sideways, the disc distorts as uneven loads are applied. Excessive loads can cause intervertebral discs to bulge or prolapse. Vertebral arches on the posterior aspect of the vertebral bodies provide protection for the spinal cord which passes through the vertebral foramina framed by the vertebral bodies, pedicles and lamina. Spinal nerves enter and exit the spinal cord through the intervertebral foramina (IVF) which are bounded above and below by the pedicles of adjacent vertebrae. Spinal nerves are vulnerable to pressure from bulging or herniated discs (see Figure 10.1 on p 139).

Superior and inferior articular processes form facet joints which prevent excessive movements between vertebrae. The superior facets are concave and face medially and posteriorly; the inferior facets are convex and face laterally and anteriorly. The articular facets of L1–4 lie in the sagittal plane, favouring flexion and extension and limiting rotation. The facets change their orientation from L1 to L5 so that the facets of L5/S1 lie more in the coronal plane (i.e. they are angled more outwards). This orientation counteracts the tremendous anterior shear force that occurs at this level. The pars interarticularis lies between the superior and inferior articular processes (see Figure 10.2 on p 140).

The orientation of the facets also permits coupled movements; that is, when movement in one direction is combined with movement in another. In the lumbar spine, lateral flexion appears to be associated with rotation. However, there is no agreement as to whether the spinous process rotates towards or away from the concave side.[6–8]

The anterior and posterior longitudinal ligaments are firmly attached to the discs and guard against excessive flexion and

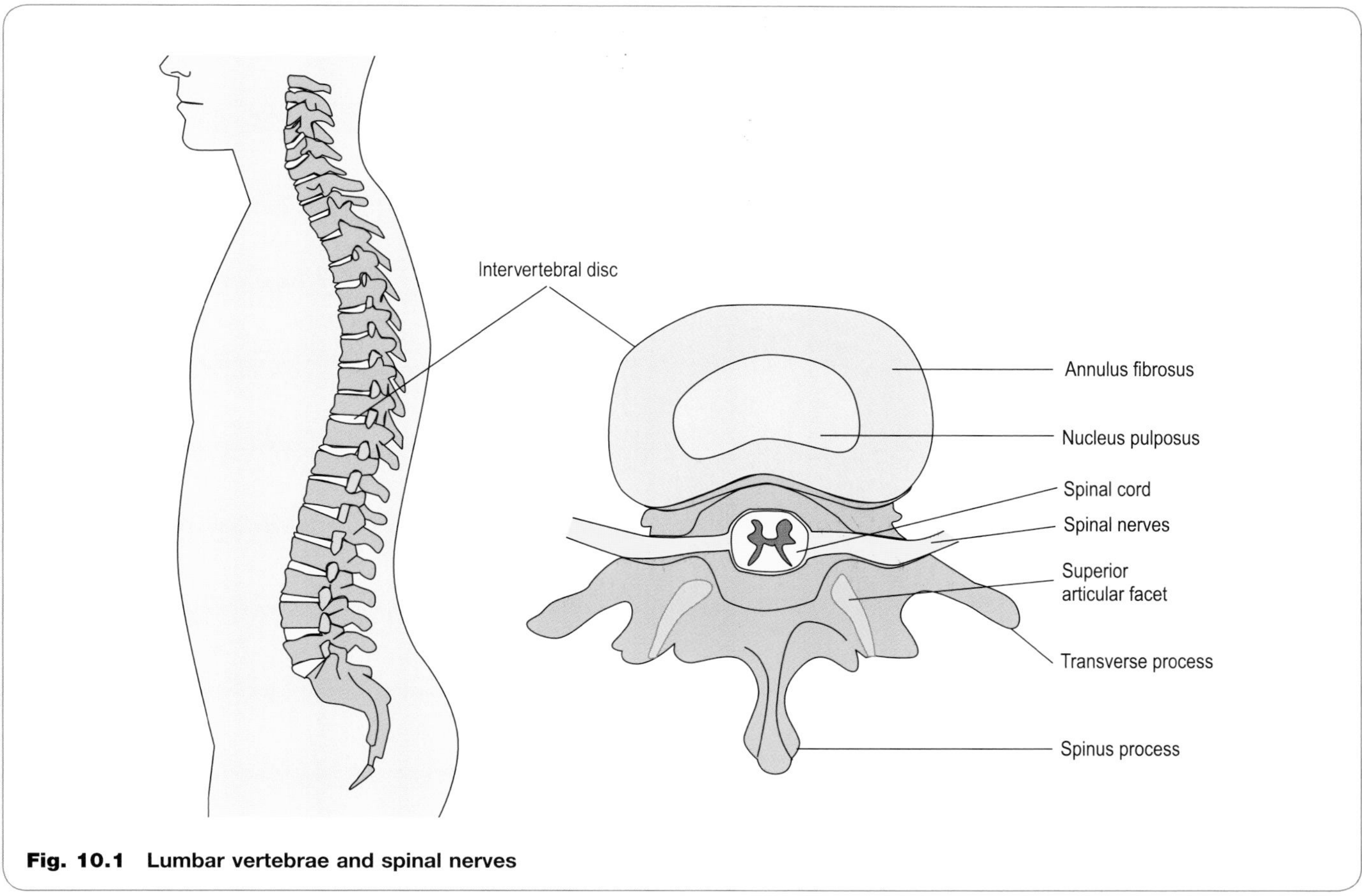

Fig. 10.1 Lumbar vertebrae and spinal nerves

extension movements of the flexible column. Movement is further limited by joint capsules and other ligaments including the ligamentum flavum, the intertransverse ligaments and the iliolumbar ligaments. The iliolumbar ligaments attach to the transverse processes of L4 and L5, the sacrum and the ilium (see Figure 10.3 on p 140).

The lumbosacral angle (the angle between the sacral base and the horizontal) is approximately 41° in the average adult.[9] The pelvic girdle is made up of the iliac bones and the sacrum. The two sacroiliac joints posteriorly and the symphysis pubis anteriorly are held together by strong ligaments (e.g. anterior and posterior sacroiliac ligament, interosseous ligaments, sacrotuberous and sacrospinous ligaments). There are no muscles that attach directly to the sacroiliac joints. The sacroiliac joint has a self-locking or close pack position; that is, the most congruent position that helps to stabilise the pelvis as weight is transferred from one leg to the other during the push-off phase of the gait cycle. Lumbar motion and sacral motion are coupled: when the lumbar spine is flexed, the sacral base tilts anteriorly (sacral nutation); when the lumbar spine is extended, the sacral base tilts posteriorly (sacral counternutation). The ilia can tilt forwards and back on the sacrum (both left and right moving together or separately). The sacrum can also move on the ilium. There is more movement in sacroiliac joints in women than in men because the pelvis is wider and flatter.

Normal biomechanics of the lumbosacral spine require the support of muscles of the lower back, abdomen and pelvic floor. (see Table 10.1 on p 141 and Figure 10.4 on p 142). When these muscles become weak or injured, loads that are normally counteracted by muscle contraction may be transmitted to deeper structures like vertebrae and discs. Moreover, the orientation of the pelvis and spinal curvature may be affected by imbalances in muscles attaching to the pelvis such as the hamstrings, quadriceps, piriformis, psoas and hip adductors (see Figure 10.5 on p 142).

ASSESSMENT OF THE LUMBAR AND SACROILIAC REGION

It is not always possible or necessary to establish definitive diagnoses for many musculoskeletal problems. It is essential, however, that clients requiring referral to other healthcare practitioners are identified. The first task of remedial massage therapists is to identify clients' suitability for remedial massage by identifying red and yellow flags. For those clients for whom remedial massage is suitable, assessments help identify the duration and severity of their conditions and the most likely tissue types involved. In some cases clients' signs and symptoms will fit patterns of common conditions but even when this is the case, it is important to remember that correlations between clinical presentations and definitive diagnoses are often low. Assess all clients, even those who come with previous medical diagnoses, not only to confirm their diagnoses but also to gather such important information as clients' preferences for treatment types and styles and the need for modification of techniques for safe and competent practice.

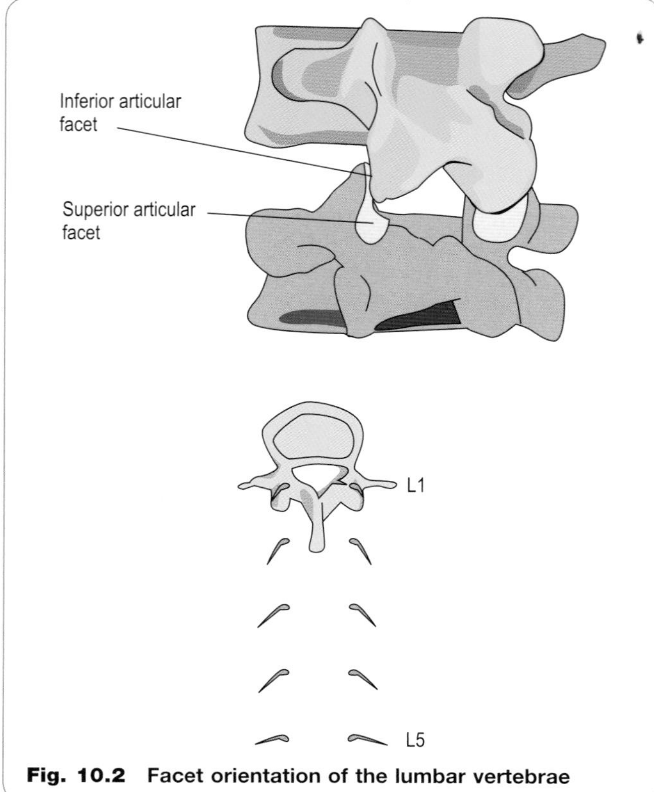

Fig. 10.2 Facet orientation of the lumbar vertebrae

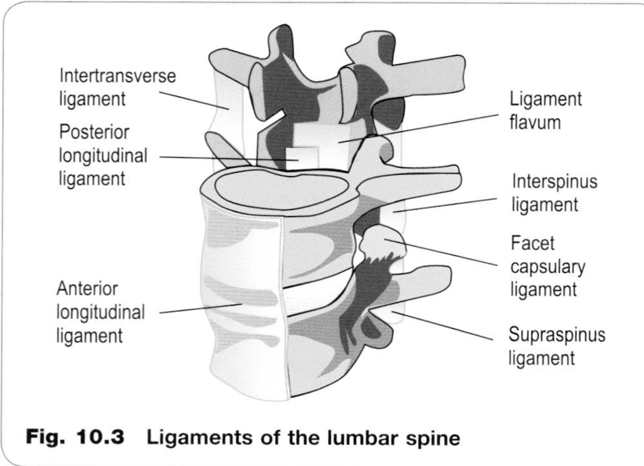

Fig. 10.3 Ligaments of the lumbar spine

Assessment procedures for remedial massage clients are discussed in detail in Chapter 2.

CASE HISTORY

- Ask clients to point to the site of pain as they may have different understandings of anatomical terms. For example 'hip' could mean iliac crest, sacroiliac joint, buttock, greater trochanter or the actual hip joint.
- Clients with low back pain, especially those with disc herniations, may prefer to stand rather than sit during the case history.
- Identify any red flags that require referral for further investigation (see Table 10.2 on p 143).

Assessment of the low back and pelvis

1. Case history
2. Outcome measures
3. Postural analysis
4. Gait assessment
5. Functional tests
   Active range of motion tests
   flexion, extension, lateral flexion, rotation
   Passive range of motion tests
   flexion, extension, lateral flexion, rotation
   Resisted range of motion tests
   flexion, extension, lateral flexion, rotation
   Resisted and length tests for specific muscle tests including
   - Piriformis
   - Iliopsoas
   - Quadratus lumborum
   - Erector spinae
   - Gluteus maximus
   - Hamstrings
   - Quadriceps
   - Abdominal muscles

   Special tests including
   - Kemp's quadrant test
   - Valsalva
   - SLR
   - Centralisation/peripheralisation
   - Patrick's test
   - Sacroiliac compression
   - Sacroiliac distraction
   - Sacral springing
   - Leg length test
6. Palpation

- Determine if the pain is likely to have a mechanical cause. (Is the pain associated with rest or activity, certain postures or time of day?) Ask clients to show you movements and positions that aggravate or relieve the pain and to be specific with descriptions of aggravating or relieving activities.
  - Mechanical pain is usually highly reactive to changes in posture, position or activity.
  - Morning pain relieved with daily activity is often associated with arthritis.
  - Current research suggests that client reports of numbness, weakness, tingling or burning do not appear to be very helpful in identifying lumbar radiculopathy.[11]
  - Pain that is not relieved by lying down, back pain at night and morning stiffness lasting more than half an hour may be helpful in identifying ankylosing spondylitis[a].[11]
  - A report of 'no pain when seated' appears to be the most useful information for the diagnosis of lumbar spinal stenosis[b].[11]
  - Pain relieved by standing may be useful for identifying SI joint pain.[11]

[a]Ankylosing spondylitis is an autoimmune disease characterised by chronic inflammation of the back and sacroiliac joints. Pain and stiffness are the main symptoms.

[b]Spinal stenosis is a narrowing of the spinal canal which causes the spinal cord and nerves to be compressed. It occurs most commonly from the degenerative changes of ageing but is also caused by disc herniation, osteoporosis or tumour.

Table 10.1 Major muscles of the low back and pelvis[10]

Muscle	Origin	Insertion	Action
Erector spinae Superficial muscles of the spinal column	Strong aponeurosis from posterior sacrum and adjacent iliac crest	Fibres ascend and divide into three columns 1. Iliocostalis – lateral column, inserts into angles of ribs 2. Longissimus – middle column, inserts into thoracic and cervical transverse processes and mastoid process 3. Spinalis – medial column, confined to the thoracic region, inserts into spinous processes	Extend the spine, laterally flex the spine
Deep muscles of the spinal column			
Multifidus	Sacrum, ilium, transverse processes of lumbar, thoracic and inferior four cervical vertebrae	Spinous process of vertebra above	Extend spine, laterally flex spine, stabilise vertebrae in local movements of vertebral column
Rotators	Transverse process of all vertebrae The rotators form the deepest layer in the lumbar and thoracic region	Spinous process of vertebra above	
Quadratus lumborum	Iliac crest	12th rib, L1–L4/5	Extends lower back, laterally flexes trunk
Iliopsoas	Psoas major and minor originate from T12 to L4/5 Iliacus originates from the superior iliac fossa	Lesser trochanter of the femur	Flexes hip Trunk flexor Assists in lateral flexion of the trunk and internal rotation of hip
Piriformis	Anterior surface of sacrum	Greater trochanter of femur	Laterally rotates and abducts hip
Gluteus maximus	Medial iliac crest and posterior inferior sacrum	Iliotibial band of the tensor fasciae latae and gluteal tuberosity of the femur	Extends and laterally rotates the hip joint
Hamstring muscles	Ischial tuberosity	Tibial condyle, pes anserine tendon, fibula head and deep fascia of the leg	Flex the knee; extend and laterally rotate the hip joint
Quadriceps femoris	Anterior inferior iliac spine, linea aspera, greater trochanter, gluteal tuberosity	Tibial tuberosity via the patella ligament	Flexes the hip joint and extends the knee
Rectus abdominis	Pubic crest and pubic symphysis	Cartilage of ribs 5–7, xiphoid process	Flexes lumbar spine, compresses abdomen
External oblique	Inferior 8 ribs	Iliac crest and linea alba	Laterally flexes spine, rotates spine, compresses abdomen, flexes spine
Internal oblique	Iliac crest, inguinal ligament and thoracolumbar fascia	Cartilage of last 3 or 4 ribs and linea alba	Laterally flexes spine, rotates spine, compresses abdomen, flexes spine
Transversus abdominis	Iliac crest, inguinal ligament, lumbar fascia, cartilages of inferior 6 ribs	Xiphoid process, linea alba and pubis	Compresses abdomen
Pelvic floor muscles Levator ani • Pubococcygeus • Iliococcygeus	 Pubis Ischial spine	 Coccyx, urethra, anal canal, perineum Coccyx	Supports and maintains position of pelvic viscera, resists increased intra-abdominal pressure
Coccygeus	Ischial spine	Lower sacrum and upper coccyx	Supports and maintains position of pelvic viscera, resists increased intra-abdominal pressure

(Note: Gluteus medius, gluteus minimus, obturator internus and externus, gemellus superior and inferior and quadratus femoris are discussed in Chapter 18.)

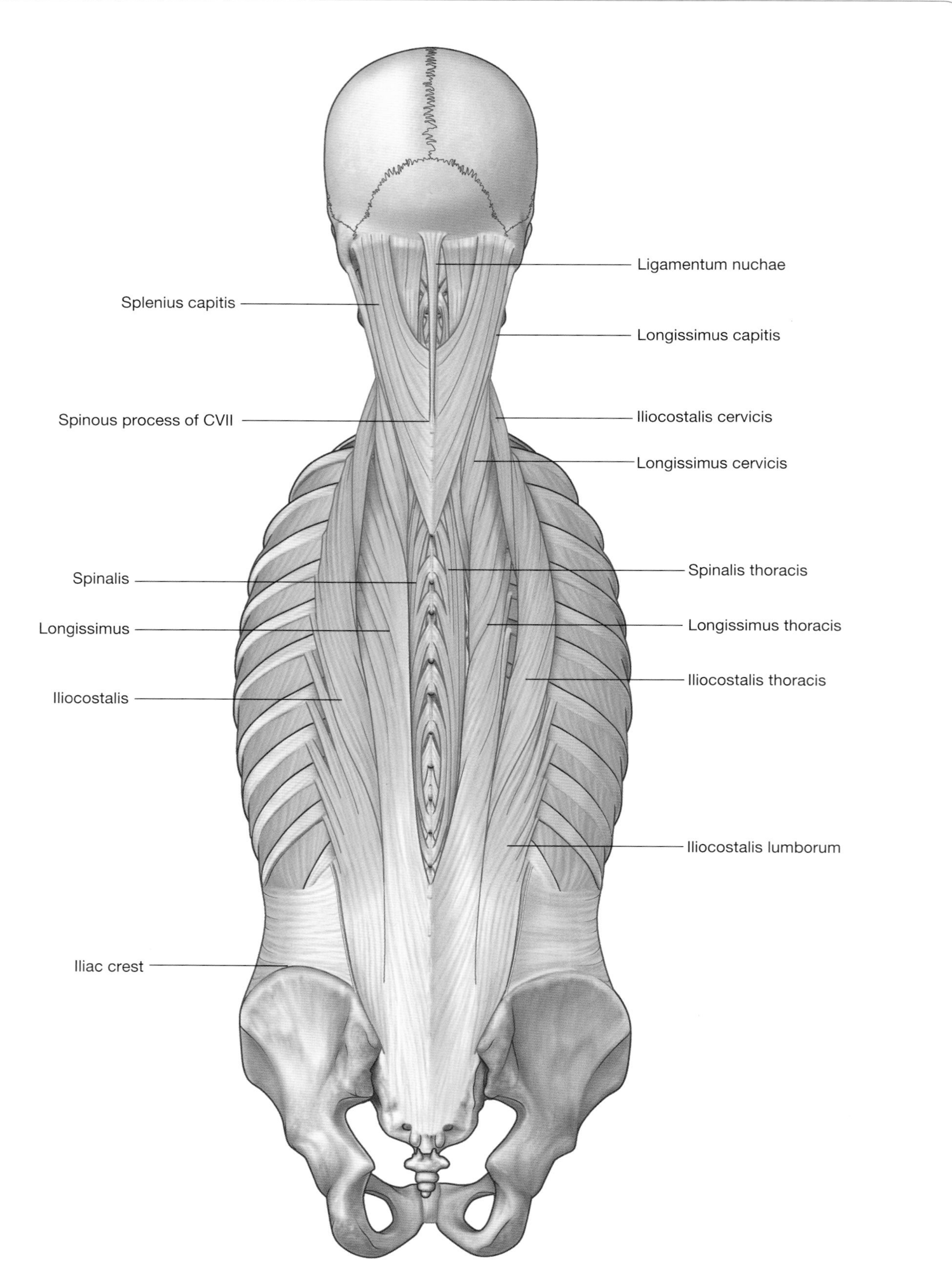

Fig. 10.4 Erector spinae group

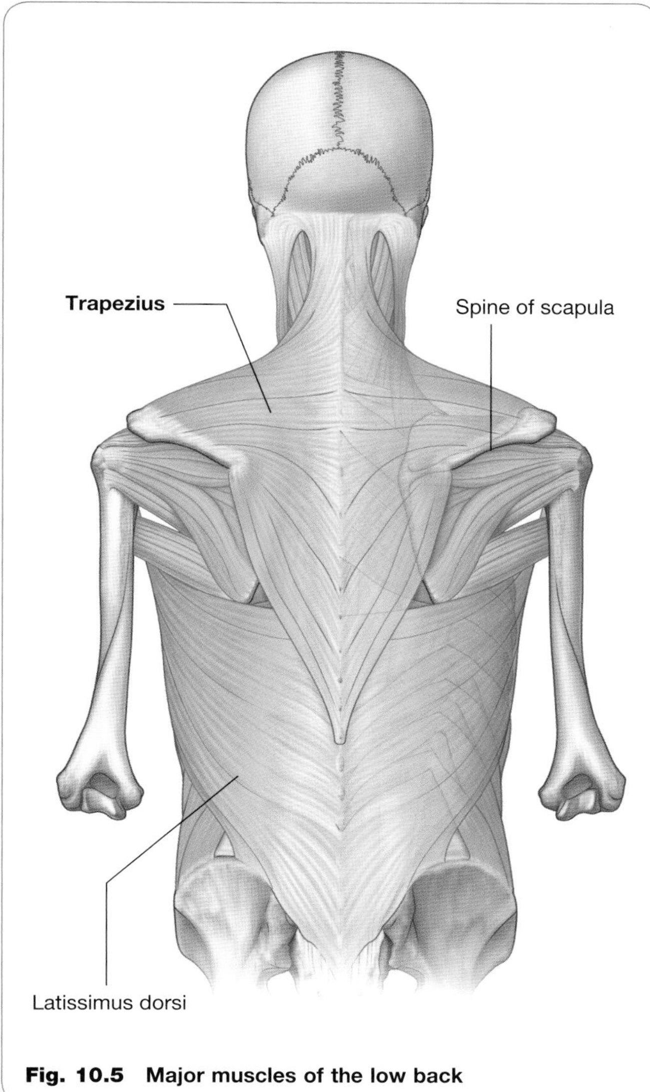

Fig. 10.5 Major muscles of the low back

- Determine if the pain is likely to be associated with visceral function, neurogenic, vascular or psychosocial issues (yellow flags).
  - Pain from the kidney, gall bladder or prostate is not usually aggravated by activity or relieved by rest, whereas mechanical back pain may be relieved by lying down.
  - Neurogenic back pain from a spinal cord tumour or from a primary or secondary vertebral bone tumour is generally constant and remains unchanged by postural position.
  - Symptoms of vascular claudication are aggravated by walking and relieved by standing still or resting.
- Sacroiliac joint sprain causes local pain that may radiate to the low back and buttock. The pain can be sharp and stabbing, aggravated by movement and relieved by lying down. It may be difficult to differentiate sacroiliac joint sprain from a condition originating in the lumbar spine. Clients with sacroiliac joint dysfunctions experience pain most intensely around one or both sacroiliac joints with or without referral to the lateral thigh. Focal tenderness on palpation of the sacroiliac joints and positive special tests can also help differentiate.

Table 10.2 Red flags for serious conditions associated with acute low back pain

Red flags for acute low back pain	Possible condition
Symptoms and signs of infection (e.g. fever) Risk factors for infection (e.g. underlying disease, immunosuppression, penetrating wound)	Infection
History of trauma Minor trauma (if >50 years, history of osteoporosis, taking corticosteroids)	Fracture
Past history of malignancy Age >50 years Failure to improve with treatment Unexplained weight loss Pain at multiple sites Pain at rest	Cancer
Absence of aggravating factors	Aortic aneurysm Other serious condition
Widespread neurological symptoms and signs in the lower limb (e.g. gait abnormality, saddle area numbness) ± urinary retention, faecal incontinence	Cauda equina syndrome (a medical emergency and requires urgent hospital referral)

Adapted from the Acute Musculoskeletal Pain Guidelines Group[4] and the New Zealand Guidelines Group.[12]
Note that acute pain in this context refers to pain of less than three months' duration.

OUTCOME MEASURES

Outcome measures are specifically designed questionnaires that are used to assess clients' level of impairment and to define benefits of treatment. The benefit is assessed in terms of client-perceived changes to health status. Common outcome measures for low back pain and disability are the Oswestry Disability Index and Roland-Morris Low Back Pain and Disability Questionnaire.

POSTURAL ANALYSIS

- Scoliosis and hyperlordosis are common conditions affecting the lumbar spine and pelvis and should not be missed.
- Soft doughy lipomata (fatty masses) appearing as lumps in the area of the low back may be a sign of spina bifida (non-union of the vertebral arch at the spinous process).
- A hairy patch (faun's beard) in conjunction with a lipoma further suggests an underlying bony pathology.
- Birth marks or excessive port wine marks should be carefully investigated since they suggest underlying bony pathology (spina bifida).
- A step defect is a visible or palpable step from one spinous process to the next. This most commonly occurs at L5/S1 and suggests spondylolisthesis.

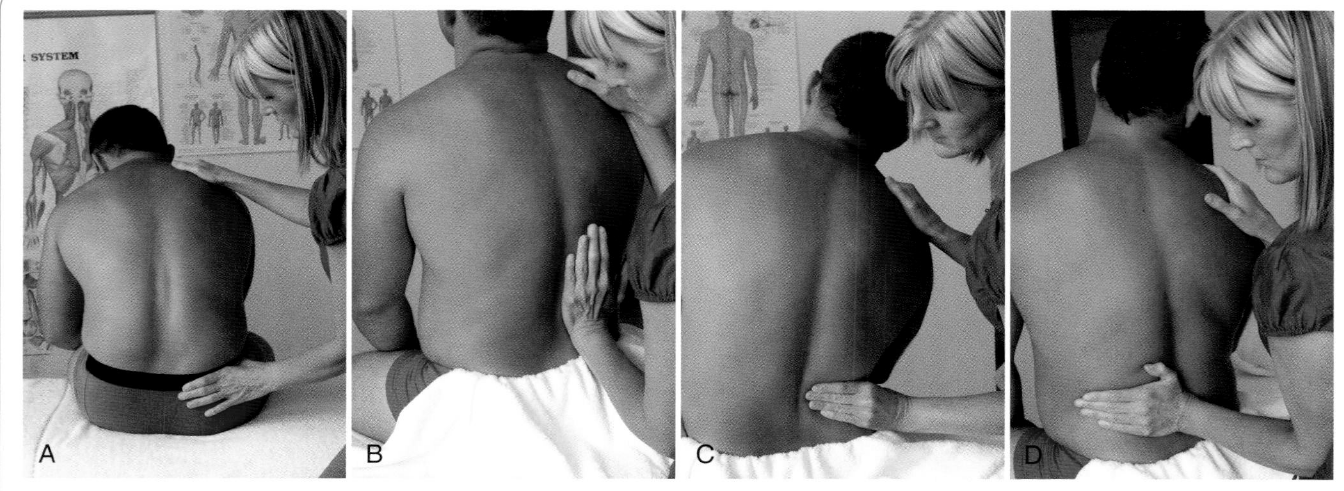

Fig. 10.6 Performing PROM of the lumbar spine. A: Flexion; **B:** Extension; **C:** Lateral flexion; **D:** Rotation.

GAIT ASSESSMENT

Many conditions of the lumbosacral spine and sacroiliac joints will affect the symmetry and rhythm of normal gait (see Chapter 2). In lower-crossed syndrome, for example, changes in movement patterns with hip extension, hip abduction and trunk flexion are often observed.[13]

FUNCTIONAL TESTS

Thoracolumbar range of motion tests have repeatedly been shown to be very reliable although their diagnostic accuracy[c] remains unclear.[11] Findings of functional tests should be correlated with case history, postural and gait analysis and other functional assessments and interpreted in this context.

Active range of motion (AROM)

FLEXION (60°)[d]

- Trunk flexion mostly occurs in the hip joints with only a very small amount occurring in the lumbar spine.
- The lumbar spine flattens but does not reverse to a kyphosis as it does in the cervical spine.
- Instruct clients to return to the erect position if they experience any pain. Special care is required with disc clients as flexion may aggravate symptoms. Ask all clients to bend forward slowly and only as far as they can without pain.

EXTENSION (25°)

- Extension will produce increased pain for a range of clients including those with spondylolisthesis or hyperlordosis and may also be painful for disc clients.

LATERAL FLEXION (SIDEBEND) (25°)

- Stabilise the iliac crest with one hand and gently guide the client with the other hand on their shoulder.
- Compare both sides and observe the coupling of the lumbar spine facet joints (lateral flexion associated with slight vertebral rotation).

ROTATION (30°)

- Stabilise the pelvis by placing one hand on each side. Ask the client to turn their shoulders to the left and then the right as far as they can comfortably go. Alternatively, ask clients to stand with their thighs against the treatment table or sit on the table and then to turn their shoulders left and right as far as they comfortably can.

Passive range of motion (PROM)

PROM of the lumbar spine is difficult to perform because of the weight of the trunk, and as a result many remedial massage therapists do not routinely perform PROM tests of the lumbar spine. However, PROM can be performed with the client seated and the practitioner placing their forearm across the top of the shoulders to guide the movements. The other hand rests on the lumbar spine to palpate the movement (see Figure 10.6).

Resisted range of motion (RROM)

With the client seated, ask them to try to bend forward, backwards, to the side and to rotate their trunk against your resistance. Use the same contacts described for PROM.

Tests for specific muscles associated with low back conditions[15, 16]

Test the major muscles of the lumbar spine and pelvis for length and strength. Make bilateral comparisons where possible and always consider other reasons for apparent muscle imbalances such as age, underlying pathology and lifestyle.

---

[c]Diagnostic accuracy refers to the degree of agreement between a clinical test and a reference standard. It is usually expressed in terms of sensitivity, specificity and likelihood ratios (see Chapter 2).[11]

[d]Reese and Bandy (2002) reviewed published data on joint ranges of motion and suggest that the normative values for the lumbar spine are 60° flexion, 30° extension, 30° lateral flexion and 6° rotation.[14]

1. PIRIFORMIS

Resisted test

Resisted external (lateral) rotation of the hip can be performed in a variety of positions to suit the comfort of the client and practitioner. One option is for the client to sit on the treatment table with their knees bent over the side. Kneel beside the client. One hand contacts the medial lower leg above the ankle; the other contacts the lateral aspect of the knee. Tap the medial lower leg and ask the client to push against that hand; that is, to externally rotate their hip against your resistance. Figure 10.7 shows the test in the prone position.

Length test

A tight piriformis muscle holds the hip in lateral rotation. Clients may have a *toe out* gait and on postural analysis stand with their foot excessively turned outwards. A test for piriformis contracture is to ask the client to lie prone, knee flexed to 90°, and to let their foot drop to the side. A tight piriformis will limit medial rotation which is suggested if the foot fails to drop to 30–40°.

Clinical significance

The sciatic nerve exits the sciatic notch and runs underneath the piriformis muscle. In 15% of the population the sciatic nerve passes through the piriformis[17, 18] and muscle spasm or contracture can press on the nerve and cause sciatic neuritis (piriformis syndrome) (see Figure 10.9). If straight leg raising has produced pain, numbness or tingling in the low back, posterior thigh and/or lower leg, straight leg raising is performed a second time with the hip externally rotated (i.e. foot turned out). If the posterior thigh and leg pain is relieved in the second test, piriformis syndrome is suggested. Although not a common cause of posterior thigh and leg pain compared with nerve compression originating from the lumbosacral spine, piriformis syndrome can usually be simply and effectively treated when identified.

2. ILIOPSOAS

Resisted test

The client lies supine. Stand contralaterally. Place one hand on the contralateral ASIS to stabilise the pelvis. With the other hand, slightly abduct and externally rotate the client's leg and raise it to 40° flexion. Ask the client to hold their leg in this position. Tap the client's medial tibia and ask the client to push up against your hand as if they were lifting their leg towards their opposite shoulder against your resistance (see Figure 10.10).

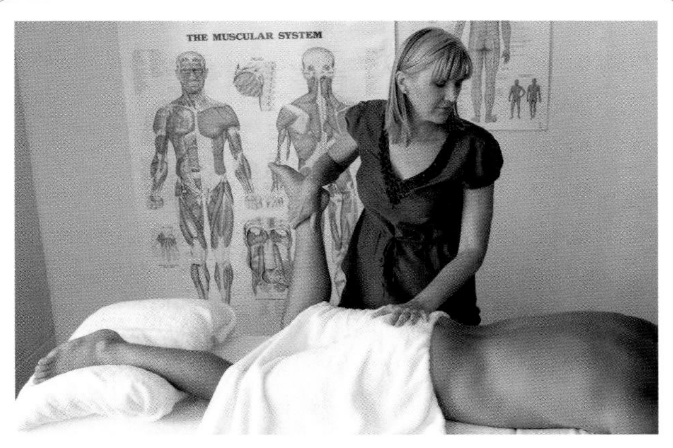

Fig. 10.7 Resisted test for piriformis

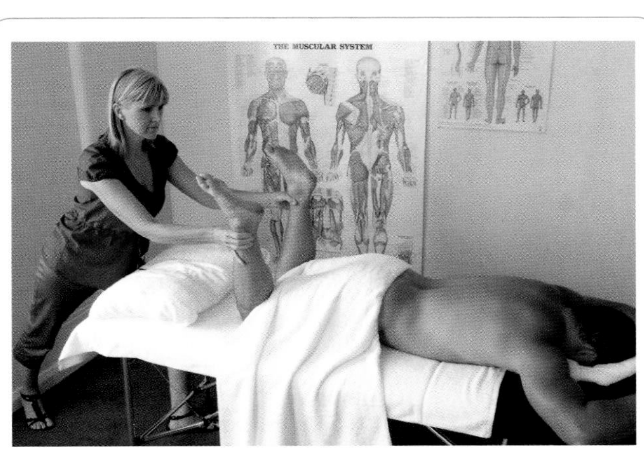

Fig. 10.8 Piriformis length test

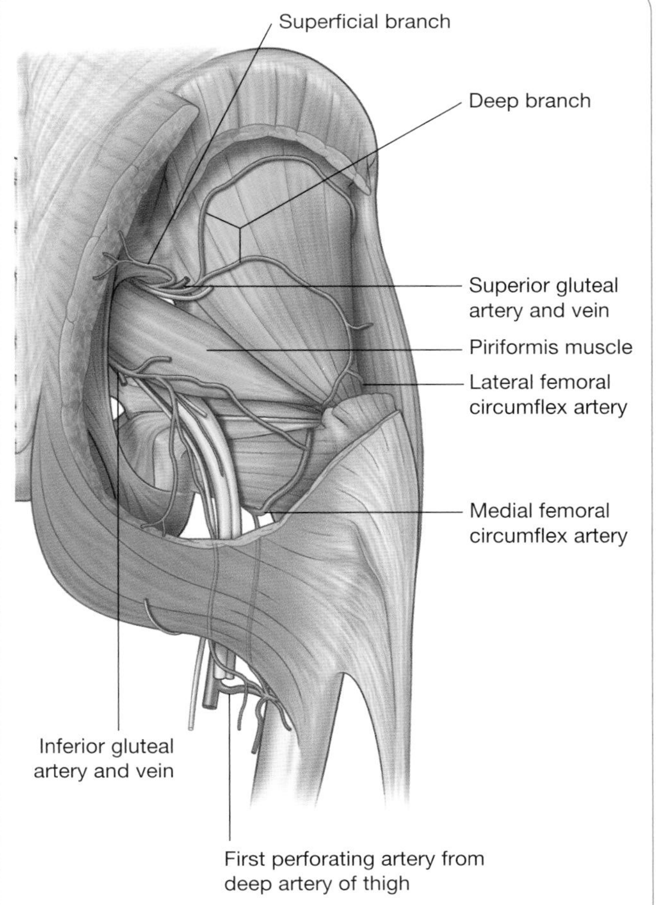

Fig. 10.9 Relationship between piriformis muscle and the sciatic nerve

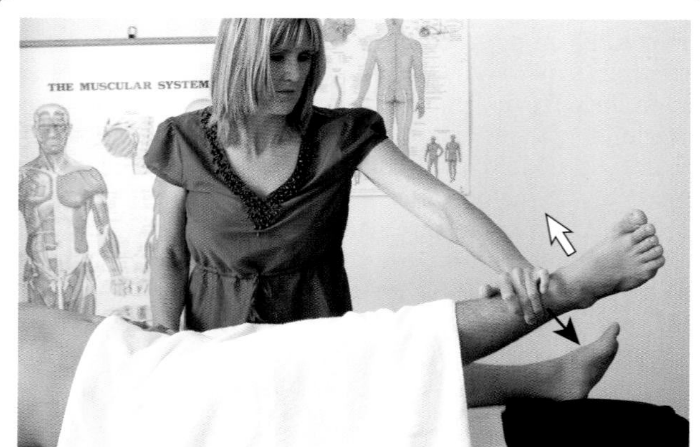

Fig. 10.10 Resisted test for iliopsoas

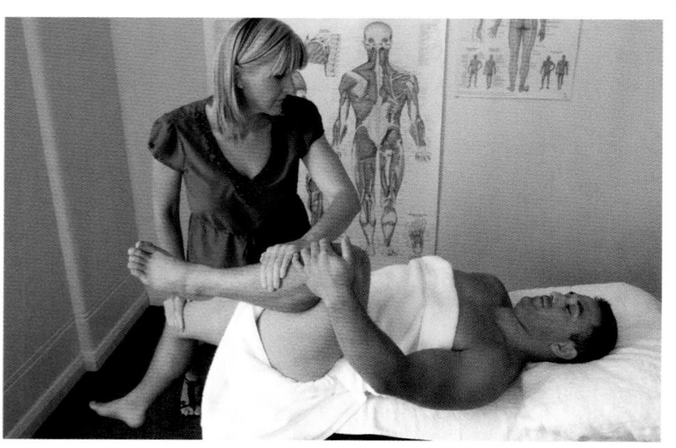

Fig. 10.11 Thomas test for iliopsoas contracture

Length test

The Thomas test is used to test the length of the iliopsoas. The client should be wearing a gown or loose clothing and the technique requires appropriate draping. The client sits on the edge of the foot of the table and rolls back bringing both knees to their chest in the process. Ask the client to hold their knees to their chest with their arms. The client slowly releases one leg and lets it fall over the end of the table, while maintaining the original degree of hip flexion on the other leg (see Figure 10.11). A shortened iliopsoas will prevent the thigh dropping to the level of the table.

The following variation of the Thomas test is easier for the client because it can be performed in the usual supine position and therefore minimises the position changes required during assessment. The client flexes the hip and knee on the opposite side to the one being tested and holds their knee against their chest. The test is positive if the straight leg lifts off the table during this manoeuvre indicating a flexion contracture of the iliopsoas muscle.

Clinical significance

A unilateral contracted iliopsoas may contribute to scoliosis; a bilaterally contracted iliopsoas may contribute to hyperlordosis – two very common postural observations in remedial massage.

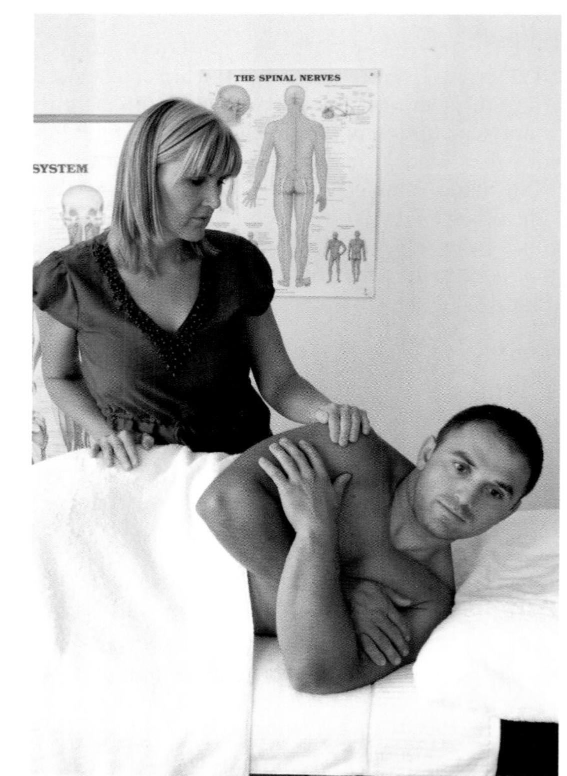

Fig. 10.12 Resisted test for quadratus lumborum

3. QUADRATUS LUMBORUM

Strength test

The client lies on their side with their arms crossed across the chest. Hold the client's feet to prevent them from lifting off the table. Ask the client to raise their shoulders and trunk off the table (sidebend the trunk) without using their arms (see Figure 10.12).

Length test

Postural observation may reveal a pelvic tilt (i.e. elevated iliac crest/hip hike) and a concave scoliosis on the side of the shortened quadratus lumborum.[19] Contracture restricts trunk sidebending towards the opposite side.

Clinical significance

A unilateral contracted quadratus lumborum may contribute to scoliosis: the pelvis is normally elevated and the lumbar spine concave on the contracted side.[20] Bilaterally contracted quadratus lumborum may contribute to hyperlordosis.

4. ERECTOR SPINAE

Strength test

The client lies prone and clasps their hands behind their back. Ask the client to lift their head and shoulders off the table (see Figure 10.13 on p 147).

Length test

The client sits with legs extended and the pelvis vertical and flexes forward towards the knees. In the normal flexible adult

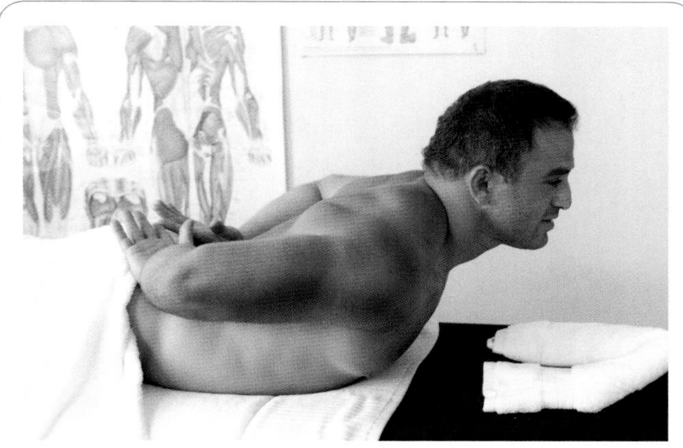

Fig. 10.13 **Strength test for erector spinae**

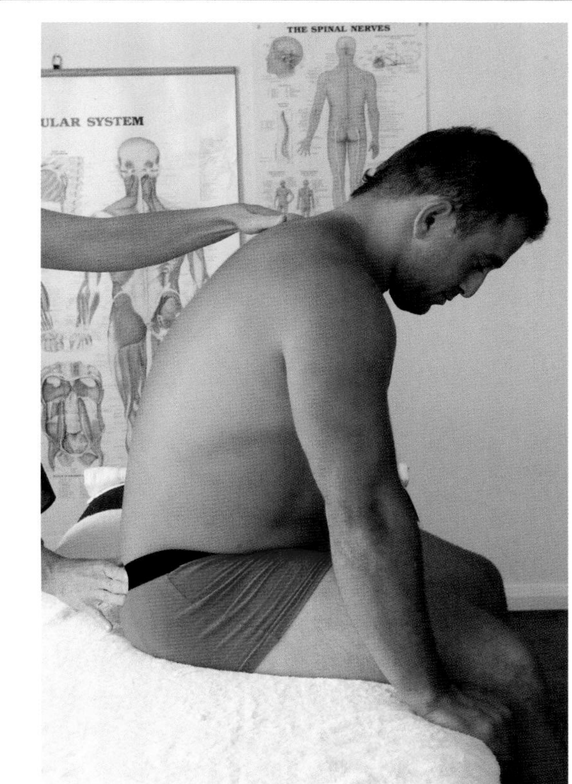

Fig. 10.14 **Erector spinae length test**

the distance between their forehead and their knees will be about 10 cm. Next, the client sits on the table with their legs bent over the side. If trunk flexion is greater in the sitting position then short hamstrings are suggested (see Figure 10.14). (Note: Clients with a history of disc problems may not be able to flex their lumbar spine without pain. Use the See-Move-Touch principle in all testing procedures.)

Clinical significance

Erector spinae muscles are usually short and tight on the concave side of a scoliosis. Bilateral erector spinae muscles may be contracted in clients with hyperlordosis.

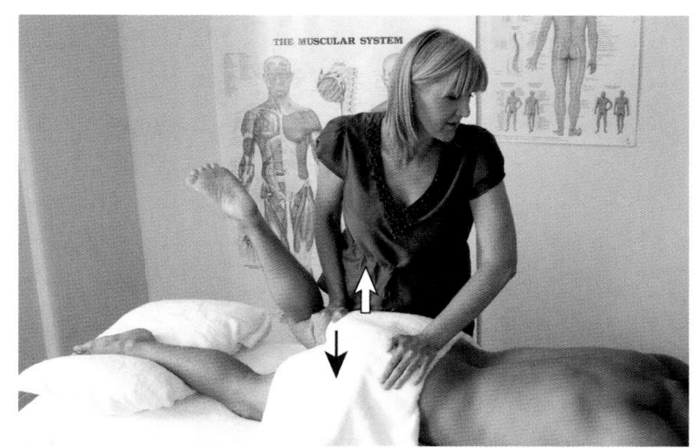

Fig. 10.15 **Resisted test for gluteus maximus**

5. GLUTEUS MAXIMUS

Resisted test

The client lies prone, flexes one knee to 90° and tries to raise the thigh (on the same side) off the table against resistance (see Figure 10.15).

Length test

The client lies supine and takes their knee towards the opposite shoulder. Normal adult clients should be able to flex their hips to 110–120°. (Note: sign of the buttock: Elevate the client's straight leg until restriction is encountered and then flex the knee and increase hip flexion. Cases where passive hip flexion with the knee flexed is more limited or painful than straight leg raising is a red flag and requires referral for further examination to eliminate such pathologies as infection, osteomyelitis of the upper femur, septic sacroiliac arthritis, ischiorectal abscess and fractured sacrum.)[21]

Clinical significance

The gluteus maximus muscle is an important stabiliser of the lumbo-pelvic region, especially of the sacroiliac joint.[22] For example, severe weakness is associated with hip extensor gait (when the hip is thrust forward and the trunk extended after heel strike). Gluteus maximus weakness is associated with overuse of hamstring muscles in abnormal hip extension firing patterns.[23] Iliotibial band syndrome is also associated with imbalances between gluteus maximus, tensor fasciae latae, hamstring and quadriceps muscles.

6. HAMSTRINGS

Resisted test

Resisted knee flexion can be tested prone, sitting or supine. In the prone position, the client flexes their knee to 90°. Place one hand on the client's gluteal region and the other on the calf just proximal to the ankle. Instruct the client to bring their heel to their buttock against your resistance (see Figure 10.16).

Length test

The Sit and Reach Test is used to test the length of the hamstrings. The client sits with their legs straight out in front of them and reaches forward towards their toes. Normal

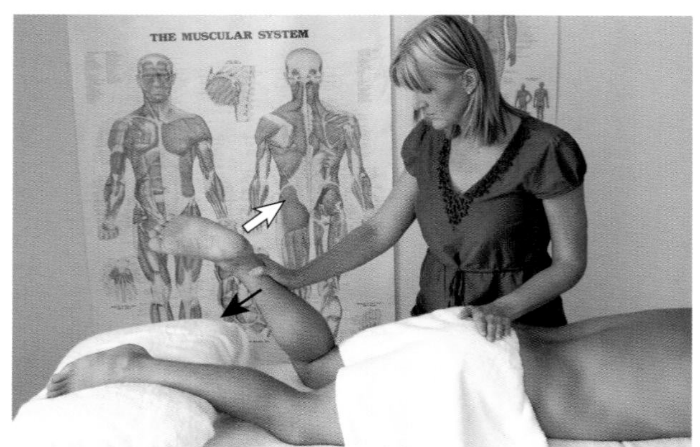

Fig. 10.16 Resisted test for hamstrings

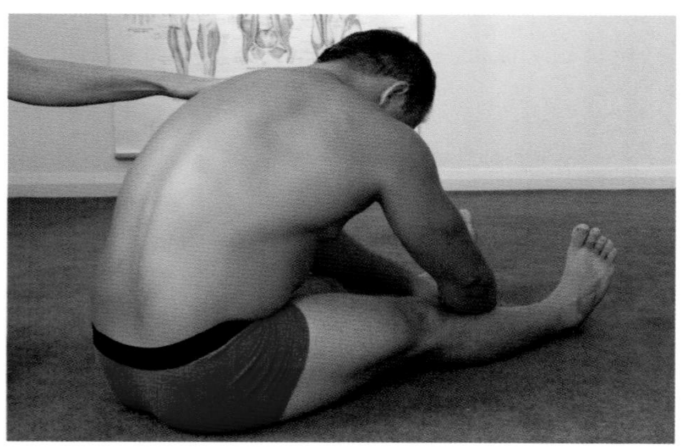

Fig. 10.17 Length test for hamstrings: Sit and Reach test

hamstring length enables the client to touch their toes. Note that the Sit and Reach test also tests the flexibility of the lumbar spine (see Figure 10.17).

Straight leg raising also tests the length of the hamstrings. Clients with normal length hamstrings can usually achieve 80° elevation.

Clinical significance

Variations from normal hamstring strength or length alter the biomechanics of the hips, sacroiliac joints, spine and knees. Hamstring muscles may be weak compared to quadriceps muscles in hyperlordosis. Weak hamstrings may also cause heavy heel strike in gait. Tight hamstrings are associated with posterior pelvic tilt and abnormal hip extension firing patterns.[23, 24] Imbalance between hamstring, tensor fasciae latae, gluteus maximus and quadriceps is implicated in iliotibial band syndrome.

7. QUADRICEPS

Resisted test

Resisted knee extension can be tested supine, sitting or prone. In the sitting position, the client flexes their knee to 90°. Place one hand on the client's tibia just proximal to the knee and the

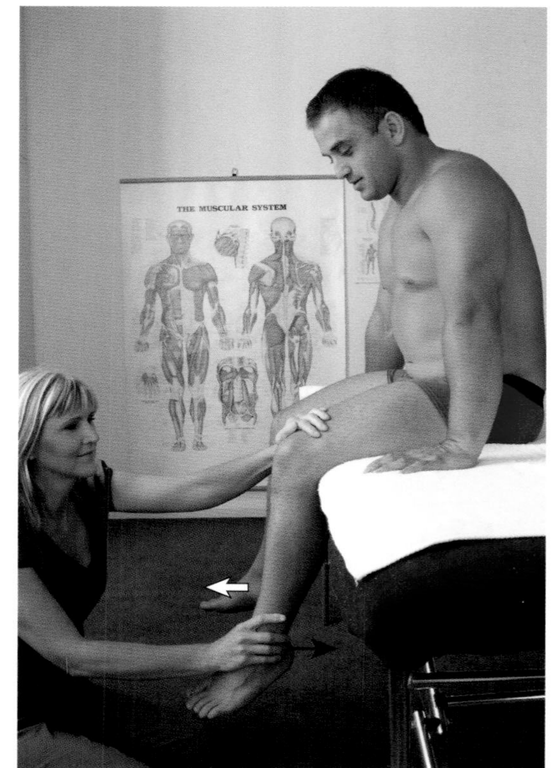

Fig. 10.18 Resisted test for quadriceps

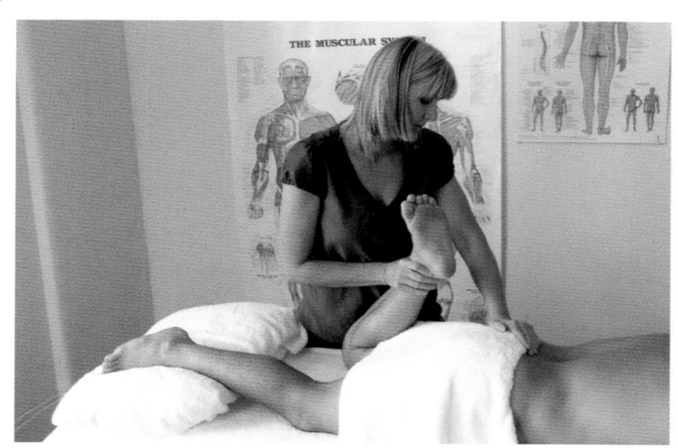

Fig. 10.19 Length test for quadriceps femoris

other just proximal to the ankle. Instruct the client to try to straighten their leg against your resistance (see Figure 10.18).

Length test

The client lies prone and flexes their knee. Normally, the client's heel will reach their buttocks (see Figure 10.19).

Clinical significance

Variations from normal quadriceps strength or length alter the biomechanics of the hips, sacroiliac joints, spine and knees. Quadriceps muscles may be short and tight compared with

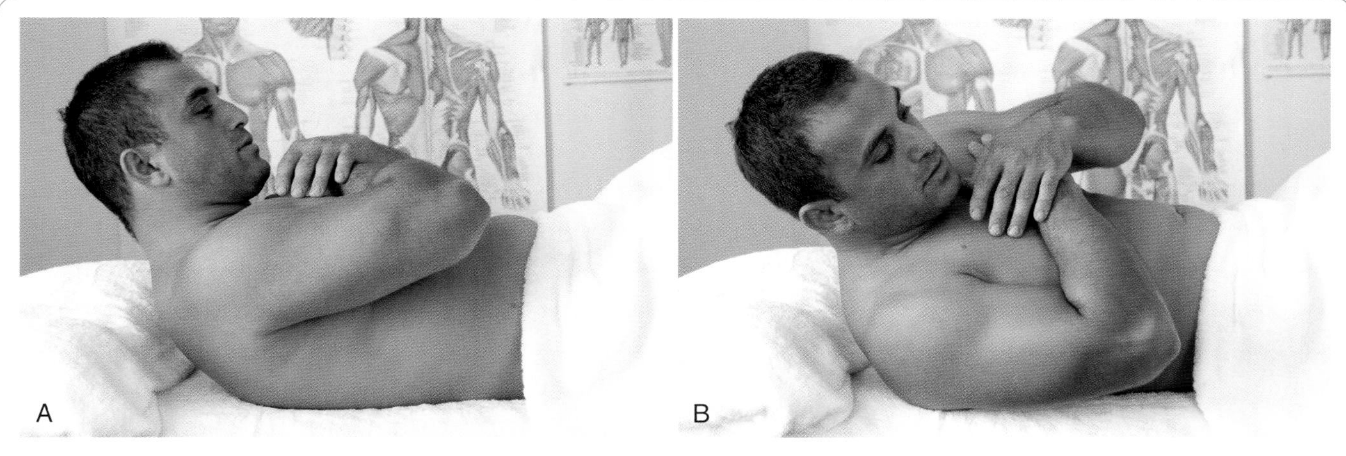

Fig. 10.20 Strength tests for abdominal muscles. A: Rectus abdominis; **B:** Oblique muscles.

hamstrings in clients with hyperlordosis. Weak quadriceps may be associated with hypolordosis. Weak quadriceps can cause abnormal hip rotation in the acceleration phase of gait or back knee gait (manually pushing the knee into extension in stance phase).

8. ABDOMINAL MUSCLES

RECTUS ABDOMINIS

Strength test

The client lies supine and tilts their pelvis posteriorly or performs a partial sit-up with knees bent and feet on the floor.

INTERNAL AND EXTERNAL OBLIQUES

Strength test

The client lies supine and tilts their pelvis posteriorly or performs a partial diagonal sit-up (i.e. elbow reaches towards opposite knee) with knees bent and feet on the floor (see Figure 10.20).

TRANSVERSUS ABDOMINIS

Transversus abdominis compresses the abdomen wall. To test its strength, instruct the client to draw in their navel to flatten their abdomen.

Length test

Although unlikely to be encountered in clinic, shortened abdominal muscle would restrict trunk extension.

Clinical significance

Weakness of any part of the core may predispose to low back injury. Weakness of rectus abdominis is often observed in hyperlordotic postures.

PELVIC FLOOR MUSCLES

Pelvic floor muscles are part of the core muscles that stabilise the lumbar spine during movement. A test for pelvic floor muscle strength that is often used is the ability to stop the flow of urine completely and rapidly. Refer clients with pelvic floor muscle weakness to a physiotherapist or exercise therapist.

Special tests

Special tests aim to isolate and identify the client's condition and in so doing often reproduce symptoms. Clients should be instructed to perform tests within their pain tolerance. Ask clients to indicate the exact location of symptoms and confirm that they are the same as those described in the case history.

KEMP'S QUADRANT TEST

The client is standing and extends and laterally flexes their trunk (ask the client to run their hand down the back of their leg). This manoeuvre compresses the posterolateral elements of the spine; that is, the facet joints and the posterolateral disc (see Figure 10.21 on p 150).

VALSALVA

The client is seated. Ask the client to close their mouth, pinch their nostrils closed and forcibly exhale. (Demonstrate this manoeuvre for the client.) The Valsalva manoeuvre raises the intrathecal pressure. Pain in the low back or pain radiating down the leg(s) suggests pathology such as disc derangement. (Note: this test is not recommended for people with uncontrolled or acute hypertension or for diabetics with potential retinopathy.)

STRAIGHT LEG RAISE (SLR)

This test is designed to reproduce back and/or leg pain. The client is supine and draped appropriately. Slowly raise the client's leg with one hand supporting the calcaneus and the other hand placed on top of the knee or on the ipsilateral anterior superior iliac spine (see Figure 10.22 on p 150). Ask the client to report any pain as soon as it is felt and when this occurs note the degree of elevation (normal hip flexion is approximately 80°). Pain usually arises from hamstring tightness or pressure on the sciatic nerve. To distinguish between these two possibilities, lower the leg a few degrees and dorsiflex the foot. Pain on dorsiflexion indicates sciatica. Pain on SLR that is experienced in the opposite leg could suggest a space-occupying lesion in the back (e.g. disc herniation, infection or tumour).

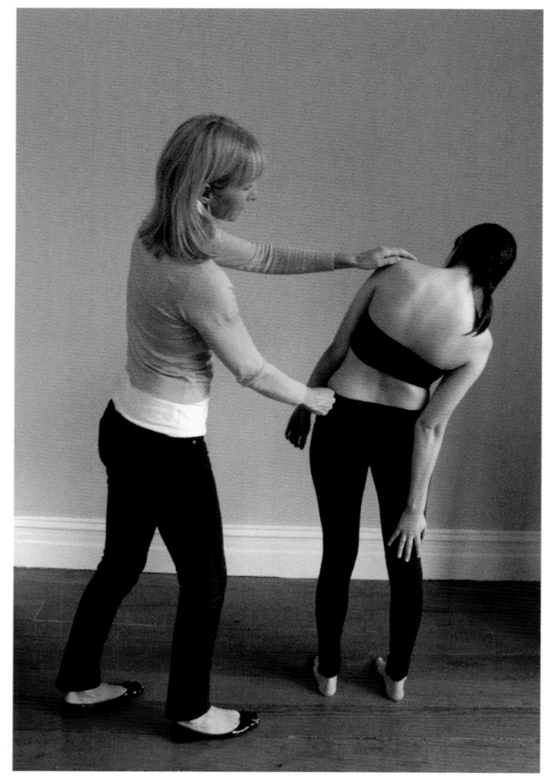

Fig. 10.21 **Kemp's test**

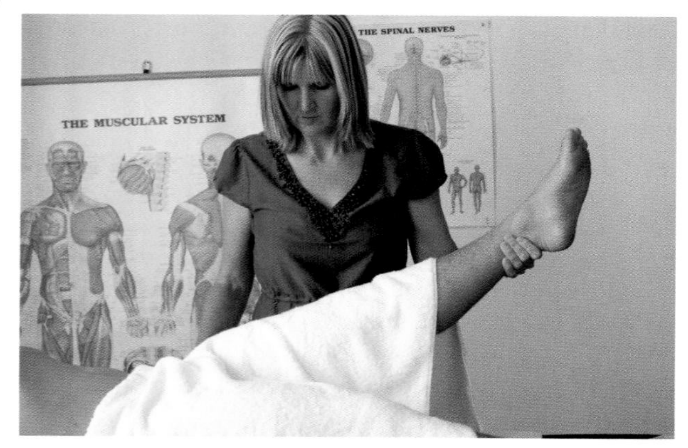

Fig. 10.22 **Straight Leg Raise**

CENTRALISATION/PERIPHERALISATION

Centralisation (the movement of symptoms from distal or lateral regions to more central regions) is useful in identifying painful lumbar discs.[11] Instruct the client to extend their back as far as possible, return to neutral and then repeat the movement up to 10 times. If pain centralises (e.g. changes from pain in the low back, buttock, posterior thigh and calf to pain in the low back and buttock) a bulging lumbar disc is indicated. Stop the movement if the pain peripheralises. (Note: A small group of clients tend to centralise with lateral flexion; a minority with flexion.)

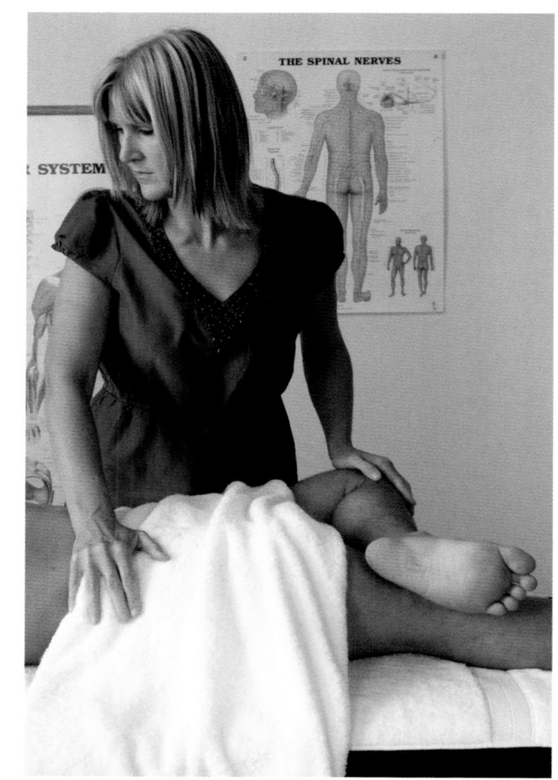

Fig. 10.23 **Patrick's test**

Note: If a client has calf pain it is important to eliminate deep venous thrombosis (DVT). Symptoms may include pain, tenderness and swelling in the calf. Bilateral supine gastrocnemius stretch may reproduce local vein pain but the test is not definitive. History of recent surgery or travel may be the best indicator. Compartment syndrome should also be considered if there is unexplained or unidentified calf pain. Refer clients with calf pain which seems out of proportion for that which is expected, paraesthesia or muscle weakness and/or signs of loss of blood flow to the leg and foot.

PATRICK'S TEST

The client is supine with the leg on the involved side in the figure 4 position (i.e. hip flexed, abducted and externally rotated and the foot placed across the opposite leg). Stand ipsilaterally. Pain in the inguinal area suggests hip pathology. With the palm of the cephalad hand on the contralateral anterior superior iliac spine, gently apply pressure on the flexed knee with the palm of the other hand (see Figure 10.23). Increased pain on this manoeuvre may suggest SI pathology.

Note that all sacroiliac pain provocation tests demonstrate fair to moderate reliability and moderate diagnostic utility for identifying sacroiliac joint pain.[11]

SACROILIAC COMPRESSION

The client is lying on their side. Place one hand on top of the other over the uppermost aspect of the lateral ilium and apply

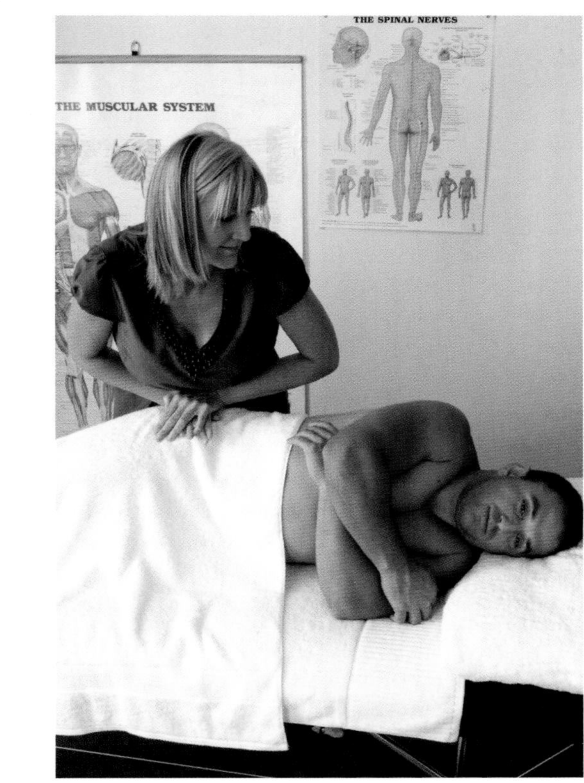

Fig. 10.24 Sacroiliac joint compression

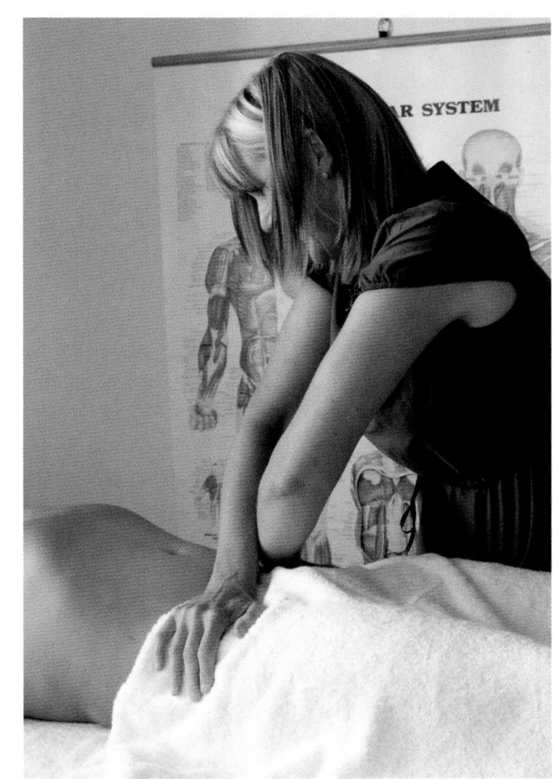

Fig. 10.25 Sacroiliac joint distraction

pressure towards the floor to compress the sacroiliac joints (see Figure 10.24). If the client experiences increased pain on this manoeuvre, SI pathology may be indicated.

SACROILIAC DISTRACTION

The client lies supine. Face the client and place the palm of each hand on the contralateral anterior superior iliac spine. If pain is reported when gentle lateral pressure is applied, sacroiliac pathology is suggested (see Figure 10.25).

SACRAL SPRING TEST

Springing directly over the sacrum (sometimes called the *sacral thrust test*) and over both sacroiliac joints may reproduce symptoms in sacroiliac joint lesions. A positive spring test along with positive sacral compression and distraction tests demonstrates good diagnostic utility for detecting sacroiliac lesions (see Figure 10.6).[11]

LEG LENGTH

With the client standing, the practitioner measures the distance from the anterior superior iliac spine to the most inferior point of the medial malleolus and compares with the other side (see Figure 10.27 and box on p 152). If clinical symptoms are present, referral for a standing scanogram (an X-ray of the hips, knees and ankles when the client is standing) may be required for a more accurate measurement.

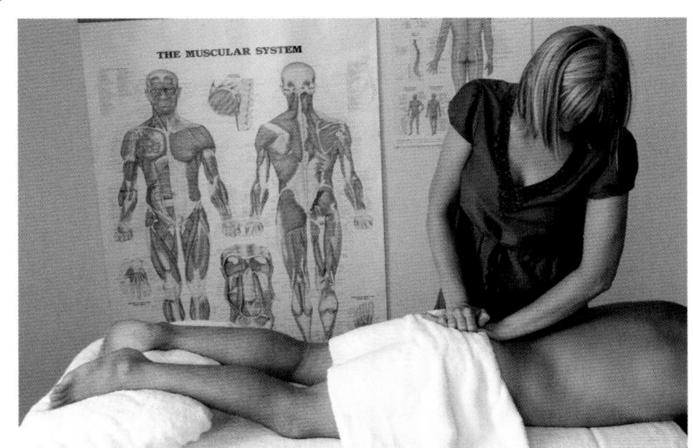

Fig. 10.26 Sacral spring test

PALPATION

In the prone position:

- Palpate the space between the spinous processes of L4 and L5 which is at the level of the L4/5 disc and also level with the top of the iliac crests. The spinous processes mark the level of the actual vertebral body as spinous processes extend directly posteriorly in the lumbars (compare the thoracic spinous processes which extend inferiorly and posteriorly).

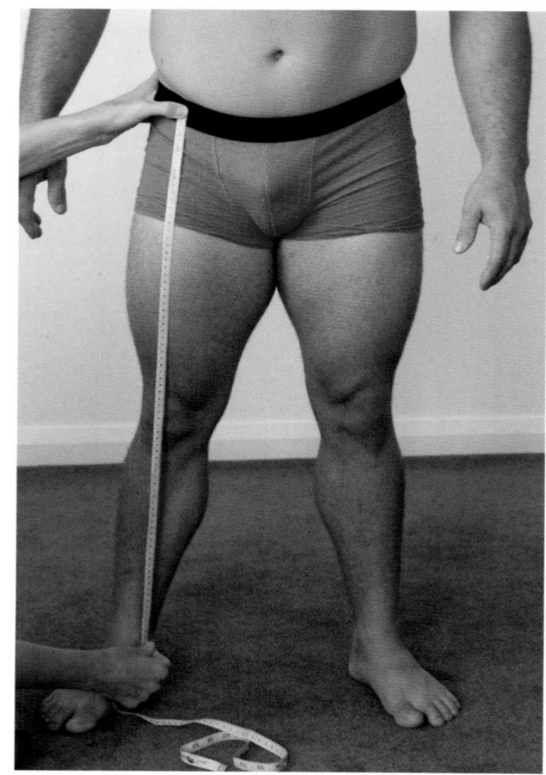

Fig. 10.27 Measuring leg length

- Palpate the spinous process of L5/S1.
- Palpate the smaller spinous processes of the sacrum. S2 spinous process is level with the PSISs.
- Gaps between the lumbar or sacral spinous processes or absence of spinous processes may indicate spina bifida.
- A step defect may be observed from one spinous process to the next. This most commonly occurs at L5/S1 and suggests spondylolisthesis.
- Palpate the iliac crests.
- Palpate the supraspinous ligaments. The interspinous ligaments located underneath the supraspinous ligaments are not directly palpable.
- Feel for muscle spasm in the erector spinae muscles either side of the spinous processes.
- Look for muscle spasm and fatty nodules in the gluteal muscles.
- Palpate the sacral triangle from the posterior superior iliac spines to the top of the gluteal cleft. Pain may be due to ligamentous sprain at the posterior superior iliac spine or the sacrotuberous or sacrospinous ligaments.
- The sciatic nerve runs under or through the piriformis muscle approximately midway between the ischial tuberosity and greater trochanter. The sciatic nerve may be more easily palpated when the client is lying on their side with their hip flexed. (Caution with hip flexion in clients with a history of disc pathology.)

In the supine position:

- Palpate abdominal muscles. To observe the abdominal muscles ask the client to cross their arms over their chest and perform a partial sit-up. (Caution: do not ask a client to perform this action if it is likely to induce back pain.)
- Palpate the inguinal area. Sources of pain in this region include inflamed inguinal nodes, the hip joint, a psoas spasm or a psoas abscess.

Leg length inequality

1. Anatomical (true) shortness

Causes include:

- growth asymmetry
- fracture (tibia, fibula, calcaneus, femur)
- epiphyseal injury
- hip disorder (e.g. Perthes' disease, slipped capital femoral epiphysis)
- degenerative joint disease of the hip, knee or ankle
- neuromuscular (e.g. cerebral palsy, poliomyelitis)
- flat foot (usually pronating) on the same side
- osteomyelitis

2. Functional (apparent) shortness

Causes include:

- imbalance of pelvic and lumbar musculature, ligaments and fascia (e.g. posterior iliac rotation on the same side/anterior iliac rotation on the opposite side, forward sacral torsion to the same side/backward sacral iliac rotation on the opposite side, forward sacral torsion to the same side/backward sacral torsion to the opposite side, lumbar convexity to the opposite side, short hamstrings or tensor fasciae latae).

Short leg tests

Client standing: measure from the ASIS to the most inferior point of the medial malleolus.

REMEDIAL MASSAGE TREATMENT

Assessment of the low back provides essential information for developing and negotiating treatment plans, including:

- client's suitability for remedial massage therapy
- duration of the condition (i.e. acute or chronic)
- severity of the condition (i.e. grade of injury; mild, moderate or severe pain)
- type(s) of tissues involved
- priorities for treatment if more than one injury or condition is present
- whether the signs and symptoms suggest a common condition of the low back
- special considerations for individual clients (e.g. client's preference for treatment types and styles, special population considerations).

Treatment options must always be considered in the context of the best available evidence for treatment effectiveness. Use clinical practice guidelines where they exist (see Chapter 3). Further research is required to prove effectiveness of many low back treatments. Findings of current research are summarised in Table 10.3.

Despite its long tradition, massage therapy remains grossly under-researched.[25] There has been an increase in research

Table 10.3 Summary of evidence for the effectiveness of treatments for acute low back pain[4]

Evidence of effectiveness	• Staying active • Patient information (written) • Heat wrap therapy (not routinely available in Australia)
Mixed results (more research is needed)	• Muscle relaxants • Anti-inflammatory drugs • Spinal manipulation
Inconclusive	• Acupuncture • Back exercises • Back schools • Bed rest • Cognitive behaviour therapy • Injection therapy • Massage • Topical treatments • Traction • TENS

over the past few years with increasing evidence for the effectiveness of massage in several areas, especially for anxiety and back pain.[26] For example, Furlan et al[2] conducted a systematic review of 13 randomised trials (1596 participants) and concluded that 'massage might be beneficial for patients with subacute (lasting 4 to 12 weeks) and chronic (lasting longer than 12 weeks) non-specific low back pain, especially when combined with exercise and education'.

MUSCLE STRAIN

Muscle strains can occur from traumas including falls, car accidents and sports injuries. They also occur from overuse and repetitive microtrauma as can occur after long periods of unaccustomed activity. Strains usually occur in the paraspinal muscles which support the spine in all its movements.

Assessment

HISTORY

The client complains of low back pain after a fall, accident or sports injury or after a period of unaccustomed activity (e.g. shovelling, horse riding). Pain can be experienced immediately or within the next 24–48 hours (delayed onset muscle soreness). Pain is associated with activity and generally relieved with rest.

POSTURAL ANALYSIS

Muscle spasm in the lumbar paravertebral muscles and functional scoliosis may be evident.

Key assessment findings for muscle strain

- History of trauma or repetitive overuse
- Functional tests
  - AROM positive
  - RROM positive for affected muscle(s)
  - Resisted and length tests positive for affected muscle(s)
- Palpation positive for pain, spasm, myofibril tears/scar tissue

GAIT ANALYSIS

Gait may be guarded.

FUNCTIONAL TESTS

AROM: limited in one or more directions.
PROM: mild to no pain except at end of range when muscle is stretched.
RROM: painful.
Resisted and length tests positive for involved muscles.
Special tests: negative.

PALPATION

Muscle spasm is usually evident. The client reports tenderness or pain on palpation of the affected muscle.

Overview of treatment of muscle strains

A typical remedial massage treatment for mild to moderate muscle strains of the low back includes:

- Swedish massage to the back, pelvis, posterior and anterior lower limbs.
- Remedial techniques, including:
  - deep gliding frictions along the muscle fibres (see Figure 10.28 on p 154)
  - cross-fibre frictions (see Figure 10.28 on p 154)
  - soft-tissue releasing techniques
  - deep transverse friction at the site of muscle injury
  - heat therapy (see Chapter 3)
  - trigger point therapy (see Chapter 6)
  - myofascial release (see Chapter 8).

A range of remedial massage techniques for muscles of the low back and pelvis is illustrated in Table 10.4.

- Address any underlying conditions or predisposing factors (e.g. scoliosis or thoracic hyperkyphosis).

CLIENT EDUCATION

Educate clients about the importance of maintaining a physical fitness program and of developing appropriate levels of fitness before activities are commenced. Where possible, clients should take an increasingly active role in their treatment through rehabilitation and health promotion activities.

Home exercise program

A program of progressive rehabilitation should accompany remedial massage treatment. Aim for maximum strength and full length of all major muscles. Unresolved strains can contribute to recurrence and to the development of more serious back injuries. Introduce stretching exercises as soon as possible and progress to isometric exercises within the client's pain tolerance. Clients may be referred for manipulation of the lower back.

NON-SPECIFIC LOW BACK PAIN

Non-specific low back pain refers to low back pain that is not associated with a specific condition such as fracture, disc herniation or spondylosis. The term encompasses strains (described above), sprains and low back pain originating from

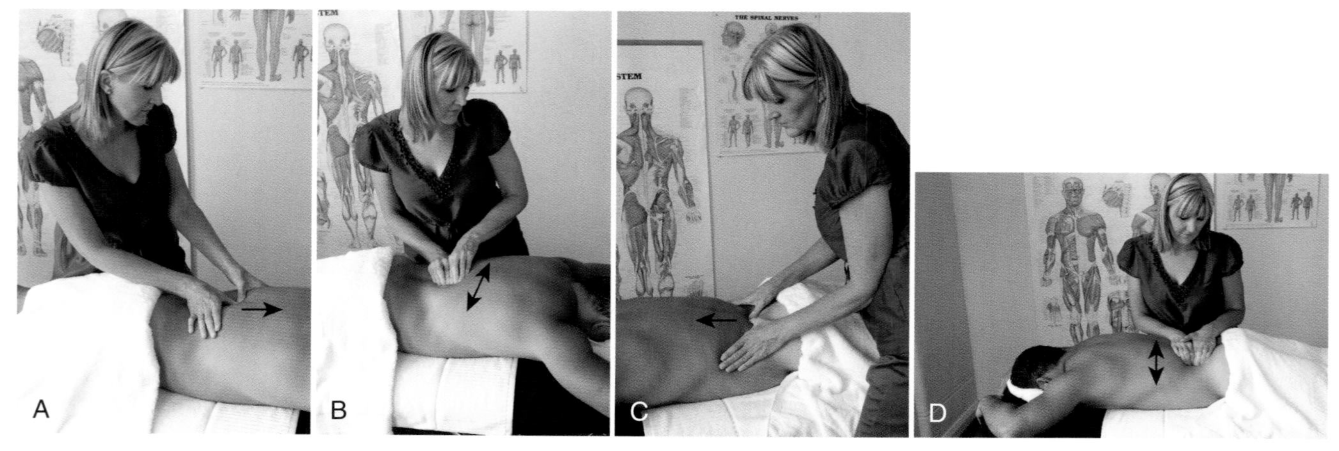

Fig. 10.28 (a) Deep gliding frictions and (b) cross-fibre frictions of lumbar erector spinae: (c) deep gliding frictions and (d) cross-fibre frictions of quadratus lumborum

the facet (zygapophyseal) joint and/or joint capsule. Non-specific low back pain accounts for about 85–95% of clients with low back pain[2] and anecdotal evidence suggests that such clients respond well to remedial massage therapy. Non-specific low back pain may originate from trauma, overuse or unaccustomed exercise leading to muscle strain and facet joint ligamentous sprain. Clients are most often young adults and there is no underlying spinal pathology. There is usually no radiation of pain.

Key assessment findings for non-specific low back pain

- Client is usually a young adult; history of trauma or repetitive overuse.
- Functional tests
  - AROM positive
  - PROM positive for ligamentous sprains
  - RROM positive for muscle strains
  - Resisted test and muscle length tests positive for affected muscles
  - Special tests – Kemp's positive in lumbar facet syndrome
- Palpation positive for tenderness ± pain at site of strain, sprain or subluxation

Assessment

HISTORY

Clients report a history of direct trauma, overuse, fatigue or repetitive microtrauma over hours or days. The pain is often described as dull and aching although it may be sharp. The pain is usually easily localised. The onset of pain is immediate or shortly after injury. Clients also describe decreased mobility and muscle spasm. Clients are usually young adults and often describe having recently undertaken an unaccustomed activity (e.g. playing social cricket).

FUNCTIONAL TESTS

AROM: limited and painful in one or more directions (pain in one direction suggests muscle strain; pain in many directions suggests joint capsule injury or a combination of muscle and joint injury). More pain on extension suggests lumbar facet syndrome.
PROM: painful when sprained ligaments are stretched. Ligamentous sprain is suggested when AROM tests are painful and RROM tests are negative.
RROM: painful for affected muscles.
Resisted and length tests: positive for affected muscles.
Special tests: are negative except for Kemp's test which may be positive for lumbar facet syndrome.

PALPATION

Clients report tenderness on palpation at the site of muscle strain or ligament sprain.

Differential diagnosis

Rule out non-mechanical causes of back pain including haematoma, abdominal aortic aneurysm and visceral referred pain (appendicitis, peritonitis, kidney pathology).[27]

Overview of treatment and management

A typical remedial massage treatment for mild or moderate non-specific low back pain includes:

- Swedish massage therapy to the back, pelvis, posterior and anterior lower limbs.
- Remedial massage therapy, which includes techniques for muscle injury/muscle imbalances such as deep gliding frictions along the muscle fibres, cross-fibre frictions, active and passive soft tissue releasing techniques, deep transverse friction, trigger point therapy and muscle stretches (see Table 10.4).
  - Apply myofascial releasing techniques for myofascial restrictions. Thermotherapy may be beneficial. Techniques such as longitudinal and rotational tractions of the

Table 10.4 Remedial massage techniques for major muscles of the low back and pelvis

Muscle	Soft tissue release	Trigger point	Stretch	Client education[19]	Home stretch
Piriformis	The client lies prone. Apply pressure into ipsilateral piriformis with thumb, fingers, elbow or palm. Flex the client's knee to 90°. Passive release: hold the client's foot or hold the medial aspect of the calf with forearm and slowly move the client's leg medially and laterally to the client's full range of motion (internally and externally rotating the hip) while pressure is maintained on the piriformis. Active release: contact the ipsilateral piriformis as above while the client performs the same movement unassisted.		The client lies in the prone position, knee flexed to 90° and foot dropped out to the side. Stabilise the middle of piriformis with the cephalad palm, fingers pointing towards the sacrum. The other hand holds the medial aspect of the lower leg proximal to the ankle. CRAC: The client tries to bring their foot back to the middle of the table against your resistance for 7 seconds and then takes their foot as far laterally as possible. The client should stretch to their comfortable tolerance. Knee injury clients are contraindicated.	Place a pillow between the thighs when sleeping on the side, take regular breaks to stretch piriformis when driving long distances, change positions often if sitting for prolonged periods.	Lying supine, flex the hip to 90° and place the foot on the floor laterally to the other leg which remains straight. With one hand on the pelvis on the flexed leg side push down towards the floor; the other hand pulls the bent leg towards the floor until a stretch is felt in the piriformis muscle.

Continued

Table 10.4 Remedial massage techniques for major muscles of the low back and pelvis—cont'd

Muscle	Soft tissue release	Trigger point	Stretch	Client education[19]	Home stretch
Iliopsoas	Active release: Client lies supine with knee flexed and foot on the table. Apply pressure to ipsilateral psoas with fingers. (Caution is required in locating psoas which is deep to abdominal organs.) The technique should only be performed if the client can tolerate it (i.e. no more than 7 out of 10 on a pain scale). Ask client to slowly slide their heel along the table while pressure is maintained on the muscle. 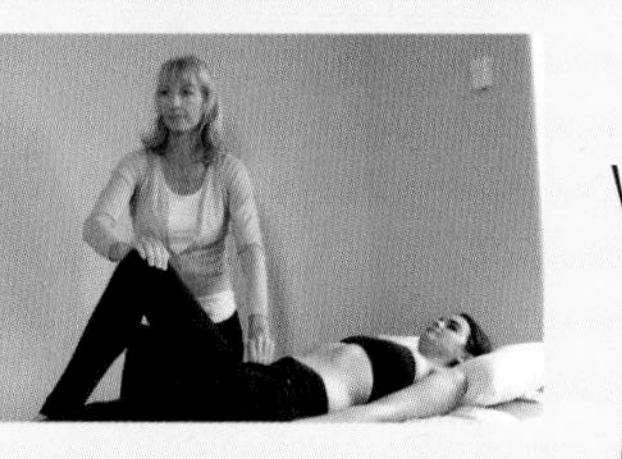	Trigger points are inaccessible. Remedial massage treatment focuses on stretching techniques only. 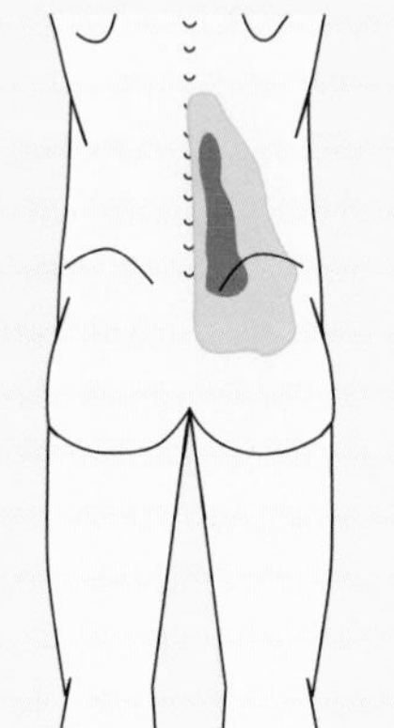	i) Use contracture testing position with buttock close to the edge of the foot of the table. The client flexes the contralateral knee and holds it with their hands. Use one hand to assist the client to hold this position. The other hand contacts the ipsilateral thigh proximal to the knee. The client tries to lift their knee against your resistance for 7 seconds, after which they try to stretch the iliopsoas by lowering their leg towards the floor. ii) The client is supine, close to the side of the table. The client flexes the contralateral knee and places their foot on the table. Face caudally and stand with the lateral thigh against the table. Contact the opposite ASIS to stabilise the pelvis. The client holds the sides of the table and drops their ipsilateral leg over the side of the table (the client has to be close enough to the side of the table so that the hip can extend). Your other hand contacts the ipsilateral thigh just proximal to the knee. The client tries to lift their knee against your resistance for 7 seconds, after which you try to stretch the iliopsoas by lowering their leg towards the floor. iii) The client is prone and flexes their knee to 90°. (If the psoas is tight the lumbar spine will dip towards the table.) Stand ipsilaterally and place one hand on the client's sacrum, the other under the knee, approaching from the medial side and stabilising the calf and foot with their forearm. Elevate the knee until the muscle stretch is felt, making sure that the pelvis remains on the table. The client tries to take their thigh to the table against your resistance for 7 seconds and then tries to elevate the thigh as far as possible to stretch the muscle. 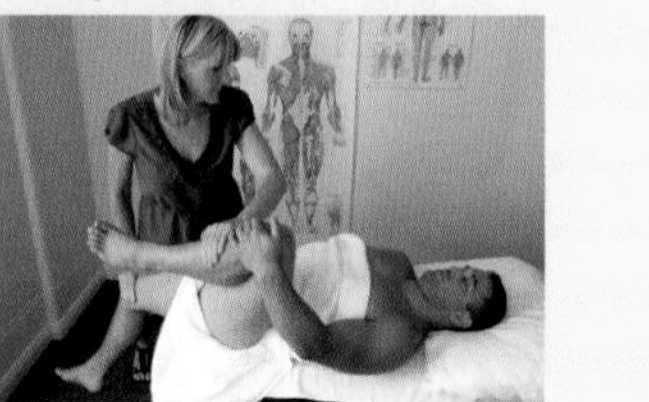	Avoid prolonged sitting with knees flexed to 90°. Sit on a seat that slants forward to avoid holding iliopsoas in a sustained contracted position.	The client kneels on the floor with one knee bent and the leg to be stretched behind. The client gently lunges forward until a stretch is felt in the front of their hip. Hold for 30 seconds. 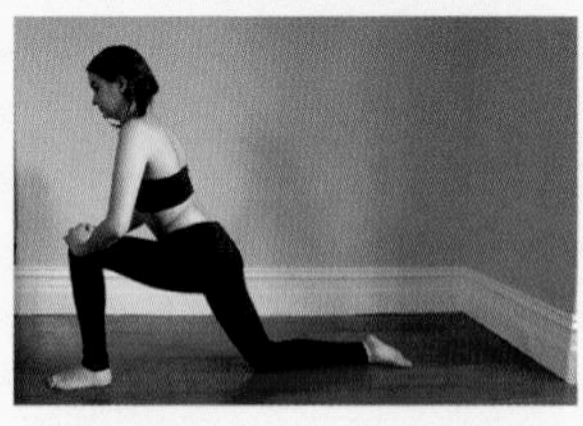

Table 10.4 Remedial massage techniques for major muscles of the low back and pelvis—cont'd

Muscle	Soft tissue release	Trigger point	Stretch	Client education[19]	Home stretch
Quadratus lumborum	Apply pressure with palms or fingers to the quadratus lumborum muscles and ask client to breathe in slowly against resistance. This can be performed in the prone position or sitting.	Deep Deep Superficial	i) Any movement that flexes or laterally flexes the trunk stretches the quadratus lumborum. For example, lying on one side over 3 or 4 pillows will stretch the quadratus lumborum.[16] ii) The client is supine holding onto the sides of the table. Cross one leg over the other at the ankles, keeping both legs extended. Holding the crossed ankles with both hands, slowly walk the client's feet in an arc towards the lower foot side. PNF stretch can be performed in this position with the client trying to bring their crossed legs back to the middle of the table against the practitioner's resistance (arms or hip). iii) The client is supine with one knee crossed over the other. Drop both knees to the side of the top knee.	Shock-absorbing and supportive footwear for good foot and ankle biomechanics, a heel lift in cases of true short leg, a firm mattress, placing a pillow under the thighs when sleeping supine.	Trunk flexion and sidebend stretches.

Continued

Table 10.4 Remedial massage techniques for major muscles of the low back and pelvis—cont'd

Muscle	Soft tissue release	Trigger point	Stretch	Client education[19]	Home stretch
Erector spinae	Active release: with the client sitting on the table and their feet on the floor, place the proximal phalanges of the fingers on the erector spinae either side of the spine at the thoracolumbar junction or above. The client slowly bends forward (may hold the side of the table) as your knuckles strip inferiorly along the erector spinae. (Do not use this technique on clients whose symptoms increase with lumbar flexion.) 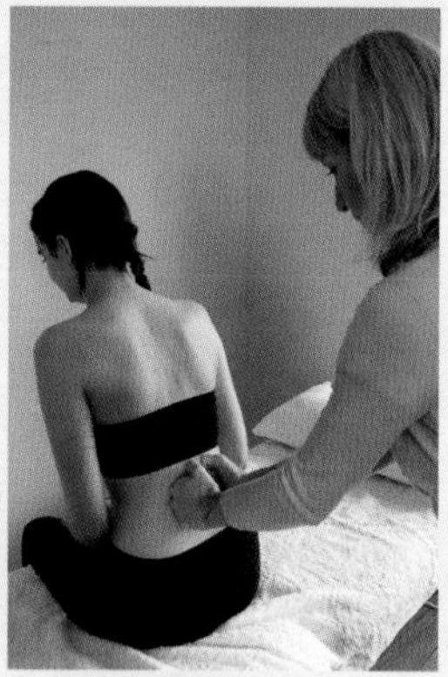	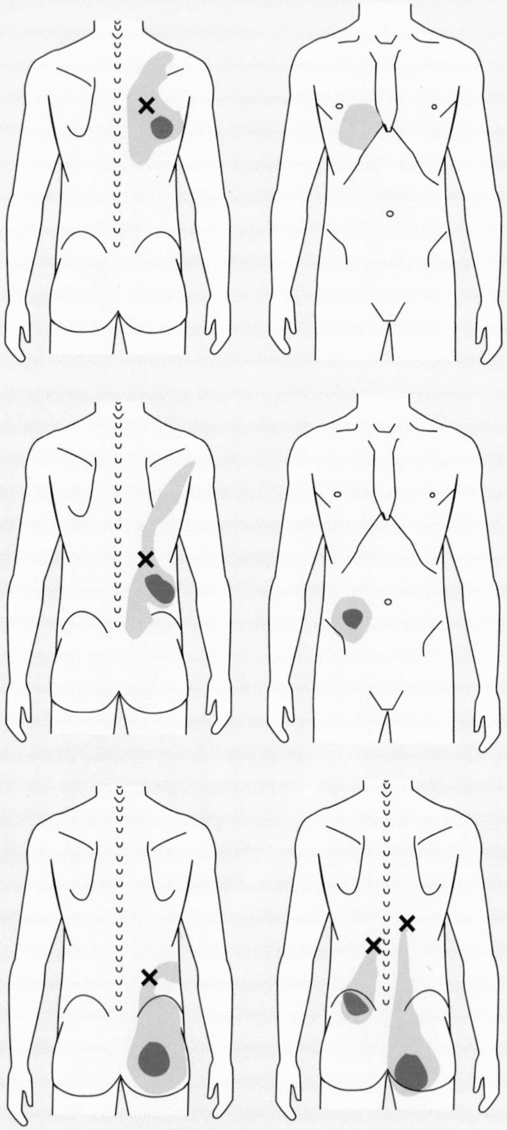	Trunk flexion stretches are usually performed actively. i) Sitting with legs extended and leaning forward until the stretch is felt. ii) Lying supine, client brings their knees to their chest as far as possible. iii) Kneeling on the floor, sitting back on their feet, the client takes their head towards the floor until the stretch is felt.	Use shock-absorbing and supportive footwear, avoid high-heeled shoes, correct lifting techniques.	Same as treatment stretches.

Table 10.4 Remedial massage techniques for major muscles of the low back and pelvis—cont'd

Muscle	Soft tissue release	Trigger point	Stretch	Client education[19]	Home stretch
Gluteus maximus	Active release: the client is sidelying and flexes and extends their bent upper leg while pressure is applied to the gluteus maximus.		The client is supine and takes their knee to the opposite shoulder (contraindicated for disc clients or any client who experiences pain on the movement). Provide resistance for 7 seconds as the client's knee moves back to the starting position. The knee is then actively or passively taken further towards the opposite shoulder.	Avoid prolonged sitting, use a small pillow behind the knees when sleeping supine.	i) The client is supine and takes one knee to the opposite shoulder. ii) The client lies supine with knees flexed and feet flat on the floor and places one foot across the other knee. They interlock their fingers around the thigh of the uncrossed leg and use their arms to draw their thigh towards their chest.

Continued

Table 10.4 Remedial massage techniques for major muscles of the low back and pelvis—cont'd

Muscle	Soft tissue release	Trigger point	Stretch	Client education[19]	Home stretch
Hamstring	The client lies in the prone position. Passive: using elbows/knuckles of one hand, glide along the muscle fibres or apply pressure at the site of the muscle lesion while the other hand holds the ankle and flexes and extends the client's leg. Active: as above but the client flexes and extends their leg unassisted. 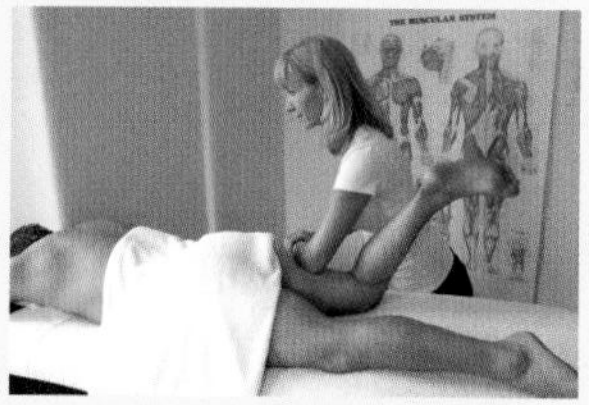	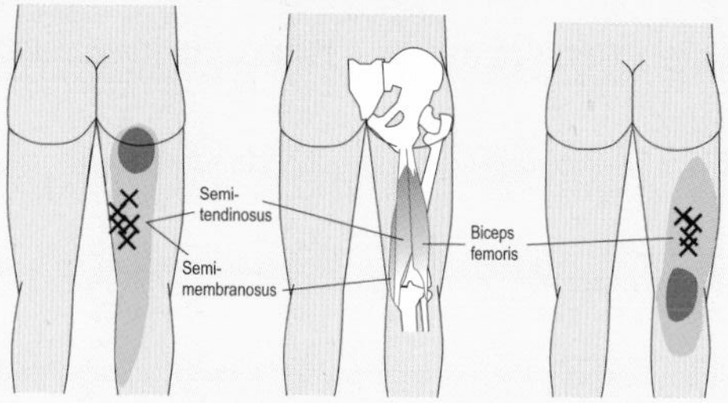	The client lies supine and raises their leg until they feel the muscle stretch. Using hands or shoulder, the practitioner resists the client as they attempt to return their leg to the table. Hold the resistance for 7 seconds after which the client tries to raise their leg further within the pain-free range. Repeat three times.	Use chairs that match the client's leg length and have a well-rounded and padded edge. Use a foot stool when seated. Take frequent breaks during long-distance driving.	There are a number of ways to stretch the hamstrings including: i) The client sits with their legs straight out in front of them or with one leg bent. The foot of the bent leg is placed on the floor alongside the thigh of the other leg and the knee rests on the floor. The client reaches forward towards their toes. ii) The client kneels with one leg straight out in front. The client leans forward from their hips towards their toes.
Quadriceps	Active: The client sits with their legs over the side of the table. Ask the client to slowly straighten and bend their leg as you apply pressure to the muscle lesion with fingers, thumbs or knuckles to glide along the muscle fibres.	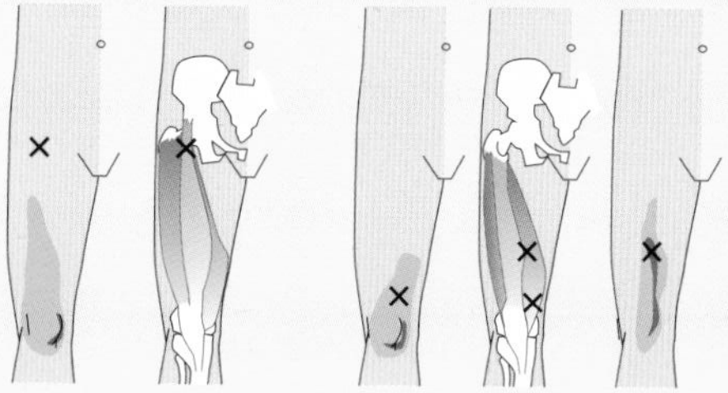	Client prone. Ask client to bend one knee towards their buttocks as far as they can comfortably. At that point apply resistance while the client tries to straighten their leg for 7 seconds (the client performs an isometric contraction of the quadriceps muscle). After the contraction the client tries to take their heel to their buttocks again. Repeat three times. 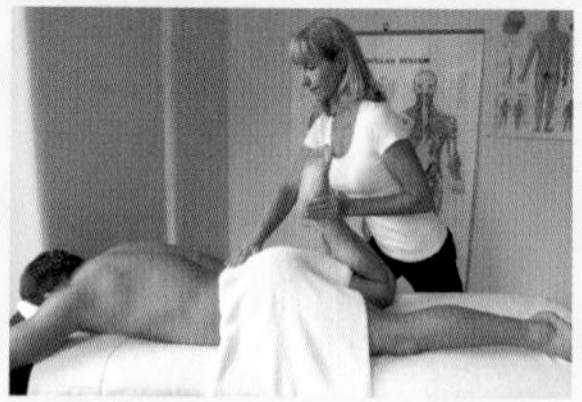	Avoid shortening and/or prolonged immobilisation of the quadriceps muscles, avoid deep knee bends and complete squats, avoid prolonged sitting with hips at 90°, avoid full flexion of the hip when sleeping on the side.	Lying prone or standing, take the heel towards the buttocks.

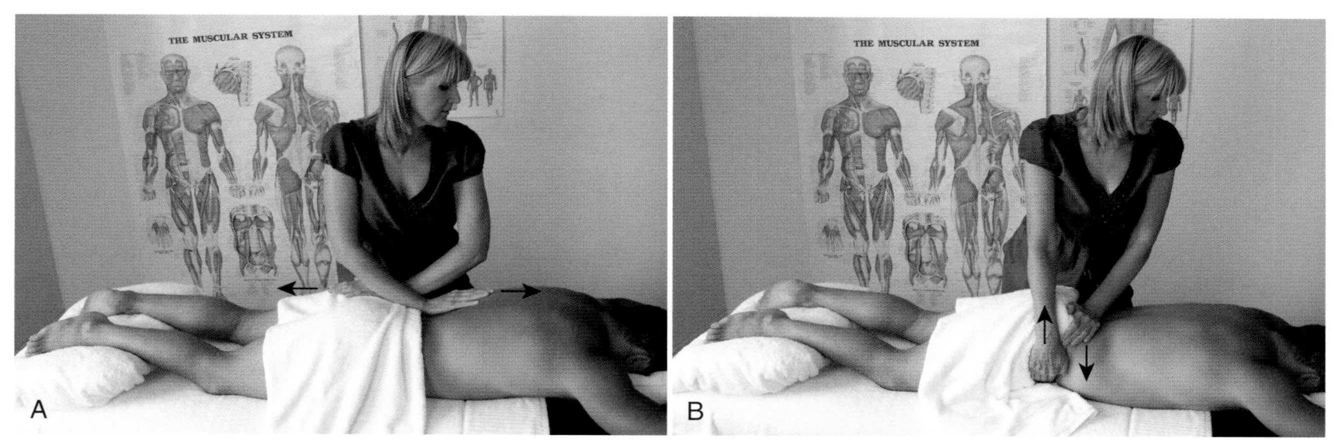

Fig. 10.29 **Longitudinal (A) and rotational (B) tractions of the lumbar spine**

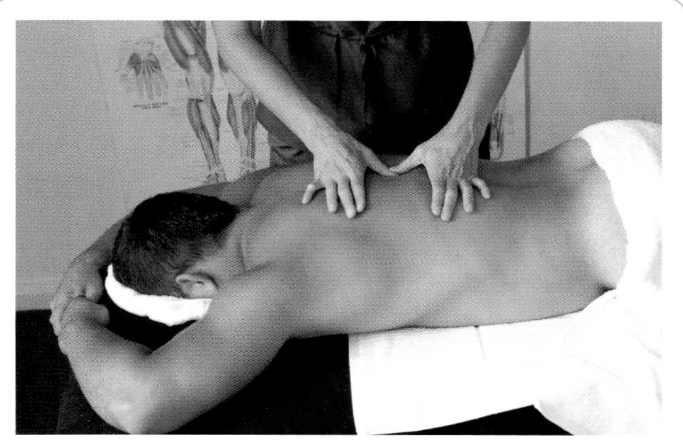

Fig. 10.30 **Multifidus and rotators release**

lumbar spine (see Figure 10.29) may be beneficial for facet joint lesions (described in detail in Chapter 7).

- Multifidus and rotators release are also useful for improving mobility of facet joints (see Figure 10.30). Work ipsilaterally. Use both thumbs together or one on top of the other. Slowly apply downward (anterior) pressure to engage muscles in the paravertebral gutter. Release muscle tightness by performing three or four small superior/inferior movements over a distance of about 1 cm, then three or four small lateral movements (i.e. deep gliding and cross-fibre frictions). Release pressure slowly and slide to a new location. Note: deep anterior pressure over the lumbar spine is contraindicated in clients with spondylolisthesis and hyperlordosis. Use with caution in clients with degenerative joint disease or history of lumbar disc herniation.

CLIENT EDUCATION

Advise clients to avoid strenuous unaccustomed activities and of the musculoskeletal benefits of regular and varied physical activity. Lifting and posture advice could help prevent future back problems. Referral to a chiropractor, osteopath or manipulative physiotherapist may be warranted for treatment of joint dysfunctions that do not resolve spontaneously. A full neurological examination is indicated in the presence of lower limb pain or other neurological symptoms.

Home exercise program

A program to stretch shortened muscles and strengthen weak ones should be instigated as soon as possible within the client's pain-free range.

Many clients with non-specific low back pain will recover within days or weeks, depending on the type of tissue injured, severity of injury and presence of complicating factors. Long-term treatment is designed to address any underlying conditions or predisposing factors to future back problems such as scoliosis or hyperlordosis and to reinforce the importance of regular and varied exercise.

DEGENERATIVE JOINT DISEASE (OSTEOARTHRITIS/DEGENERATIVE ARTHRITIS)

Degenerative joint disease (DJD) represents a range of degenerative conditions characterised by progressive loss of articular fibrocartilage and reactive changes in subchondral bone.[27] Radiographs show asymmetrical joint space narrowing, osteophytes, subchondral bone sclerosis and subluxation[28] (see Figure 10.31 on p 152). DJD is the most common form of joint disease in the elderly and it is important to note that 27–37% of people without symptoms have evidence of degenerative changes in the lumbar spine on radiographs.[27] There is usually a long history of low back pain, stiffness and limited range of motion. DJD is most common in weight-bearing joints. In the lumbar spine it occurs most often at L4–L5.

Assessment

HISTORY

Clients are usually over 50 years old. Pain is described as slowly developing, dull and aching, aggravated by activity and relieved by rest. Clients often describe stiffness, especially in the morning. Pain can vary from a dull ache to severe, sharp pain and there may be nerve pinching and radiation of pain. DJD is most common in weight-bearing joints that have been subjected to abnormal stresses (e.g. from overuse or obesity).[29]

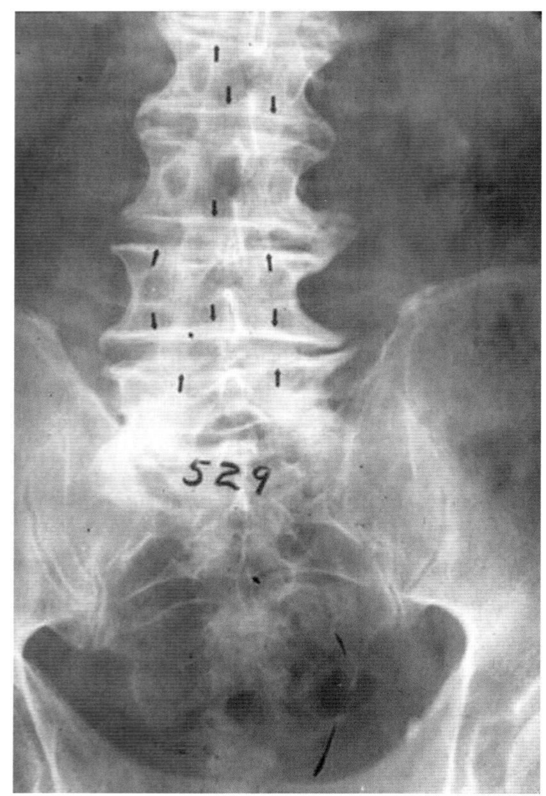

Fig. 10.31 Radiograph of degenerative joint disease of the lumbar spine

Key assessment findings for DJD

- Client usually over 50; history of dull, aching pain that worsens with activity and improves with rest, morning stiffness.
- Functional tests:
  - AROM tests positive
  - PROM tests positive
  - RROM usually negative
  - Special tests may be positive (e.g. if associated with neural compression).
- Palpation positive for tenderness.

FUNCTIONAL TESTS

AROM: limitation ± pain in some ranges depending on the structures involved (e.g. extension may be painful and/or limited by facet degeneration or IVF encroachment, flexion may be painful and/or limited by disc degeneration).

PROM: limited ± painful in lateral flexion, rotation and extension.

RROM: negative unless there is associated muscle spasm. Specific muscle tests may be positive for associated muscle spasm.

Special tests are usually negative unless DJD is causing neural compression.

PALPATION

Palpation of the lumbar spine usually reveals tenderness over the affected joints.

Differential diagnosis

- Ankylosing spondylitis: A key difference between ankylosing spondylitis and DJD is age of onset – the former usually begins between 15 and 35 years of age. Clients with ankylosing spondylitis complain of progressive morning pain and stiffness which is worse after periods of inactivity. Pain in DJD is usually relieved by rest.
- Psoriatic arthritis: psoriasis is a chronic autoimmune disease that causes red, scaly patches of inflammation and excessive skin production. Plaques frequently occur on the skin of the elbows and knees, but can affect any area including the scalp, palms of hands and soles of feet, and genitals. Between 10% and 30% of people with psoriasis develop psoriatic arthritis about 10 years after the onset of skin symptoms (i.e. typically between 30 and 50 years of age).
- Rheumatoid arthrosis (RA): Key differences between RA and DJD are age of onset (RA 30–60 years at time of onset), symmetrical involvement of joints (RA begins in bilateral proximal interphalangeal joints and metacarpophalangeal joints), associated prodrome (fever, malaise, night sweats), and ratio of females to males (3 to 1 in RA).[27]

Overview of treatment and management

Successful management of DJD depends on finding a balance between mobility and rest. This applies to treatment in the clinic and home exercise regimens. Use light pressure for the initial treatment and consider restricting treatment options to Swedish massage until the client's response to massage therapy has been assessed. Most DJD clients respond positively to Swedish massage, heat and gentle stretches. Heavy pressure and rigorous or long application of techniques can sometimes inflame arthritic joints.

Determine the type of tissue involved to guide selection of appropriate treatment techniques. Although DJD is a degenerative condition of the joints, it is often accompanied by myofascial adhesions and muscle contracture.

A typical remedial massage treatment for DJD of the lumbar spine includes:

- Swedish massage therapy to the back, pelvis and posterior lower limbs.
- Remedial massage therapy, including thermotherapy and lumbar stretches (e.g. longitudinal and rotational tractions of the lumbar spine, bilateral leg traction. Caution: use the See-Move-Touch principle, especially before applying rotational tractions) (see Figure 10.29 on p 161). Apply specific muscle techniques including trigger point therapy and muscle stretches (see Table 10.4) to treat muscle spasm/imbalance. (Caution: proceed gently with older clients and regularly check their pain levels to avoid an acute exacerbation.) Myofascial release may be beneficial for treating fascial restrictions.

CLIENT EDUCATION

Footwear with shock-absorbing soles lessens jarring impacts when walking and weight loss can help reduce symptoms. Lifting and posture advice is important. A good supportive mattress and pillow may be beneficial. Investigate work ergonomics and recommend measures to minimise impacts caused or aggravated by occupational tasks (e.g. avoiding repetitive tasks that overload the joints). Glucosamine and other nutritional supplements may be beneficial. A Cochrane review on the effect of glucosamine on osteoarthritis concluded that people with osteoarthritis who take glucosamine may experience reduced pain, improved physical function and will probably not have side effects.[30] Consider referral to a naturopath for specific dietary, herbal and nutritional support. Heat packs on affected joints may bring pain relief.

Home exercise program

Encourage clients to find a balance between activity and rest that optimises joint range of motion without inflaming joints. Recommend range of motion stretches and yoga. Clients appear to respond well to low-impact activities like aquarobics, swimming, tai chi or walking with appropriately cushioned footwear.

Address any underlying conditions or predisposing factors such as scoliosis or muscle weaknesses and contractures.

LOWER CROSSED SYNDROME

Lower crossed syndrome is a commonly observed back condition that results from a lower kinetic chain reaction of the lumbopelvis, hip, knee and ankle in which the hip flexors and back extensors shorten and tighten and the abdominal and gluteal muscles weaken (see Figure 10.32).[13] Clients may complain of chronic low back pain that is aggravated by extension and relieved by forward flexion. The pain is also aggravated by prolonged standing, wearing high-heeled shoes and activities that hyperextend the spine. There is usually no radiation of pain, although lower crossed syndrome is also associated with piriformis syndrome which may cause pressure on the sciatic nerve. The condition may result from repetitive action as may occur in gymnastics and water polo, immobilisation including sitting for prolonged periods or poorly rehabilitated previous injuries.

Key assessment findings for lower crossed syndrome

- History can include repetitive activity, poorly rehabilitated previous injury, prolonged immobilisation. Pain after prolonged standing, bending backwards; pain relieved by lumbar flexion; usually no radiation of pain.
- Postural analysis: Hyperlordotic lumbar spine.
- Functional tests:
  - AROM positive in extension
  - PROM usually negative
  - RROM may be positive for affected muscles
  - Resisted and length tests positive for affected muscles including short iliopsoas, rectus femoris, erector spinae, quadratus lumborum, tensor fasciae latae, hip adductors; weak abdominal muscles, gluteal muscles
  - Special tests negative except for Kemp's.
- Palpation positive for tenderness ± pain on anterior pressure of the lumbar spine; tightness palpable in affected muscles.

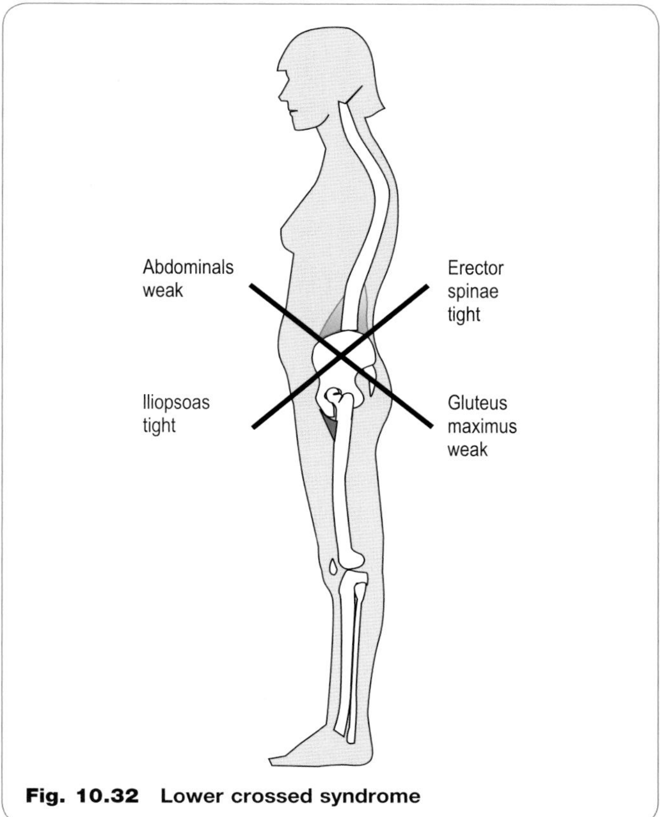

Fig. 10.32 Lower crossed syndrome

Assessment

HISTORY

Clients with lower crossed syndrome/hyperlordosis usually describe a dull aching pain that can be localised at the lower back. The pain is aggravated by extension or prolonged standing and relieved by flexion. There is usually no radiation of pain and no neurological symptoms except in cases of associated piriformis syndrome where clients may experience sciatic pain. The patient often has difficulty lying supine with legs extended and prefers to lie with knees bent.

POSTURAL ANALYSIS

Lumbar hyperlordosis is evident and may be accompanied by compensatory thoracic kyphosis.

FUNCTIONAL TESTS

AROM: lumbar extension increases pain and trunk flexion relieves it.
PROM: usually negative.
RROM: may be positive for affected muscles.
Resisted and length tests may indicate muscle weakness (e.g. abdominal muscles, gluteal muscles) and shortness (e.g. iliopsoas, erector spinae, quadratus lumborum, rectus femoris) respectively.
Special tests: Kemp's test is usually positive and all other special tests negative.

PALPATION

Anterior pressure over L3 area often reproduces the pain. Tightness of affected muscles is usually palpable.

Differential diagnosis

Lower crossed syndrome is not difficult to identify. However, it is important to identify those clients with the possible presence of spondylolisthesis. Spondylolisthesis clients may experience bilateral sciatica and/or other neurological symptoms. Some also present with a hairy tuft over the lumbosacral area and a palpable step defect.

Overview of treatment and management

The key to successful remedial massage treatment is identification and correction of muscle imbalances associated with hyperlordosis. Check for relative imbalances between abdominal muscles and lumbar extensor muscles (erector spinae and quadratus lumborum), hip flexors (iliopsoas and rectus femoris) and gluteal muscles. In most cases abdominals, gluteal muscles and hamstrings will need to be strengthened in a home exercise program and erector spinae, iliopsoas, rectus femoris and quadratus lumborum need to be stretched during treatment and at home.

A typical treatment for lower crossed syndrome includes the following:

- Swedish massage to the back, buttocks and anterior thighs. Place a pillow in front of the client's waist during prone massage to reduce the lordosis and avoid undue anterior pressure on the spine. When the client lies supine, place a pillow under their thighs.
- The aim of remedial massage is to address muscle imbalances found during assessment. Tight muscles require stretching. Trigger point therapy and soft-tissue releasing techniques are usually beneficial (see Table 10.4). Tight muscles may respond to thermotherapy. Treat fascial restrictions with myofascial releasing techniques (see Chapter 8).

CLIENT EDUCATION

Posture advice includes avoiding all postures and activities that exacerbate lumbar lordosis. For example, advise the client to bend their knees when lying on their back or on their side. Advise the client to use a footstool when sitting or place a pillow under the thighs so that their knees are higher than their hips. When standing, they should use a footstool for one leg. Thermotherapy may be beneficial. Referral for osseous manipulation may be helpful.

Home exercise program

Many clients respond well to an exercise program. Muscle stretches performed during treatment (e.g. erector spinae, quadratus lumborum, iliopsoas and rectus femoris) should be continued at home. A program to strengthen weak muscles (e.g. abdominal muscles, gluteal muscles and hamstrings) may be progressively introduced for long-term biomechanical improvements. If pelvic floor muscles are weak, refer the client to a physiotherapist for specific exercises.

Address any underlying conditions or predisposing factors such as scoliosis, overtraining or obesity. Refer for a full neurological examination if the client has lower limb pain or other neurological symptoms.

LUMBAR DISC SYNDROME

Lumbar disc syndrome is a rare presenting condition, accounting for 1–3% of clients with low back pain. A herniated disc is a fragment of the nucleus pulposus which protrudes through tears or ruptures in the annulus fibrosus. The displaced disc fragment may press on spinal nerves, often producing pain which can be severe. L4–L5 and L5–S1 account for 95% of all disc herniations.[27] A herniated disc can result from a single excessive strain or injury or from chronic overloading of the disc (see Figure 10.33).

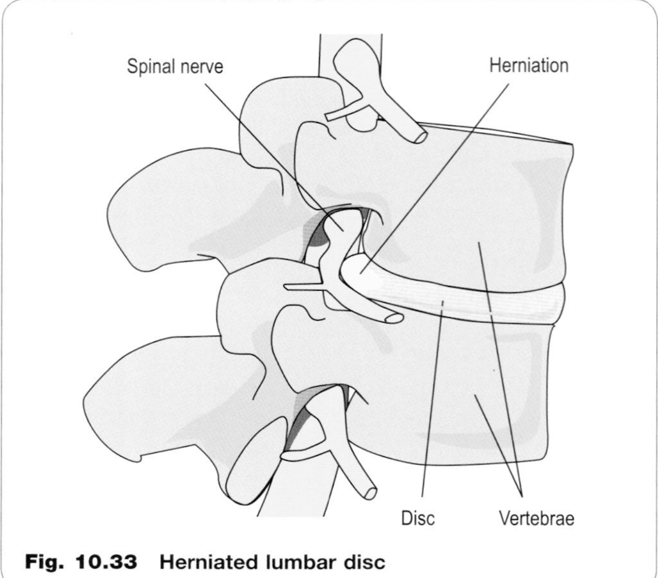

Fig. 10.33 Herniated lumbar disc

Key assessment findings for lumbar disc syndrome

- Client usually 25–45 years old; history of recent trauma, heavy lifting, or niggling low back pain; pain may be severe; dermatomal radiation of pain.
- Functional tests:
  - AROM positive, particularly for flexion
  - PROM positive, particularly in flexion
  - RROM negative unless associated muscle strain
  - Resisted and length tests usually negative unless associated muscle strain
  - Special tests: positive Valsalva, SLR, centralisation.
- Palpation positive for tenderness ± pain at the level of the lesion.

Assessment

HISTORY

Lumbar disc herniation occurs most commonly in 25- to 45-year-olds. Clients may describe a recent trauma, heavy or awkward lifting or repetitive stress trauma. Alternatively, the client may simply have leaned forward, usually to one side, when the injury occurred. These clients typically have a history of niggling low back pain. Unilateral sciatica commonly results from a herniated disc in the low back. Pain is often described as sharp and shooting and radiates in a dermatomal pattern. Symptoms include pain radiating from the buttock to the back of the leg and sometimes to the foot, burning, paraesthesia (tingling, numbness, pins and needles), sharp electric-shock pain and muscle weakness. Pain may be felt immediately or over a day or so after an episode of heavy

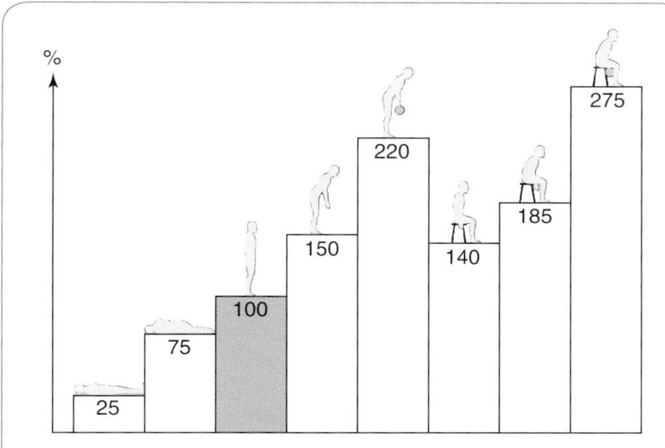

Fig. 10.34 Pressure on lumbar discs in various postures

or awkward lifting. Pain is aggravated by sitting, bending forward, coughing, sneezing or straining and is usually relieved by lying down (see Figure 10.34).

Features that are suggestive of lumbar disc syndrome include:

1. Severity of pain.
2. Dermatomal radiation of pain (e.g. L5/S1 disc herniation may impinge on the sciatic nerve root causing pain in the posterolateral leg and lateral foot).
3. Pain on Valsalva, SLR; pain centralises with repeated lumbar extension.[e]

POSTURAL ANALYSIS

The client may adopt an antalgic posture (i.e. the client leans away from the side of injury).

GAIT ANALYSIS

Clients with lumbar disc symptoms will move slowly and cautiously. In acute cases, clients may adopt an antalgic lean.

FUNCTIONAL TESTS

AROM: positive in flexion and/or any direction that increases neural compression.
PROM: positive in flexion and/or any direction that increases neural compression.
RROM: negative unless associated muscle strain.
Note: PROM and RROM tests may not be performed because of the potential to put further pressure on the disc.
Special tests: Valsalva, SLR and centralisation are often positive. A positive SLR in conjunction with changes in reflexes, muscular strength and sensation suggest that lumbar radiculopathy is highly likely.[11] If pain centralises during repeated lumbar extension a bulging lumbar disc is indicated.[11]

PALPATION

The client commonly reports tenderness to palpation at the level of the lesion (usually over L4–S1). Spasm is usually palpated in muscles associated with adaptive contracture to guard against further pressure on the disc.

[e]In a small number of clients, pain centralised in a direction other than extension.

Differential diagnosis

- Cauda equina syndrome can result when a large central disc herniation presses on the cauda equina with effects on bowel and bladder function. It is a very rare (less than 1% of low back pain clients) but serious condition that requires urgent medical attention. The most significant finding leading to diagnosis is urinary retention. (Ask all disc clients if they have had any recent difficulty with urination or defecation.[27])
- Central or lateral canal stenosis refers to narrowing of the spinal canal caused by bone and/or soft tissue encroachment (e.g. congenital defects, spondylosis, thickening of the ligamentum flavum). Narrowing of the spinal canal can lead to compression of the spinal cord. Clients present with an inconsistent pattern of back and leg pain that is increased by activity and relieved by rest. Symptoms may be relieved by extension and flexion of the lumbar spine.
- Piriformis syndrome refers to sciatic neuritis caused when mechanical or chemical irritants infiltrate the epineurium of the nerve as a result of piriformis contracture. Although not a common cause of posterior thigh and leg pain, the piriformis is easily assessed and treated. It may be caused by trauma to the gluteal region or excessively tight external hip rotators. A positive SLR test with hip neutral and a negative SLR with hip in external rotation suggest piriformis syndrome.

Overview of treatment and management

Because of its severity most clients with acute lumbar disc herniation immediately consult a medical practitioner, chiropractor, osteopath or physiotherapist. All clients with severe pain (i.e. pain above 7 or 8 out of 10 on a pain scale) should be referred for further investigation and treatment. The aim of treatment in the acute phase is usually to control pain, reduce nerve compression, prevent any further nerve compression and to teach clients how to protect and stabilise their lower back. Clients are advised to stay as active as possible within their pain-free range. Gentle intermittent mobility such as pottering around the house is encouraged. The sooner the client moves about, the better the prognosis. Within the first week the client could try to walk up to 20 minutes for every 3 hours spent supine.[27] In the acute phase many clients adopt an antalgic posture (usually trunk flexed and sidebent). As soon as the client can achieve lumbar lordosis without pain it should be encouraged (e.g. by using lumbar supports). Clients may be able to tolerate the Mackenzie back exercises if, when lying prone, extending a straight leg decreases or centralises their pain (see Appendix 10.1). Clients should avoid any movement that peripheralises pain both during treatment and in home exercise programs.

Typical remedial massage treatments for acutely inflamed lumbar discs include cryotherapy, acupressure, Reiki and reflexology. Note that anti-inflammatory or analgesic medication and muscle relaxants are often prescribed, but there is conflicting evidence that oral or injectable non-steroidal anti-inflammatory drugs (NSAIDs) are effective compared to placebo or no treatment for acute low back pain.[4] Instruct clients to contact their medical practitioner should they require urgent care.

Most clients seek remedial massage for treatment of subacute or chronic back pain. However, even a history of disc herniation in the absence of presenting symptoms is sufficient to require modificaton of remedial massage techniques because of the recurrent nature of the condition. A typical treatment for subacute lumbar disc herniation includes:

- Swedish massage to the back, buttocks and posterior thighs. Pillows should be arranged to maintain pain-free lumbar lordosis if possible. (Caution: even Swedish massage strokes aggravate symptoms in some clients.) Initial treatments should be short until the client's tolerance to massage in the prone position has been ascertained.
- Remedial massage therapy includes gentle bilateral leg traction within the client's painfree range. Remedial massage therapy for muscle strains/muscle imbalance includes deep gliding frictions along the muscle fibres, cross-fibre frictions and soft-tissue releasing techniques. Use the See-Move-Touch principle (see Chapter 2) and avoid techniques that could produce symptoms or aggravate the condition, particularly when performing trigger point therapy and muscle stretches. Incorrect or inappropriate stretches (especially into flexion) may aggravate the condition. For example, caution should be applied when performing a hamstring muscle stretch on a client with a recent history of pain on lumbar flexion. Note also that some practitioners suggest that spasm in the quadratus lumborum and lumbar erector spinae muscles creates a positive splinting for the lower back and therefore should not be completely released in the case of acute disc clients or clients with a history of disc damage. Thermotherapy and fascial releasing techniques are often used.

CLIENT EDUCATION

Posture and lifting advice may be helpful. Encourage clients to maintain good lumbar posture at work, at home, while driving and undertaking all activities of daily living. Advise clients to get in and out of bed by rolling onto their side without twisting their lumbar spine, bending knees and using their arms to push their trunk upright, making sure their pelvis remains perpendicular to the spine. Clients should avoid sitting, forward bending (even the slight forward bending required to brush teeth), lifting and any activities or positions that aggravate symptoms. If clients do lift, they must use appropriate lifting techniques (e.g. tighten core muscles when lifting, bend their knees, hold the load close to their body). Advise clients about the use of shock-absorbing soles when walking, about supportive mattresses and about weight loss if appropriate.

Refer clients to a chiropractor, osteopath or manipulative physiotherapist for spinal manipulation. Refer clients to an appropriate healthcare practitioner for identified yellow flags. Clients may also be referred for nutritional advice, for acupuncture and for exercise therapy. Always refer clients at six weeks post injury who have muscle weakness or who fail to respond to treatment.

Home exercise program

Muscle stretches and core strengthening exercises are recommended when they can be performed within the client's pain-free range and without aggravating symptoms. As the client recovers, conditioning and proprioceptive training for the trunk and lower limbs can be progressively introduced. Pilates core strengthening programs and swimming could be useful for long-term prevention of pain and relapse.

The long-term aim of treatment of lumbar disc herniation is to educate and encourage clients to resume their normal activities. Remedial techniques are designed to maintain or improve good biomechanics. Most cases of lumbar disc herniation resolve spontaneously as the herniated material is reabsorbed. However, recurrences are not uncommon and have been associated with the presence of yellow flags.[4] Early assessment and intervention of yellow flags is essential.

SPONDYLOLISTHESIS

Spondylolisthesis is the forward slipping of a vertebra on the vertebra below. The term derives from the Greek words *spondylos* for vertebra and *olisthesis* for slippage or displacement. The slippage is most commonly due to a pars interarticularis defect (a separation of the vertebral body and the arch). Ninety per cent occur at L5. The cause of the condition is unclear although structural forces are involved. One widely accepted theory for the mechanism of the defect is that mechanical stresses cause a stress fracture of the pars interarticularis. The prevalence of spondylolisthesis is 5–7% in Caucasians and 40% in Inuit populations (possibly due to the vertical papoose fashion of carrying infants). For this reason, clients are sometimes advised to avoid vertical pouches or upright walkers for infants. Onset can occur after walking begins although the most common age is between 10 and 15 years. It is more common in people who have high levels of physical activity such as diving, gymnastics, weight lifting or pole vaulting where hyperextension and jarring stresses can occur.

Radiographs of spondylolisthesis show:

- anterior slippage of the vertebrae
- discontinuation of the posterior longitudinal ligament line
- oblique views have a 'collar on the Scotty dog' (see Figure 10.35 on p 167).

Grading of spondylolisthesis is based on the percentage of forward slip of one vertebra (usually L5) compared to the vertebra below (usually S1) (see Figure 10.36 on p 167). The higher the grade, the greater the instability.

- Grade 1: up to 25%
- Grade 2: up to 50%
- Grade 3: up to 75%
- Grade 4: up to 100%.

Key assessment findings for spondylolisthesis

- History of pain after prolonged standing, bending backwards; pain relieved by lumbar flexion; ± bilateral sciatica or other neurological symptoms.
- Postural observation: hyperlordosis ± hairy tuft over lumbosacral area.
- Functional tests:
  - AROM positive in extension; pain reduced in flexion
  - PROM positive in extension; pain reduced in flexion
  - RROM usually negative
  - Special tests negative except for Kemp's test.
- Palpation; anterior pressure over L5/S1 is positive; ± step defect.

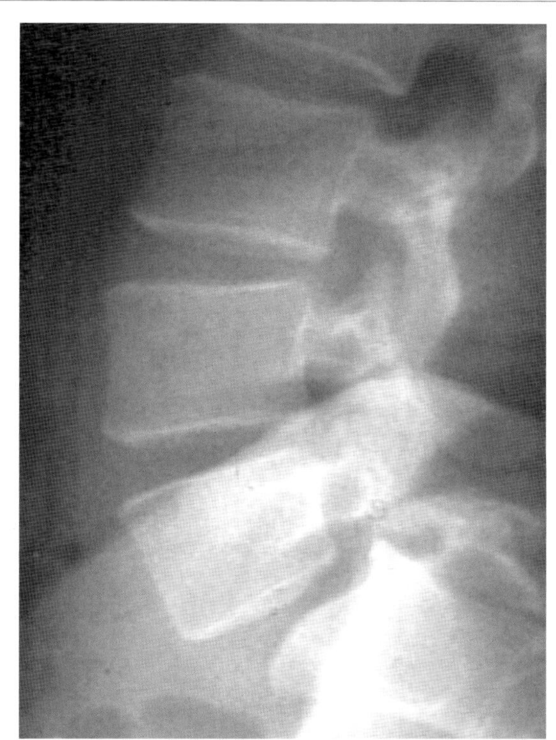

Fig. 10.35 Radiograph of spondylolisthesis

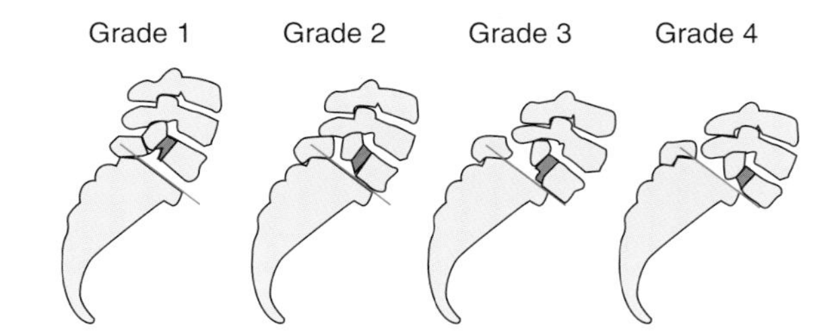

Fig. 10.36 Grades of spondylolisthesis

Assessment

HISTORY

Clinical presentations vary and clients are often asymptomatic. Clients may complain of low back pain, sciatica and other neurological symptoms. Note that spondylolisthesis is the most common cause of bilateral sciatica. The pain may be sharp and severe. Severe symptoms or neurological symptoms differentiate spondylolisthesis from an uncomplicated hyperlordotic posture.

POSTURAL ANALYSIS

A hyperlordotic lumbar spine is commonly observed. There may be a hairy tuft (faun's beard) over the lumbosacral area.

FUNCTIONAL TESTS

AROM: Pain and neurological symptoms usually increase with extension and decrease with flexion.
PROM: Pain and neurological symptoms usually increase with extension and decrease with flexion.
RROM: Usually negative.
Special tests: Kemp's test is usually positive.

PALPATION

Clients report tenderness and/or pain over L5–S1 (or region of slippage) and caution is required when applying anterior pressure to the area. Sometimes a 'step deformity' is palpable (i.e. the anteriority of the spinous process above palpates as a hollow or dip in the spine).

Differential diagnosis

A less common cause of low back pain with bilateral sciatica is a central disc bulge exerting pressure on both sciatic nerves. Spondylolisthesis may be distinguished from lower crossed/hyperlordosis syndrome by the presence of neurological symptoms, a palpable step-defect and a hairy tuft over the lumbosacral spine.

Overview of treatment and management

All clients with spondylolisthesis should be assessed by a medical practitioner, chiropractor, osteopath or physiotherapist. In most cases, remedial massage treatment will be provided in conjunction with other treatment (e.g. spinal manipulation, exercise therapy). This is potentially a very serious condition. Great attention is required to avoid lumbar extension in all phases of treatment. For example, incorrect pillow placement when the client is prone could increase lumbar lordosis and exert anterior pressure on the displaced vertebra. When the client is supine, ensure that the client lie with their knees flexed or place pillows under their knees to increase lumbar flexion. Posture and exercise advice for managing spondylolisthesis is similar to that for hyperlordotic (lower crossed posture), including avoiding all activities that extend the spine and cultivating flexion activities such as bringing knees to chest.

A typical treatment for spondylolisthesis includes the following:

- Swedish massage therapy to the low back and buttocks (pillow in front of the client's waist when prone: pillow under their thighs when supine). Avoid any strokes that place anterior pressure on the area of slippage.
- Remedial massage techniques include deep gliding friction, cross-fibre friction, trigger point, or active and passive release for affected muscles. Use only those techniques that can be performed without inducing lumbar extension (e.g. avoid deep massage on the multifidus and rotator muscles). Fascial releasing techniques for fascial restrictions are commonly used. Stretching techniques that flex the lumbar spine are beneficial (e.g. client supine, bilateral knees to chest). Thermotherapy may be beneficial.

CLIENT EDUCATION

Advise the client to avoid all lumbar extension: consider sleeping position and mattress, workstation ergonomics, sitting with knees higher than hips, when standing for a long time putting one foot on a foot rail. Provide lifting advice (disc degeneration occurs at the level of the spondylolisthesis more rapidly than at any other level of the spine). Advise clients to avoid high-heeled shoes, use shock-absorbing soles and discuss weight loss if appropriate. Refer clients to a chiropractor, osteopath or manipulative physiotherapist for vertebral and sacral manipulation. Clients with spondylolisthesis should always be co-managed with a general medical practitioner, chiropractor, osteopath or physiotherapist. Some clients have reported benefit with acupuncture.

Home exercise program

Clients with spondylolisthesis may benefit from isometric strengthening of core stabilisers, and stretching low back extensor and hip flexor muscles, conditioning and proprioceptive training for the trunk and lower limbs, and painfree range of motion exercises.

Remedial massage therapy should continue with increasing reliance on home exercise programs and client self-help. Any underlying conditions, predisposing or complicating factors like scoliosis or sports and training programs that emphasise hyperextension should be addressed.

SACROILIAC SYNDROME

The sacroiliac joint is subject to mechanical lesions, including sprains and movement dysfunctions. Normally the sacroiliac joints have very little movement. Ligamentous laxity is a contributing factor during pregnancy when sacroiliac movements are enhanced by the action of the hormone relaxin, producing a 4 mm increase in the width of the symphysis pubis. Pain of mechanical origin is usually unilateral and can be aggravated by movements that stress the joint. There are usually no neurological symptoms. Note that pain in this area can also be referred from the lower lumbar spine or hip joint. It is also a common site for secondary malignant deposits or Paget's disease.

Assessment

HISTORY

The client usually describes a dull ache, although occasionally sacroiliac sprains can produce sharp stabbing pain. The most intense pain is reported over the sacroiliac joint itself but pain may refer to the buttock, groin or posterior thigh although it rarely extends below the knee. In clients with inflammatory sacroiliitis there is often a history of buttock pain that alternates from one side to the other. It is usually not relieved by lying down, is worse at night and is associated with stiffness in the back. Pain relieved by standing appears to be a useful indicator for sacroiliac joint sprain.[11]

Key assessment findings for sacroiliac syndrome

- History of recent trauma, repetitive overuse or stress of the low back and pelvis, pregnancy; unilateral SI pain ± radiation to buttock, groin, posterior thigh. Pain relieved by standing.
- Functional tests:
  - AROM: positive, especially flexion and extension of the pelvis
  - PROM: may be positive, especially flexion and extension of the pelvis
  - RROM: usually negative
  - Special tests: Patrick, SI compression and distraction, leg length, sacral springing may be positive.
- Palpation positive for tenderness ± pain over SI joint.

POSTURAL ANALYSIS

Mechanical sacroiliac lesions may be associated with scoliosis, leg length inequality and musculoskeletal compensations that may be identified during postural observation.

FUNCTIONAL TESTS

AROM: positive when weight bearing, moving from sitting to standing, walking, flexion or extension of the pelvis.
PROM: may be positive with flexion or extension of the pelvis.
RROM: usually negative unless there are associated muscle imbalances.
Specific muscle tests: resisted tests and muscle length tests may be useful for identifying associated muscle imbalances.
Special tests: Pain provocation tests such as the Patrick test, compression and distraction tests and sacral springing demonstrate fair to moderate reliability; some have moderate diagnostic usefulness.[11]

PALPATION

With the client supine, place the palms of the hands on the anterior superior iliac spines and palpate for symmetry (i.e. the distances between the anterior superior iliac spines and the umbilicus, the height of the anterior superior iliac spines from the table) (see Figure 10.37).

In the prone position, gently rock the sacrum from side to side and up and down. Palpate the sacroiliac joints for tenderness.

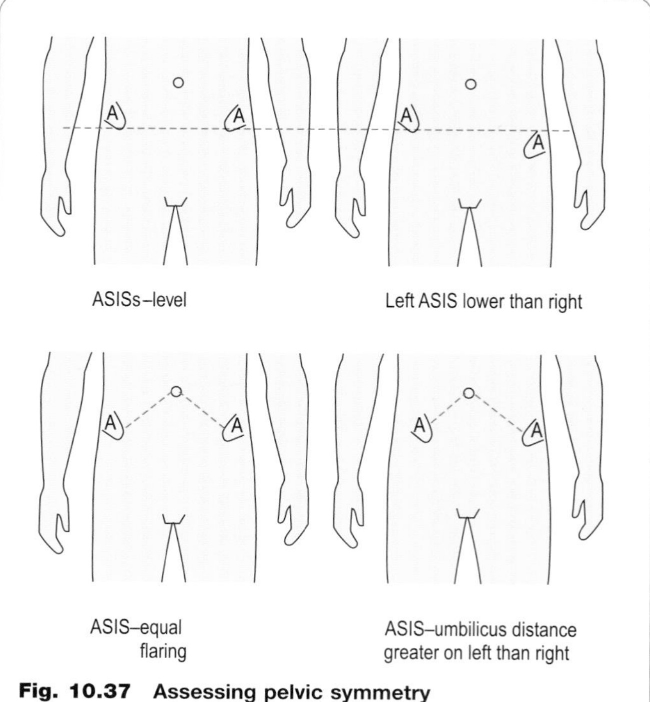

Fig. 10.37 Assessing pelvic symmetry

Overview of treatment and management

A typical remedial massage treatment for SI sprain includes the following:

- Swedish massage to the lumbosacral area (including the gluteal muscles and piriformis muscle) and posterior thighs.
- Remedial massage therapy, which includes prone sacroiliac joint mobilisations and supine pelvic rocking (anterior/posterior, superior/inferior and medial/lateral) within the client's pain-free range (to avoid stretching sprained ligaments).

PRONE SACROILIAC JOINT MOBILISATIONS

The client is prone and the pelvis is covered with a towel. Stabilise the sacrum with your caudal hand, fingers pointed superiorly; the cephalad palm contacts over the gluteal area on one side, fingers pointing inferiorly so that your hands are either side of the sacroiliac joint. Apply gentle pressure inferiorly with the caudal hand. Reverse the hand positions and apply gentle pressure with the caudal hand in a superior direction. Repeat both movements on the other sacroiliac joint (see Figure 10.38).

SUPINE PELVIC ROCKING

The client is supine, pelvis and lower limbs covered with a towel. Face towards the head of the table and contact the client's anterior superior iliac spines with each hand. Apply gentle posterior pressure to the anterior superior iliac spine on one side, release the pressure, and then apply posterior pressure on the other. Pressure can also be applied one side at a time superiorly and inferiorly and medially and laterally (see Figure 10.39 on p 170).

- Tapotement can be applied directly over the sacrum and SI joints.
- Cross-fibre frictions to iliolumbar ligaments and sacrotuberous ligament (see Figure 10.40 on p 170).
- Thermotherapy may be beneficial.
- Treat any muscle imbalance with specific muscle techniques such as trigger point therapy, soft-tissue releasing techniques and stretches to specific muscles, including piriformis, quadratus lumborum, gluteus maximus, hamstrings and hip adductors (see Table 10.4). Myofascial releasing techniques may be beneficial for treating fascial restrictions. Hip joint articulation and a lymphatic pump from the feet may indirectly mobilise the sacroiliac joints.

LYMPHATIC PUMP

The client lies supine, legs extended. Hold the ankle of one leg and apply gentle pulsing pressure towards the client's head. (The leg acts as a lever to gently rock the pelvis posteriorly on one side.) Repeat seven times, at a rate of one pulse a second. Next apply gentle pulsing tractions to the leg so that the pelvis gently rocks anteriorly on that side. Repeat the whole sequence (seven pushes and seven tractions) on the

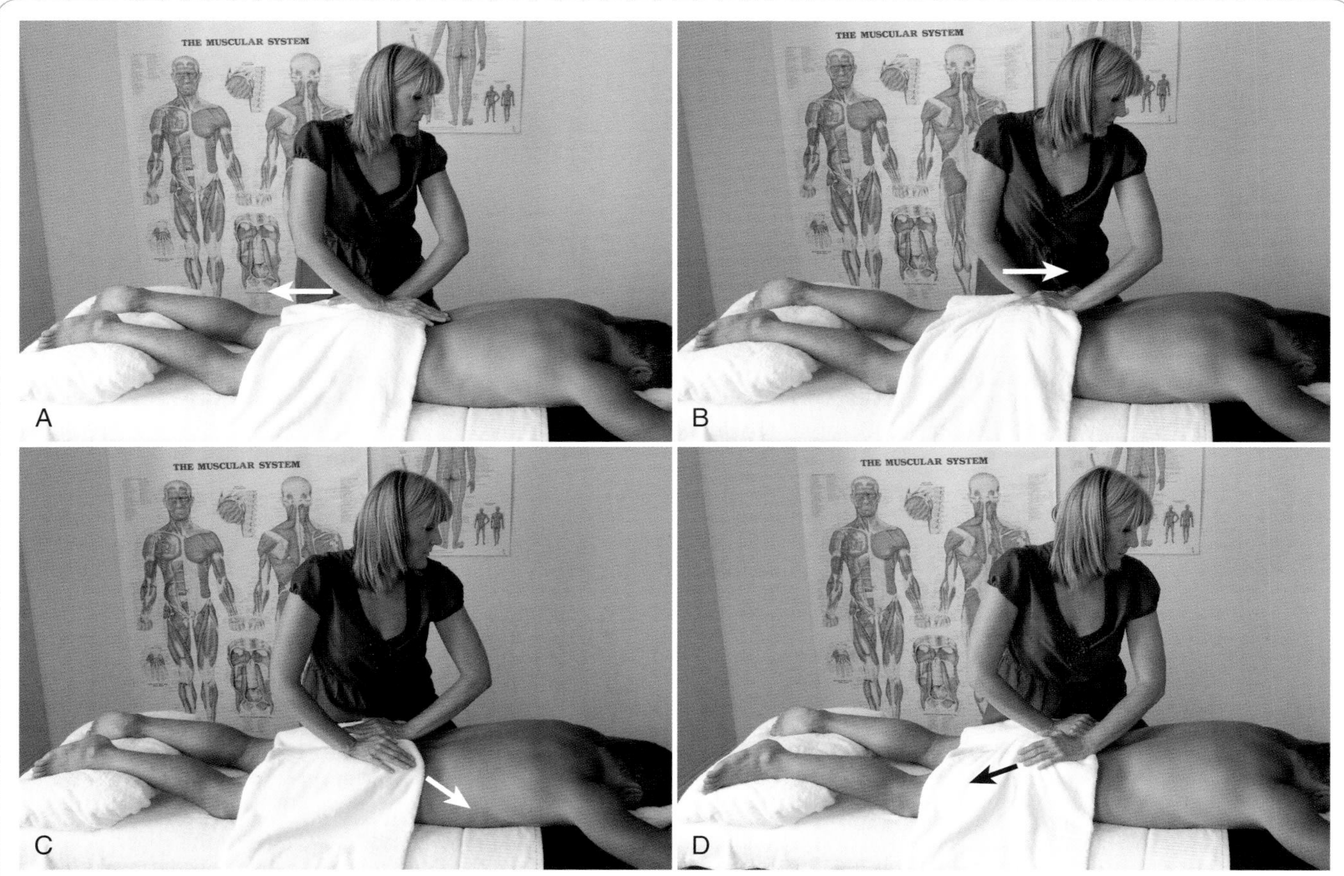

Fig. 10.38 Prone sacroiliac mobilisation

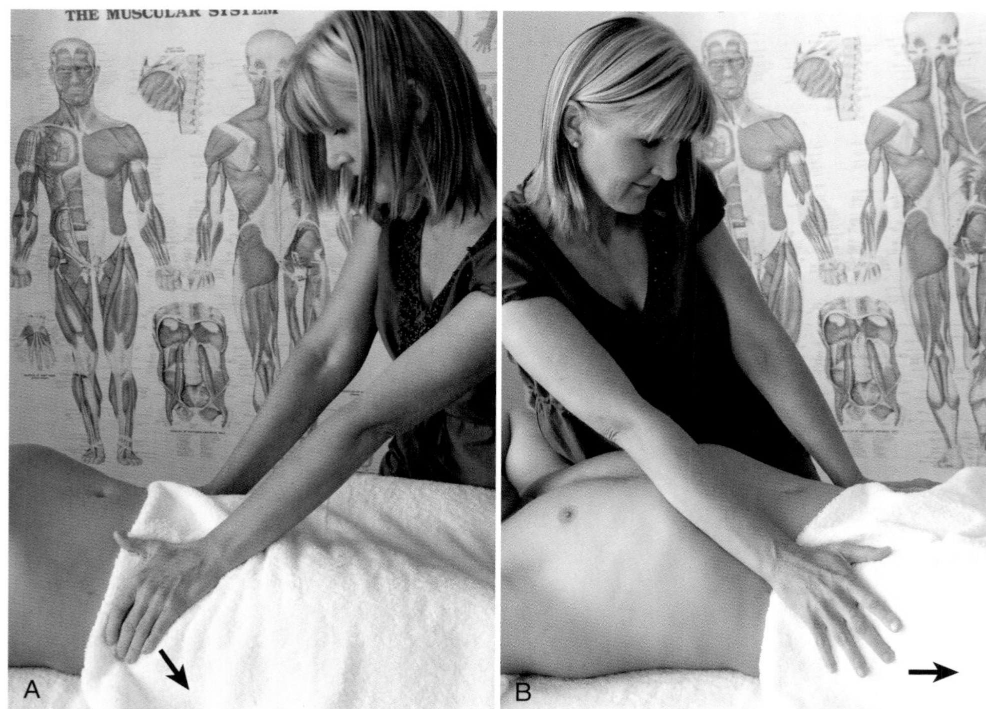

Fig. 10.39 **Supine pelvic rocking**

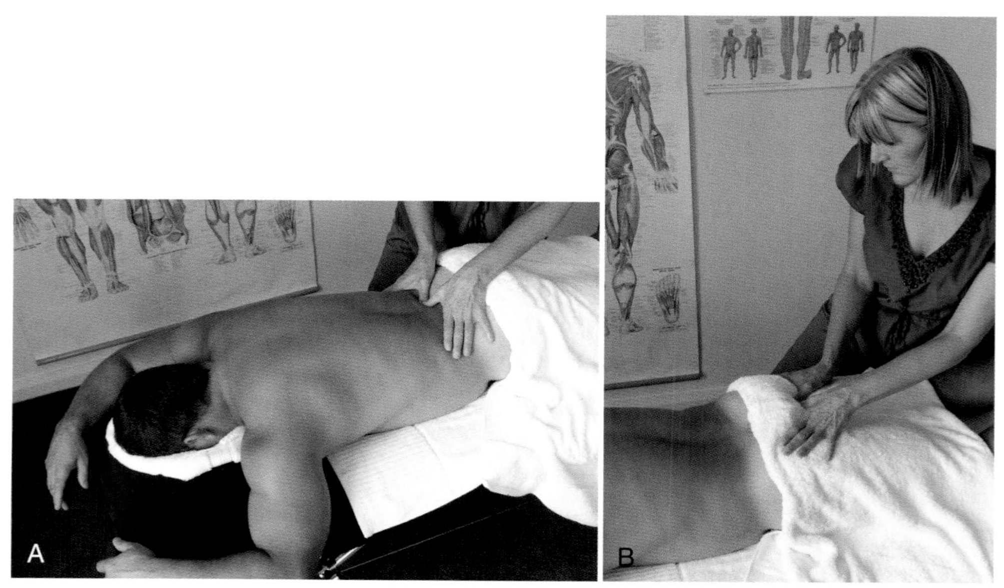

Fig. 10.40 **Cross-fibre frictions to A:** iliolumbar ligaments and **B:** sacrotuberous ligaments

other leg and then repeat the sequence holding both legs at once (see Figure 10.41).

CLIENT EDUCATION

Refer for osseous manipulation and for a heel lift in cases of anatomical short leg. Advise clients to avoid cross-legged sitting. Minimise impacts caused or aggravated by occupation (e.g. avoiding repetitive tasks that overload the joints). Using footwear with shock-absorbing soles lessens jarring impacts when walking, and losing weight can reduce symptoms. A home exercise program should be introduced to strengthen and stretch muscles as indicated.

Address any underlying conditions or predisposing factors (e.g. scoliosis or hyperlordosis).

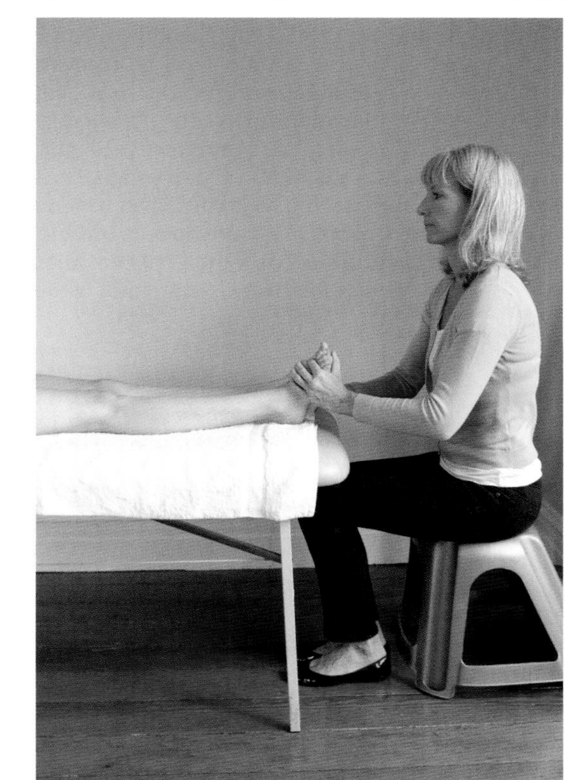

Fig. 10.41 Lymphatic pump

KEY MESSAGES

- Low back pain has a high prevalence in the community and is a common presenting condition to remedial massage clinics.
- Most (85–95%) of low back pain is non-specific; that is, a specific pathoanatomical cause cannot be located.
- Assessment of clients with low back conditions involves history, outcome measures, postural analysis, gait analysis, functional tests (including resisted tests and muscle length tests for specific muscles of the low back and lower limbs) and special tests for the low back.
- Assessment findings may indicate the type of tissue involved (contractile or inert), duration of condition (acute or subacute) and severity.
- Assessment findings may indicate a common presenting condition such as
  - muscle strains
  - non-specific low back pain
  - degenerative joint disease
  - lower crossed syndrome
  - lumbar disc herniation
  - spondylolisthesis
  - sacroiliac syndrome.
- Although serious conditions of the low back are rare, clients with such conditions will present for remedial massage from time to time. Caution is required when treating all clients with low back pain, especially when there are indications of lumbar disc herniation and spondylolisthesis. Be conservative in treatment: if in doubt, refer.
- Incorporate the best available evidence in therapy planning.
- Short-term treatments tend to focus on presenting symptoms; long-term treatments tend to focus on potential contributing factors (e.g. lifestyle factors, underlying structural features or underlying disease processes).
- Educating clients about likely causal and predisposing factors is an essential part of remedial massage therapy, particularly for potentially catastrophic and incapacitating conditions of the low back like disc herniation and spondylolisthesis.

APPENDIX 10.1

McKenzie self-treatments for sciatica[31]

'If your problem is worse with bending forward, after sitting, or in the morning, a few exercises originally developed by a physical therapist Robin McKenzie from New Zealand, may also be helpful — the sphinx, cobra, and standing back extension. The sphinx and cobra can be performed a few times a day. Carry out 10–12 repetitions slowly. If it hurts in your low back, but not in your leg that is fine. If however, leg pain increases then stop the exercise. The standing back extension manoeuvre can be performed a few times every 20 minutes when you have been sitting.

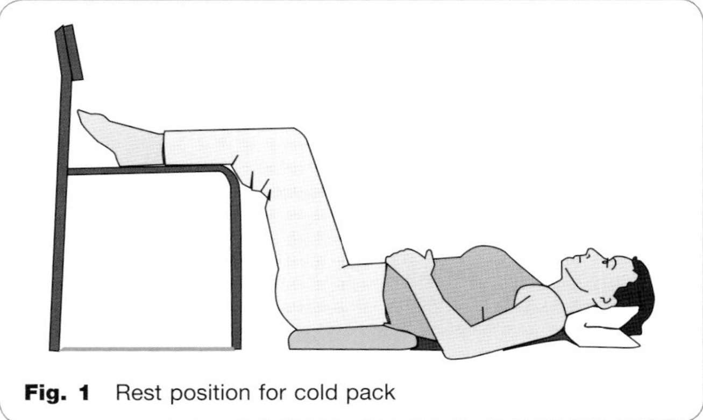

Fig. 1 Rest position for cold pack

Fig. 2 Sphinx

Since your nerves are behind your disc bending forward usually squeezes the bulging disc into the spinal nerve roots. Therefore, it is important to avoid slouching or slumping forward when sitting, standing or bending for things. McKenzie realized that it is also helpful to 'milk' the disc forward of the nerve roots by performing a variety of back bending or extension exercises. These may be uncomfortable in your back, BUT after a few repetitions you should feel that your leg symptoms are lessening. Scientific studies have proven that this is a good sign and means the exercises are right for you. If however, you feel your leg symptoms worsening then you are not ready for these movements yet.'

Review questions

1. A 20-year-old man has played a social game of cricket on the weekend, his first game since he left school. He woke the next day with low back pain that was very uncomfortable and made it hard for him to sit at his desk at work. On examination, Valsalva, SLR and compression are negative. His postural observation is unremarkable. A provisional assessment could be:
   a) Non-specific low back pain
   b) Hyperlordosis of the lumbar spine
   c) Spondylolisthesis
   d) Lumbar disc syndrome
2. A 23-year-old client has low back pain that is worse at the end of the day after she has been standing at work. She gets most relief when she lies on her back and brings her knees up to her chest. The pain does not refer beyond the low back and there are no neurological symptoms. A provisional assessment could be:
   a) Non-specific low back pain
   b) Lower crossed/hyperlordosis syndrome
   c) Spondylolisthesis
   d) Degenerative joint disease
3. Straight leg raising (SLR) test is used to distinguish between:
   a) Lumbar disc and degenerative joint disease
   b) Sciatica and hip flexor tightness
   c) Sciatica and hamstring tightness
   d) Degenerative joint disease and sciatica
4. The most common level for a lumbar disc herniation to occur is:
   a) L4/L5 b) L3/L4
   c) L1/L2 d) L5/S1
5. The Valsalva test of the lumbar spine is used to indicate the presence of:
   a) a space-occupying lesion such as a disc prolapse
   b) paravertebral muscle strain
   c) lumbar facet syndrome
   d) spondylolisthesis
6. A client has low back pain that is aggravated by lumbar extension and relieved by forward flexion. He has a hairy tuft over the lumbosacral spine. He describes radiating pain down the back of both thighs. A likely assessment is:
   a) lumbar facet syndrome
   b) spondylolisthesis
   c) lower crossed/hyperlordosis syndrome
   d) lumbar disc syndrome
7. Name three signs and symptoms that could suggest a lumbar disc prolapse.
8. Briefly describe the precautions you would take when treating a client with spondylolisthesis.
9. A patient is observed to have a hyperlordotic spine. List three muscles that may be short and tight.
10. a) What is the clinical significance of a tight piriformis muscle?
    b) Draw or describe a test for piriformis muscle length.
11. Draw or describe a home stretch for the following muscles:
    a) iliopsoas
    b) quadratus lumborum
    c) quadriceps femoris
12. List three red flags for acute lumbar pain.

REFERENCES

1. Deyo RA, Rainville J, Kent D. What can the history and physical examination tell us about low back pain? JAMA 1992;268:760–5.
2. Furlan AD, Imamura M, Dryden T, et al. Massage for low-back pain. Cochrane Database Syst Rev [serial on the Internet]. 2008;(4)CD001929.
3. Statistics ABS. Musculoskeletal conditions in Australia: a snapshot 2004–5. Online. Available: www.abs.gov.au/ausstats/abs@.nsf/mf/4823.0.55.001; 2006.
4. Australian Acute Musculoskeletal Pain Guidelines Group. Evidence-based management of acute musculoskeletal pain: a guide for clinicians. Bowen Hills, Queensland: Australian Academic Press; 2004.
5. Deyo RA, Weinstein JN. Low back pain. N Engl J Med [Research Support, U.S. Gov't, P.H.S.Review]. 2001;344(5):363–70.
6. Ebrall P. Assessment of the spine. Philadelphia: Churchill Livingstone; 2004.
7. Legaspi O, Edmond S. Does the evidence support the existence of lumbar spine coupled motion? A critical review of the literature. J Orthop Sports Phys Ther 2007;37(4):169–78.
8. White A, Panjabi M. Clinical biomechanics of the spine. 2nd edn. Philadelphia: Lippincott Williams and Wilkins; 1990.
9. Fritz S, Grosenbach M. Mosby's Essential Sciences for Therapeutic Massage. 3rd edn. St Louis, MI: Mosby Elsevier; 2009.
10. Tortora G, Grabowski S. Principles of anatomy and physiology. Stafford, Qld: John Wiley; 2002.
11. Cleland J, Koppenhaver S. Netter's orthopaedic clinical examination: an evidence-based approach. 2nd edn. Philadelphia: Saunders; 2011.
12. New Zealand Guidelines Group. New Zealand Acute Low Back Pain Guide. Online. Available: www.nzgg.org.nz/guidelines/0072/acc1038_col.pdf; 2004.
13. Chaitow L. Muscle energy techniques. 2nd edn. Edinburgh: Churchill Livingstone; 2001.
14. Reese N, Bandy W. Joint range of motion and muscle length testing. Philadelphia: W.B. Saunders; 2002.
15. Kendall McCreary E, Provance P, McIntyre Rodgers M, et al. Muscles, testing and function, with posture and pain. 5th edn. Philadelphia PA: Lippincott Williams and Wilkins; 2005.
16. Hislop H, Montgomery J. Daniels and Worthingham's muscle testing: Techniques of manual examination. 8th edn. Oxford: Saunders Elsevier; 2007.
17. Brukner P, Khan K. Clinical Sports Medicine. 3rd edn. North Ryde, NSW: McGraw-Hill; 2010.
18. Pokorny D, Jahoda D, Veigl D, et al. Topographical variations of the relationship of the sciatic nerve and the piriformis muscle and its relevance to palsy after total hip arthroplasty. Surg Radiol Anat 2006;28(1): 88–91.
19. Simons D, Travell J, Simons L. Myofascial pain and dysfunction: the trigger point manual. Vol 1: upper half of body. 2nd edn. Philadelphia: Williams and Wilkins; 1999.
20. Knutson G, Owens E. Erector spinae and quadratus lumborum muscle endurance tests and supine leg-length alignment asymmetry: an observational study. J Manipulative Physiol Ther 2005;28(8): 575–81.
21. Vizniak N. Physical assessment. Burnaby, BC: Professional Health Systems; 2008.
22. Gibbons S, editor. The anatomy of the deep sacral part of the gluteus maximus and the psoas muscle: a clinical perspective. The 5th Interdisciplinary World Congress on Low Back Pain; 7–11 November 2004; Melbourne.
23. Fritz S, Chaitow L, Hymel GM. Clinical massage in the healthcare setting. St Louis, MI: Mosby Elsevier; 2008.
24. McCarthy J, Betz R. The relationship between tight hamstrings and lumbar hypolordosis in children with cerebral palsy. Spine 2000;25(2):211–13.
25. Ernst E. Evidence-based massage therapy: a contradiction in terms? In: Rich GJ, editor. Massage therapy the evidence for practice. Edinburgh: Mosby; 2002, pp. 11–25.
26. Ernst E. Massage therapy: Is its evidence-base getting stronger? Complement Health Pract Rev 2007;12(3):179–83.
27. Carnes M, Vizniak N. Quick reference evidence-based conditions manual. 3rd edn. Burnaby, BC: Professional Health Systems; 2009.
28. Yochum T, Rowe L. Essentials of skeletal radiology. 3rd edn. Baltimore: Lippincott Williams and Wilkins; 2005.
29. Swagerty D, Hellinger D. Radiographic assessment of osteoarthritis. Am Fam Physician 2001;64(2): 279–87.
30. Towheed TE, Maxwell L, Anastassiades TP, et al. Glucosamine therapy for treating osteoarthritis. Cochrane Database Syst Rev [serial on the Internet]. 2005;(2):CD0029.
31. Liebenson C. McKenzie self-treatments for sciatica. Journal of bodywork and movement therapies. 2005;9:40–2.

The thoracic region

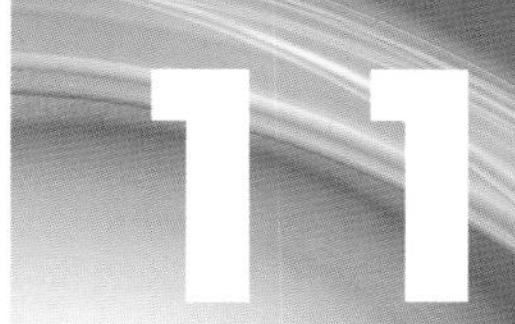

The content of this chapter relates to the following Units of Competency:

HLTREM503C Plan remedial massage treatment strategy
HLTREM504C Apply remedial massage assessment framework
HLTREM502C Provide remedial massage treatment
HLTREM510B Provide specialised remedial massage treatment

Health Training Package HLT07

Learning Outcomes

- Assess clients with conditions of the thoracic region for remedial massage, including identification of red and yellow flags.
- Assess clients for signs and symptoms associated with common conditions of the thoracic spine; treat and/or manage these conditions with appropriate remedial massage therapy.
- Develop treatment plans for clients with conditions of the thoracic region, taking into account assessment findings, duration and severity of the condition, likely tissue types, clinical guidelines, the best available evidence and client preferences.
- Develop short- and long-term treatment plans to address presenting symptoms, underlying conditions and predisposing factors, and to progressively increase the self-help component of therapy.
- Adapt remedial massage therapy to suit individual client needs based on duration and severity of injury, the client's age and gender, the presence of underlying conditions and co-morbidities, and other considerations for special population groups.

INTRODUCTION

Conditions of the thoracic spine are a less common presenting condition in remedial massage clinics than conditions of the lumbar or cervical spine. They are characterised by hypomobility and consequently play an important role in other conditions including those of the shoulder, neck and chest. For example, clients with neck pain of more than 30 days' duration have been observed to have a high probability of rapid improvement if treated with thoracic manipulation.[1] It is reasonable to expect that remedial massage techniques that improve the mobility of the thoracic spine will also be beneficial particularly in the treatment of chronic neck and shoulder pain.

FUNCTIONAL ANATOMY REVIEW

There are 12 vertebrae in the thoracic spine with 12 pairs of ribs extending laterally from the vertebral column. Thoracic intervertebral discs are typically thin. The facet joints are small and flat and lie in the coronal plane allowing only slight movement at each segment. The rib cage and sternum provide added stability for the thoracic spine during movement. During load-bearing tasks, increased thoracic pressure from contractions of the diaphragm and deep abdominal and intercostal muscles adds further stability.

TYPICAL VERTEBRAE – T2–T8

The body of a typical thoracic vertebra is bean-shaped. Each rib head attaches to two contiguous vertebral bodies and the intervertebral fibrocartilage between them. The tubercles of the ribs attach to the transverse processes of the lower vertebrae. The spinous processes are long, slender and pointed and project inferiorly so that their tips are located at the level of the intervertebral discs below (see Figure 11.1 on p 174).

SPECIAL FEATURES OF T1 AND T9–12

T1 resembles cervical vertebrae with its horizontal and prominent spinous process. T9 may have no demi-facets; T10 usually has an entire articular facet on either side, partly on the pedicles. The shape and size of the vertebral bodies of T11 and T12 are more like lumbar vertebrae. Their rib facets are large and lie mainly on the pedicles.

Thoracic spine mobility is significantly limited by the rib cage. Movements in one plane are invariably accompanied by one or more coupled movements because of the structural and anatomical features of the thoracic spine. In particular, rotation of the thoracic vertebrae is associated with ipsilateral lateral flexion; movement of the thorax into right rotation is accompanied by posterior rotation of the ipsilateral ribs. Right lateral flexion is accompanied by anterior rotation of the ipsilateral ribs.[2]

There are three layers of muscles in the thoracic region (see Figure 11.2 on p 175). The superficial layer consists of middle and lower trapezius, rhomboids and latissimus dorsi muscles. The strap-like *erector spinae* form the middle layer of muscles. Muscles of the deep layer connect vertebra to vertebra and rib to rib. Major muscles of the mid and upper back are described in Table 11.1.

ASSESSMENT

The aims of remedial massage assessment of the thoracic region are:

- determining the suitability of clients for massage (red flags)
- determining duration (acute or subacute) and severity of injury, and types of tissues involved
- determining if symptoms fit patterns of common conditions.

Assessment procedures for remedial massage clients are discussed in detail in Chapter 2.

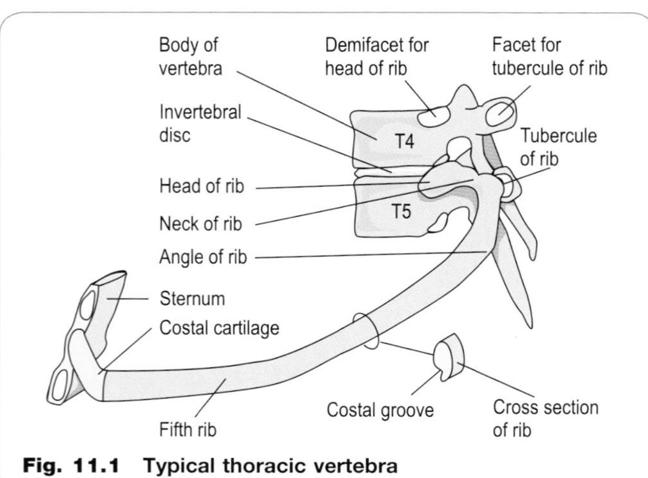

Fig. 11.1 Typical thoracic vertebra

Assessment of the thoracic region

1. Case history
2. Outcome measures
3. Postural analysis
4. Gait analysis
5. Functional tests
   Active range of motion tests
   flexion, extension, lateral flexion, rotation
   Passive range of motion tests
   flexion, extension, lateral flexion, rotation
   Resisted range of motion tests
   flexion, extension, lateral flexion, rotation
   Specific muscle tests including
   Erector spinae
   Latissimus dorsi
   Rhomboids
   Middle and lower trapezius
   Serratus anterior
   Special tests including
   Adam's test
   Deep breathing
   Elevated arm stress test (Roo's test)
   Springing
6. Palpation

Table 11.1 Muscles of the mid and upper back

Muscle	Origin	Insertion	Action
Erector spinae			As a group, extend the vertebral column
Iliocostalis thoracics	Angles of ribs 7–12	Angles of ribs 1–6, transverse process of C7	
Longissimus thoracic	Transverse and accessory processes of L1–5, anterior layer of thoracolumbar fascia	Transverse processes of T1–12, and lower nine or 10 ribs	
Spinalis thoracics	Spinous processes of L1–2, T11–T12	Spinous processes of T1–4/8	
Latissimus dorsi	An aponeurosis from T6–T12, all lumbar vertebrae and the posterior half of the iliac crest	Floor of biceps groove of humerus	Internally rotates, adducts and extends the humerus
Rhomboid major	T2–T5	Medial border of scapula between spine and inferior angle	Adducts and elevates the scapula
Rhomboid minor	C7 and T1	Medial border at spine of scapula	
Middle trapezius	Spinous processes of T1–T5	Acromion and spine of scapula	Adducts the scapula
Lower trapezius	Spinous processes of T6–T12	Spine of scapula	Rotates the scapula (along with upper fibres)
Serratus anterior	Outer ribs 1–8 or 9	Anterior surface of medial border of scapula	Abducts the scapula

(Note: Upper trapezius and levator scapulae are discussed in Chapter 12; intercostal muscles are discussed in Chapter 14.)

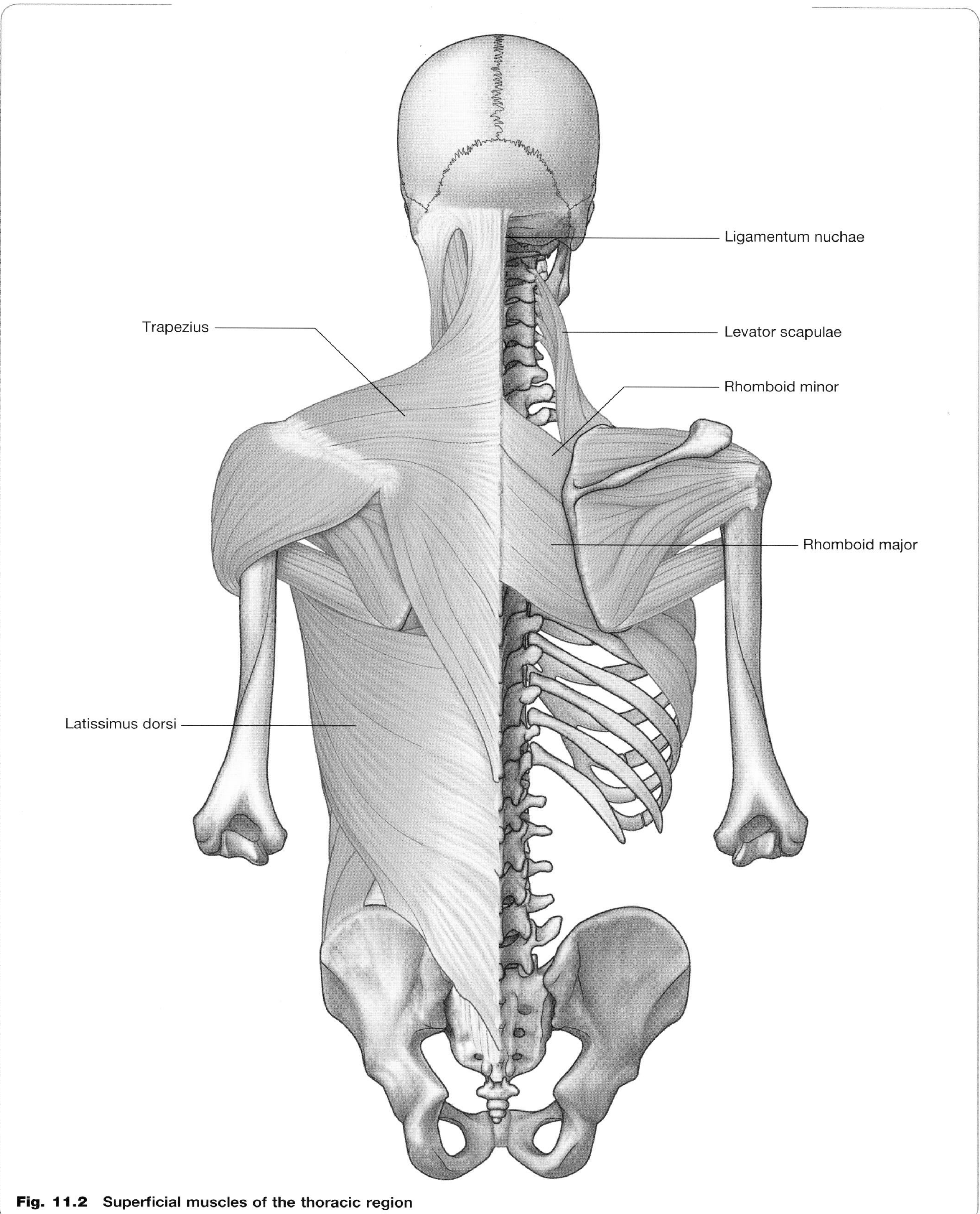

Fig. 11.2 Superficial muscles of the thoracic region

Table 11.2 Red flags for serious conditions associated with acute thoracic spine

Red flags for acute thoracic pain	Possible condition
Minor trauma (if >50 years, history of osteoporosis and taking corticosteroids) Major trauma	Fracture
Fever Night sweats Risk factors for infection (e.g. underlying disease process, immunosuppression, penetrating wound)	Infection
Past history of malignancy Age >50 years Failure to improve with treatment Unexplained weight loss Pain at multiple sites Pain at rest Night pain	Tumour
Chest pain or heaviness Movement, change in posture have no effect on pain Abdominal pain Shortness of breath, cough	Other serious condition

Adapted from the Acute Musculoskeletal Pain Guidelines Group[3] and the New Zealand Guidelines Group[4]
Note that acute pain in this context refers to pain of less than three months' duration.

CASE HISTORY

- Identify any red flags that require referral for further investigation (see Table 11.2).
- Ask clients to point to the site of pain as they may have different understandings of anatomical terms. For example *shoulder pain* could mean pain in the rhomboid region, scapula, upper trapezius, deltoid (anterior, middle or posterior) or shoulder joint pain.
- Determine if the pain is likely to have a mechanical cause. (Is the pain associated with rest or activity, certain postures or time of day?) Ask clients to demonstrate movements and positions that aggravate or relieve pain and to be specific with descriptions of aggravating or relieving activities.
- Mechanical pain is usually highly reactive to changes in posture, positions or activity.
- Morning pain relieved with daily activity is often associated with arthritis.
- Determine if the pain is likely to be associated with visceral, neurogenic, vascular or psychosocial functions (yellow flags).
- Pain from the gallbladder, liver or stomach is not usually aggravated by activity or relieved by rest, whereas mechanical back pain may be relieved by lying down.
- Neurogenic back pain from a spinal cord tumour or from a primary or secondary vertebral bone tumour is generally constant and remains unchanged by postural position.

OUTCOME MEASURES

Outcome measures are specifically designed questionnaires that are used to assess clients' levels of impairment and to define benefits of treatment. The benefit is assessed in terms of client-perceived changes to health status. The Patient Specific Scale is an example of outcome measures that could be used to assess conditions affecting the thoracic region.

POSTURAL ANALYSIS

Common conditions of the thoracic spine include:

- scoliosis
- hyperkyphosis: look for postural hyperkyphosis (e.g. upper crossed syndrome), lower cervical/upper thoracic region (dowager's hump) and Scheuermann's disease
- flattened thoracic curvature (*dishing*) usually between the scapulae (T2 to T7). (This appears to be an increasingly observed postural distortion, perhaps due to prolonged sitting or work stations with poor ergonomic design.)

GAIT ANALYSIS

Conditions of the thoracic region are less likely to affect the symmetry and rhythm of normal gait than those affecting the lumbar and pelvic regions or the weight-bearing lower limbs. However, changes in the centre of gravity and other adaptations to unlevel shoulders and forward or tilted head position will be evident.

FUNCTIONAL TESTS

Thoracic range of motion is tested with the client seated on the massage table, arms crossed in front of the body. This stabilises the pelvis, enabling thoracic movement to be more accurately assessed. Active, passive and resisted range of motion are often tested in one plane before moving to the next; however they are dealt with discretely here for illustrative purposes. For example active, passive and resisted thoracic flexion can be tested first, followed by active, passive and resisted thoracic extension tests.

Active range of motion (AROM)

FLEXION

- Stand behind the client.
- Instruct the client to bend forward slowly as far as they can without pain.

EXTENSION

- Stand at the side of the client and place a hand on the spine at T12 level. Ask the client to bend backwards from the contact point as far as they comfortably can.

LATERAL FLEXION (SIDEBEND)

- Ask the client to take their shoulder towards the hip on the same side. Stabilise the iliac crest with one hand and gently guide the client with the other hand on their shoulder as they laterally flex the trunk.
- Compare both sides and observe the coupling of the thoracic spine facet joints and posterior ribs.

ROTATION

Ask the client to turn their shoulders to the left and then the right as far as they are comfortably able.

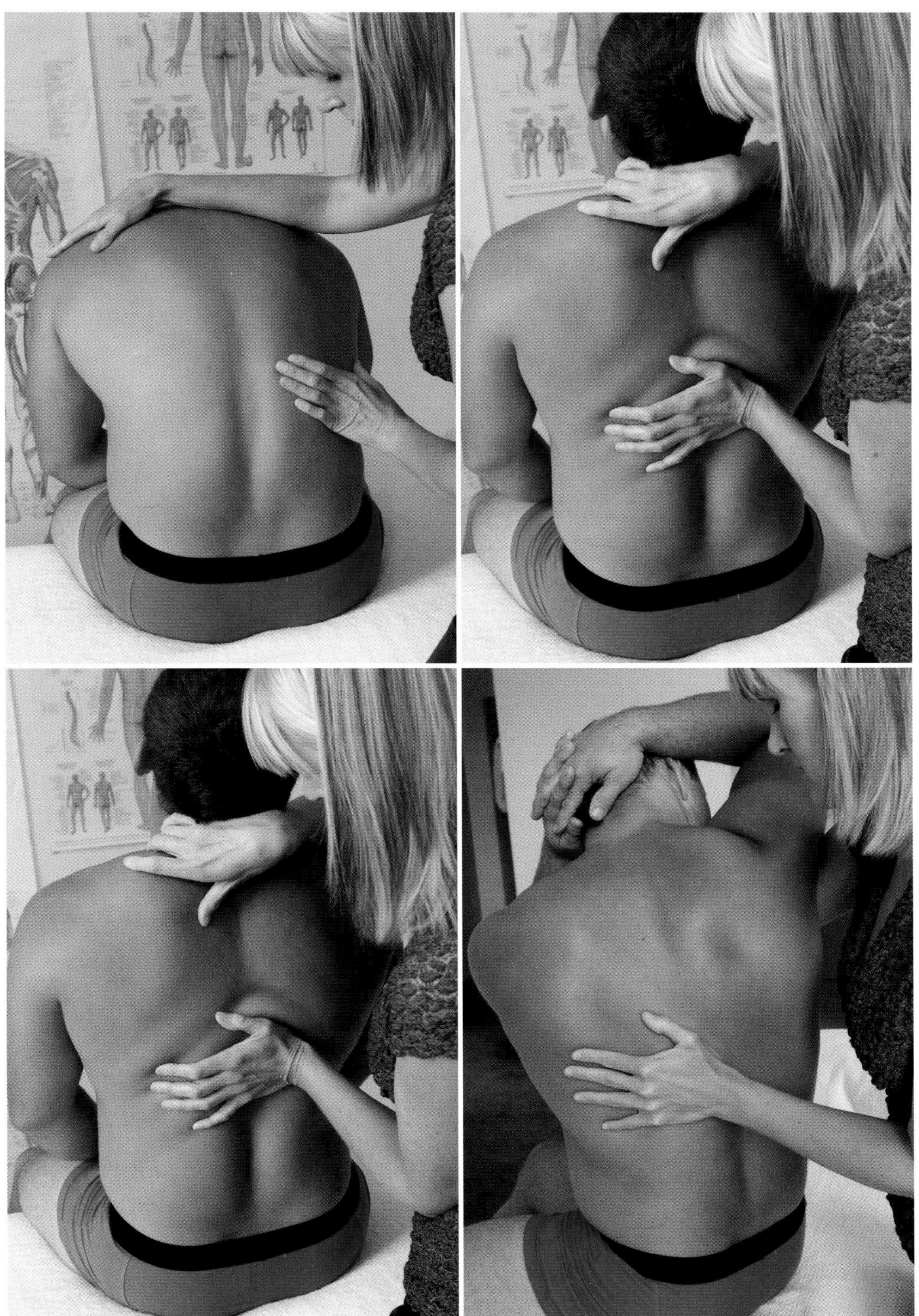

Fig. 11.3 PROM tests of the thoracic spine

Passive range of motion (PROM)

Passive range of motion of the thoracic spine can be performed with the client seated. Place your forearm across the top of the client's shoulders to guide the movements. Your other hand rests on the middle thoracic spine as the client's trunk is flexed, extended, laterally flexed and rotated. Next your spinal contact is moved to the upper thoracic spine and the movements are repeated (see Figure 11.3).

Resisted range of motion (RROM)

The six ranges of motion of the thoracic spine tested in AROM are also tested against resistance. Resisted range of motion tests

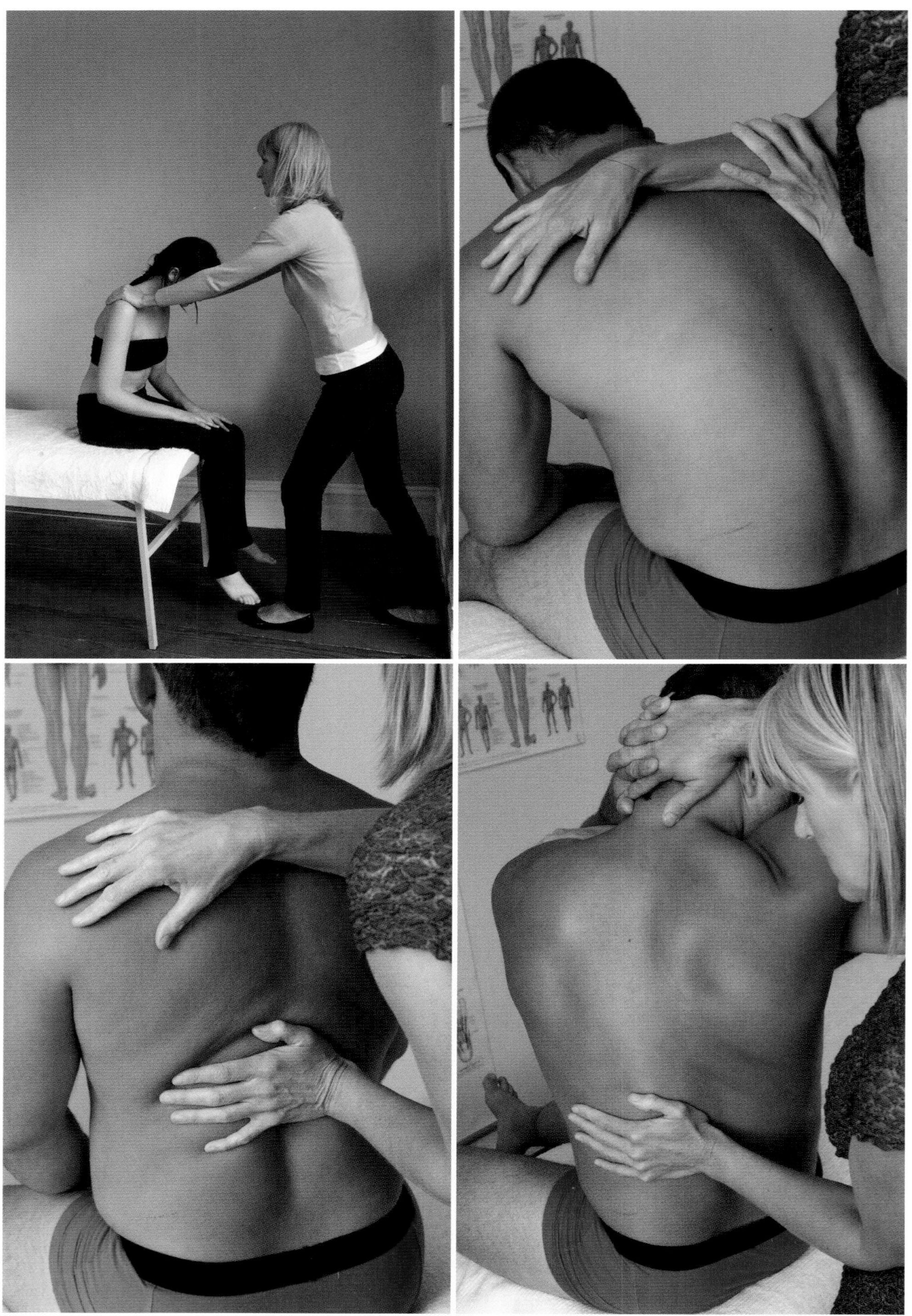

Fig. 11.4 RROM tests of the thoracic spine

are best performed with the client sitting on the treatment table to minimise extraneous muscle recruitment (see Figure 11.4).

Resisted and length tests for specific muscles

Tests for specific muscles usually follow positive resisted range of motion tests or indications from other assessments including postural analysis where muscle imbalances may be identified. Muscle imbalances arise from muscle contractures and weaknesses. Mobilisers (e.g. upper trapezius) tend to tighten and shorten; stabilisers (e.g. lower trapezius, serratus anterior) tend to weaken and lengthen.[5]

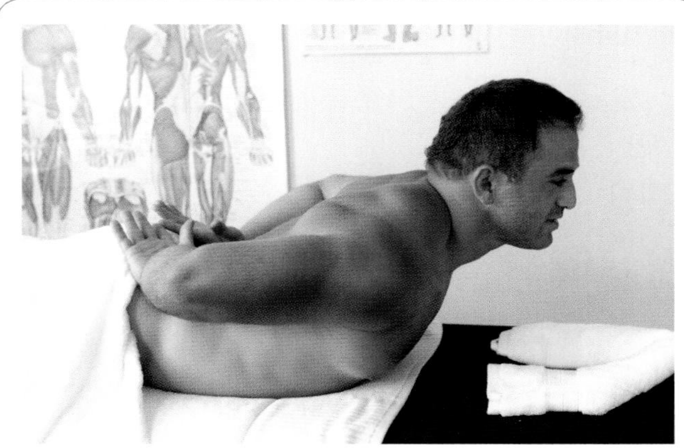

Fig. 11.5 Erector spinae strength test

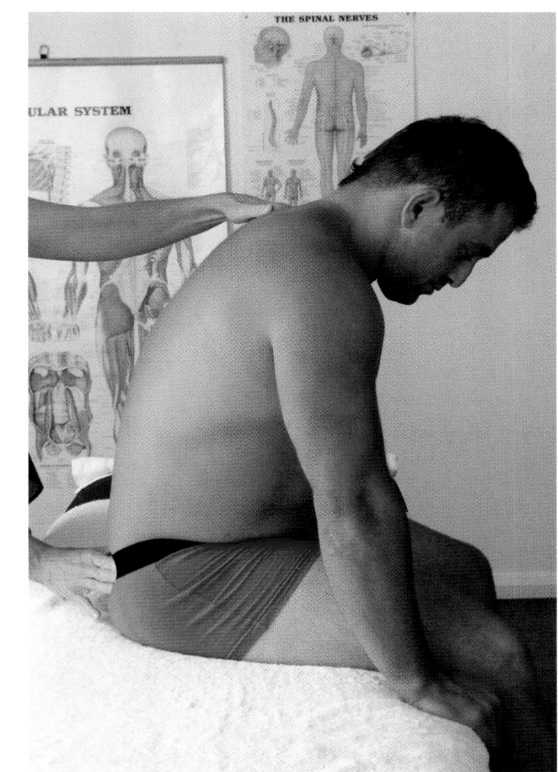

Fig. 11.6 Erector spinae length test

ERECTOR SPINAE

Strength test

Resisted trunk extension. The client lies prone and is instructed to raise their chest off the table without using their arms (see Figure 11.5).

Length test

Lumbar and thoracic erector spinae can be tested by having the client sit on the end of the table, feet flat on the floor, and bend their trunk forward towards the floor. Normally there should be 10 cm or less between the client's head and their knees[6] (see Figure 11.6 on p 179). (Note: posterior tilting of the pelvis during trunk flexion suggests short hamstrings.)

Clinical significance

Ererctor spinae may be relatively weak in the thoracic spine in hyperkyphotic postures. Unilateral contractures are common in scoliosis.

LATISSIMUS DORSI

Resisted test

Stand behind the client whose extended arm is adducted and internally rotated. Instruct the client to hold this position as you try to move the arm diagonally forward (into flexion and abduction).

Alternatively, clients reproduce the action of performing a 'lat pull-down' at the gym. The elbow is flexed and the upper arm raised up to 90° and abducted to 45°. Resist as the client tries to bring their elbow downwards and backwards (see Figure 11.7).

Length test

The client lies supine and brings their arms into full flexion. Clients with shortened latissimus dorsi will not be able to rest their arms on the table above their heads. The length of latissimus dorsi can also be tested in the same position by observing the client's low back when their arm is raised overhead. An increased arch in the low back suggests latissimus dorsi shortening (see Figure 11.8 on p 180).

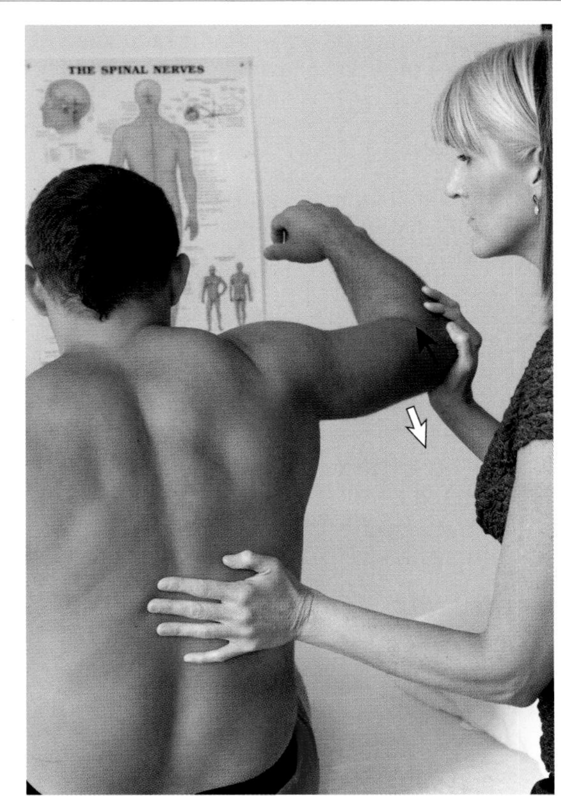

Fig. 11.7 Resisted tests for latissimus dorsi

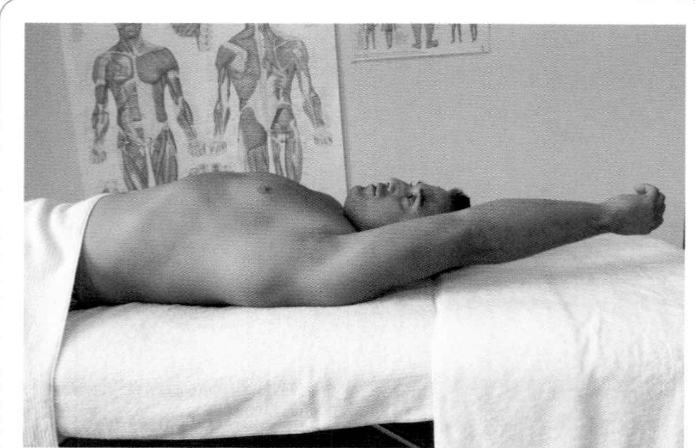

Fig. 11.8 Length test for latissimus dorsi

Clinical significance

Bilateral shortening brings the shoulders forward and increases thoracic kyphosis.

RHOMBOID MAJOR AND MINOR

Resisted test

Stand behind the client. The client takes their flexed elbow behind their back and adducts it as far as possible. Instruct the client to hold this position. Apply downward pressure with one hand on the client's shoulder. At the same time, with the other hand, try to push the elbow into flexion and abduction (see Figure 11.9).

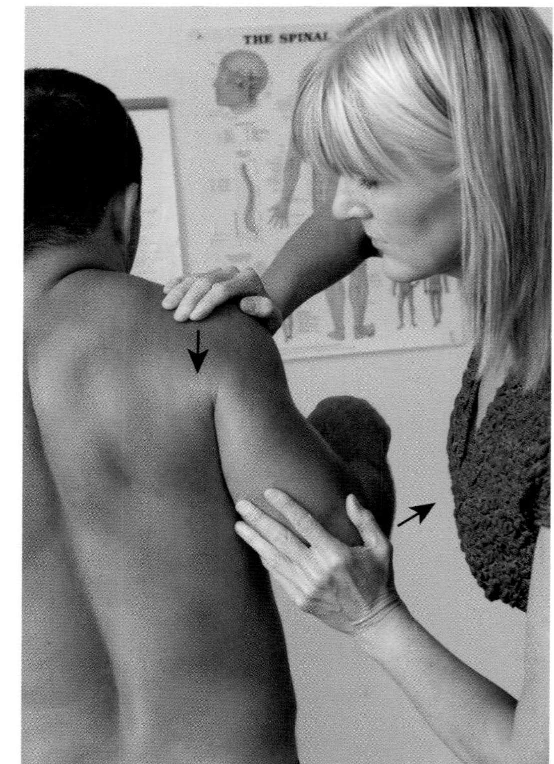

Fig. 11.9 Resisted test for rhomboid muscles

Length test

Shortened rhomboid muscles will adduct and elevate the scapula. This presentation is rarely observed in clinical practice.

Clinical significance

Lengthened and weakened rhomboids are commonly observed in upper crossed syndrome and in clients who spend frequent hours working at a desk, particularly sitting at a computer. There may be little reason in clinical practice to stretch the rhomboids. A more common need is to strengthen the rhomboids, lower trapezius and serratus anterior muscles in order to depress and adduct the scapula thereby improving clients' postures.

MIDDLE AND LOWER TRAPEZIUS

Resisted test

To test the middle fibres the client is prone and instructed to abduct their straight arm to 90°, thumbs pointed up to the ceiling. Place one hand on the client's forearm and the other on the client's back over the trapezius muscle. Instruct the client to hold this position as you apply pressure towards the floor. Repeat this procedure with the client's arm abducted to 135° to test the lower fibres (see Figure 11.10 on p 181).

Length test

Middle and lower trapezius contracture is rarely observed in clinical practice. Shortened middle trapezius muscles adduct and depress the scapula.

Clinical significance

Lengthened and weakened middle and lower trapezius are commonly observed in upper crossed syndrome.

SERRATUS ANTERIOR

Resisted test

With the client lying supine, direct them to raise their straight arm vertically in front of them (so that the shoulder is flexed to 90°) and to thrust their arm upward to lift their scapula off the table. The client resists as you apply downward pressure to the client's fist (see Figure 11.11 on p 181).

Note that the appearance of winging of the scapula in postural observation or when the client attempts a wall push-up also indicates serratus anterior weakness.

Length test

Serratus anterior contracture is rarely observed in clinical practice.

Clinical significance

Serratus anterior weakness is commonly observed in upper crossed syndrome.

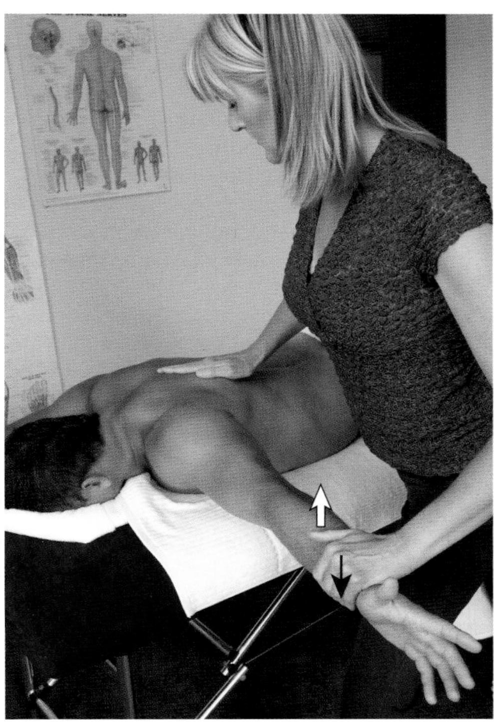

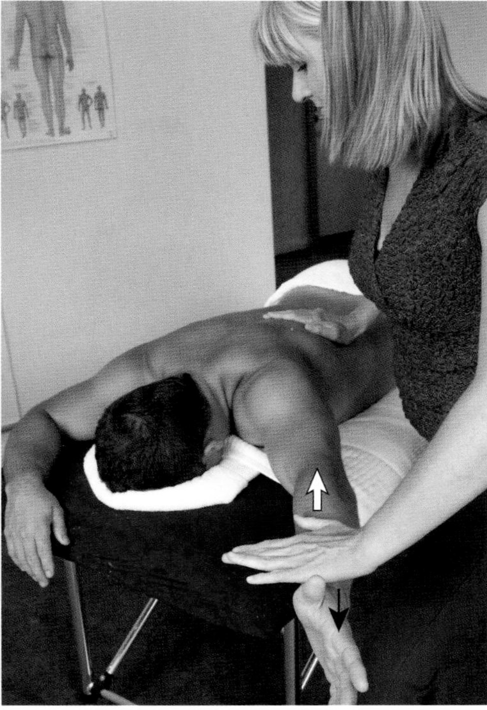

Fig. 11.10 Resisted tests for middle and lower trapezius

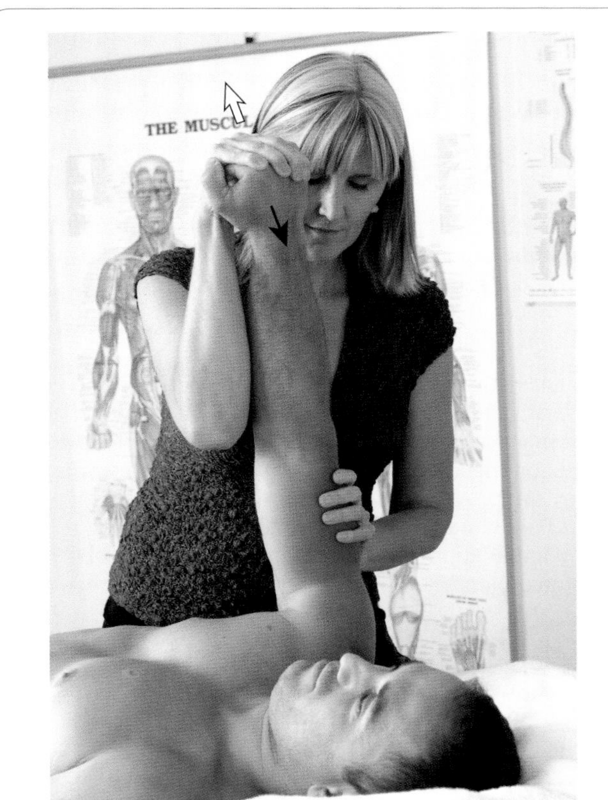

Fig. 11.11 Resisted test for serratus anterior

Special tests

Instruct clients to perform tests within their own pain tolerance. If clients experience pain while performing a special test, ask them for the exact location of the pain and confirm that it is the same pain as the one described in the case history.

Adam's test

The client stands and slowly bends forward to touch their toes. Stand behind and observe the symmetry of the ribs during trunk flexion. An abnormal rib hump on one side observed during trunk flexion indicates structural scoliosis (see Figure 11.12 on p 182).

Deep breathing

Instruct the client to remain still while taking a few deep breaths. Pain on deep breathing suggests a rib subluxation or fracture, intercostal or other respiratory muscle strain or a respiratory condition.

Elevated arm stress test (Roo's test)

The patient is seated with their arms abducted to 90° and their elbow flexed to 90° (the stop sign position). Ask the client to open and close their fists for 3 minutes at a rate of twice a second. Resulting numbness, tingling or weakness may indicate thoracic outlet syndrome. (Note: these effects may occur in less than 3 minutes.)

Springing

Springing over different regions of the thoracic spine indicates tender or painful areas. It may be useful in identifying regions

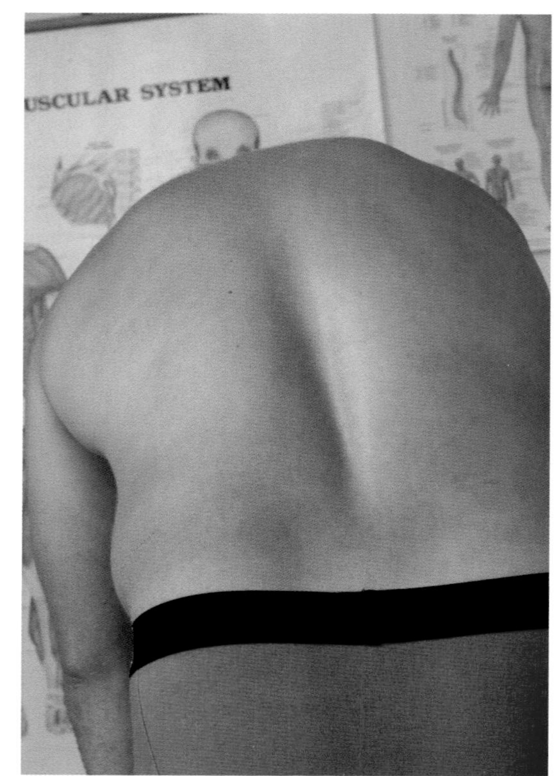

Fig. 11.12 Adam's test

of hypomobility, for example in Scheuermann's disease. Springing in the thoracic region involves applying gentle pressure to the spinous processes, facet joints and rib heads. Begin with springing over the spinous processes of the thoracic spine, starting at T12 and moving up to T1. Next spring over the facet joints bilaterally. (Note that thoracic spinous processes project posteriorly and inferiorly so that the tip of each spinous process is level with the facet joints of the vertebra below. For example, the spinous process of T1 is level with the facet joints of T2. It is also important to remember that the most prominent vertebra below the neck is C7 not T1.) The head of each rib inserts anteriorly to the facet joints at that level. This means that the rib head of right rib 4 inserts anteriorly to the right facet joints of T4. This makes direct palpation of the rib heads impossible. Instead, spring the rib angles bilaterally. The rib angles are the most posterior section of each rib, or the highest part of the rib when the client is prone. Move laterally from the spinous processes to the highest part of the rib to spring each rib angle.

PALPATION

Pain produced on palpation helps determine the type of tissue involved in the lesion. Palpate the borders of the scapulae and compare the orientation of the scapulae bilaterally. Note any asymmetry in scapula winging, the levels of the inferior angle or the distances of the medial border from the spine.

To palpate rib alignment place four fingertips in four consecutive intercostal spaces and slide from the spine laterally as far as possible. Start at the floating ribs and work up the rib cage. If the space between two consecutive ribs narrows considerably the intercostal muscles at that location are typically contracted and the ribs are often misaligned.

To palpate erector spinae place eight consecutive fingertips lateral to the lower thoracic spine. Palpate each section of the erector spinae muscle by moving the fingertips laterally across the strap of muscle and then return to the medial edge of the muscle. Continue palpating sections of the erector spinae muscles from the lower to the upper thoracic spine. Repeat on the other side.

Palpate middle and lower trapezius muscles from the lower thoracic spinal insertion using the fingertip sectioned approach described above. Palpate the fibres laterally and superiorly from the lower thoracic spine to the spine of the scapulae. Deep to the trapezius muscle palpate the rhomboids moving from the spine to the medial border of the scapulae.

Palpate infraspinatus in the infraspinatus fossa moving from the medial border laterally. Palpate the supraspinatus belly in the supraspinatus fossa, moving from the medial border of the scapula above the spine of the scapula, across to the medial aspect of the acromium. The levator scapulae insertion is palpable at the medial border of the scapula above its spine. Compare both sides. Latissimus dorsi forms the posterior wall of the axilla where it is easily palpated.

REMEDIAL MASSAGE TREATMENT

Assessment of the thorax provides essential information for development and negotiation of treatment plans, including:

- client's suitability for remedial massage therapy
- duration of the condition (i.e. acute or chronic)
- severity of the condition (i.e. grade of injury: mild, moderate or severe pain)
- type(s) of tissues involved
- priorities for treatment if more than one injury or condition is present
- whether the signs and symptoms suggest a common condition of the thoracic region
- special considerations for individual clients (e.g. clients' preferences for treatment types and styles, special population considerations).

Treatment options must always be considered in the context of the best available evidence for treatment effectiveness and clinical practice guidelines where they exist. Little research is available on the effectiveness of physical interventions to the thoracic spine. According to the Australian Acute Musculoskeletal Pain Guidelines Group, one small study suggests that spinal manipulation is effective compared to placebo in thoracic spinal pain.[3]

MUSCLE STRAIN

Muscle strains usually result from trauma such as accidents, falls and sports injuries. They are not common in the thoracic region because the stability provided by the rib cage protects thoracic muscles from sudden and excessive overload. Strains can also occur as a result of overuse or unaccustomed activity, such as may occur when starting an upper body weights program.

Key assessment findings for muscle strain

- History of trauma or repetitive overuse
- Postural analysis
- Functional tests:
  - Active range of motion positive
  - Passive range of motion may be positive at end of range from passive muscle stretching
  - Resisted tests positive
  - Resisted and length tests positive for affected muscles
  - Special tests usually negative
- Palpation positive for pain and spasm/myofibril tears

Assessment

HISTORY

The client complains of pain occurring after a trauma (e.g. accident, fall or sports injury) or after a period of unaccustomed activity like pruning a hedge. Pain is related to activity and is relieved by rest.

POSTURAL ANALYSIS

Muscle spasm may be evident on postural observation.

FUNCTIONAL TESTS

AROM: limited and painful usually.
PROM: may be painful at end of range of motion due to passive muscle stretching.
RROM: positive.
Resisted tests and length tests are painful for affected muscle(s).
Special tests: usually negative.

PALPATION

Tenderness and/or pain may be elicited over the affected muscle. Spasm or myofibrial tear may be palpable.

Overview of treatment and management of muscle strain

A typical remedial massage treatment for mild or moderate thoracic muscle strain includes:

- Swedish massage to the back, neck, shoulders and chest.
- Remedial massage techniques for muscle strains including:
  - deep gliding frictions along the muscle fibres
  - cross-fibre frictions
  - soft tissue releasing techniques
  - deep transverse friction
  - trigger point therapy
  - thermotherapy (see Chapter 3).
  - myofascial release (see Chapter 8).

Remedial massage techniques for muscles of the thoracic spine are illustrated in Table 11.3.

Note: Muscles of the thoracic spine are often tight and lengthened (e.g. rhomboid muscles in clients who spend excessive hours working at a desk). For such muscles, avoid techniques that work along the line of the fibre, which could encourage further muscle lengthening. Cross-fibre techniques are recommended to reduce muscle tightness without lengthening the muscle.

CLIENT EDUCATION

Advise clients to avoid aggravating activities in the early phases of healing. Educate the client about likely causative and predisposing factors and ways to avoid recurrence, including maintaining a physical fitness program and developing appropriate levels of fitness before activities are commenced. Referral for osseous manipulation may be beneficial. Longer-term treatment should be designed to address any underlying conditions or predisposing factors to future back problems.

Home exercise program

As soon as the client can tolerate movement they should begin stretching the muscle and progressively introduce isometric strengthening exercises and a weights program. The aim is to achieve maximum strength and full length of the injured muscle and to restore muscle balance in the body.

THORACIC FACET SYNDROME

Thoracic facet syndrome refers to subluxation of the facet (zygapophyseal joint) and/or sprain of the surrounding ligaments or joint capsule. Clients are often young adults who develop acute pain in the region of the facet or rib attachment following unaccustomed exercise or trauma. In older clients there may be an underlying hypomobility of the thoracic spine.

Assessment

HISTORY

The client complains of pain originating from the facet (zygapophyseal joint) which may be experienced locally and in the region of the rib head attachments to the spine. If referral exists it is typically along the curve of the ribs inferiorly and laterally. Referred pain may also be experienced in the costochondral junctions. The pain may be sharp and aggravated by movement, coughing and deep breathing. There is often a history of a recent episode of thoracic twisting, such as may occur during a boxing session at the gym. Conditions characterised by hypomobility of the thoracic spine may increase

Key assessment findings for thoracic facet syndrome

- Client is usually a young adult; history of recent trauma or repetitive overuse; pain may be acute and refer along the ribs
- Functional tests:
  - AROM positive
  - PROM positive
  - RROM positive if associated muscle strain
  - Resisted tests and length tests positive for associated muscle strain
  - Special tests usually negative (± pain on deep breathing)
- Palpation positive for tenderness ± pain at site of strain, sprain or subluxation

Table 11.3 Remedial massage techniques for muscles of the thoracic region

Muscle	Soft tissue release	Trigger point	Stretch	Client education[7]	Home exercise
Erector spinae	Active release: with the client sitting on the table and their feet on the floor, place knuckles of both hands either side of the spine on the erector spinae at the thoracolumbar junction or above. The client slowly bends forward, holding the side of the table, as your knuckles glide deeply inferiorly along the erector spinae. (Do not use this technique on clients whose symptoms increase with lumbar flexion.)	A: Iliocostalis thoracis B: Iliocostalis thoracis C: Iliocostalis lumborum D: Longissimus thoracis	Trunk flexion stretches: i) Sitting and leaning forward until the stretch is felt ii) Kneeling on all fours and arching the thoracic spine (cat posture in yoga) (Note: thoracic erector spinae may be long and weak and require strengthening)	Posture correction (e.g. lumbar support when sitting), correct ergonomics at workstation	Stretching: same as in treatment stretches Strengthening: Instruct the client to lie prone with their head in neutral. Ask the client to bring their arms straight up above their head in the fully abducted position. Keeping elbows and knees straight, gently raise one leg and the opposite arm slightly off the ground to activate the erector spinae muscles. Hold for 3 seconds then lower. Raise the alternate arm and leg. Hold for 3 seconds and lower. Repeat up to 5 times.

Table 11.3 Remedial massage techniques for muscles of the thoracic region—cont'd

Muscle	Soft tissue release	Trigger point	Stretch	Client education[7]	Home exercise
Latissimus dorsi	**One option for an active release:** The client sits on the table, feet on the floor, and adducts one arm to 90° and flexes the elbow to 90° (stop sign position). Grasp the posterior border of the axilla as the client slowly extends and adducts their upper arm. 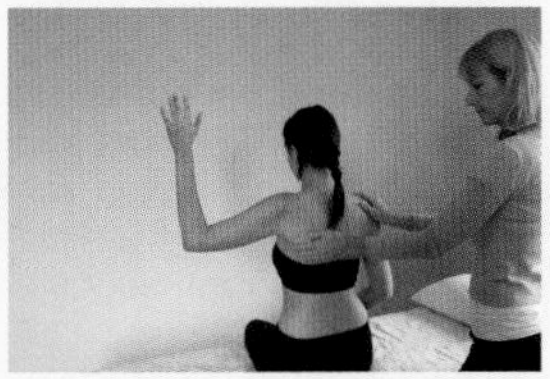	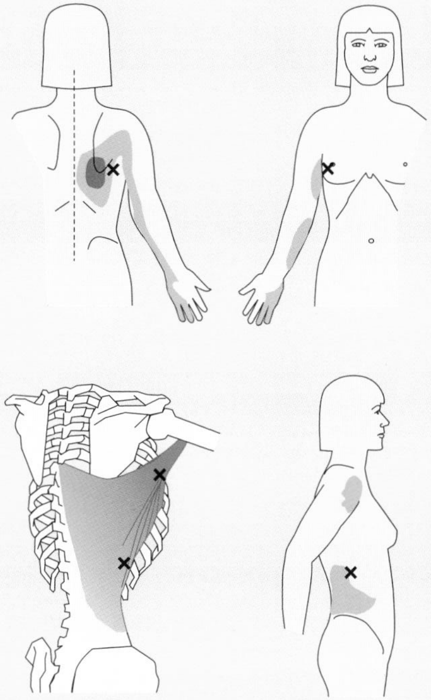	Kneeling and sitting on feet, lean forward towards the floor, stretching both arms overhead 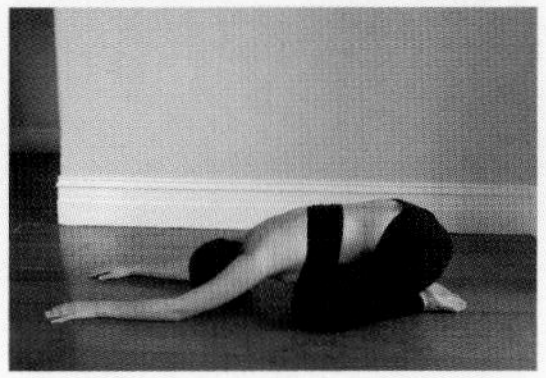	Use a footstool to avoid reaching high for heavy objects	The Mouth Wrap-around test. Turn head 45°. Reach around back of head to corner of mouth. 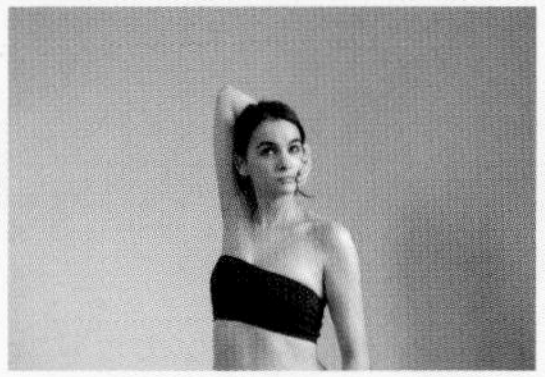 Arms overhead and sidebending the trunk stretches the latissimus dorsi muscle. 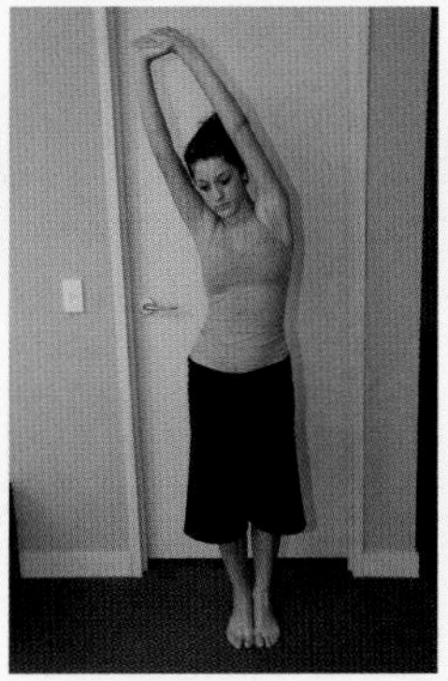

Continued

Table 11.3 Remedial massage techniques for muscles of the thoracic region—cont'd

Muscle	Soft tissue release	Trigger point	Stretch	Client education[7]	Home exercise
Rhomboids	Active release techniques should not be used to lengthen an already long muscle. Use cross-fibre and diagonal fibre techniques only. The client is seated, feet on the floor. The client slowly protracts and retracts the scapula as you apply cross-fibre or diagonal fibre strokes to the rhomboids.		Rhomboid muscles present more commonly as lengthened and weakened than overcontracted. Consequently there is little need to stretch the muscle. Should a stretch be required, protraction and depression of the scapula would be required. The 'cat posture' (i.e. kneeling on all fours and arching the back) stretches the rhomboids.	Correct rounded shoulder posture	Strengthen the rhomboids by pulling the scapulae together. This exercise is often combined with the doorway stretch for pectoralis major.

Table 11.3 Remedial massage techniques for muscles of the thoracic region—cont'd

Muscle	Soft tissue release	Trigger point	Stretch	Client education[7]	Home exercise
Middle and lower trapezius	Active release techniques should not be used to lengthen an already long muscle. Use cross-fibre and diagonal fibre techniques only.	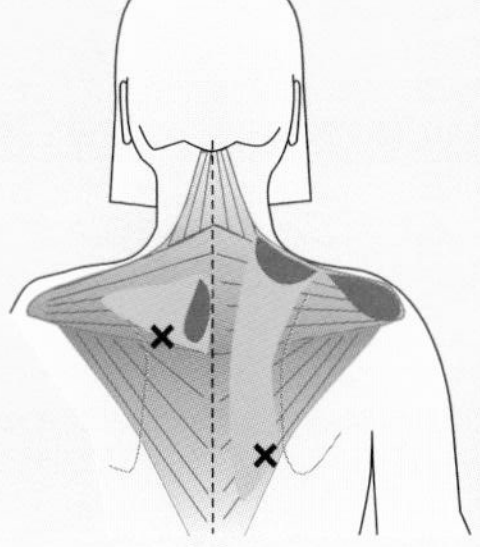	Middle and lower trapezius muscles present more commonly as lengthened and weakened than overcontracted. Consequently there is little need to stretch the muscle. The 'cat posture' stretches the middle and lower trapezius. 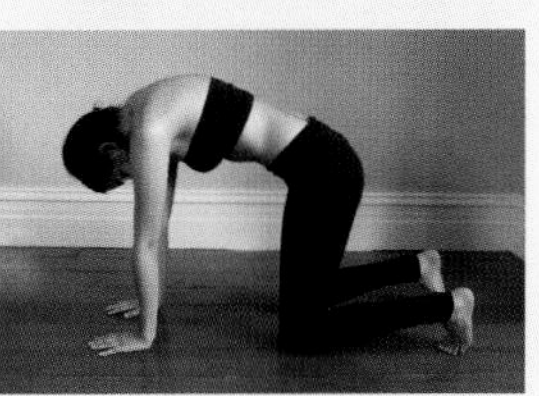 The lower trapezius is also stretched by kneeling and sitting on feet, lean forward towards the floor, stretching both arms overhead. 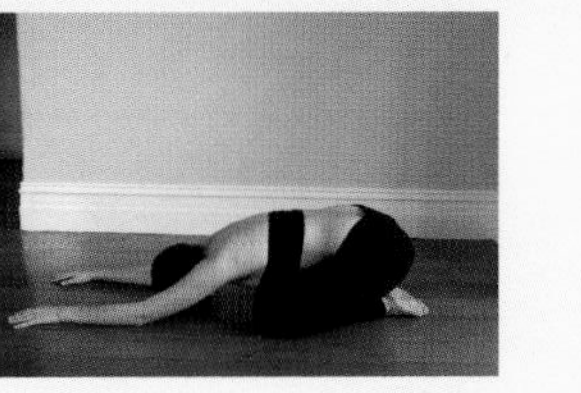	Using an elbow rest if arms need to be held out in front of the body for prolonged periods; adjust workstation so that the chair is pulled close to the table and the client can lean back on the chair.	The middle trapezius stretch stretches middle and lower fibres of trapezius. Strengthening exercises can be performed prone, with the arms horizontally for middle trapezius and overhead for lower trapezius, and then using the back muscles to elevate the arms, head and trunk. 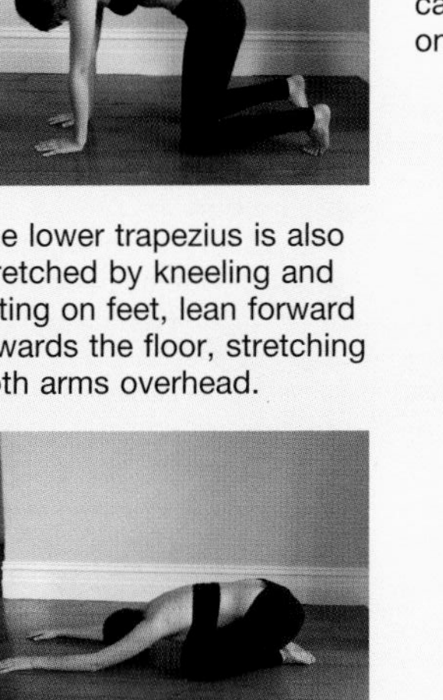

Continued

Table 11.3 Remedial massage techniques for muscles of the thoracic region—cont'd

Muscle	Soft tissue release	Trigger point	Stretch	Client education[7]	Home exercise
Serratus anterior	Active release techniques should not be used to lengthen an already long muscle. Use cross-fibre and diagonal fibre techniques only.	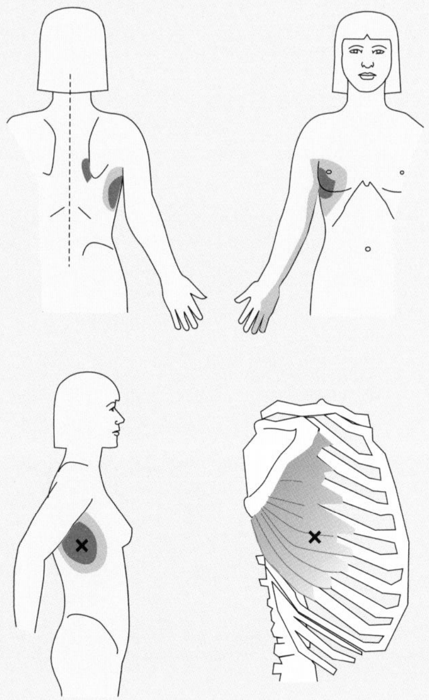	There is little need to stretch serratus anterior in clinical practice. To stretch serratus anterior (e.g. after ischaemic pressure to release a trigger point) the client lies on their side, rests their upper hand on their hip and lets their elbow drop behind their back. 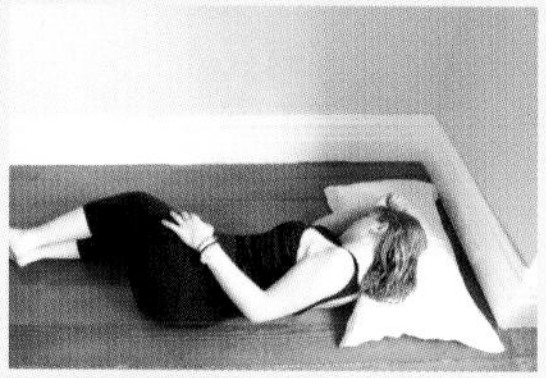	Avoid overuse (e.g. paradoxical breathing, push-ups, chin-ups)[6]	Wall push-ups with the scapula retracted strengthen serratus anterior. Also lying supine, arm raised to 90° flexion, holding weight, protract the scapula. 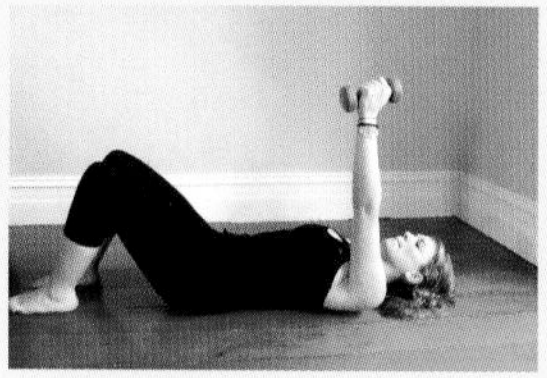

susceptibility to facet syndrome from trauma, repetitive overuse or unaccustomed or prolonged activity.

FUNCTIONAL TESTS

AROM: limited and painful, especially on extension. Pain in more than one direction suggests joint capsule injury.
PROM: limited and painful, especially on extension.
RROM may be painful if there is an associated muscle strain.
Resisted tests and length tests may be painful for local muscle strain.
Special tests are negative except that associated rib subluxation may cause pain on coughing and deep breathing.

PALPATION

Tenderness ± pain may be elicited over the affected facet joint or rib head. There is often a palpable intercostal contracture between adjacent ribs. This can occur posteriorly, laterally or anteriorly.

Differential diagnosis

The most important condition to rule out is rib fracture. A history of trauma and slow resolution of the symptoms suggests this diagnosis. X-rays are required to confirm the presence of a fracture. Lung pathology must also be ruled out. Any history of smoking, fever, weight loss or intractable pain that is not relieved by rest requires medical referral.

Overview of treatment and management

A typical remedial massage treatment for thoracic facet syndrome/rib subluxation includes:

- Swedish massage therapy to the back and chest.
- Remedial massage therapy. The remedial massage technique that is most appropriate at the primary ligamentous site is deep transverse friction applied to the rib head attachment or costochondral joint. Work within the client's pain tolerance, instructing the client to breathe deeply. Work intermittently and alternate with other techniques.
  - Associated intercostal contractures should be located and treated, usually with fingertip deep transverse friction between the approximated ribs. The goal is to release the contracture and to restore normal spacing between ribs. Other techniques for muscle contractures include deep gliding frictions along the muscle fibres, cross-fibre frictions, active and passive soft tissue releasing techniques, trigger point therapy and muscle stretches. Massage to the chest may be beneficial. Apply myofascial releasing techniques for myofascial restrictions. Thermotherapy may be beneficial.
- Thoracic mobilisation techniques are recommended for facet joint lesions (see Chapter 7):
  - thoracic longitudinal mobilisation
  - thoracic diagonal mobilisation
  - thoracic rocking
  - arm overhead rib mobilisation
  - rib rotation.

CLIENT EDUCATION

Advise clients to avoid such aggravating activities as extension or rotation, particularly in the early phases of healing. Referral for osseous manipulation may be beneficial. Longer-term treatment should be designed to address any underlying conditions or predisposing factors to future back problems.

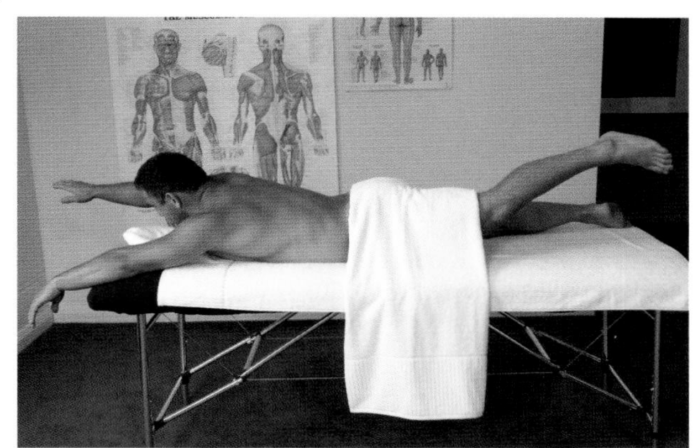

Fig. 11.13 Strengthening exercise for erector spinae

Home exercise program

As soon as the client can tolerate movement they should begin stretching exercises, including trunk lateral flexion away from the side of injury. Progressively introduce strengthening exercises including the erector spinae muscles (see Figure 11.13).

ERECTOR SPINAE STRENGTHENING EXERCISES

Instruct the client to lie prone with their head in neutral and bring their arms straight up above their head in the fully abducted position. Keeping their elbows and knees straight, the client gently raises one leg and the opposite arm slightly off the ground to activate the erector spinae muscles. This position is held for 3 seconds and then released. The client raises the other arm and leg and holds for 3 seconds before lowering to the ground. This sequence is repeated up to 5 times.

DEGENERATIVE JOINT DISEASE (OSTEOARTHRITIS/DEGENERATIVE ARTHRITIS)

Degenerative joint disease (DJD) represents a range of degenerative conditions characterised by progressive loss of articular cartilage and reactive changes in subchondral bone. By the time DJD is evident in the thoracic spine it is usually also present in the lower lumbar spine, lower cervical spine and weight-bearing joints. In younger clients DJD may develop after a previous significant trauma.

Assessment

HISTORY

The client is typically middle aged, elderly or has a history of a previous significant trauma. The condition is chronic with episodes of acute exacerbation. The pain may be worse on rising, during periods of inactivity or excessive activity due to the presence of low-grade inflammation. There is generalised reduction in thoracic range of motion with the client reporting stiffness and occasional sharp pain. Clients often report an increase in the severity of symptoms in cold weather.

Key assessment findings for thoracic DJD

- Client usually over 50 years old; history of dull, aching pain, morning stiffness, pain that worsens with activity and improves with rest
- Functional tests:
  - AROM positive
  - PROM positive
  - RROM usually negative
  - Special tests usually negative
- Palpation positive for tenderness ± pain

FUNCTIONAL TESTS

AROM: limited ± painful in some directions.
PROM: limited ± painful in some directions.
RROM: usually negative.
Resisted and length tests for specific muscles usually negative.
Special tests: usually negative (springing may reveal reduced mobilitiy and a hard end-feel).

PALPATION

The client may report tenderness and/or pain on palpation of the affected joints.

Differential diagnosis

Osteoporosis may occur independently although it is frequently concurrent with DJD. Further tests such as X-rays and bone density scans may be required.

Overview of treatment and management

DJD is a progressive degenerative condition. Acute exacerbations require anti-inflammatory measures such as cryotherapy, anti-inflammatory medications or gels. Treatment often includes gentle thoracic range of motion stretches, especially extension stretches, within the client's pain threshold. Thoracic extension exercises such as the doorway stretch (see Figure 11.14) can be recommended to arrest the progression of hyperflexion. (Note: Variations on the doorway stretch are also used to stretch pectoralis major and biceps brachii. It is recommended here primarily to extend the thoracic spine.)

Although degenerative joint disease mainly affects spinal cartilage, the surrounding ligaments and muscles often become contracted and hypertonic.

A typical remedial massage treatment for mild or moderate thoracic DJD includes:

- Swedish massage therapy to the back, neck, shoulders and chest.
- Remedial massage therapy. Apply friction techniques (transverse and longitudinal) to the ligamentous structures. Muscular hypertonicity can be reduced with a range of remedial massage techniques including (see Table 11.3):
  - deep gliding frictions along the muscle fibres
  - cross-fibre frictions
  - active and passive soft-tissue releasing techniques
  - trigger point therapy
  - muscle stretches.
- Thermotherapy may be beneficial in the absence of an acute episode.

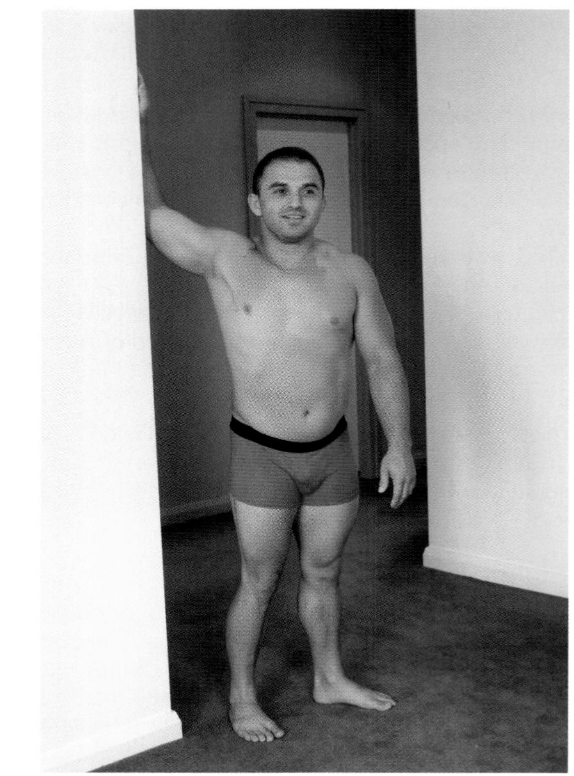

Fig. 11.14 Doorway stretch

- Gentle thoracic mobilising techniques are recommended (see Chapter 7). Be careful to not overwork the area with sustained or overly deep techniques to avoid inflaming the area:
  - compression
  - rhythmic compressions
  - thoracic rocking
  - thoracic longitudinal mobilisation
  - thoracic diagonal mobilisation.
- Myofascial release techniques are reportedly very successful for the thoracic region (see Chapter 8).

CLIENT EDUCATION

Clients should avoid any activity that has a high impact on the spine. For example, it is better to go for a brisk walk than for a run. Wearing shock-absorbing footwear is also advisable. Encourage clients to remain active within their pain threshold. Supplements such as glucosamine may benefit the spinal joints.[8] According to an Australian Institute of Health and Welfare report, osteoarthritis sufferers commonly take glucosamine, omega-3 fatty acid and calcium.[9]

Home exercise program

Generalised thoracic range of motion stretches with particular emphasis on thoracic extension should be performed within the client's pain-free range. Progressively introduce strengthening exercises for the erector spinae muscles (see Figure 11.13) and other thoracic muscles as indicated.

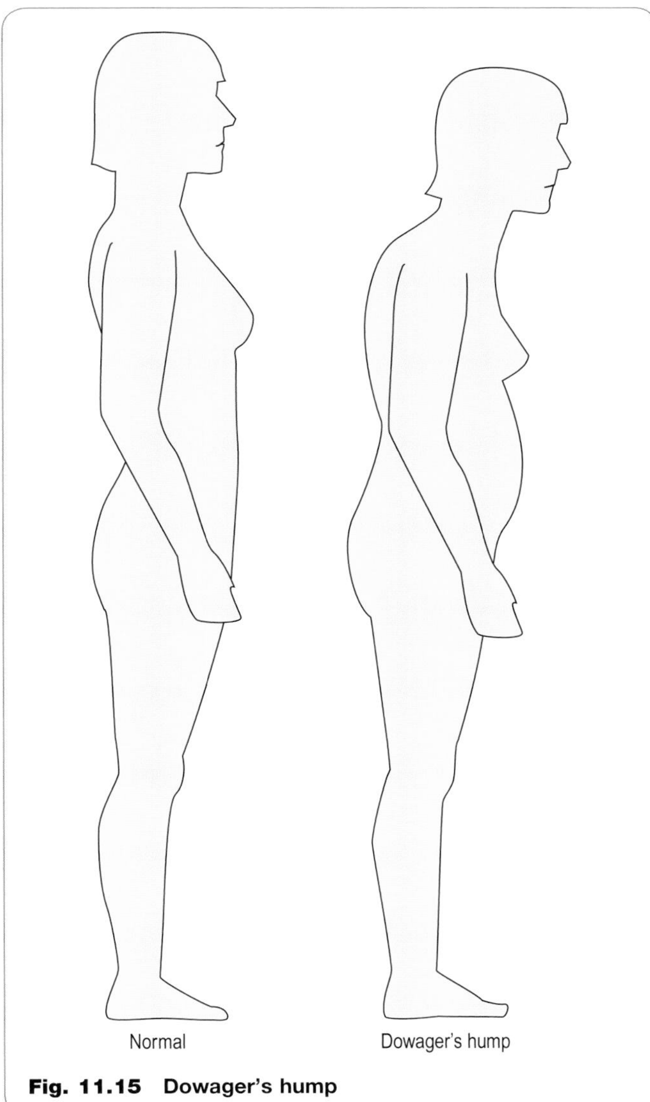

Fig. 11.15 Dowager's hump

HYPERKYPHOSIS OF THE UPPER THORACIC SPINE (DOWAGER'S HUMP)

Dowager's hump is a spinal deformity characterised by hyperkyphosis of the upper thoracic spine. It is most frequently observed in post-menopausal women (hence its name) and is associated with osteoporotic bone loss.

Assessment

HISTORY

There are usually no symptoms unless a fracture has occurred. Clients typically express concern at their increasing kyphosis. There is frequently a family history of osteoporosis or early menopause.

POSTURAL ANALYSIS

The most significant indicator is the presence of increased thoracic kyphosis from C7 to the upper thoracic spine.

> **Key assessment findings for upper thoracic hyperkyphosis**
>
> - Clients are usually post-menopausal women; usually no symptoms unless fracture occurs
> - Postural analysis: hyperkyphosis of the upper thoracic spine
> - Functional tests:
>   - AROM: limited especially in extension
>   - PROM: limited especially in extension
>   - RROM: usually negative
>   - Special tests: negative
> - Palpation: associated muscles fibrotic

FUNCTIONAL TESTS

AROM: limited, especially in extension.
PROM: limited, especially in extension.
RROM: may be positive for associated muscle strain.
Resisted tests and length tests may be positive for affected muscles.
Special tests: negative.

PALPATION

Palpation may reveal contractures of associated muscles, particularly the upper trapezius muscles.

Differential diagnosis

An osteoporotic compression fracture of the anterior body of a thoracic vertebra would be associated with significant pain. Scheuermann's disease, which is also characterised by hyperkyphosis, most commonly affects the lower thoracic spine.

Overview of treatment and management

A typical remedial massage treatment for hyperkyphosis of the upper thoracic spine includes:

- Swedish massage therapy to the back, neck, shoulders and chest.
- Remedial massage therapy. Techniques designed to reduce fibrotic muscles of the upper thoracic region (specifically upper trapezius muscles, erector spinae, levator scapulae, and supraspinatus muscles) and chest (pectoralis major and minor), form the basis of the remedial massage approach (see Table 11.4):
  - deep gliding frictions along the muscle fibres
  - cross-fibre frictions
  - active and passive soft tissue releasing techniques
  - deep transverse friction
  - trigger point therapy
  - muscle stretches.
- Apply myofascial releasing techniques for myofascial restrictions.
- Thermotherapy may be beneficial.

CLIENT EDUCATION

Advise clients to use heat packs nightly draped over the upper thoracic spine and upper trapezius muscle. Refer clients for osseous manipulation of the upper thoracic spine and for hormone assessment where appropriate.

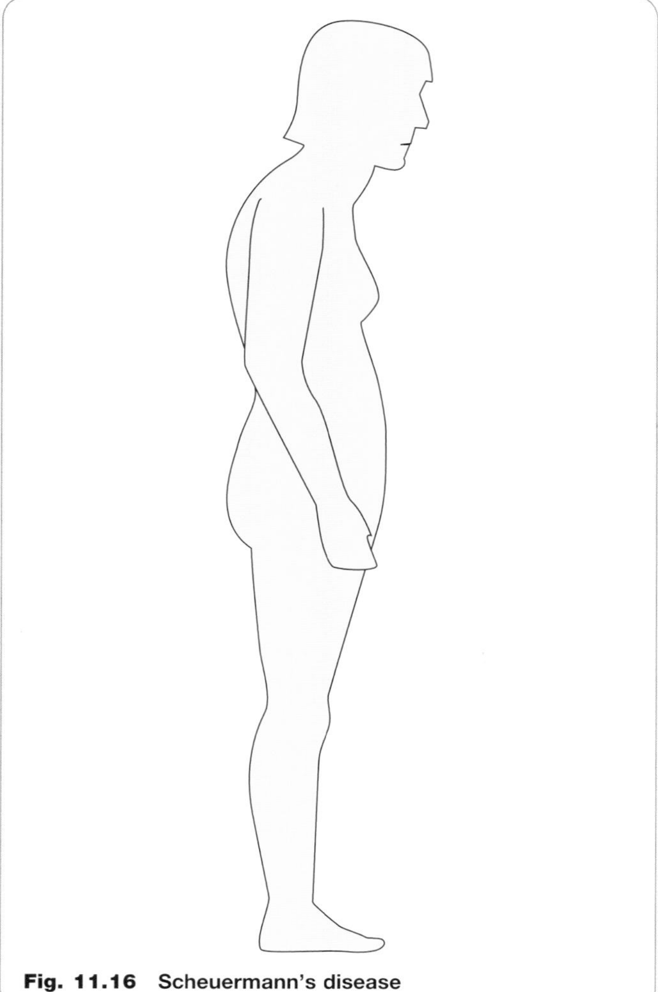

Fig. 11.16 Scheuermann's disease

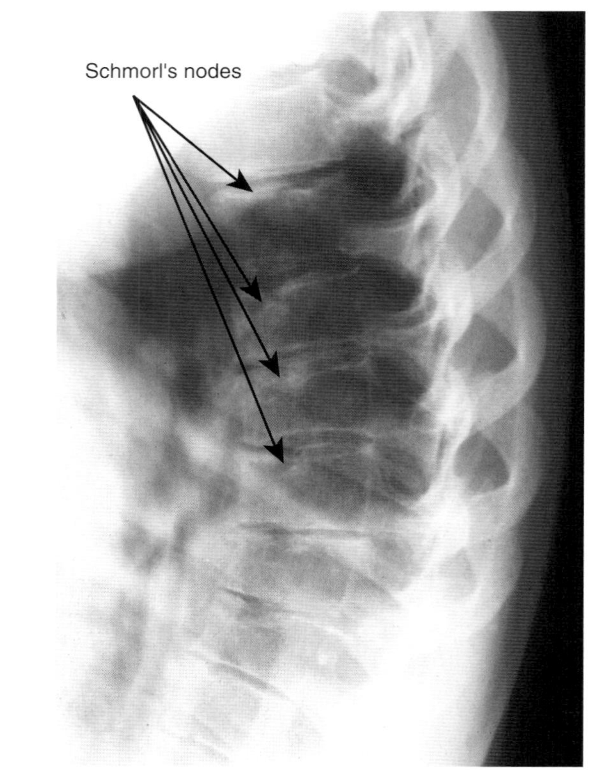

Fig. 11.17 Radiographs of Scheuermann's disease

Key assessment findings for Scheuermann's disease

- Clients may present at any age; disease is usually active between 13 and 17 years. Clients may experience dull aching pain ± tiredness in the mid back
- Postural analysis: hyperkyphosis usually in the mid or low thoracic spine
- Functional tests:
  - AROM: limited especially in extension
  - PROM: limited especially in extension
  - RROM usually negative unless associated muscle strain
  - Resisted tests and length tests may be positive for affected muscles
  - Special tests: springing over affected vertebrae reveals limited mobility
- Palpation: There may be tenderness above and below the hyperkyphotic area

Home exercise program

The doorway stretch (see Figure 11.14) is recommended to extend the upper thoracic spine and open the chest. Another useful stretch is to roll a towel and place it lengthways along the spine just below the hump. The client lies supine on the rolled towel for at least 10 minutes a day. Erector spinae strengthening exercises may also be useful (see Figure 11.13).

SCHEUERMANN'S DISEASE (VERTEBRAL EPIPHYSITIS)

Scheuermann's disease is a disorder of the vertebral epiphysis characterised by anterior vertebral wedging, irregular endplates and loss of vertebral disc height.[10] It is usually limited to several vertebrae, most often in the lower thoracic spine. It is a self-limiting condition with an active phase in the teenage years (13–17 years). Its ratio of males to females is 2 : 1. The cause of the condition is unclear although a hereditary component appears to be involved.

Assessment

HISTORY

Scheuermann's disease affects adolescents between 13 and 17 years of age although clients can present at any age. Clinical presentations vary. There may be no symptoms or the client may experience dull, aching pain and/or tiredness in the mid back, especially during the active phase. Pain is usually aggravated by activity and relieved by rest. X-rays are required to confirm the diagnosis of Scheuermann's disease. The vertebral bodies are wedge-shaped and endplates are sclerotic and irregular (Schmorl's nodes) (see Figure 11.16 on p 192). Clients with Scheuermann's disease have an increased incidence of DJD and spondylolisthesis in the lumbar spine.

POSTURAL ANALYSIS

Hyperkyphotic deformity of the thoracic spine, especially the lower thoracic spine, is evident. Scoliosis is present in 20–40% of clients.[11] Anterior head carriage is commonly observed.

FUNCTIONAL TESTS

AROM: limited ± pain, especially in extension.
PROM: limited ± pain, especially in extension.
RROM: usually negative unless there is associated muscle strain.
Resisted tests and length tests may be positive for affected muscles.
Special tests: Springing positive for hypomobility and hard end-feel.

PALPATION

Tenderness may be elicited by palpating the vertebrae directly above or below the hyperkyphotic area. Associated muscles may be fibrotic.

Differential diagnosis

Exclude gibbus spine (interruption of normal thoracic kyphosis from previous osteoporotic fracture).

Overview of treatment and management

A typical remedial massage treatment for Scheuermann's disease includes:

- Swedish massage therapy to the back, neck, shoulders and chest.
- Remedial massage therapy. Muscle imbalances are addressed (see Table 11.3):
  - deep gliding frictions along the muscle fibres
  - cross-fibre frictions
  - active and passive soft tissue releasing techniques
  - deep transverse friction
  - trigger point therapy
  - muscle stretches.
- Thoracic spine mobilisation to encourage flexibility in the region (see Chapter 7):
  - compression
  - rhythmic compressions
  - thoracic rocking
  - thoracic longitudinal mobilisation
  - thoracic diagonal mobilisation.
- Apply myofascial releasing techniques for myofascial restrictions.
- Thermotherapy may be beneficial. Heat increases the blood supply to the region and helps relax the ligamentous and muscular contractures. Heat packs also assist pain relief.

CLIENT EDUCATION

Advise clients to be vigilant with posture (avoid slouching in flexion). Practise thoracic extension activities (e.g. the doorway stretch, backstroke swimming) as much as possible. Advise clients about correct lifting techniques. Clients should be referred for spinal manipulation.

Home exercise program

Place a rolled towel along the entire length of the thoracic spine. Lie on the towel for at least 10 minutes per day in order to oppose the increased kyphosis.

Daily extension exercises of the thoracic spine are recommended to increase the mobility of the affected area and to strengthen the back extensor muscles (see Figure 11.13).

OSTEOPOROSIS

Osteoporosis involves an imbalance between bone formation and reabsorption that results in loss of bone density (see Figure 11.18). As bones become fragile, the risk of fracture increases. Osteoporosis is most prevalent in the axial skeleton, pelvis and proximal long bones. It occurs predominantly in post-menopausal women or older clients and has also been associated with use of medications (e.g. glucocorticoids). Other predisposing factors include low levels of physical activity, lack of dietary calcium, particularly in the pre-teen years, smoking, alcohol consumption, family history and excessive exercise (e.g. from amenorrhoea in marathon runners).[11] Osteoporosis is of particular relevance for remedial massage therapists because of the increased risk of fracture, and deep work, particularly on the spine and ribs, is contraindicated.

Key assessment findings for osteoporosis

- Clients are usually women over 50 years old; asymptomatic unless fracture present
- Postural observation may reveal increased thoracic kyphosis
- Functional tests:
  - AROM: limited especially in extension
  - PROM: limited especially in extension
  - RROM: usually negative
  - Special tests: negative (if no fracture present)
- Palpation: no specific palpatory findings (severe pain and muscle guarding if fracture present)

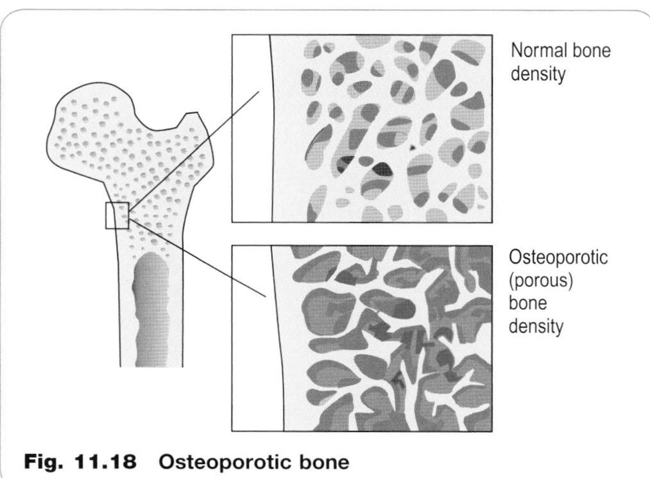

Fig. 11.18 Osteoporotic bone

Assessment

HISTORY

Osteoporosis typically affects elderly females. They are usually asymptomatic. If compression fracture has occurred, clients complain of sharp pain.

POSTURAL ANALYSIS

An increased thoracic kyphosis may be present.

FUNCTIONAL TESTS

AROM: limited, especially in extension.
PROM: limited, especially in extension.
RROM: usually negative.
Special tests: only positive if fracture present.

PALPATION

There are no specific palpatory findings associated with osteoporosis. However, a reactive splinting response and pain may be elicited if a compression fracture is present.

Note that osteoporosis may be associated with other conditions such as Cushing's syndrome, hyperthyroidism, rheumatoid arthritis, disuse and medication use (e.g. glucocorticosteroids, anti-convulsives). Refer clients with associated symptoms for further investigation.

Overview of treatment of a client with a history of osteoporosis

The primary concern when treating osteoporotic clients is the risk of fracture, especially of the ribs. The pressure of all techniques should be light.

A typical remedial massage treatment for an osteoporotic client includes the following:

- Swedish massage therapy to the thoracic region, in particular the erector spinae. It is crucial to massage without putting undue strain on the skeleton. Always massage the muscles in accordance with the client's pain threshold but no anterior pressure on the thorax should be applied. Anterior pressure may inadvertently cause a fragile spine or ribs to spontaneously fracture.
- Remedial massage therapy is directed to reactive contractures within the surrounding muscle and ligamentous tissues. For example, remedial massage for erector spinae, intercostals and rhomboid muscle contracture could include gentle applications of gliding frictions along the muscle fibres, cross-fibre frictions, active and passive soft tissue releasing techniques, trigger point therapy and muscle stretches (see Table 11.3). Avoid all deep techniques. Gentle myofascial releasing techniques may be particularly beneficial and heat therapy may be used.

CLIENT EDUCATION

Osteoporosis requires monitoring by the client's medical practitioner. Periodic bone density scans are required, as well as advice regarding mineral supplements and hormone replacement medication. Clients may choose to consult a naturopath for nutritional support.

Home exercise program

Gentle doorway stretches (see Figure 11.14) are helpful to counteract the thoracic kyphosis. Strengthening exercises for the back and leg muscles are particularly important to reduce the risk of falls and fractures. For example, erector spinae strengthening exercises may be prescribed (see Figure 11.5).

SCOLIOSIS

Scoliosis refers to a lateral curvature of the spine.[a] It is present in 2–4% of children between 10 and 16 years of age.[12] There are two major types of scoliosis:

1. **Structural (idiopathic) scoliosis.** This is a curvature of the spine of unknown cause. It is relatively fixed and does not straighten on forward bending of the trunk (Adam's test is positive if rib hump does not straighten on lumbar flexion). It is often associated with vertebral and rib abnormalities and can be so severe as to require bracing and surgery. Adolescent scoliosis; that is, scoliosis appearing between 10 years and skeletal maturity, accounts for 90% of cases and it occurs six times more often in females than in males. Scoliosis screenings in schools are designed to detect adolescent scoliosis. Structural scoliosis may also be due to such congenital conditions as hemivertebra and Klippel-Feil syndrome[b], and in rare cases associated with tumour, spinal fracture and metabolic and neuromuscular disorders.[11] As with many conditions, the earlier and more severe the onset, the poorer the prognosis. Curves are measured on radiographs and these measurements have been used to determine those clients requiring bracing and to monitor the progression of the scoliosis (see Figure 11.19 on p 195). A Cochrane Review of two studies concluded that there appears to be low-quality evidence in favour of using braces.[13] A study by Goldberg et al[14] examined the incidence of surgery for adolescent scoliosis by comparing one group of patients who received bracing and another group who did not. The authors could not find any statistical difference between the groups from surgery rates. The role of specific asymmetrical exercises in idiopathic scoliosis has also been investigated. In one study specific asymmetrical exercises increased electromyographic amplitudes of paraspinal muscles in the concavity of spinal curves.[15] Such exercises may be useful in the treatment of scoliosis.
2. **Functional scoliosis.** This is a temporary curvature that may be associated with pelvic tilt and muscle imbalance due to work, sport or other activity. This type of scoliosis straightens on forward bending of the trunk (Adam's test is negative). It is correctable with massage, spinal manipulation, exercises and in some cases orthotics.

Assessment

HISTORY

In structural scoliosis, the client initially presents as an adolescent or young adult. There may be mild back pain that does not usually refer. Scoliosis may not be associated with symptoms in the early stages but over time stiffness and pain in the

[a]Scoliosis affects all spinal curves (not only thoracic curves). Discussion of scoliosis is included in the thoracic chapter because presence of a left thoracic curve (90% of thoracic curves are to the right) is a red flag for referral for further examination.
[b]Klippel-Feil syndrome results from the congenital fusion of any two cervical vertebrae. The neck appears short and webbed and has restricted range of motion.

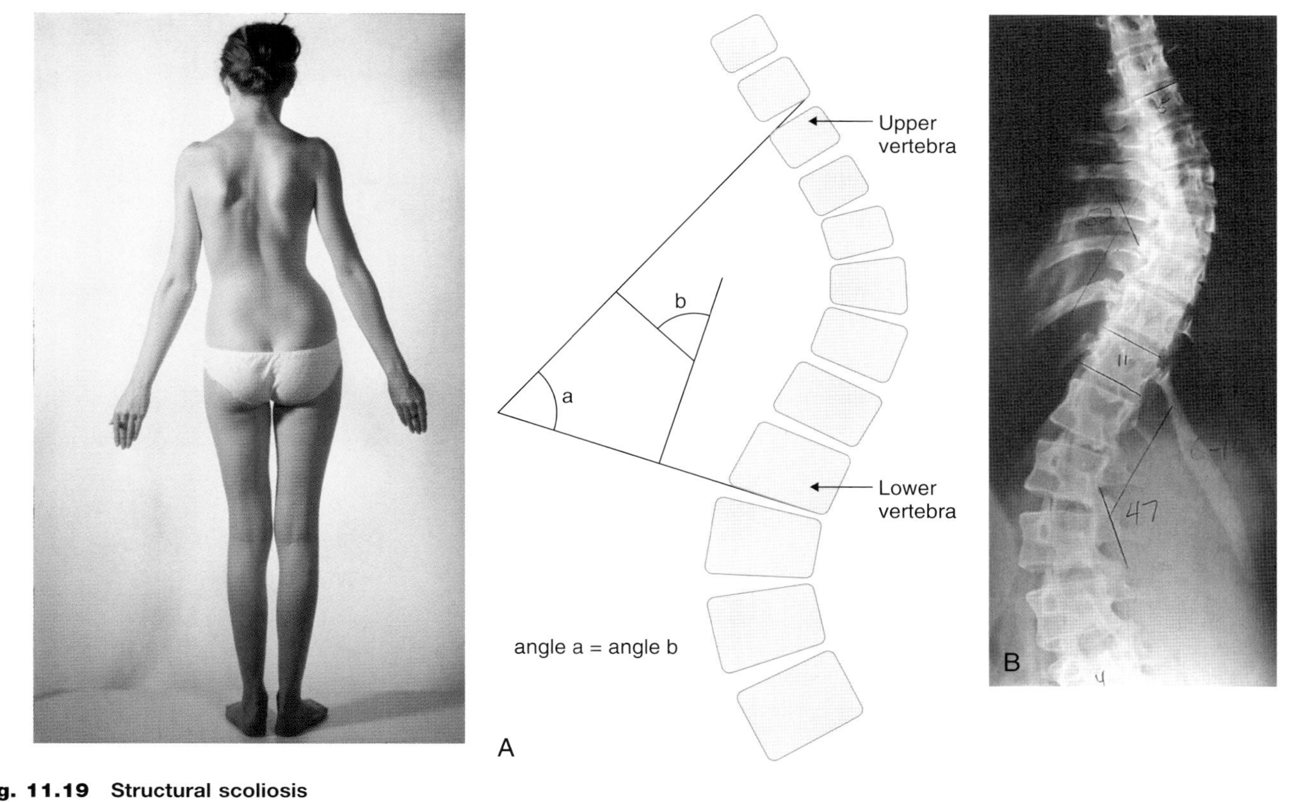

Fig. 11.19 Structural scoliosis

spine are common. Clients may also present with neck pain and headache. Functional scoliosis can occur at any stage and is associated with muscular pain and spasm.

POSTURAL ANALYSIS

Scoliosis is identified on postural observation. Scolioses are often described by the direction of curvature. For example, a left thoracic scoliosis describes a thoracic spine that curves to the left (i.e. the thoracic spine is convex on the left). Curves may be C-shaped or S-shaped. Note that 90% of curves are right thoracic (i.e. the thoracic spine curves to the right).

Key assessment findings for scoliosis

- Structural scoliosis: client is usually an adolescent or young adult; functional scoliosis can present at any age: mild to moderate back pain and associated muscle pain
- Postural analysis: scoliosis present
- Functional tests:
  - AROM: limited ± pain in some directions
  - PROM: limited ± pain in some directions
  - RROM: may be positive for affected muscles
  - Resisted and length tests may be positive for affected muscles
  - Special tests: Adam's test is positive in structural scoliosis
- Palpation: muscle hypertonicity is usually present on the convex side of the curve

FUNCTIONAL TESTS

AROM: limited in some directions.
PROM: limited in some directions.
RROM: may be positive for affected muscle groups.
Resisted muscle tests and length test may be positive for affected muscles.
Special tests: Adam's test helps differentiate between structural and functional scoliosis. Structural scoliosis does not straighten on forward flexion whereas functional scoliosis does. Leg length inequality may be present.

PALPATION

The muscles on the convex side of the curve are usually hypertonic. Palpating the spinous processes from T1 to L5 traces the lateral curvatures.

Differential diagnosis

The onset of scoliosis is usually insidious and progressive. Severe pain, a left thoracic curve or the presence of neurological signs and symptoms are red flags for a possible secondary cause of scoliosis.[12]

Overview of treatment and management

In cases of idiopathic scoliosis, radiographic assessment determines treatment. One way of measuring scoliosis is by the Cobb method: lines are drawn from the top of the most tilted vertebra above the apex of the curve and from the bottom of the most tilted vertebra below the apex. Two lines are drawn perpendicular to these lines. The angle between the

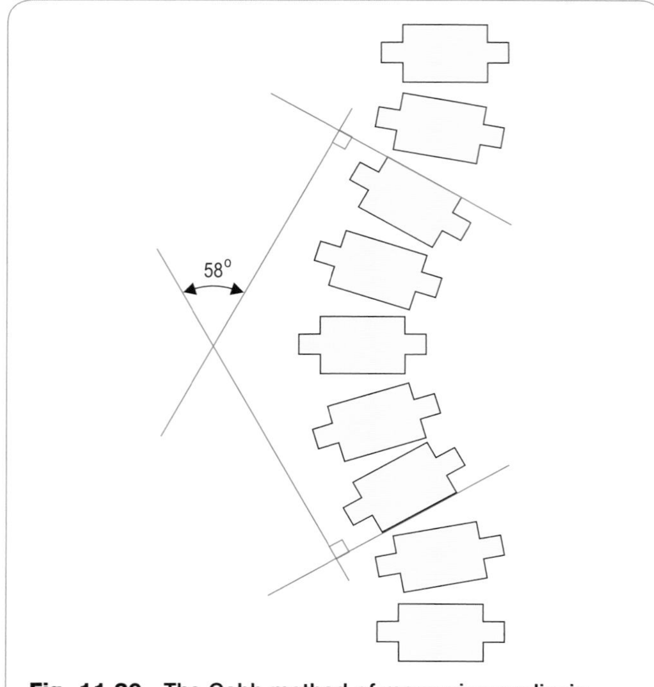

Fig. 11.20 The Cobb method of measuring scoliosis

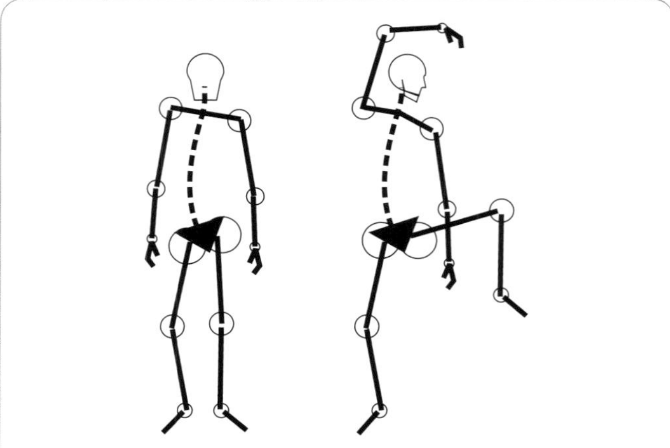

Fig. 11.21 The Scoliosis technique: exaggerating the C-curve

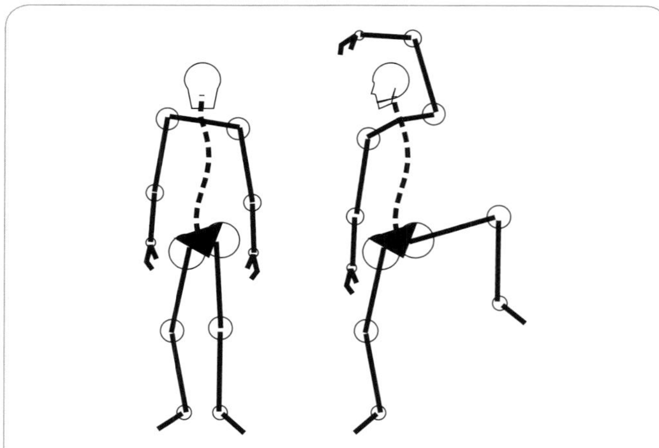

Fig. 11.22 The Scoliosis technique: exaggerating the S-curve

intersection of the perpendicular lines is the Cobb angle. Clients with curves that are greater than 35° require referral (see Figure 11.20).

A typical remedial massage treatment for structural or functional scoliosis includes:

- Swedish massage therapy to the back, neck, lower limbs and chest.
- Remedial massage therapy to correct muscle imbalances where possible, reduce pain and increase range of motion. For muscle contractures remedial massage therapy includes (see Table 11.3):
  - deep gliding frictions along the muscle fibres, especially on the concave side
  - cross-fibre frictions, especially on muscles on the convex side
  - active and passive soft tissue releasing techniques
  - deep transverse friction
  - trigger point therapy
  - muscle stretches.
- Manual traction of the spine (e.g. using leg traction techniques) may be beneficial. Apply myofascial releasing techniques for myofascial restrictions. Thermotherapy may be beneficial.
- The scoliosis technique may be useful for structural scoliosis. The technique is performed in two parts. The aim of the first part is to exaggerate the curvature and to stimulate neural input to the central nervous system. In the second part, the curvature is reversed and muscle-lengthening techniques are applied.

SCOLIOSIS TECHNIQUE:

i) C-shaped curve

1. The client lies prone. The client is instructed to exaggerate the curve by flexing the knee on the side of concavity, stretching the arm overhead on the side of convexity, and turning the head towards the concavity (see Figure 11.21). In this position, massage the paraspinal muscles on the side of concavity. Use cross-fibre techniques only for approximately 3–5 minutes.
2. Reverse the arm and leg positions to the opposite sides to minimise the curve. Continue massaging the same muscle groups using longitudinal gliding (lengthening the fibres) for approximately 5 minutes. (Massage the same muscles as in the previous step on the concave side of the curve only.)

ii) S-shaped curve

1. The client lies prone. Instruct the client to exaggerate the curves by flexing the knee on the side of lumbar concavity, stretching the arm overhead on the side of thoracic convexity and turning the head towards the thoracic concavity (see Figure 11.22). Use cross-fibre techniques for approximately 3–5 minutes massaging muscles on the convex side of the curves only.
2. Reverse arm and leg positions to the opposite sides to minimise the curve. Continue massaging the same

muscle groups but using longitudinal gliding (lengthening the fibres) for about 5 minutes. Massage the same muscles as in the previous step.

CLIENT EDUCATION

Advise clients about the importance of maintaining and improving range of motion and of avoiding any activities that are likely to add excessive load to the spine such as heavy lifting or wearing hard-soled shoes on hard surfaces. Refer clients with structural scoliosis who have not reached skeletal maturity or who have not been previously assessed. Refer to a chiropractor, osteopath or physiotherapist for consideration of a heel lift if true leg length inequality is suspected. Clients may also be referred for spinal manipulation and for treatment with a Feldenkrais practitioner[c].

Home exercise program

It is important that all clients with scoliosis undertake an exercise program to help correct muscle imbalances. Stretching exercises for contracted muscles (concave side) and strengthening exercises for weak muscles (convex side) are required. Breathing exercises will help maintain maximum chest expansion. Spinal traction exercises may be considered.

THORACIC OUTLET SYNDROME (ANTERIOR SCALENE SYNDROME)

Thoracic outlet syndrome refers to compression on the neurovascular bundle at the thoracic outlet (see Figure 11.23). Symptoms include numbness or paraesthesia in the upper limb. The condition may arise as a consequence of previous shoulder or lower cervical trauma, the presence of a cervical rib or anomalous or excessively toned or contracted scalene, pectoralis minor and/or subclavian muscles. Sleeping with the arm overhead and having a rounded shoulders posture may predispose people to this syndrome.

Assessment

HISTORY

The client commonly reports constant numbness and/or paraesthesia on the medial side of the arm and hand on the affected side. Pain may occur at night and wake the client from sleep. Thoracic outlet syndrome is also associated with occipital headache. Venous causes are less common and, if present, can lead to swelling in the upper limb. Arterial compression can lead to pallor and sensitivity to cold.

POSTURAL ANALYSIS

The client often has head forward carriage and rounded shoulders.

FUNCTIONAL TESTS

- AROM and PROM of the lower cervical, upper thoracic or shoulder may reproduce or aggravate symptoms.
- RROM tests may be positive in affected muscles.
- Resisted and length tests may be positive in affected muscles.
- Special tests: Elevation arm stress test (Roo's test) is positive.

PALPATION

The anterior scalene, and pectoralis minor muscles may be hypertonic and tender to palpation.

Differential diagnosis

Cervical radiculopathy can also mimic the neurological symptoms of thoracic outlet syndrome. Refer all clients with suspected thoracic outlet syndrome to a chiropractor, osteopath or physiotherapist for assessment before commencing massage therapy.

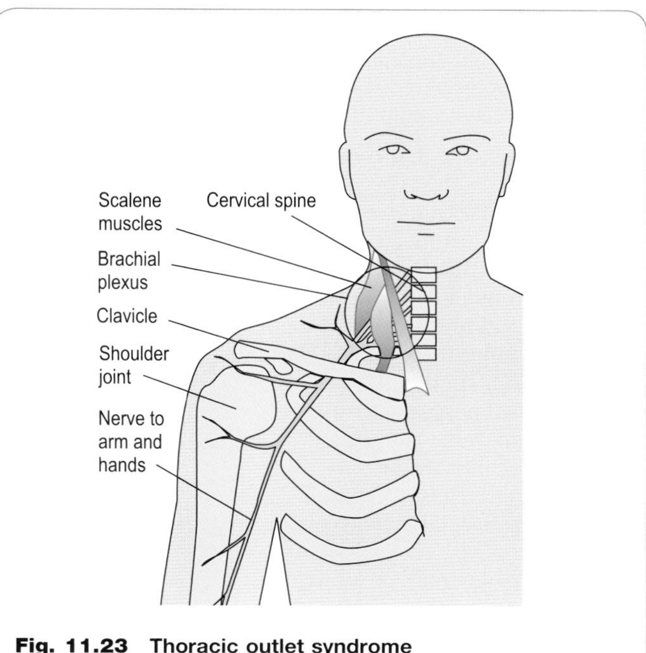

Fig. 11.23 Thoracic outlet syndrome

Key assessment findings for thoracic outlet syndrome

- History of unilateral numbness/paraesthesia in the upper limb; nocturnal pain often wakes clients from sleep
- Postural analysis: head forward position, rounded shoulders
- Functional tests
  - Cervical, thoracic and shoulder AROM and PROM may cause further neurovascular compression and reproduce or aggravate symptoms
  - RROM may be positive for affected muscles
  - Resisted tests and length tests may be positive for specific muscles
  - Special tests: Elevated arm stress test is positive
- Palpation: tenderness and hypertonia in scalenes, pectoralis minor

[c]The Feldenkrais Method was developed by Moshe Feldenkrais in the 1960s. Gentle exercises are used to increase self-awareness of movement and then to re-educate the body's movement patterns.

Overview of treatment and management

Remedial massage therapy may be used as an adjunct to other physical therapies. A typical remedial massage treatment for thoracic outlet syndrome includes:

- Swedish massage therapy to the upper back, neck, chest and upper limb.
- Remedial massage techniques, which are designed to address muscle imbalance that could be causing or aggravating the condition. For example, remedial massage therapy for hypertonic anterior scalene, pectoralis minor and other tight cervical muscles could include (see Table 12.4):
  - deep gliding frictions along the muscle fibres
  - cross-fibre frictions
  - active and passive soft tissue releasing techniques
  - deep transverse friction
  - trigger point therapy
  - muscle stretches.
- Apply myofascial releasing techniques for myofascial restrictions.
- Thermotherapy may be beneficial.

CLIENT EDUCATION

Advise clients about postural corrections for forward head carriage and rounded shoulders and to avoid sleeping with arms overhead.

Home exercise program

An exercise program to stretch contracted muscles (e.g. anterior scalenes, pectoralis minor and other cervical muscles) and to strengthen upper trapezius and rhomboids will help correct posture and may relieve neurovascular compression at the thoracic outlet.

KEY MESSAGES

- Assessment of clients with conditions of the thoracic region involves history, outcome measures, postural analysis, gait analysis, functional tests (including resisted tests and length tests for specific muscles) and special tests for the thoracic region (e.g. Adam's test, deep breathing, Roo's test).
- Assessment findings may indicate the type of tissue involved (contractile or inert), duration of condition (acute or subacute) and severity.
- Assessment findings may indicate a common presenting condition (thoracic facet syndrome, DJD, dowager's hump, Scheuermann's disease, scoliosis and thoracic outlet syndrome).
- Assessment findings also indicate client perception of injury and preferences for treatment.
- Consider Clinical Guidelines, available evidence, clinical efficacy and client preferences when planning therapy.
- Although serious conditions of the thoracic region are rare, clients with such conditions will present for remedial massage from time to time. Caution is required when treating all clients with pain in the thoracic region, especially when there is a history of trauma, previous malignancy or other indications of potentially serious disease, including fever and chest pain.
- Educating clients about likely causal and predisposing factors is an essential part of remedial massage therapy. Over time, increase the client self-help component of treatment wherever possible to reduce likelihood of recurrence and/or to promote health maintenance and illness prevention.

Review questions

1. The term *idiopathic* means:
   a) induced by treatment
   b) congenital
   c) unknown cause
   d) of genetic origin
2. A dowager's hump refers to:
   a) an increased kyphosis at the C7 to T3 level
   b) an increased kyphosis at the T9 to L2 level
   c) a flattened kyphosis between the shoulder blades
   d) a hairy tuft over the lower lumbar spine
3. A patient presents with lower right rib cage pain three days after being injured in a game of football. The pain is sharp, localised and continuing to be very painful. He is unable to take a deep breath without pain. Palpation of the injury site is very tender and there is evidence of reflex muscle guarding. A provisional diagnosis would be:
   a) subluxated rib
   b) fractured rib
   c) herniated thoracic disc
   d) intercostal muscle strain
4. An adolescent client is observed to have a moderate to severe scoliosis. An appropriate treatment would be:
   a) Swedish massage, trigger point therapy, muscle stretches and the scoliosis technique
   b) referral to a medical practitioner for further assessment
   c) Swedish massage only
   d) Swedish massage and a weights program
5. Schmorl's nodes on an X-ray are often associated with:
   a) Scheuermann's disease
   b) structural scoliosis
   c) degenerative joint disease of the thoracic spine
   d) Tietze's syndrome
6. The most common cause of chest pain in a 25-year-old athlete is:
   a) referred pain from the thoracic spine
   b) rib subluxation
   c) rib stress fracture
   d) pectoralis major trigger point
7. a) What is Scheuermann's disease?
   b) What group of the population does it most affect?
   c) Name one test or observation that would make you suspect Scheuermann's disease.
   d) What recommendations would you make to a client with Scheuermann's disease?
8. Describe or draw a resisted muscle test for each of the following muscles:
   a) latissimus dorsi
   b) rhomboid muscles
   c) serratus anterior
   d) middle trapezius

Review questions—cont'd

9. A client presents with a history of numbness and pins and needles on the inside of her left arm. During the night she is often woken from sleep with arm pain. The arm elevated stress test brings pins and needles to her arm and hand. The client could have:
   a) dowager's hump
   b) thoracic outlet syndrome
   c) a fractured rib secondary to osteoporosis
   d) degenerative joint disease in the upper thoracic spine
10. Degenerative joint disease in the thoracic spine is associated with:
    a) osteophytic lipping
    b) disc degeneration
    c) muscle spasm
    d) all of the above
11. In assessing rib pain how would you differentiate a rib fracture from an intercostal muscle strain?
12. The following diagram represents a stretch for which muscle(s)?
    a) middle trapezius
    b) pectoralis major
    c) latissimus dorsi
    d) serratus anterior

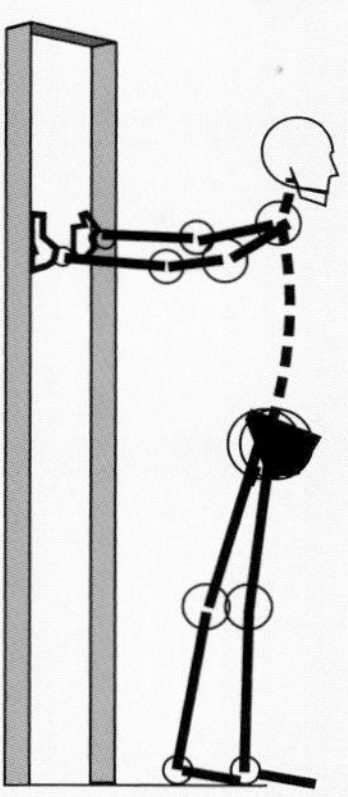

REFERENCES

1. Cleland J, Koppenhaver S. Netter's orthopaedic clinical examination: an evidence-based approach. 2nd edn. Philadelphia: Saunders; 2011.
2. Boyling J, Jull G, editors. Grieve's modern manual therapy: the vertebral column. London: Churchill Livingstone; 2005.
3. Australian Acute Musculoskeletal Pain Guidelines Group. Evidence-based management of acute musculoskeletal pain: a guide for clinicians. Bowen Hills, Qld: Australian Academic Press; 2004.
4. New Zealand Guidelines Group. New Zealand acute low back pain guide. Online. Available: www.nzgg.org.nz/guidelines/0072/acc1038_col.pdf; 2004.
5. Chaitow L. Muscle energy techniques. 2nd edn. Edinburgh: Churchill Livingstone; 2001.
6. Reiman MP, Manske R. Functional testing in human performance. Champaign, IL: Human Kinetics; 2009.
7. Simons D, Travell J, Simons L. Myofascial pain and dysfunction: The trigger point manual. Volume 1 Upper half of body. 2nd edn. Philadelphia: Williams & Wilkins; 1999.
8. Towheed TE, Maxwell L, Anastassiades TP, et al. Glucosamine therapy for treating osteoarthritis. Cochrane Database Syst Rev [serial on the Internet]. 2005; (2):CD002946.
9. Australian Institute of Health and Welfare. A picture of osteoarthritis in Australia. Online. Available: www.aihw.gov.au/publications/phe/apooia/apooia.pdf; 2007.
10. Yochum T, Rowe L. Essentials of skeletal radiology. 3rd edn. Baltimore: Lippincott Williams and Wilkins; 2005.
11. Carnes M, Vizniak N. Quick reference evidence-based conditions manual. 3rd edn. Burnaby, BC: Professional Health Systems; 2009.
12. Reamy B, Slakey J. Adolescent idiopathic scoliosis: review and current concepts. Am Fam Physician 2001;64(1):111–16.
13. Negrini S, Minozzi S, Bettany-Saltikov J, et al. Braces for idiopathic scoliosis in adolescents. Cochrane Database Syst Rev 2010;(1):CD006850.
14. Goldberg CJ, Moore DP, Fogarty EE, et al. Adolescent idiopathic scoliosis: the effect of brace treatment on the incidence of surgery. Spine 2001;26(1):42–7.
15. Schmid AB, Dyer L, Boni T, et al. Paraspinal muscle activity during symmetrical and asymmetrical weight training in idiopathic scoliosis. J Sport Rehabil 2010;19(3):315–27.

12 The cervical region

The content of this chapter relates to the following Units of Competency:

HLTREM503C Plan remedial massage treatment strategy
HLTREM504C Apply remedial massage assessment framework
HLTREM502C Provide remedial massage treatment
HLTREM505C Perform remedial massage health assessment

Health Training Package HLT07

Learning Outcomes

- Assess clients with conditions of the cervical region for remedial massage, including identification of red and yellow flags.
- Assess clients for signs and symptoms associated with common neck conditions and treat and/or manage these conditions with appropriate remedial massage therapy.
- Develop treatment plans for clients with neck conditions, taking assessment findings, duration and severity of the condition, likely tissue types, clinical guidelines, best available evidence and client preferences into account.
- Develop short- and long-term treatment plans to address presenting symptoms, underlying conditions and predisposing factors, and to progressively increase the self-help component of therapy.
- Adapt remedial massage therapy to suit individual client needs based on duration and severity of injury, the client's age and gender, the presence of underlying conditions and co-morbidities, and other considerations for special population groups.

INTRODUCTION

Neck complaints are common presenting conditions in remedial massage clinics and have a high incidence of recurrence. It is estimated that 50–80% of adults will experience neck pain at some time in their lives.[1] Most people with neck pain can continue their usual activities, but between 5% and 10% of people will find their neck pain disabling. Acute or repetitive neck injuries account for about 85% of all neck pain.[2] Chronic neck pain (i.e. neck pain of more than 6 months' duration) is estimated to affect around 14% of the general population.[2] Apart from serious causes of neck pain (less than 1% of cases),[3] it is not necessary to know the exact cause of the neck condition before treating the client. Anecdotal evidence supports the benefits of remedial massage therapy for many cases of neck pain and a sound knowledge of the underlying anatomical structures and their relationships is required for safe and competent practice.

FUNCTIONAL ANATOMY REVIEW

The biomechanics of the cervical spine are complex, involving three-dimensional spinal coupling movements (i.e. movement in one plane of motion accompanied by movements in other planes) and unequal movements from one vertebra to the next in any range.[4] The proximity of vital structures such as the spinal cord, cranial nerves and arteries means that changes in cervical biomechanics can potentially influence their function. The cervical vertebrae are characterised by transverse foramina which transmit the vertebral arteries, veins and sympathetic plexus in the transverse processes of C1–C7 (the vertebral foramen of C7 is small and sometimes absent). C1 and C2 are specialised vertebrae. There is little or no rotation at the atlanto-occipital junction and little to no lateral flexion at C1/C2. C1 (the atlas) is a ring of bone which supports the skull. Its superior articular facets are elliptical and concave and articulate with the occipital condyles to create the nodding movement of the head. Its transverse processes are large and wide and palpable behind the mandible just below the ear. The vertebral foramen is divided by the transverse ligament into a posterior compartment which houses the spinal cord and an anterior compartment containing the dens of the C2 (the axis).The axis with its large dens or odontoid process forms a pivot around which the atlas and head rotate. The weight of the head is transferred to the cervical spine through the lateral atlanto-axial articulations of C2 (see Figure 12.1 on p 201). The spinous processes of C2–C6 are bifid. C2 spinous process is palpated immediately below the external occipital protuberance.

The first of the eight cervical nerves emerges between the skull and the atlas and except for the eighth each nerve emerges above the corresponding vertebra (i.e. C3 spinal nerve exits above C3). The eighth nerve emerges below C7 and thereafter spinal nerves emerge below their corresponding vertebrae (see Figure 12.2). C7 with its long spinous process is known as the vertebra prominens.

Major muscles of the cervical region are summarised in Table 12.1 (see also Figure 12.3). Muscle balance in the cervical region can be affected by traumas and stresses applied directly to the head and neck and habitual postures like forward head carriage. Cervical musculature also reflects musculoskeletal adaptations to conditions of the thoracolumbar spine, pelvis and lower limbs including scoliosis or leg length inequality.

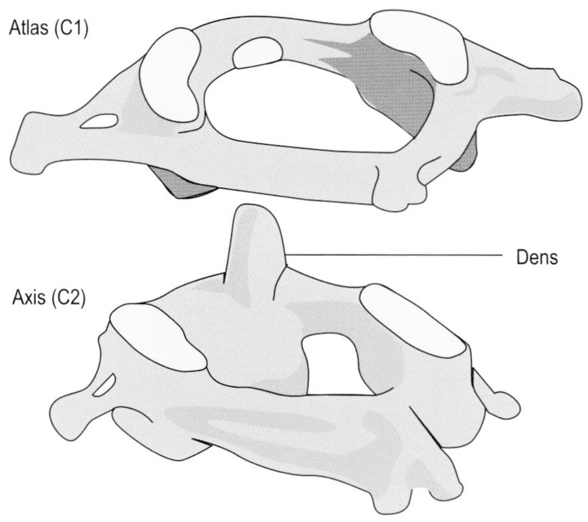

Atlas (C1)

Dens

Axis (C2)

Fig. 12.1 Cervical vertebrae

ASSESSMENT

Chapter 2 presents details of assessment procedures for remedial massage therapy clients. Assessment procedures are designed to:

- determine the suitability of clients for massage (red flags)
- determine the duration (acute or subacute) and severity of the condition, and the types of tissues that could be involved
- determine if the client's symptoms fit patterns of common conditions.

CASE HISTORY

Identify any red flags that require referral for further investigation (see Table 12.2). For example, a client involved in a recent car accident should be referred for further assessment as symptoms may not appear immediately.

- Features that alert practitioners to the possible presence of serious underlying conditions include the nature and mode of pain onset and its intensity.

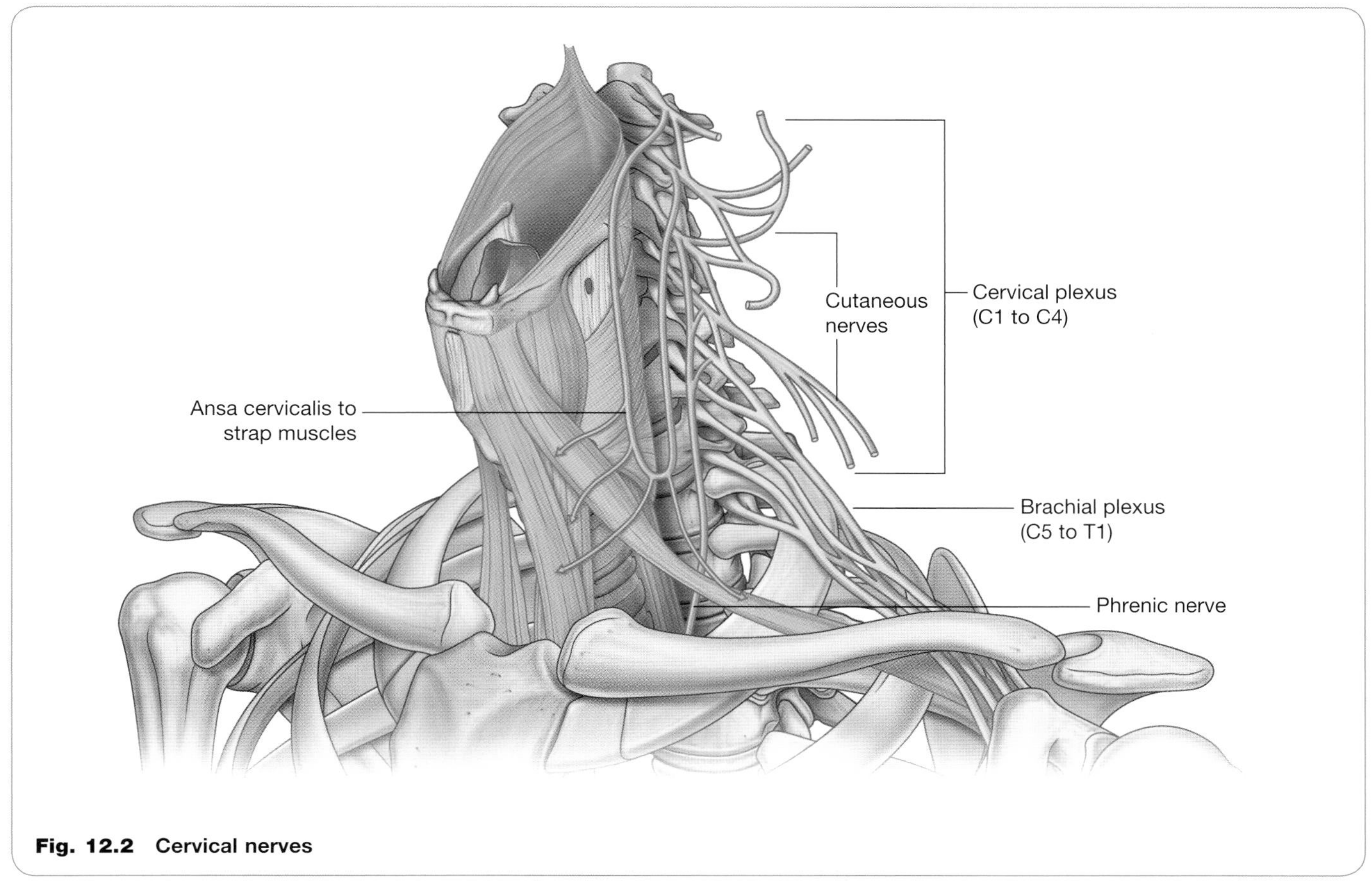

Fig. 12.2 Cervical nerves

Table 12.1 Muscles of the neck

Muscle	Origin	Insertion	Action
Upper trapezius	External occipital protuberance, superior nuchal line, nuchal ligament and spinous process of C7	Acromion process, lateral clavicle, spine of scapula	Ipsilateral lateral flexion and contralateral rotation of the neck and head, elevates scapula
Sternocleidomastoid	Mastoid process and lateral half of superior nuchal line	Anterior manubrium and medial third of the clavicle	Ipsilaterally lateral flexion and contralateral rotation of the head and neck
Levator scapulae	Transverse processes of C1–C4	Superomedial border of scapula	Elevation and retraction of the scapula; ipsilateral lateral flexion and rotation of the neck
Sub-occipital muscles			
Inferior oblique	C2 spinous process	C1 transverse process	Rotation of atlas (turns head ipsilaterally)
Superior oblique	C1 transverse process	Occipital bone	Extension and lateral flexion of the head
Rectus capitis posterior major	C2 spinous process	Occipital bone	Extension of head, ipsilateral rotation of head
Rectus capitis posterior minor	Posterior tubercle of C2	Occipital bone	Extension of the head As a group, they act to stabilise the head. They also extend and rotate the head at the atlanto-occipital joint to make small, precise head movements.
Posterior cervical muscles			Mainly extension of the head and neck by the longer and more vertical muscles; rotation of the head and neck by the deeper more diagonal fibres[5]
Splenius capitis	Nuchal ligament, spinous processes of C7–T3/4	Mastoid process	
Spenius cervicis	Spinous processes of T3–T6	Transverse processes of C1–2/3	
Longissimus capitis	Articular processes of C4/5–C7, transverse processes of T1–T4/5	Mastoid process	
Longissimus cervicis	Transverse processes of T1–T5	Transverse processes of C2–C6	
Iliocostalis cervicis	Angles of ribs 3–6	Transverse processes of C4–C6	
Spinalis cervicis (spinalis capitis, is medial part of semispinalis capitis)	Nuchal ligament, spinous process of C7	Spinous process C2	
Semispinalis cervicis	Transverse processes of T1–T5/6	Spinous processes C2–C5	
Semispinalis capitis	(Overlies semispinalis cervicis) Articular processes of C4–C6, transverse processes of T1–T6	Between the nuchal lines	
Multifidus	Articular processes of C4–C7 (cross two to four vertebrae)	Spinous processes of C2–C5	
Scalenus anterior	Transverse processes of C4–C6	Scalene tubercle and superior border rib 1	Ipsilateral lateral flexion and contralateral rotation of the neck; elevates rib 1
Scalenus medius	Transverse processes of C2–C7	Superior surface of rib 1	
Scalenus posterior	Transverse processes of C5–C6	Outer surface of rib 2	Lateral flexes neck ipsilaterally and contralaterally rotates the neck; elevates rib 2

- Severe neck pain, regardless of its cause, is an important risk factor for chronicity.[3]
- According to the Canadian C-Spine Rule (see Figure 12.4), all high-risk clients should be referred for radiographic examination. Clients are considered high risk if they are more than 65 years of age, if the mechanism of injury was dangerous (e.g. head injuries from diving, falls from a height greater than 1 metre or falls down five or more stairs) or if the client reports paraesthesia in the extremities.[6]
- Ask clients to point to the site of pain as they may have different understandings of anatomical terms.
- Determine if the pain is likely to have a mechanical cause. (Is the pain associated with rest or activity, certain postures or time of day?) Ask clients to demonstrate movements and positions that aggravate or relieve their pain and to be specific with descriptions of aggravating or relieving activities.
- Mechanical pain is usually highly reactive to changes in posture, positions or activity.

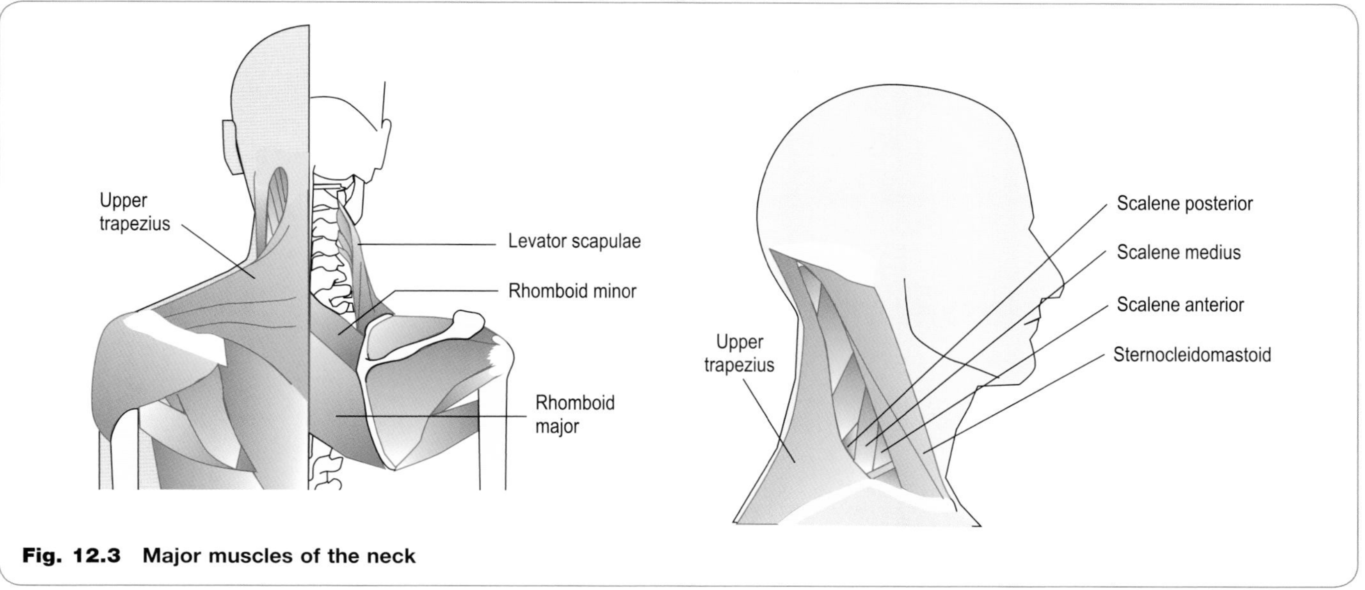

Fig. 12.3 Major muscles of the neck

Table 12.2 Red flags for serious conditions associated with acute neck pain

Red flags for acute neck pain	Possible condition
Symptoms and signs of infection (e.g. fever, night sweats) Risk factors for infection (e.g. underlying disease, immunosuppression, penetrating wound)	Infection
History of trauma Minor trauma (if taking corticosteroids)	Fracture
Past history of malignancy Age >50 years Failure to improve with treatment Unexplained weight loss Dysphagia, headache, vomiting	Cancer
Neurological symptoms in the limbs	Neurological condition
Cerebrovascular symptoms or signs, anticoagulant use	Cerebral or spinal haemorrhage
Cardiovascular risk factors; transient ischaemic attack	Vertebral or carotid aneurysm

Adapted from the Acute Musculoskeletal Pain Guidelines Group[3] and the New Zealand Guidelines Group[7]
Note that acute pain in this context refers to pain of less than three months' duration.

- Morning pain relieved with daily activity is often associated with arthritis.
- Determine if the pain is likely to be associated with visceral function, neurogenic, vascular or psychosocial causes (yellow flags).
- Pain from glandular fever, rheumatoid arthritis or neurogenic pain from a tumour, for example, are not usually aggravated by activity or relieved by rest, whereas mechanical neck pain may be relieved by lying down.

Assessment of the cervical region

1. Case history
2. Outcome measures
3. Postural analysis
4. Functional tests
   Active range of motion tests
   Flexion, extension, lateral flexion, rotation
   Passive range of motion tests
   Flexion, extension, lateral flexion, rotation
   Resisted range of motion tests
   Flexion, extension, lateral flexion, rotation
   Resisted and length test for specific muscles including
   - Upper trapezius
   - Sternocleidomastoid
   - Levator scapulae
   - Suboccipital muscles
   - Posterior cervical muscles
   - Scalene muscles

   Special tests including
   - Cervical compression
   - Cervical distraction
   - Valsalva
5. Palpation

OUTCOME MEASURES

Outcome measures are questionnaires that are specifically designed to assess clients' level of impairment and to define benefits of treatment. The benefit is assessed in terms of client-perceived changes to health status. The Vernon-Mior Neck Disability Questionnaire is frequently used to assess clients' perceptions of neck pain.

POSTURAL ANALYSIS

- Viewed laterally, the ear should be in line with the shoulder. A protruding chin could indicate compensation to balance the body's centre of gravity, short occipital muscles and weak deep neck flexors in upper crossed syndrome. Is the chin retracted (military posture)?

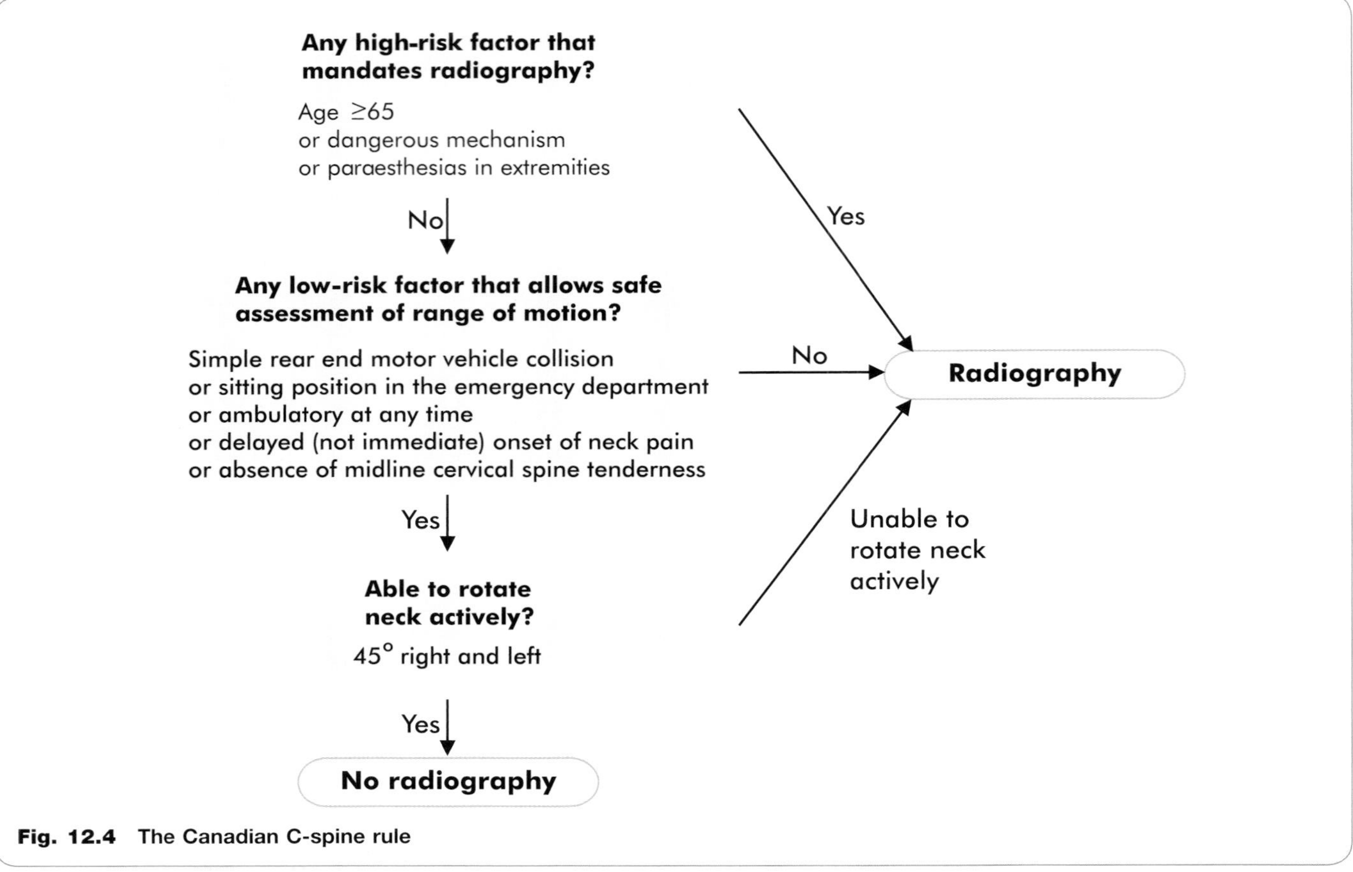

Fig. 12.4 The Canadian C-spine rule

- View the client from behind and observe head tilt or rotation. (Note that approximately 50% of cervical flexion and extension takes place between the occiput and C1; approximately 50% of rotation occurs in the C1–C2 spinal segment.) When the client is observed anteriorly the chin should be in line with the sternum.
- Habitual posture deviations may result from postural compensations (e.g. scoliosis, lumbar hyperlordosis or thoracic hyperkyphosis), hearing and visual adaptations.

FUNCTIONAL TESTS

As discussed in Chapter 2, many clinical tests lack validity and reliability. However, physical examination, including functional tests, may alert practitioners to potentially serious conditions and help determine whether symptoms are of local or referred origin (e.g. limited cervical range of motion and tenderness may indicate the presence of a local cause of pain[3]). Functional tests also provide information about clients' perceptions of their conditions and their preferences for assessment and treatment styles.

a) Active range of motion

FLEXION (50°)[8]

- Stand in front of the client and ask them to take their chin towards their chest as far as they comfortably can.
- The client should be able to touch their chin to their chest.

EXTENSION (60°)

- Ask the client to look up to the ceiling as far as they comfortably can.
- The client should be able to extend their neck so that their face is parallel to the ceiling.

LATERAL FLEXION (SIDEBEND) (45°)

- Ask the client to take their ear towards their shoulder as far as they comfortably can.
- The client should be able to tilt their ear to their shoulder approximately 45°.

ROTATION (80°)

- Ask the client to look over their shoulder as far as they comfortably can.
- The client should be able to rotate their neck so that their chin is almost in line with their shoulder.

b) Passive range of motion

Lie the client supine to relax the neck muscles. Great care is needed when performing cervical passive range of motion tests. Perform all neck movements slowly and gently and only ever after you have observed the client's ability to perform active ranges of motion (the See-Move-Touch principle discussed in Chapter 2). Note the end-feel at the end of each range of motion (see Figure 12.5 on p 205).

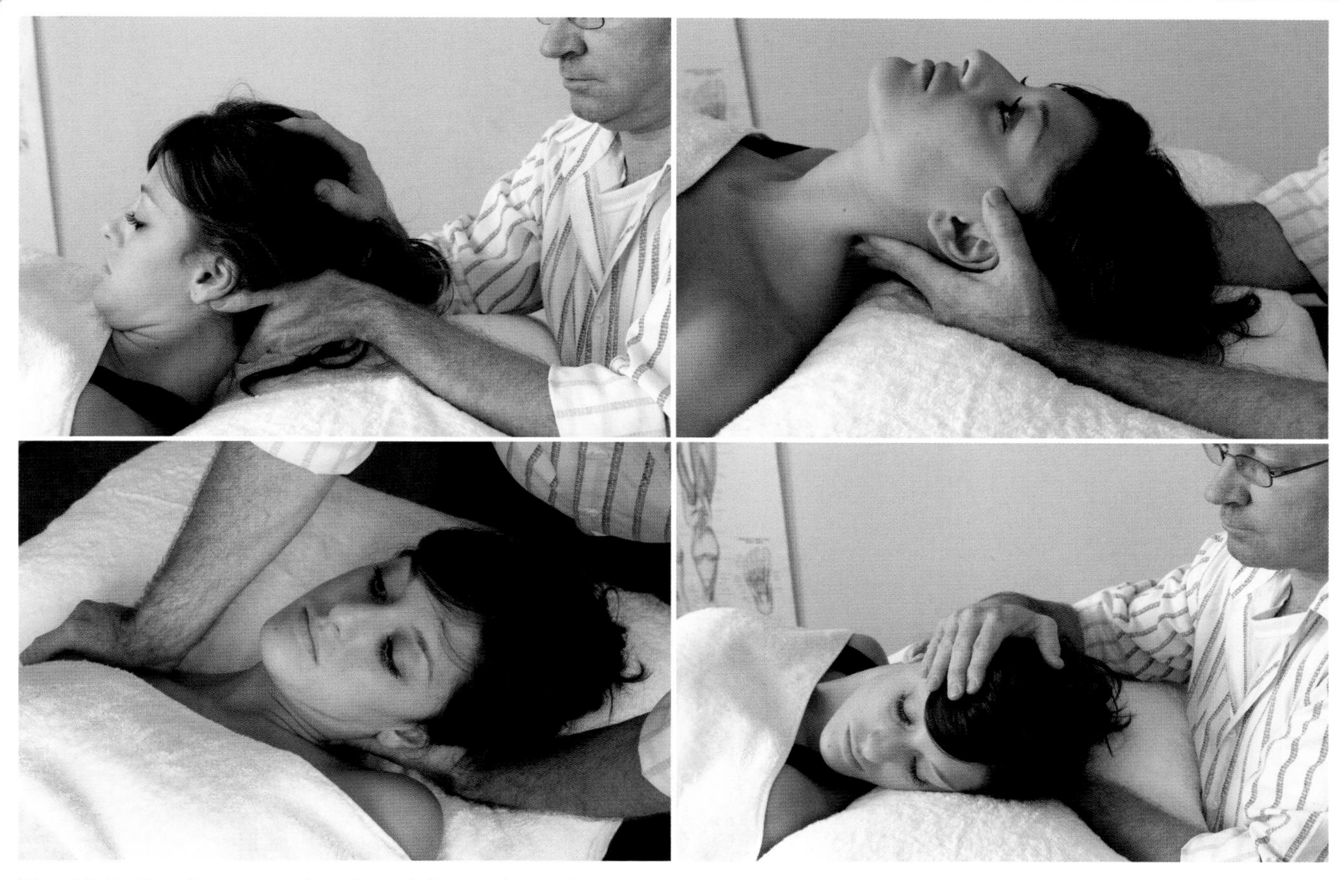

Fig. 12.5 **Passive range of motion of the cervical spine**

FLEXION

- Cup the client's occiput and gently flex the client's neck.

EXTENSION

- When the client is positioned with shoulders level with the top of the table, the neck can be gently extended. Alternatively, the neck can be passively extended by lifting the neck towards the ceiling.

LATERAL FLEXION

- Place one hand on the client's shoulder and with the other cup the occiput. Gently laterally flex the client's neck with the cupped hand.

ROTATION

- Cup the client's occiput and gently rotate the neck to one side and then the other.

c) Resisted range of motion

Resisted range of motion (RROM) tests are designed to identify muscle groups that may be contributing to the client's condition. Resist the movement as the client flexes, extends, laterally flexes and rotates their head. The client may be seated or lying supine. These tests are usually carried out in conjunction with passive range of motion tests. For example, passive rotation of the neck can be followed immediately by resisted rotation before testing another movement in another plane. If any RROM tests are positive, resisted tests for specific muscle tests are required to identify individual muscles.

d) Tests for specific muscles associated with neck conditions

For any tests involving joint movements remember to take into account individual anatomical variation and the influence of age, lifestyle and underlying pathology on movement. Comparing both sides provides important information about individual clients.

1. UPPER TRAPEZIUS

Resisted test

Test upper trapezius by resisting extension or lateral flexion of the head and neck. The tests can be performed with the client sitting or standing. One possible test is described here.

With the client seated, place one hand on the client's shoulder and the other on the ipsilateral side of their head. Ask the client to take their ear towards their shoulder against your resistance (apply sufficient pressure so that the contraction is isometric, i.e. no head movement actually occurs) (see Figure 12.6 on p 206).

Length test

Clients with shortened upper trapezius muscles will be unable to take their chin to their chest or to laterally flex their

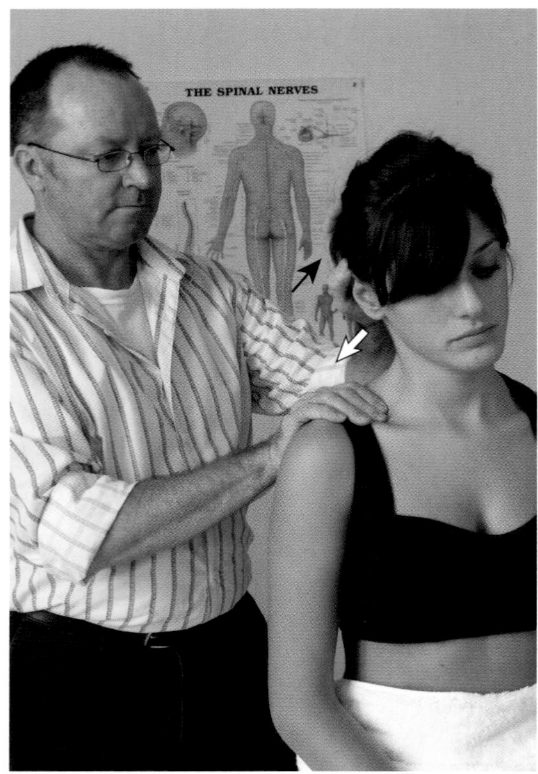

Fig. 12.6 Resisted test for upper trapezius

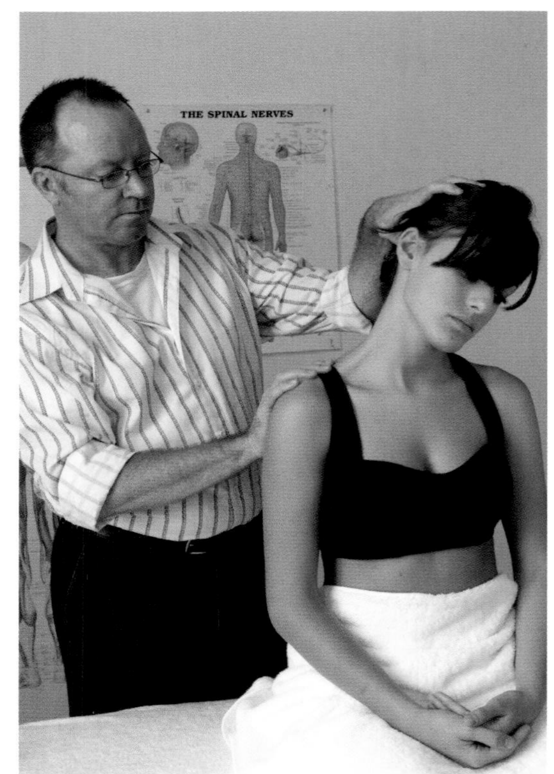

Fig. 12.7 Length test for upper trapezius

neck to 45° (see Figure 12.7). Rotating the head ipsilaterally helps isolate upper trapezius from other posterolateral extensors of the neck.

Clinical significance

Shortening of upper trapezius may occur as a result of habitual rounded shoulder posture or chin protraction, as a compensation for hyperkyphotic postures and in chronic stress. Upper trapezius strains are commonly associated with other conditions of the cervical spine, such as cervical degenerative joint disease (DJD) or facet syndrome.

2. STERNOCLEIDOMASTOID

Resisted test

Sternocleidomastoid can be assessed by resisting flexion, ipsilateral lateral flexion or contralateral rotation of the head and neck. The tests can be performed with the client sitting, standing or supine. One test is described here.

The client lies supine with their head turned slightly to one side. Place one hand across the client's forehead and ask the client to try to take their chin to their chest. Resist this movement by applying gentle pressure to the client's forehead. Adjust the pressure so that the contraction is isometric; that is, no head movement actually occurs (see Figure 12.8).

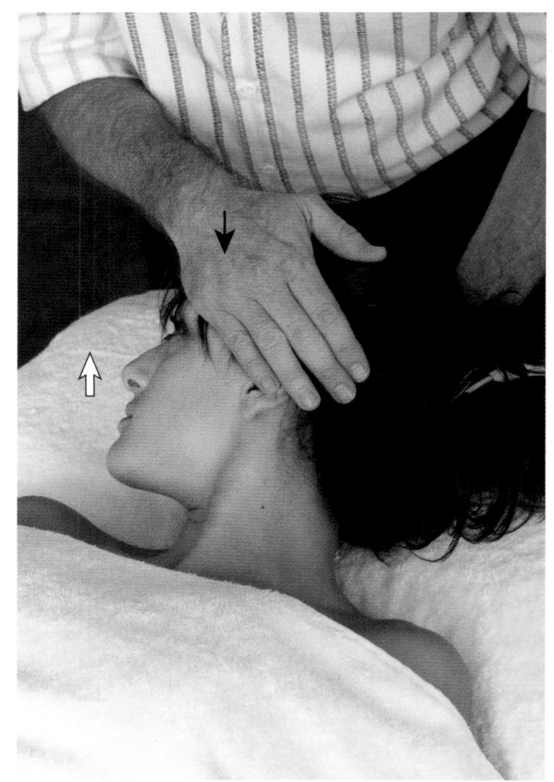

Fig. 12.8 Resisted test for sternocleidomastoid

Length test

Clients with shortening of bilateral sternocleidomastoid muscles will have limited extension of the head and neck. Unilateral contraction of sternocleidomastoid limits contralateral lateral flexion and ipsilateral rotation.

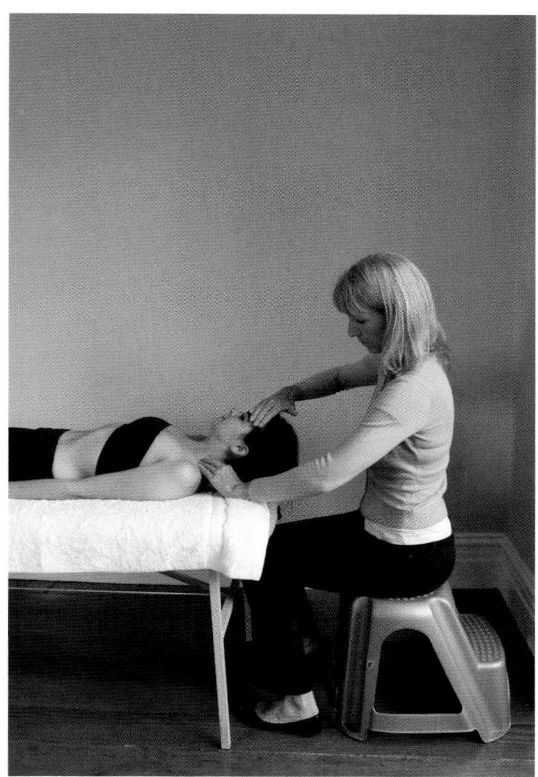

Fig. 12.9 **Palpating the attachment of anterior scalene**

Clinical significance

Sternocleidomastoid is often implicated in whiplash injuries and in torticollis. Caution is always required when treating injuries of sternocleidomastoid because of its proximity to the carotid artery. Sternocleidomastoid muscle also overlies the cervical lymphatic chain and may be affected by lymph adenopathy such as can occur in upper respiratory tract infections and glandular fever.

Note: Anterior scalene is also tested with sternocleidomastoid during resisted flexion and lateral flexion of the neck. It is distinguished from sternocleidomastoid by palpation to its attachment at the first rib (see Figure 12.9).

3. LEVATOR SCAPULAE

Resisted test

Levator scapulae can be assessed by resisting scapulae elevation, neck extension, lateral flexion or rotation of the neck. One method involves standing behind the seated client, placing hands on the client's shoulders and resisting as they try to shrug their shoulders (see Figure 12.10). (This test will also test upper trapezius.)

Length test

Clients with habitually elevated shoulders could have chronic contracture of levator scapulae. Shortening of levator scapulae could also result in limited neck flexion, lateral flexion or rotation. The client reaches behind their back to the opposite hip, laterally flexes and rotates their neck to the opposite side, and then flexes their neck as far as they comfortably can (see Figure 12.11).

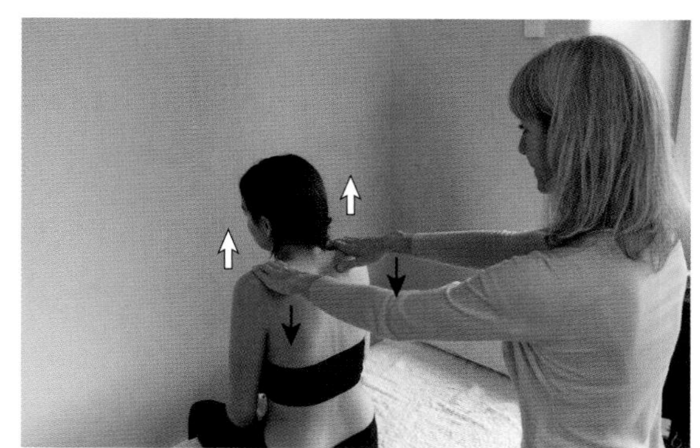

Fig. 12.10 **Resisted test for levator scapulae**

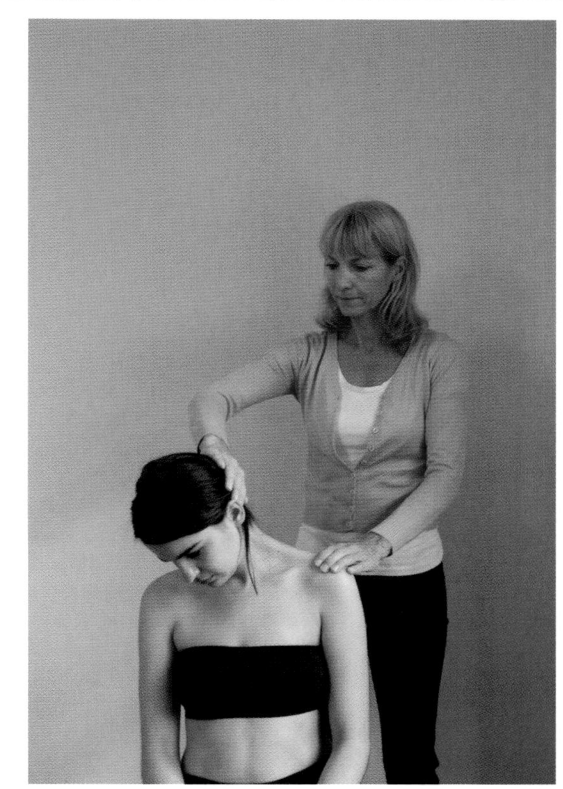

Fig. 12.11 **Length test for levator scapulae**

Clinical significance

Levator scapulae is commonly tight and short in upper crossed syndrome.

4. SUBOCCIPITAL MUSCLES

It is difficult to isolate the suboccipital muscles in functional tests. Their strength is assessed along with other muscles by resisting extension, lateral flexion or ipsilateral rotation of the head at the atlanto-occipital joint. Contractures of suboccipital muscles could limit neck flexion, and contralateral lateral flexion or rotation. Suboccipital muscles are commonly associated with cervicogenic headache (see Figure 12.12 on p 208).

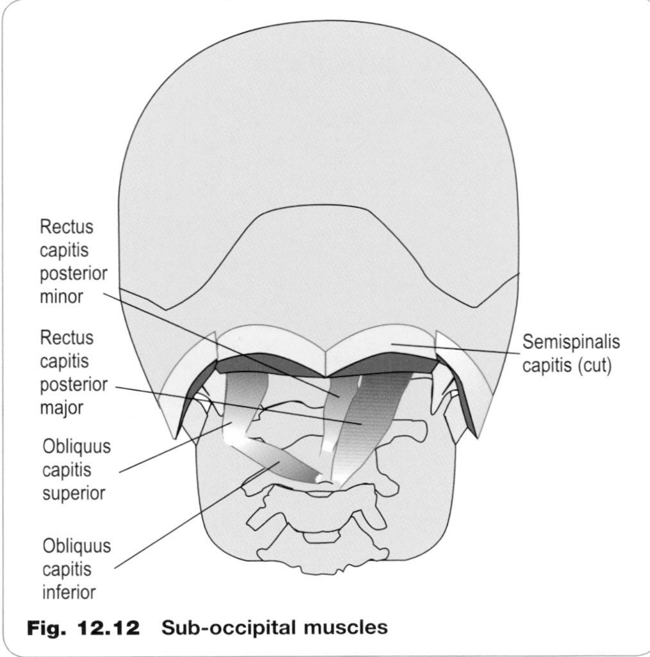

Fig. 12.12 Sub-occipital muscles

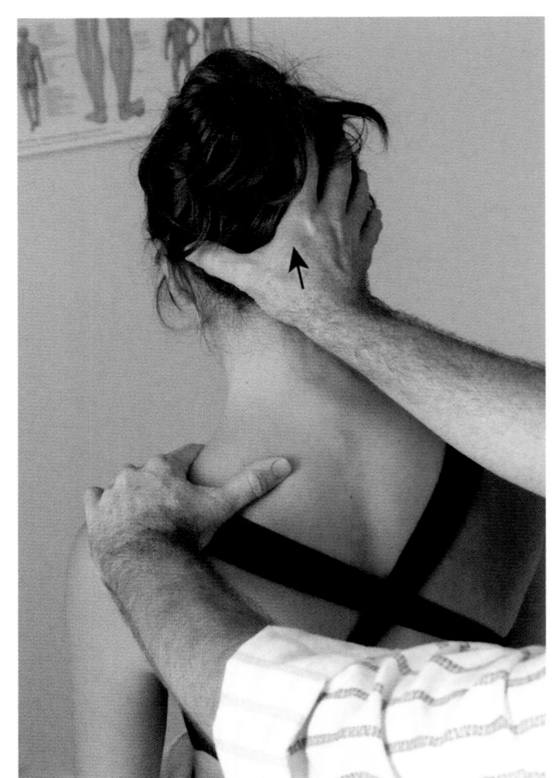

Fig. 12.13 Resisted test for posterolateral neck extensors

5. POSTERIOR CERVICAL MUSCLES

Resisted test

The posterior cervical muscles (i.e. splenius capitis and cervicis, longus colli and capitis, iliocostalis cervicis, longissimus cervicis and capitis, spinalis cervicis and capitis, semispinalis cervicis and capitis, and multifidus) are not distinguishable on resisted tests. Resisted posterolateral neck extension tests splenius capitis and cervicis, semispinalis capitis and cervicis and cervical erector spinae muscles (see Figure 12.13). Note upper trapezius, also a posterolateral neck extensor, is distinguished by turning the client's face away from the side being tested.[9] Palpation may also distinguish individual muscles (e.g. upper trapezius is superficial; fibres of splenius capitis and cervicis are diagonal compared to the more vertical fibres of the erector spinae).

Length test

Contractures of posterior cervical muscles could limit neck flexion and contralateral lateral flexion or rotation.

Clinical significance

Shortened posterior cervical muscles are commonly observed in upper crossed syndrome and may be implicated in cervicogenic headache.

6. SCALENE GROUP

Resisted test

The scalene muscles are difficult to isolate by resisted test. They are generally tested by resisting ipsilateral lateral flexion (± contralateral rotation) (see Figure 12.14). Anterior scalenus also flexes the neck and can be tested by resisting anterolateral neck flexion although this also tests sternocleidomastoid.

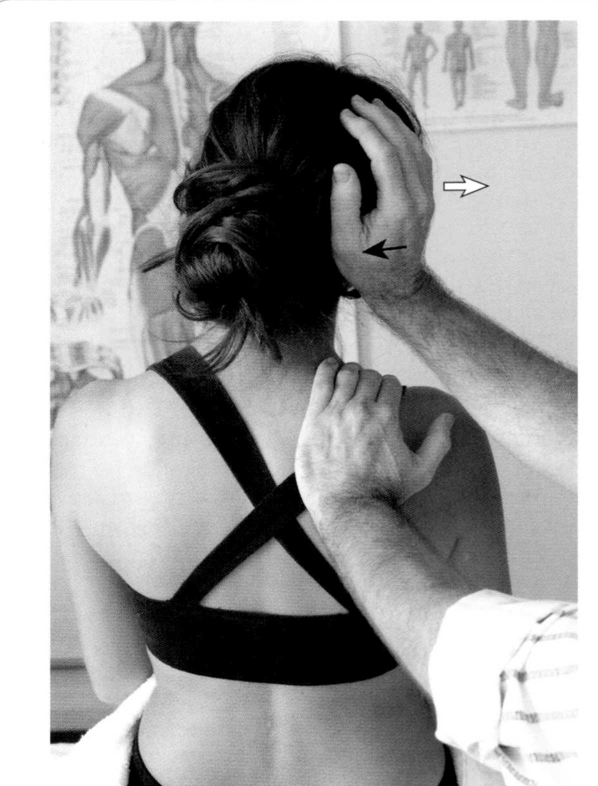

Fig. 12.14 Resisted test for scalene muscles

Length test

Clients with contracture of one or more of the scalene muscles will have limited contralateral lateral flexion and ipsilateral rotation of the neck.

e) Special tests

Special tests are designed to reproduce the client's pain and/or other symptoms. They are always performed within the client's pain tolerance and stopped as soon as symptoms appear. If symptoms are experienced while performing a special test, ask the client for the exact location of the symptom and confirm that it is the same symptom described in the case history.

CERVICAL COMPRESSION

With the client seated, interlock your fingers or place one hand over the other on top of the client's head and slowly and gently apply downward pressure (see Figure 12.15). (Stop immediately the onset or aggravation of symptoms is reported.) Pain may be felt locally or referred to the upper extremity according to the neurological level of the pathology. A positive compression test could indicate narrowing of the intervertebral foramen and nerve root compression or facet joint lesion.

CERVICAL DISTRACTION

Stand behind the seated client and cup the occiput in the palms under the mastoid processes, fingers pointing superiorly. Vertical traction is applied by slowly and gently lifting the head towards the ceiling (see Figure 12.16). A positive distraction test indicates ligamentous damage (e.g. after whiplash injury or facet joint sprain). Distraction may also relieve pressure on a nerve root or facet joint. (Note: avoid covering hearing aids with palms. Earrings should be removed.)

VALSALVA

Ask clients if they experience pain or symptoms when they cough, sneeze or laugh. Alternatively, ask clients to hold their breath and bear down. Valsalva raises intrathecal pressure and may elicit local or referred pain for a particular neurological level if a space-occupying lesion such as a herniated disc or tumour is present in the canal. (Note: Valsalva is not recommended for clients with uncontrolled or acute hypertension or with diabetics with potential retinopathy.)

Note: The Canadian C-spine Rule (see Figure 12.4) and the NEXUS Low-Risk criteria have been consistently shown to be superior to clinical examination.[10] They are simple guidelines for determining clients requiring referral.

NEXUS LOW-RISK CRITERIA

Cervical spine radiography is indicated for patients with trauma unless they meet all of the following criteria:

1. No posterior midline cervical spine tenderness
2. No evidence of intoxication
3. Normal level of alertness
4. No focal neurological deficit
5. No painful distracting injuries

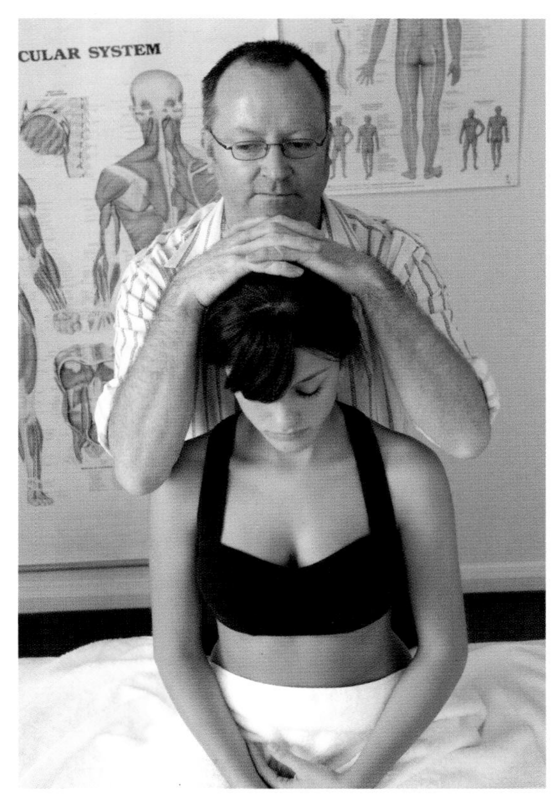

Fig. 12.15 Cervical compression test

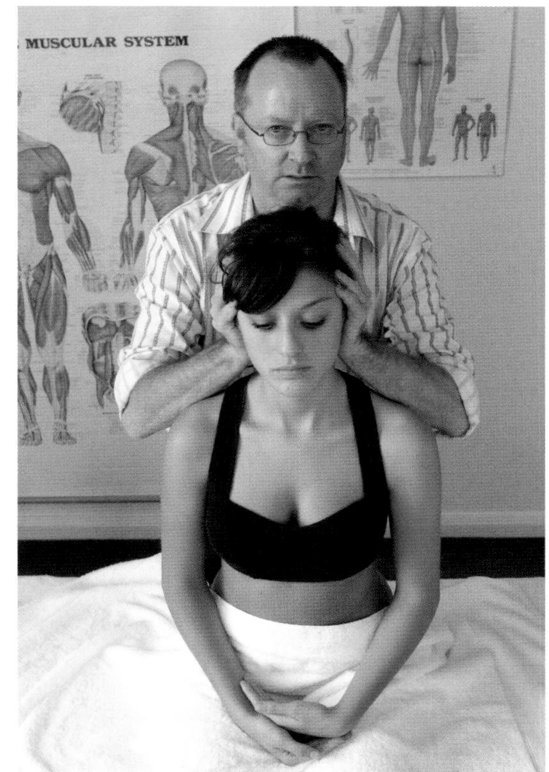

Fig. 12.16 Cervical distraction test

PALPATION

Pain produced on palpation helps confirm the location of the lesion and determine the type of tissue(s) involved. The neck is best palpated with the client supine or prone to relax the cervical musculature.

Prone

Palpate the mastoid processes, superior nuchal line and external occipital protuberance of the occiput. The spinous processes of C2–C7 are palpable in the midline. C7 and T1 spinous processes are larger than the others. C1 transverse processes are palpable inferior and slightly anterior to the mastoid processes. Transverse processes of C2–C7 are palpable if the neck muscles are relaxed. Facet joints, which lie about 2.5 cm from the midline, are sometimes palpable under the trapezius and paraspinal muscles.

Trace the upper trapezius muscle from its proximal attachments to its insertion at the acromion. Palpate the levator scapulae attachment at the superomedial aspect of the scapula under the trapezius muscle. Trace the muscle fibres from the scapula to the transverse processes of C1–C4. Palpate the paraspinal muscles in the space between the spinous and transverse processes.

Supine

The sternocleidomastoid attaches with the trapezius across the base of the occiput to the mastoid processes. With the client supine and head turned to the opposite side, the muscle is easily palpated. A chain of lymph nodes lies along the medial border of the sternocleidomastoid. Lymph nodes are usually not palpable unless they become enlarged and tender (e.g. if the client has an upper respiratory tract infection). The carotid pulse can be palpated in the carotid artery on the anterior border of the sternocleidomastoid muscle above the hyoid bone and lateral to the thyroid cartilage. (Caution: do not palpate both carotid pulses at the same time.) Parotid glands partially cover the angles of the mandible. They are normally only palpable when they are swollen.

With the client supine, use the fingertips of both hands to palpate the spinous processes of C2–C7 in the midline. Palpate the deep posterior cervical muscles and note the diagonal fibres of splenius capitis and cervicis. Palpate multifidi from the articular processes of the last four cervical vertebrae to the spinous processes of the vertebrae two to four levels above. Turn the head slightly to palpate the suboccipital muscles between the inferior nuchal line and the C1 transverse process and spinous processes of C1 and C2.

REMEDIAL MASSAGE TREATMENT

Assessment of the cervical region provides essential information for development and negotiation of treatment plans, including:

- client's suitability for remedial massage therapy
- duration of the condition (i.e. acute or chronic)
- severity of the condition (i.e. grade of injury; mild, moderate or severe pain)
- type(s) of tissues involved
- priorities for treatment if more than one injury or condition is present
- whether the signs and symptoms suggest a common condition of the cervical region
- special considerations for individual clients (e.g. client's preference for treatment types and styles, special population considerations).

Treatment options must always be considered in the context of the best available evidence for treatment effectiveness and clinical practice guidelines where they exist. Findings of current research are summarised in Table 12.3.

A systematic review of manual therapies (including spinal manipulation, mobilisation and non-manipulative manual therapy but excluding trigger points and manual traction) found moderate- to high-quality evidence that subjects with chronic uncomplicated neck pain of mechanical origin showed clinically important improvement from spinal manipulation at 6, 12 and up to 104 weeks post treatment. However, the current evidence did not support the same level of benefit from massage.[11] A further systematic review by Haraldsson et al[12] was also unable to draw a conclusion about the effectiveness of massage for improving neck pain because of the wide range of massage techniques and comparison treatments used, and the variability of quality of the 19 trials in the review. Clearly there is an urgent need for more high-quality studies into the effectiveness of massage therapy to support its wide public use.[13]

Table 12.3 Summary of evidence for the effectiveness of treatments for acute neck pain[3]

Evidence of effectiveness	• Advice to stay active • Gentle neck exercises introduced early after injury • Exercises performed at home are as effective as tailored outpatient programs
Insufficient evidence (more research is needed)	• Acupuncture • Opioids • Insufficient evidence that paracetamol is more effective than placebo, natural history or other measures for acute neck pain • Cervical manipulation • Cervical passive mobilisation • Electrotherapy • Gymnastics • Regular breaks from computer work compared to irregular breaks • Multidisciplinary treatment • Muscle relaxants • Neck school • Non-steroidal anti-inflammatory drugs (NSAIDs) • Patient education • Spray and stretch therapy • Traction • TENS
Evidence of no benefit	• Soft collars

MUSCLE STRAIN

Muscle strains (*pulled muscles*) can occur from traumas including falls, motor vehicle accidents and sports injuries. They are usually the result of extreme stretching that causes myofibrils to tear. Strains also occur from overuse, fatigue and repetitive microtrauma; for instance when the neck is held in an awkward position for long periods. Exposure to a draught has also been implicated. Pain is associated with activity and relieved by rest.

Assessment

HISTORY

The client complains of neck pain after a fall, motor vehicle accident or sports injury or after holding the neck in an awkward position for a long time (e.g. holding a telephone between neck and shoulder, reading in bed, falling asleep in an awkward position, straining to read a monitor). Pain can be experienced immediately or within the next 24–48 hours (delayed onset muscle soreness). Pain is associated with activity and generally relieved with rest.

POSTURAL ANALYSIS

The neck may be held in an antalgic position and movements may be guarded.

FUNCTIONAL TESTS

AROM: limited in one or more directions.
PROM: mild to no pain except at end of range when the muscle is passively stretched.
RROM: painful.
Resisted and length tests positive for involved muscles.
Special tests: negative.

PALPATION

Muscle spasm is usually evident. The client reports tenderness or pain on palpation of the affected muscle.

Overview of treatment of muscle strains

A typical remedial massage treatment for mild to moderate muscle strains of the neck includes:

- Swedish massage to the neck, upper back, shoulders, head (± chest).
- Remedial techniques including:
  - deep gliding frictions along the muscle fibres
  - cross-fibre frictions
  - soft tissue releasing techniques
  - deep transverse friction at the site of muscle injury
  - heat therapy (see Chapter 3)
  - trigger point therapy (see Chapter 6).
    (A range of remedial massage techniques for muscles of the cervical region are illustrated in Table 12.4.)
- Myofascial release (see Chapter 8).

Address any underlying conditions or predisposing factors (e.g. scoliosis or thoracic hyperkyphosis).

CLIENT EDUCATION

Advise clients to avoid aggravating activities. For example, using a headset will leave the client's hands free for other tasks when talking on the phone. Clients should avoid sleeping in the prone position. Pillows should support the neck without distorting the normal lordotic cervical curve.

Home exercise program

A program of progressive rehabilitation should accompany remedial massage treatment. Aim for maximum strength and full length of all major muscles. Unresolved strains can contribute to recurrence and to the development of compensatory muscle imbalance. Introduce stretching exercises as soon as possible and progress to isometric exercises within the client's pain tolerance. Clients may be referred for spinal manipulation.

Key assessment findings for muscle strain

- History of trauma or prolonged awkward position
- Functional tests
  - AROM positive in one or more directions
  - PROM may be positive at end of range due to passive muscle stretching
  - RROM positive for affected muscle(s)
  - Resisted and length tests positive for affected muscle(s)
- Palpation elicits pain; spasm ± myofibril tears palpable

NON-SPECIFIC NECK PAIN (INCLUDING CERVICAL SPRAIN, STRAIN AND VERTEBRAL SUBLUXATION)

Non-specific neck pain may arise from minor trauma, unaccustomed exercise, sudden unguarded movement or overuse and is associated with muscle strain, ligament sprain and facet syndrome. Facet syndrome is the term used to describe any injury or condition affecting the cervical facet joints (zygapophyseal joints). It can refer pain to the cranium, cervical spine, shoulder and upper back. It is estimated that cervical facet involvement could occur in 26–65% of neck pain complaints.[2] Non-specific neck pain can resolve spontaneously in days or weeks.

Assessment

HISTORY

Clients are usually young adults who complain of pain, stiffness and limited range of motion following trauma, overuse,

Key assessment findings for non-specific neck pain

- Client is usually a young adult; history of trauma or repetitive overuse
- Functional tests:
  - AROM positive in one or more directions
  - PROM positive if facet joints involved
  - RROM positive if muscle strain involved
  - Resisted tests and muscle length tests may be positive for affected muscles
  - Special tests usually negative
- Palpation positive for tenderness ± pain at site of strain, sprain or subluxation

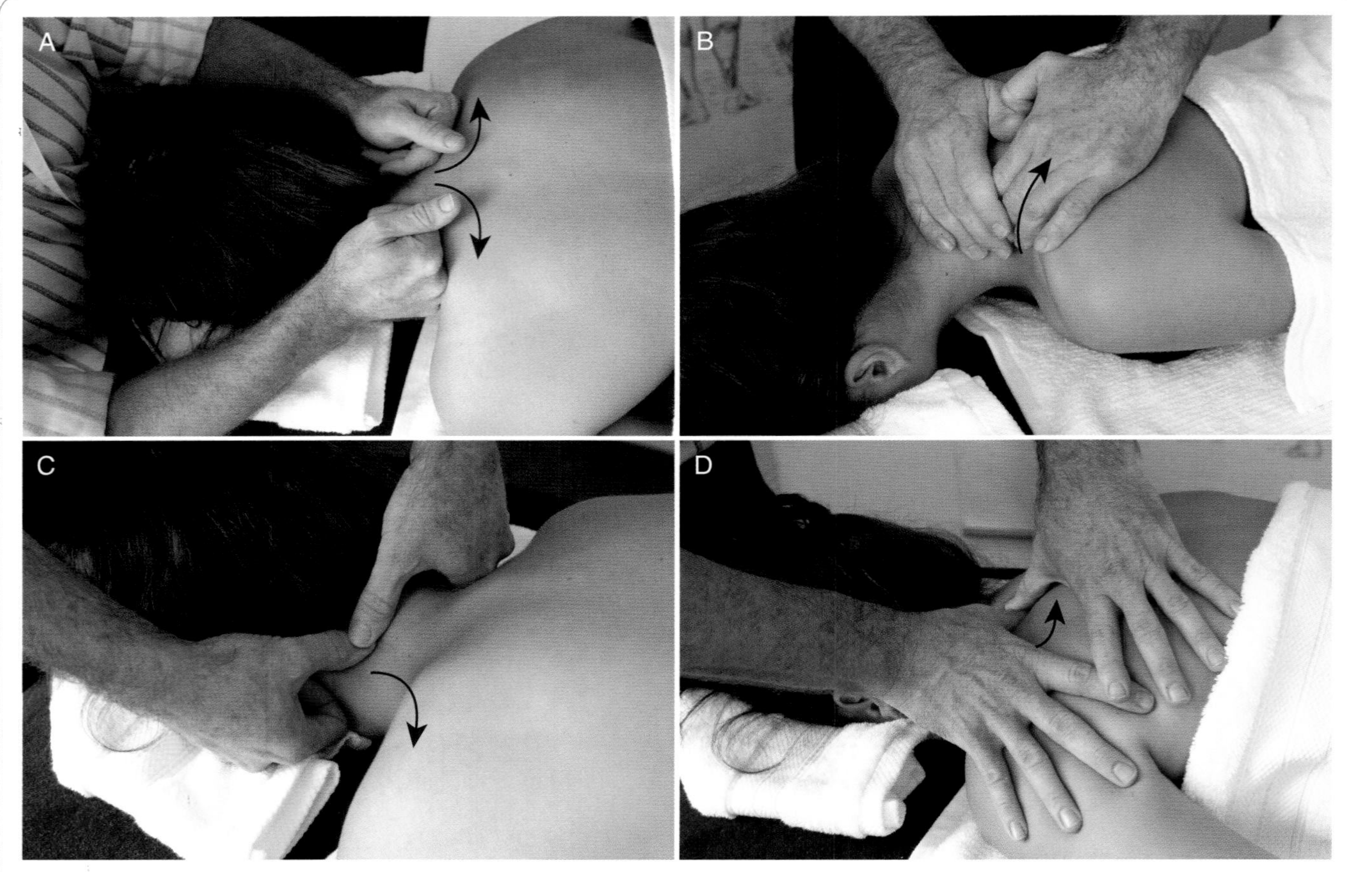

Fig. 12.17 Upper trapezius (A) deep gliding, (B) cross-fibre frictions; levator scapulae (C) deep gliding, (D) cross-fibre frictions

fatigue or repetitive microtrauma over hours or days. The pain is usually localised, although an upper cervical lesion may produce headache and lower cervical lesion may radiate pain to the shoulder or upper back. There is usually no neurological involvement.

FUNCTIONAL TESTS

AROM: limited and painful in one or more directions (pain in one direction suggests muscle strain; pain in many directions suggests joint capsule injury or a combination of muscle and joint injury).[2] Increased pain on extension and rotation suggests facet syndrome.

PROM: may be limited and painful if facet joints, ligaments or joint capsule involved. Increased pain on extension suggests facet joint involvement. (Note that ligament sprains are uncommon.)

RROM: may be positive if muscles have been strained.

Resisted and length tests may be positive if muscles have been strained.

Resisted and length tests usually indicate muscle strain.

Special tests are usually negative although cervical compression can produce local pain.

PALPATION

Local tenderness is often reported at the site of injury. Muscle spasm is palpable and occasionally local swelling is present.

Differential diagnosis

Rule out cervical disc syndrome and cervical radiculopathy by history and functional tests. Reports of weakness, numbness, tingling, burning or arm pain have generally been found to be unhelpful in identifying cervical radiculopathy. The most useful diagnostic symptoms for cervical radiculopathy appear to be those that are most bothersome in the scapular area, and those that improve with neck movement.[10]

Overview of treatment and management

A typical remedial massage treatment for mild or moderate non-specific neck pain includes:

- Swedish massage therapy to the neck, upper back, shoulder and head (± chest).
- Remedial massage techniques depending on the type of tissue(s) involved. For example, remedial massage therapy for muscle tissue injury/muscle imbalances could include (see Table 12.4):
  - deep gliding frictions along the muscle fibres (see Figure 12.17)
  - cross-fibre frictions (see Figure 12.17)
  - active and passive soft tissue releasing techniques
  - deep transverse friction
  - trigger point therapy
  - muscle stretches.

Table 12.4 Remedial massage techniques for muscles of the cervical region

Muscle	Soft tissue release	Trigger point	Stretch	Client education[5]	Home stretch
Upper trapezius	Passive: the client lies supine. Cup the occiput in one hand. Using knuckles, fingers or thumb of the other hand glide from occiput to acromion as the client's head is laterally flexed with the other hand. Active: The client is seated and the practitioner uses a pincer grip to hold the upper trapezius muscle between the acromion and C7. Maintaining this contact, ask the client to take their head slowly towards their shoulder. 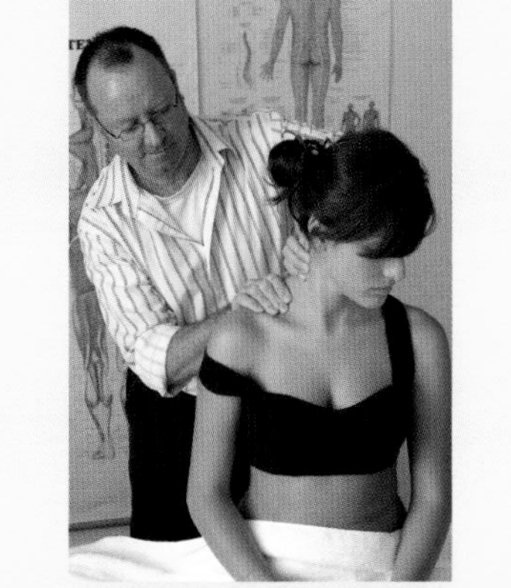	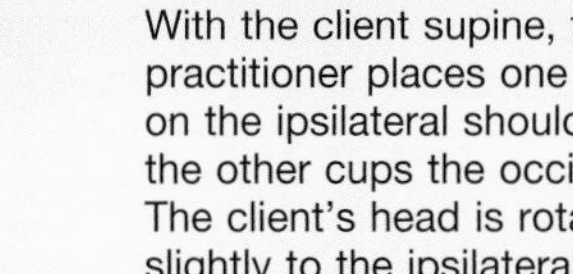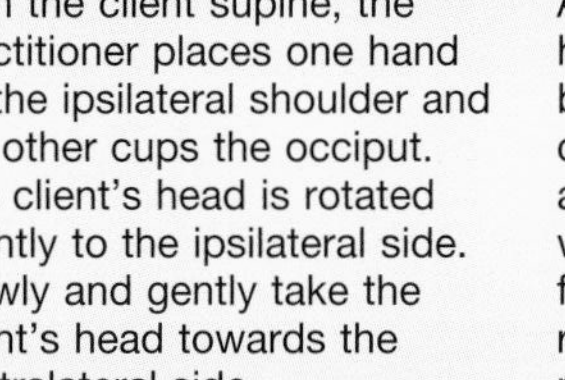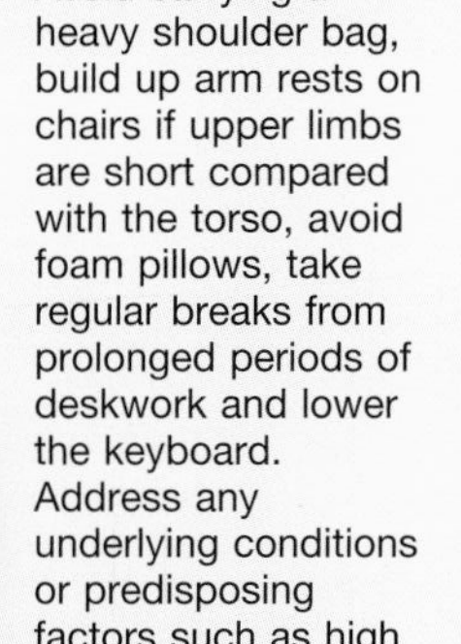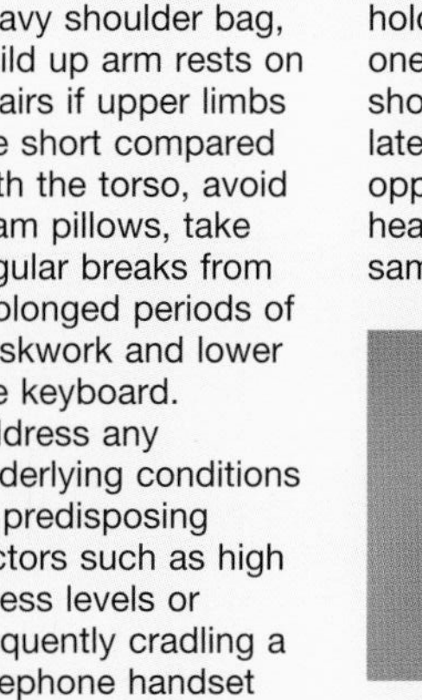	With the client supine, the practitioner places one hand on the ipsilateral shoulder and the other cups the occiput. The client's head is rotated slightly to the ipsilateral side. Slowly and gently take the client's head towards the contralateral side. 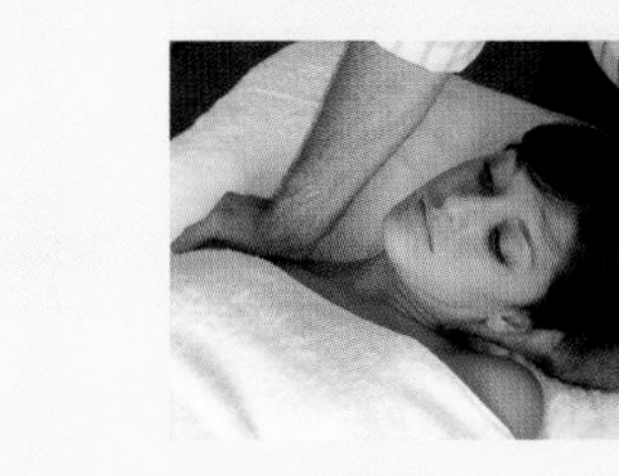	Avoid carrying a heavy shoulder bag, build up arm rests on chairs if upper limbs are short compared with the torso, avoid foam pillows, take regular breaks from prolonged periods of deskwork and lower the keyboard. Address any underlying conditions or predisposing factors such as high stress levels or frequently cradling a telephone handset between the ear and shoulder.	The client sits in a chair and holds the side of the seat with one hand to anchor the shoulder. Next the client laterally flexes their neck to the opposite side and rotates their head towards the same side. 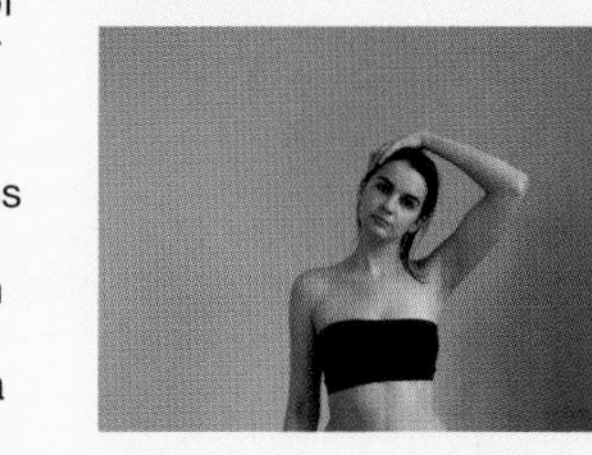
Sternocleidomastoid	A number of variations are possible, including the following passive release: The client is supine. Cup the occiput with the contralateral hand. The fingers of the other hand contact the ipsilateral sternocleidomastoid. Glide down the muscle as the head is laterally flexed with the other hand. 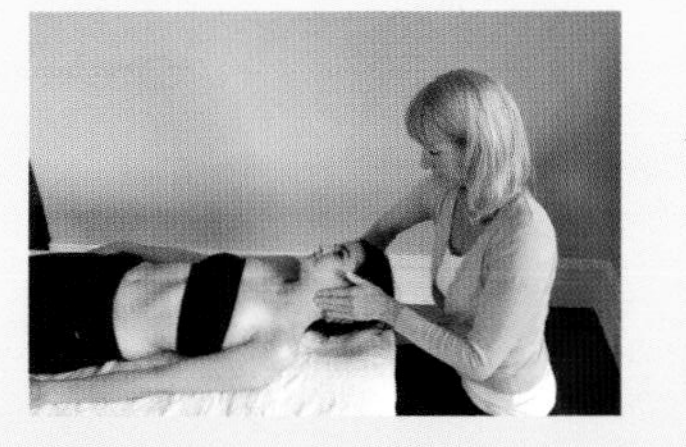	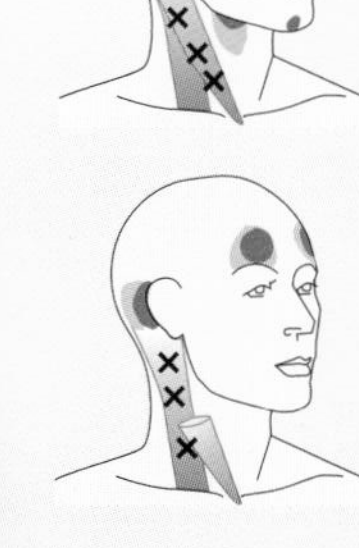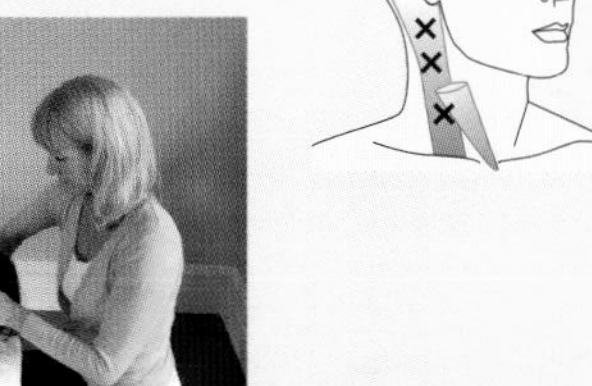	With the client supine or seated, gently laterally flex their neck to the opposite side or rotate their neck to the same side. 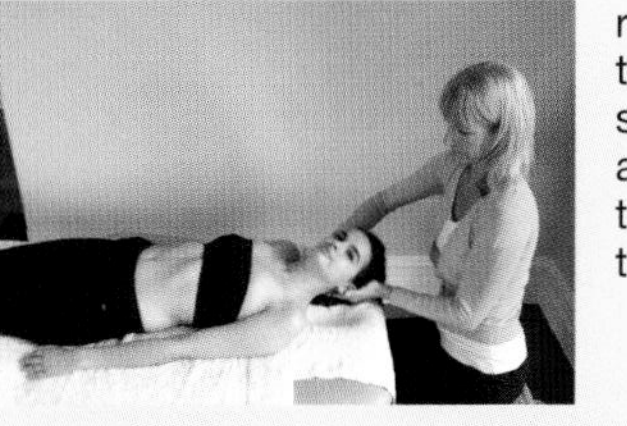	Avoid prolonged neck flexion, use a lumbar support to correct slumping in a chair with head forward, avoid lying in bed reading with the head turned towards one side, use a headset to avoid tilting the head to one side to a telephone receiver.	Laterally flexing away from the affected muscle or rotating the neck towards it will stretch the sternocleidomastoid muscle. 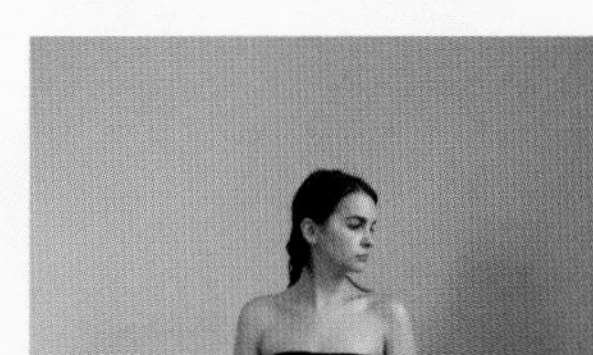

Continued

Table 12.4 Remedial massage techniques for muscles of the cervical region—cont'd

Muscle	Soft tissue release	Trigger point	Stretch	Client education[5]	Home stretch
Levator scapulae	A number of variations can be performed including the following: The practitioner stands behind the seated client and holds the scapula attachment of the muscle as the client slowly moves their head towards their opposite axilla. 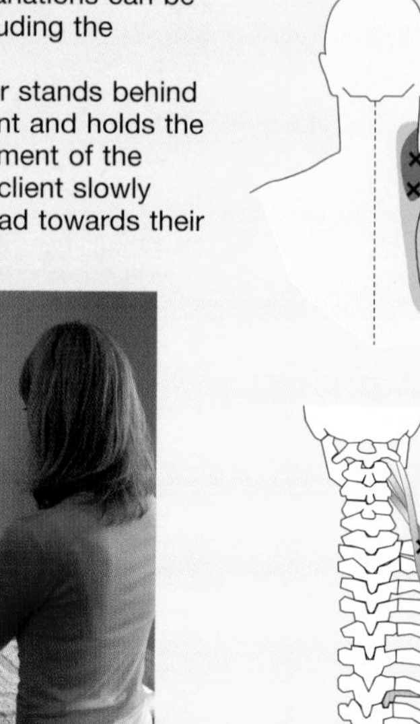	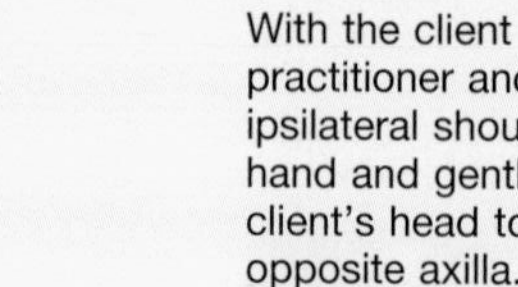 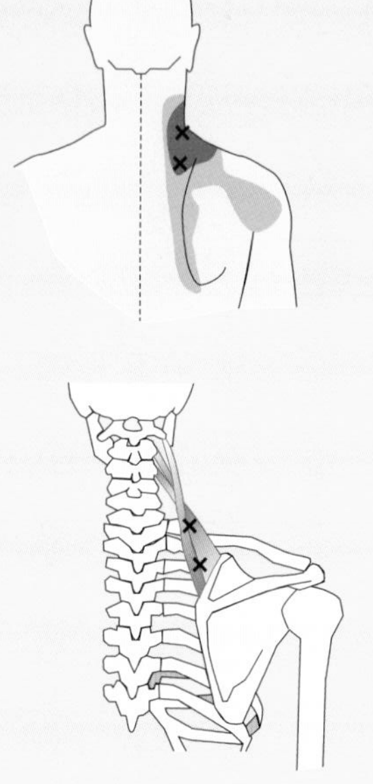	With the client supine, the practitioner anchors the ipsilateral shoulder with one hand and gently takes the client's head towards the opposite axilla. 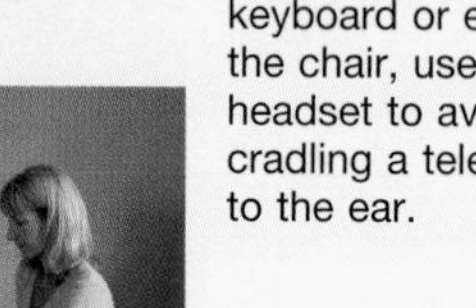	Use a document or book stand when reading to reduce neck flexion, for deskwork lower the keyboard or elevate the chair, use a headset to avoid cradling a telephone to the ear.	The client sits, holding the bottom of the seat of the chair or sitting on their hand to stabilise the shoulder. The muscle is stretched by contralateral lateral flexion and ipsilateral rotation of the neck (i.e. the client takes their head towards the axilla on the unaffected side). 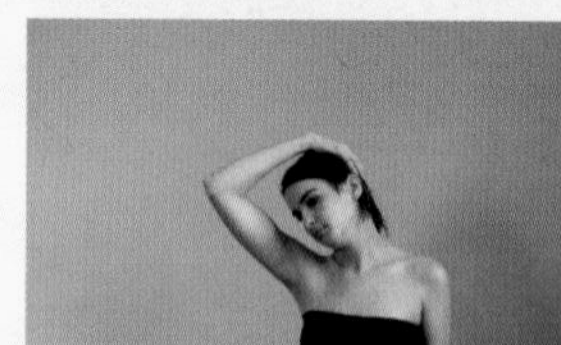
Suboccipital muscles	A number of variations can be performed, including the following: With the client seated, the practitioner places both thumbs under the occiput and instructs the client to slowly flex and extend their head. Repeat with thumbs at different positions under the occiput. 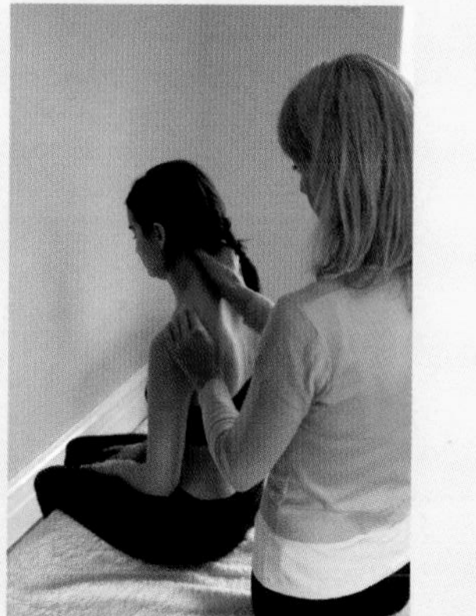		With the client seated or supine, gently flex their neck. Contralateral rotation can also be used to stretch the more diagonal muscles. 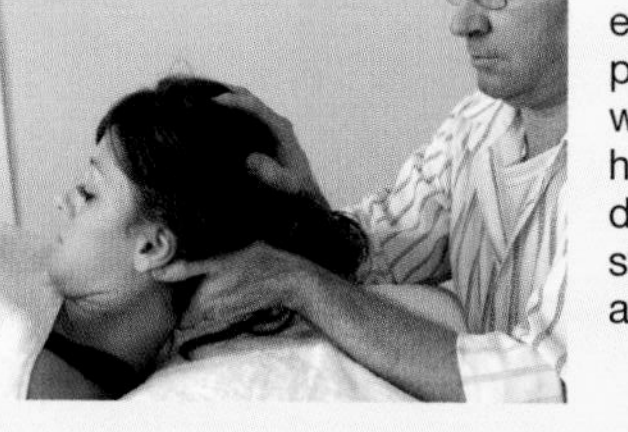	Avoid forward head posture, keep the neck warm (e.g. wearing scarves or jackets with hoods), avoid prolonged neck extension (e.g. painting a ceiling, working under a hoist), using a document or book stand when working at a desk.	The client interlocks their fingers behind the head and gently pulls their head forward towards the chest. 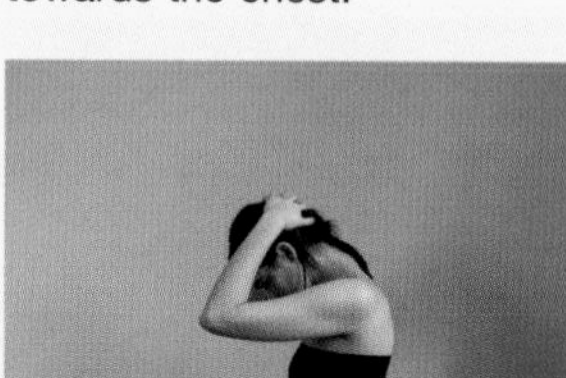

Table 12.4 Remedial massage techniques for muscles of the cervical region—cont'd

Muscle	Soft tissue release	Trigger point	Stretch	Client education[5]	Home stretch
Posterior cervical muscles	A number of variants can be performed, including the following: The client lies supine. Facing the client, spread the fingers of one hand on the paraspinal muscles between the transverse and spinous processes of C1 to C7 on the contralateral side. Either passively or actively, the client's head is rotated across the finger contacts.		The posterior cervical muscles can be stretched by flexing the head and neck. The client can be seated or supine. For the supine stretch the practitioner crosses their arms under the client's head and places their hands on the client's shoulders. The client's head is gently flexed when the practitioner slowly raises their crossed arms. Ensure that the head and neck are controlled at all times during the stretch.	Avoid prolonged neck flexion, use a document or book stand when reading to reduce neck flexion, for deskwork elevate the monitor, sit upright on an exercise bike (i.e. avoid holding low handle bars), use a lumbar support when sitting to improve head and neck posture.	The client interlocks their fingers behind the head and gently pulls their head forward towards the chest.

Continued

Table 12.4 Remedial massage techniques for muscles of the cervical region—cont'd

Muscle	Soft tissue release	Trigger point	Stretch	Client education[5]	Home stretch
Scalene muscles	A number of variations can be performed including the following: With the client seated, the practitioner uses fingers, thumb or knuckle along the scalene as the client laterally flexes their neck to the opposite side. 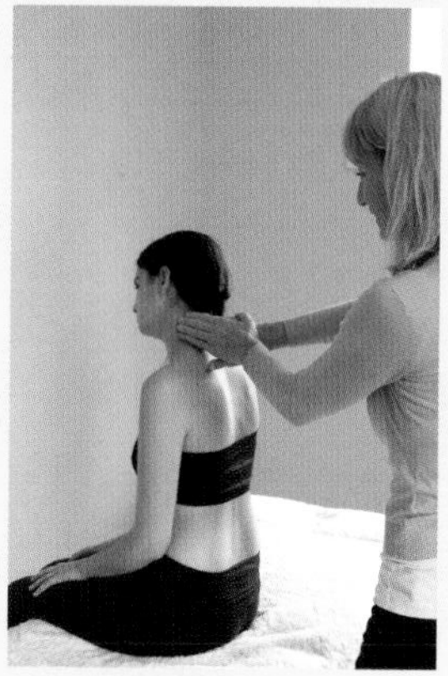	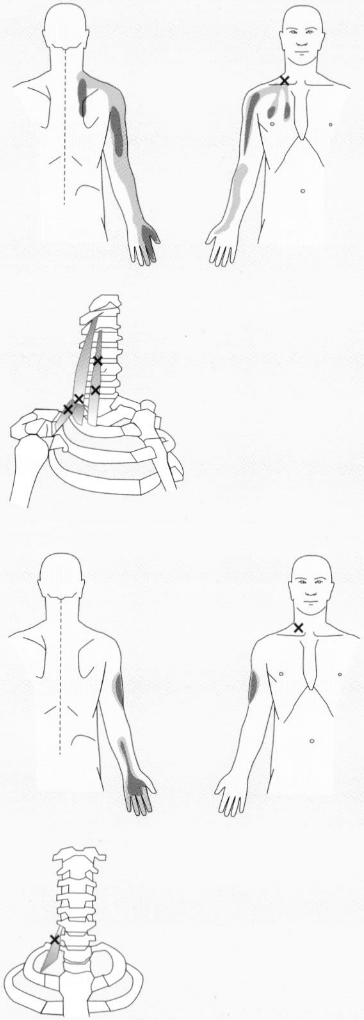	With the client seated or supine, gently laterally flex their neck. From this position gently rotate their head towards or away from the affected side. 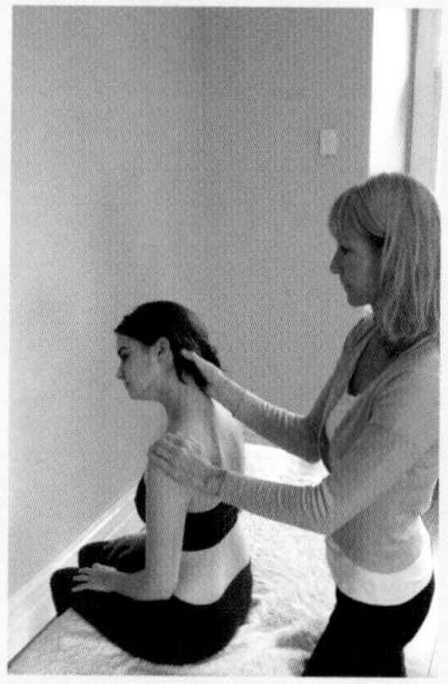	Keep the neck warm, use a supportive pillow when sleeping, use elbow rests when seated and use a hands-free telephone or a headset.	The client laterally flexes their neck to their comfortable limit and holding that position turns their head to look downwards or upwards 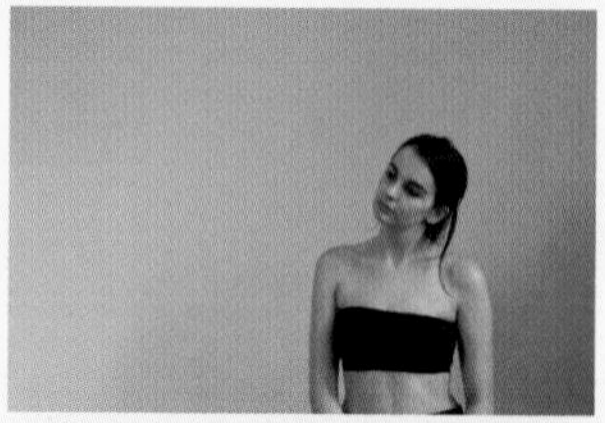 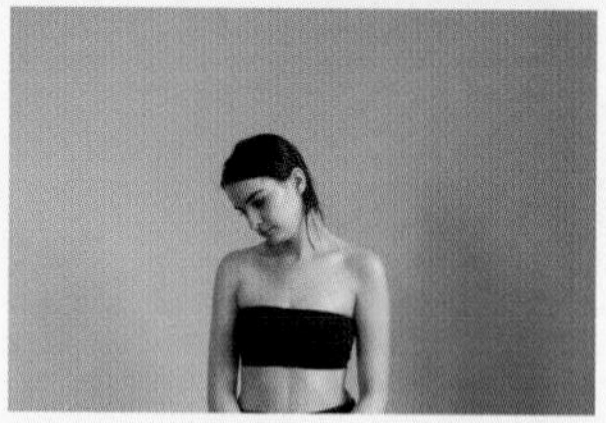

- Use myofascial releasing techniques for myofascial restrictions.
- Thermotherapy may be beneficial.

For facet joint lesions passive joint articulation for the cervical spine and deep multifidus work may be beneficial. Joint articulations include cervical lateral flexion, rotation, extension, horizontal traction, stair-step, facet rotation and facet lateral flexion (see Chapter 7). (Note: if ligament sprain is involved cervical distraction is contraindicated.)

MUTIFIDUS RELEASE

With the client lying supine, sit at the head of the table. Place fingertips of both hands either side of the spine between the spinous process and transverse processes of C6 or C7. Apply anterior pressure to contact the multifidus muscles in the deepest muscle layer. Maintain the pressure and apply small frictions (about 1 cm) along the line of the fibres and then across the fibres for several seconds. Release the pressure and move to the vertebra above. Repeat the frictions, working the multifidus muscles at each level up the cervical spine. Muscle spasm is palpable around the subluxated facet joints and is often tender. Always work within the client's pain tolerance (see Figure 12.18).

CLIENT EDUCATION

Advise clients about cervical posture including the importance of thoracolumbar posture. Advise clients about lumbar supports, and ways to improve the ergonomics of work stations and activities of daily living including using supportive pillows. Pillows placed behind the neck (not only behind the head) support the cervical spine. Pillows should be malleable enough to take the weight of the head without distorting the normal lordotic cervical spine. Alternatively, a rolled towel may be placed behind the neck and its height adjusted until the position is comfortable. If neck pain is the result of unaccustomed activity advise the client of the importance of a regular fitness program to prepare for sports or demanding physical work. Clients may benefit from referral to a chiropractor, osteopath or physiotherapist for spinal manipulation.

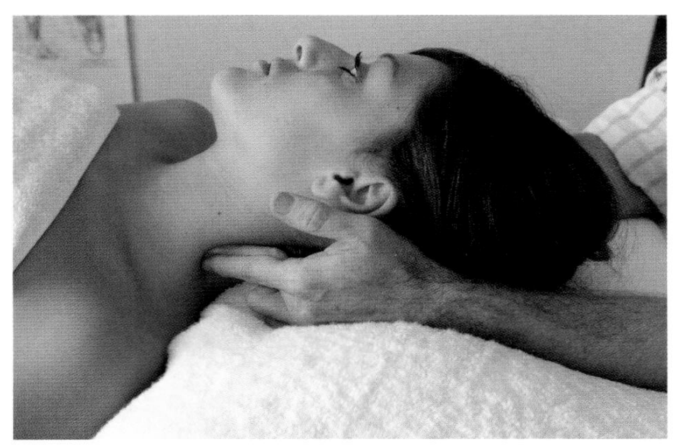

Fig. 12.18 Multifidus release

Home exercise program

Home exercises usually begin by stretching the affected muscles within pain tolerance. As function returns muscle strengthening exercises are progressively introduced as required.

DEGENERATIVE JOINT DISEASE (OSTEOARTHRITIS/DEGENERATIVE ARTHRITIS)

Degenerative joint disease (DJD) is a non-inflammatory disease characterised by progressive loss of articular cartilage and its related components.[14] DJD is the most common form of joint disease and in the cervical spine most commonly affects C5–C6. It may be the result of sustained muscle spasm, vertebral subluxation, injuries and overuse. Clients are usually over 50 years old or have a history of a previous significant trauma such as a whiplash injury. X-rays show loss of disc height, loss or reversal of cervical lordosis, osteophytes and subchondral bone/endplate sclerosis (see Figure 12.19). However, 45% of radiographic evidence of DJD is found in asymptomatic adults. Neurological symptoms may occur especially in arms and hands.

Assessment

HISTORY

Clients are usually over 50 years old or have a history of a previous significant trauma. Typically clients report a recurrent dull ache in the neck that developed slowly or after a

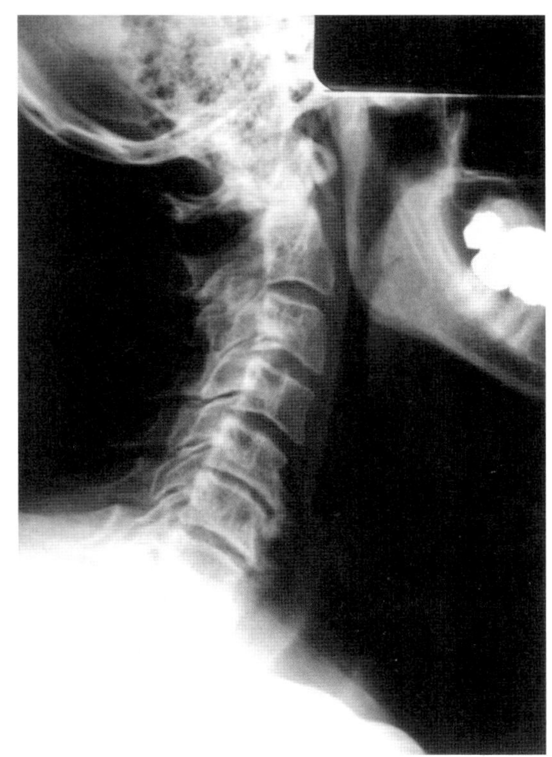

Fig. 12.19 Radiograph of cervical degenerative joint disease

Key assessment findings for DJD

- Client is usually over 50; history of dull, aching pain that worsens with activity and improves with rest, morning stiffness
- Functional tests:
  - AROM tests positive
  - PROM tests positive (capsular pattern)
  - RROM tests usually negative
  - Special tests may be positive (e.g. if DJD is associated with neural compression)
- Palpation positive for tenderness and hard end-feel. Fibrotic muscle may be palpable.

period of increased activity. Neck ache or pain is aggravated by repetitive use and relieved by rest. Morning stiffness is common.

FUNCTIONAL TESTS

AROM: limitation ± pain in some directions.
PROM: limitation ± pain on lateral flexion and rotation, and then extension (capsular pattern).
RROM: negative unless there is associated muscle strain.
Special tests are usually within normal limits unless spinal canal stenosis or disc degeneration is present.

PALPATION

Palpation may elicit tenderness or pain at the affected site. Fibrotic muscle tissue is a common accompaniment. Crepitus and hard end-feel may be present.

Differential diagnosis

Neck pain (± neurological symptoms) increasing on flexion suggests disc herniation or damage; pain increasing on extension could suggest facet involvement or IVF encroachment.

Overview of treatment and management

Successful management depends on finding a balance between activity and rest. Too much activity may inflame the joints; too little may lead to muscle contractures, fibrosis and stiffness. It is also likely that increasing thoracic mobility is important in the management of cervical conditions, including DJD.

A typical remedial massage treatment for cervical DJD includes:

- Swedish massage therapy to the neck, upper and mid back, shoulders, head (± chest).
- Remedial massage therapy. The range of remedial massage techniques and their application will be determined by assessment results (i.e. use the See-Move-Touch principle described in Chapter 2). The most important remedial techniques for DJD are joint articulation, heat therapy and myofascial release.
- Joint articulation (see Chapter 7): Cervical horizontal traction may be beneficial. Other cervical stretches are indicated but should be performed with caution (especially with side bending, flexion and diagonal flexion).

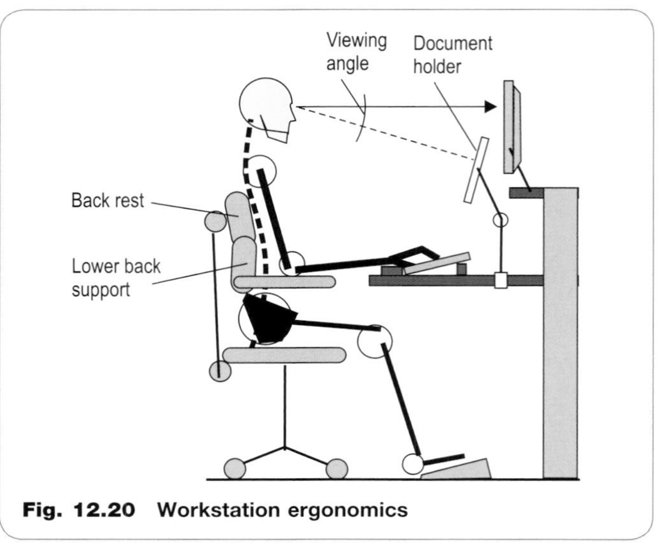

Fig. 12.20 Workstation ergonomics

- Muscle techniques: If tolerated by the client, remedial massage therapy for chronic muscle contracture or fibrositis could include (see Table 12.4):
  - deep gliding frictions along the muscle fibres
  - cross-fibre frictions
  - active and passive soft tissue releasing techniques
  - deep transverse friction
  - trigger point therapy
  - muscle stretches.

CLIENT EDUCATION

Advise clients about neck posture, including using a supportive pillow and mattress. Good ergonomics at work will help prevent repetitive overload of muscles and joints. Desk workers should check the height of their chairs, desks, keyboards and monitors as even small stresses may become significant if sustained for prolonged periods (see Figure 12.20). Glucosamine and other dietary supplements may be beneficial for people with DJD.[15] Advise clients of the importance of shock-absorbing soles to avoid jarring impacts that can be transmitted to the neck when walking. Referral to a chiropractor, osteopath or manipulative physiotherapist may result in an improvement in joint mobility and relieve pain.

Home exercise program

Begin with pain-free range of motion exercises and progressively introduce full-length sustained stretches and pain-free isometric exercises. It is best to exercise after the area has been warmed (e.g. after a warm shower or hot pack).

UPPER CROSSED SYNDROME

A common pattern of muscle imbalance and adaptation which is characterised by forward head carriage, rounded shoulders and hyperextension at the occiput and C1/2 is referred to as upper crossed syndrome. Typically, pectoralis major and minor, upper trapezius, levator scapulae and sternocleidomastoids tighten and shorten, and lower and middle trapezius, serratus anterior and rhomboids tend to weaken (see Figure 12.21 on p 219).[16]

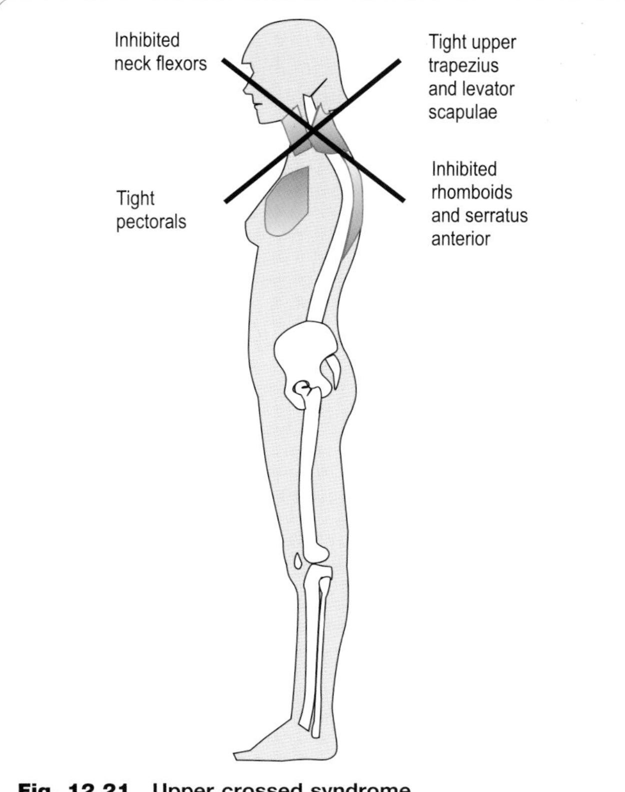

Fig. 12.21 Upper crossed syndrome

Key assessment findings for upper crossed syndrome

- History can include repetitive activity, poorly rehabilitated previous injury, prolonged immobilisation. Pain in the neck and upper back after prolonged sitting/working at a computer; pain relieved by lying down or arching upper thoracic spine backwards; usually no radiation of pain
- Postural analysis: Forward head posture, rounded shoulders and increased thoracic kyphosis
- Functional tests:
  - AROM limited ± painful
  - PROM usually negative
  - Resisted tests and length tests are positive for specific muscles including:
    - short pectoralis major and minor, upper trapezius, levator scapulae, sternocleidomastoid
    - weak lower and middle trapezius, serratus anterior and rhomboids
  - Special tests negative
- Palpation positive for tenderness ± pain at sites of mechanical overload (e.g. mid and upper thoracic spine, mid and upper cervical spine), contractures in affected muscles

Assessment

HISTORY

Clients with upper crossed syndrome often describe a dull aching pain in the neck and/or upper back. The pain is aggravated by prolonged periods of neck flexion such as working at a computer, reading or sewing. There is usually no radiation of pain and no neurological symptoms, although pain is sometimes reported in the chest, shoulders and arms. Respiratory function may also be compromised. The pain is often relieved by taking breaks from aggravating activities, lying down or extending their upper back.

POSTURAL ANALYSIS

The head is held forward of the centre of gravity line, often with the chin jutting up. Thoracic kyphosis may be exaggerated and the shoulders protracted.

FUNCTIONAL TESTS

AROM: limited ± pain in some ranges of motion (e.g. cervical extension, thoracic extension) may be observed.
PROM: may be limited by muscle shortness.
RROM: positive for affected muscles.
Specific muscle tests may indicate muscle shortness (e.g. pectoralis major and minor, upper trapezius, levator scapulae, sternocleidomastoid) and weakness (e.g. lower and middle trapezius, serratus anterior and rhomboids).
Special tests: usually negative

PALPATION

Muscle contractures are readily palpated. Pressure over areas of mechanical overload (such as the middle and upper cervical spine) may elicit tenderness or pain.

Differential diagnosis

Upper crossed syndrome is usually identified by its characteristic pattern of muscle imbalance and absence of pain radiation and neurological involvement. However, if accompanied by chest pain, underlying organic disease needs to be eliminated. All clients with neurological symptoms should be referred for further investigation.

Overview of treatment and management

Successful remedial massage treatment depends on identification and correction of muscle imbalances and client participation in corrective measures. In most cases lower and middle trapezius, serratus anterior and rhomboids will need to be strengthened in a home exercise program. Pectoralis major and minor, upper trapezius, levator scapulae and sternocleidomastoid muscles need to be stretched during treatment and at home.

A typical treatment for upper crossed syndrome includes:

- Swedish massage to the upper back, neck, chest, shoulders and head.
- Remedial massage therapy. The aim of remedial massage is to address muscle imbalances found during assessment. Tight muscles require stretching and specific muscle techniques including (see Table 12.4):
  - deep gliding frictions along the muscle fibres
  - cross-fibre frictions
  - active and passive soft tissue releasing techniques
  - deep transverse friction
  - trigger point therapy.
- Thermotherapy is usually beneficial.
- Myofascial releasing techniques are also indicated for myofascial restrictions (see Chapter 8).

- Joint articulation of cervical, and mid and upper thoracic spinal segments may be effective (see Chapter 7).

Address any underlying conditions or predisposing factors such as scoliosis or hypomobile thoracic spine. Refer any client with upper limb pain accompanied by other neurological symptoms for a full neurological assessment.

CLIENT EDUCATION

Posture advice is essential and includes avoidance of all postures and activities that cause the head to be held forward. Advise clients about lumbar supports, correct sitting posture and improving the ergonomics of the work area (see Figure 12.20 on p 218). Instruct clients to take regular breaks from activities that aggravate their condition. Clients often respond well to a corrective exercise program, but referral for osseous manipulation may be required.

Home exercise program

Muscle stretches performed during treatment (e.g. pectoralis major and minor, upper trapezius, levator scapulae and sternocleidomastoid) should be continued by the client at home (see Tables 12.5 and 14.3). A program to strengthen weak middle and lower trapezius, rhomboids and serratus anterior should be progressively introduced for long-term biomechanical improvements.

MECHANICAL/ACQUIRED TORTICOLLIS

Mechanical/acquired torticollis or wry neck is occasionally seen in remedial massage clinics. This is an acute episode of muscle spasm and vertebral subluxaton, generally brought on by sleeping face down with the neck sustained in flexion and rotation. Many cases resolve spontaneously in 7–10 days.

Assessment

HISTORY

The condition commonly affects people under the age of 30. The client reports sudden onset of severe neck pain which is easily localised and aggravated by movement, especially rotation to the side of injury. Typically, the client reports waking with acute neck pain and being unable to move their neck after sleeping face down. Other histories report onset following activities that involved prolonged cervical flexion and rotation, or after sleeping near an open window or in a room cooled by air conditioning.

Key assessment findings for mechanical/acquired torticollis

- The client is a young adult or child. History of acute neck pain following a prolonged period of cervical flexion and rotation. Typically onset on waking after sleeping in prone position. Pain usually aggravated by rotation to affected side. Usually no radiation of pain
- Posture adaptations to guard neck movement
- Functional tests (only performed within client's pain tolerance):
  - AROM: limited and painful, especially rotation to affected side
  - PROM: limited and painful, especially rotation to affected side
  - RROM: limited and painful, especially rotation to side of injury
  - Resisted tests and length tests positive for specific muscles, especially SCM
  - Special tests negative
- Palpation elicits pain at site of injury (usually C4). Muscle spasm evident in the affected SCM and associated muscles

POSTURAL ANALYSIS

Clients adopt an antalgic posture, often with their head laterally flexed towards and rotated away from the injured side. Clients turn their whole body to avoid painful neck movements.

FUNCTIONAL TESTS

It may be difficult to perform functional tests in the acute phase. Work only within the client's pain tolerance.

AROM: very limited and painful in one or more directions, usually rotation to the affected side.
PROM: limited and painful in one or more directions.
RROM: limited and painful in one or more directions.
Resisted muscle tests for specific muscles positive (usually for sternocleidomastoid).
Special tests: usually negative.

PALPATION

Palpation at the site of injury (often C4) usually elicits pain.

Differential diagnosis

Special tests (e.g. cervical compression, cervical distraction and Valsalva) usually aggravate symptoms in clients with cervical nerve root compression.

Overview of treatment and management

Clients often present for treatment within hours of the onset. Treatment could include cryotherapy, acupressure, Reiki, reflexology or anti-inflammatory medication. Massage directly on the sternocleidomastoid or other affected muscles should be brief. Minimise any strokes that increase circulation to the area. Use acupressure and trigger points therapy if it can be tolerated. In the acute phase, clients may benefit from lying on a rolled towel (height adjusted to pain-free position) placed horizontally under their neck for short periods (15–20 minutes). This position helps to restore normal cervical lordosis. Adjust the height of the rolled towel to the client's comfort. Place an ice pack over the rolled towel if required. Introduce corrective exercise therapy, beginning with gentle stretches as soon as they can be tolerated. Myofascial release techniques may be beneficial. Advise clients about sleeping positions, pillows and avoidance of aggravating activities. Refer clients for spinal manipulation. Clients may require daily or second daily treatment for the first week.

After the acute phase, a full assessment should be performed. Introduce a treatment plan to address muscle imbalances. A typical remedial massage treatment for subacute mechanical torticollis includes:

- Swedish massage therapy to the neck, upper back, shoulders and head (± chest).

- Remedial massage therapy. Remedial massage therapy for sternocleidomastoid and other neck muscles includes (see Table 12.4):
  - deep gliding frictions along the muscle fibres
  - cross-fibre frictions
  - active and passive soft tissue releasing techniques
  - deep transverse friction
  - trigger point therapy
  - muscle stretches.
- Apply myofascial releasing techniques for myofascial restrictions (see Chapter 8).
- Passive joint articulation for the cervical spine may be beneficial for facet joint lesions (see Chapter 7).
- Thermotherapy may be beneficial.

CLIENT EDUCATION

Advise clients to avoid prolonged neck postures, especially flexion and rotation and sudden neck movements. Encourage good sleeping postures (i.e. avoid sleeping prone) and use of pillows that support cervical lordosis. Thermotherapy may be beneficial. Clients may require spinal manipulation by a chiropractor, osteopath or physiotherapist to restore normal biomechanics and prevent relapse.

Home exercise program

Begin with stretches to affected muscles as soon as they can be tolerated and progressively introduce stretches to other cervical muscles and strengthening exercises as required. Upper thoracic and shoulder muscles (e.g. arm swings, scapula retraction) may be incorporated as soon as they can be tolerated.

CERVICAL DISC SYNDROME

Acute cervical disc lesions are not commonly seen in remedial massage clinics. Cervical disc lesions account for about 36% of all spinal disc lesions and because of their severity are usually treated initially by medical practitioners, chiropractors, osteopaths and physiotherapists. About 70% of cases have C7 nerve root impingement (C6–C7) and 25% have C6 nerve root impingement (C5–C6).[2] Clients with chronic conditions may incorporate remedial massage into their overall treatment and management plans. When treating clients with a history of disc degeneration it is important to be mindful of the frequency of relapse and the vulnerability that in many cases persists even years after the initial injury.

Assessment

HISTORY

Clients are usually between 25 and 45 years old. Younger clients usually develop symptoms immediately or shortly after a direct trauma such as a diving or a motor vehicle or sports accident. Older clients may report repetitive overuse or poor posture, which can lead to intervertebral foramen narrowing from osteophyte encroachment, particularly in the presence of congenital osseous variants. Radiographs may show loss (or reversal) of cervical lordosis, osteophyte formation and decreased intervertebral disc space.

Pain and paraesthesia may radiate to the shoulders and upper limbs. Headache and tinnitus are also described. Symptoms can be so severe that clients report being unable to lie down to sleep. Pain can be sharp and shooting. It may also arise insidiously. Table 12.5 illustrates the effects of impingements on the lower cervical and first thoracic nerves.

Table 12.5 Effects of impingement on C5–T1 nerves

Nerve	Disc	Muscles affected	Sensation
C5	C4–5	Deltoid, biceps brachii	Lateral upper arm
C6	C5–6	Biceps brachii, wrist extensors	Lateral forearm and hand, thumb, index finger
C7	C6–7	Triceps brachii, wrist flexors	Middle finger
C8	C7–T1	Finger flexors, interossei	Medial forearm and hand, 4th and 5th fingers
T1	T1–2	Interossei	Medial upper arm

Key assessment findings for cervical disc syndrome

- The client is usually between 25 and 45 years old with a history of recent trauma, overuse or repetitive microtrauma. Pain may be severe. Pain and paraesthesia may radiate to shoulder and upper limb; headache may be present.
- Postural analysis: Postural adaptations to limit and guard neck movement may be present
- Functional tests
  - AROM limited in most directions, especially flexion
  - PROM limited in most directions
  - RROM may be positive if associated muscle strain or weakness
  - Resisted tests for specific muscles may indicate weakness, or associated muscle strain
  - Special tests (compression, Valsalva) positive
- Palpation may elicit local tenderness; muscle hypotonicity or hypertonicity may be evident

POSTURAL ANALYSIS

Postural adaptations may be observed. Clients often adopt an antalgic posture and minimise aggravating neck movements.

FUNCTIONAL TESTS

AROM: limited and painful especially towards the affected side.
PROM: limited and painful, especially towards the affected side.
RROM: may be positive for associated muscle weakness or strain.
Resisted and length tests may be positive for affected muscles.
Special tests: usually positive for compression, distraction, Valsalva and any test that challenges the disc.

PALPATION

Palpation usually elicits tenderness in cervical paraspinal muscles, most often on the affected side. Muscle spasm is also found in areas of compensation.

Differential diagnosis

Clients with severe pain (more than 8 out of 10 on the pain scale), with neurological symptoms or following trauma should be referred for further investigation to rule out fracture, ligament sprain or other serious condition.

Overview of treatment and management

Clients with cervical disc syndrome will have been previously assessed and treated by a medical practitioner, chiropractor, osteopath or physiotherapist. Remedial massage therapy is usually introduced in the chronic phase and can be a useful adjunct to other forms of treatment. It is important to liaise with other treating practitioners wherever possible so as to deliver the most appropriate care.

A typical remedial massage treatment for cervical disc syndrome after pain and inflammation have been controlled includes:

- Swedish massage therapy to the neck, upper back, shoulders, head (± upper limbs, chest).
- Remedial massage therapy. The selection of remedial massage techniques depends on assessment findings. Muscle strain or spasm invariably accompanies disc syndrome. Remedial massage therapy for muscle tissue injury/muscle imbalances includes (see Table 12.4):
  - deep gliding frictions along the muscle fibres
  - cross-fibre frictions
  - active and passive soft tissue releasing techniques
  - deep transverse friction
  - trigger point therapy
  - muscle stretches.
- Gentle passive cervical extension stretches may be beneficial (see Chapter 7). Horizontal traction may be beneficial (caution: horizontal traction is contraindicated in cervical ligament sprain). Other passive joint articulation may be beneficial for facet joint lesions, but all techniques must be applied with caution. Use the See-Move-Touch principle described in Chapter 2 to guide treatment.
- Myofascial releasing techniques are useful for myofascial restrictions (see Chapter 8).
- Thermotherapy may be beneficial.

Refer clients for further investigation if no significant improvement has been reported in 6 to 8 weeks, if muscle weakness is progressing or if symptoms worsen (peripheralise). Clients may also be referred for nutritional, herbal or homeopathic support.

CLIENT EDUCATION

Advise clients about cervical posture. Clients should avoid heavy lifting, sudden neck movements, and positions that aggravate their neck condition such as awkward or sustained neck positions. Advise clients about sleeping posture (avoid lying in the prone position or arms overhead) and to use a supportive pillow and mattress. Referral for osseous manipulation may be beneficial. Thermotherapy may be useful for pain relief and reducing muscle spasm.

Home exercise program

The main purpose of a home exercise program is to restore muscle balance and to strengthen the cervical muscles to reduce the risk of recurrence. All exercises should be performed within the client's pain-free range. Begin with stretches and/or isometric contractions of affected neck muscles and progressively increase to stretching and strengthening muscles of the neck, upper back, shoulders and upper limbs, and proprioceptive training. Advise clients to discontinue any exercise that aggravates symptoms.

WHIPLASH (ACCELERATION/DECELERATION) ASSOCIATED DISORDERS

Whiplash refers to an acute traumatic acceleration-deceleration injury to the cervical spine, commonly caused by rear end or side-impact motor vehicle collisions. The injury often results in a loss (or reversal) of cervical lordosis. Injuries range from mild to severe and can include ligament sprain, disc injury, vertebral subluxation, fracture and muscle tears. They are classified from Grade 0 (no complaints or physical signs) to Grade 4 (fracture or dislocation).[17]

Whiplash is the most common injury for people involved in a motor vehicle accident. It is a significant cost to the Compulsory Third Party scheme in Australia and appears to have a large effect on the ongoing health of its sufferers. In one study only 50% of the cohort had recovered at two years. Physical measures of health appeared to improve over time, although mental measures of health did not. However, the group was generally able to participate in activities and work at two years after injury.[18] To date there is insufficient evidence to draw conclusions about the effectiveness of conservative treatments of whiplash-associated disorders such as rest, ultrasound and exercises.[19] The 2007 Guidelines for the Management of Acute Whiplash-associated Disorders for Health Professionals[20] which is based on currently available evidence makes the following recommendations.

Treatments recommended

- Reassure/act as usual.
- Prescribed functional exercises.
- Return to usual activity, work alteration.
- Exercise – range of motion exercises, muscle re-education.
- Pharmacology – simple analgesics.

Treatments not routinely recommended because of insufficient evidence or lack of evidence

- Postural advice
- Passive joint mobilisation (should only be given in combination with manual and physical therapies and exercise, provided there is evidence of continuing measurable improvement)
- Manipulation
- Traction
- Acupuncture
- Multimodal treatment
- Passive modalities such as electrotherapies, heat and ice
- Surgical treatments

Treatments not recommended

(Note that treatments like cervical pillows are included in this category because no evidence exists regarding their use.)

Key assessment findings for whiplash-associated disorders

- History of acceleration-deceleration injury. Neck pain and limitation ± headache. Symptoms depend on grade of injury and structures affected.
- Postural analysis: Posture adaptations to limit and guard neck movement
- Functional tests
  - AROM positive in some directions
  - PROM positive if facets, ligaments, joint capsules involved
  - RROM positive if muscle tissue injured
  - Resisted tests and length tests for specific muscles may indicate weakness, strain or contracture
  - Special tests (including compression, distraction, Valsalva) positive in severe cases (e.g. disc involvement)
- Palpation positive for local tenderness and muscle spasm

- Cervical pillows
- Spray and stretch
- Intra-articular and intrathecal steroid injections
- Magnetic necklaces
- Immobilisation – prescribed rest for >4 days
- Immobilisation – collars for >48 hours
- Pharmacology – psychopharmacological agents
- Other interventions (e.g. Pilates, massage, etc.)

There is an urgent need for high-quality clinical trials to support or refute the large body of anecdotal clinical evidence for the efficacy of massage therapy for whiplash-associated disorders.

Assessment

HISTORY

The client usually presents with neck pain ± headache and paraesthesia, and limited neck movement following an acceleration-deceleration trauma to the cervical spine. Pain is felt immediately or shortly after injury. Some clients describe feeling sore immediately after the accident with pain and/or headache increasing over the next few hours or days. Symptoms depend on the nature of the injury and the type(s) of tissue involved. More severe cases involve ligament damage and disc degeneration, especially in the mid cervical spine. In some cases, swelling at the site of injury can make swallowing difficult or painful. It is estimated that 60% of post-whiplash pain comes from cervical facet joints, usually at C2–C3 and C5–C6 level.[2] DJD may follow in a few years.

FUNCTIONAL TESTS

AROM: limited and painful; the greater the limitation, the more severe the injury.
PROM: limited and painful in some directions.
RROM: limited and painful in some directions – pain in many directions suggest joint capsule damage; pain in a single direction suggests muscle strain.
Resisted and length tests positive for specific muscles. Sternocleidomastoid is commonly involved.
Special tests: may be positive if discs or ligaments involved. Positive compression test suggests disc involvement; pain produced by traction suggests ligamentous sprain; pain relieved by traction suggests cervical disc damage.

POSTURAL ANALYSIS

Clients may adopt an antalgic posture and minimise aggravating neck symptoms.

PALPATION

Local tenderness can be elicited at the site of injury and muscle spasm palpated in affected muscles.

Differential diagnosis

It is important to identify and refer any clients with neurological signs (Grade 3) or muscle guarding or symptoms increasing over time (Grade 4) following whiplash injury.

Overview of treatment and management

If acute inflammation is present, treatment usually includes cryotherapy, acupressure, Reiki, reflexology or anti-inflammatory medication. Advise the client to place a rolled towel behind their neck to restore cervical lordosis if a comfortable position can be found. Introduce corrective exercise therapy (e.g. gentle stretches, range of motion exercises, stabilisation exercises) as soon as tolerated by the client. Myofascial release may be beneficial. Because of the potential for serious injury, screen all whiplash clients carefully and refer clients with neurological symptoms, increasing pain and muscle guarding for further assessment.

A typical remedial massage treatment for mild or moderate whiplash-associated disorder includes:

- Swedish massage therapy to the neck, upper back, shoulders, head (± upper limbs, chest).
- Remedial massage therapy. The selection of remedial massage techniques depends on assessment results which suggest the type of tissue(s) involved. Use the See-Move-Touch principle to guide treatment (see Chapter 2). Remedial massage therapy for muscle tissue injury/muscle imbalances includes (see Table 12.4):
  - deep gliding frictions along the muscle fibres
  - cross-fibre frictions
  - active and passive soft tissue releasing techniques
  - deep transverse friction
  - trigger point therapy (A study in 2008 found that patients with whiplash showed a distinct pattern of trigger point distribution and that semispinalis capitis was more frequently affected by trigger points in whiplash patients than patients with non-traumatic chronic cervical syndrome or fibromyalgia.)[21]
  - muscle stretches.
- Gentle joint mobilisation should be introduced when tolerated, particularly extension to restore cervical lordosis (see Chapter 7). Other passive joint articulation may be beneficial for facet joint lesions, but all techniques must be applied with caution. Use the See-Move-Touch principle to guide treatment. Horizontal traction is contraindicated for ligamentous sprains.
- Apply myofascial releasing techniques for myofascial restrictions (see Chapter 8).
- Thermotherapy has been reported to be a useful analgesic and muscle relaxant.

Refer clients for spinal manipulation to restore normal biomechanics and prevent the onset of DJD.

CLIENT EDUCATION

Encourage clients to continue their daily activities as usual within pain tolerance. Advise clients about cervical posture for work and activities of daily living. Avoid heavy lifting and sudden neck movements. Activities that require awkward or prolonged neck positions should be avoided. Good sleeping posture (avoid lying in the prone position or with arms overhead) should be maintained. Shock-absorbing shoes help minimise jarring impacts transferred to the neck when walking.

Clients may require education about seat and headrest position to minimise the impact of any subsequent whiplash-associated injuries. The seat should be inclined to less than a 20° angle, the head restraint should be level with the centre of the driver's head and less than 10 cm from the back of the head.

Home exercise program

Introduce range of motion stretches and/or isometric contractions of affected neck muscles as soon as possible. All exercises should be performed within the client's pain-free range. Stretches and strengthening exercises should be progressively increased. Advise clients to discontinue any exercise/activity that aggravates symptoms.

KEY MESSAGES

- Assessment of clients with conditions of the cervical region involves history, outcome measures, postural analysis, functional tests (including resisted and length tests for specific muscles of the neck) and special tests (e.g. cervical compression, cervical distraction and Valsalva).
- Assessment findings may indicate the type of tissue involved (contractile or inert), duration of condition (acute or subacute), and severity (grade).
- Assessment findings may indicate a common presenting condition such as
  - strain of cervical muscles
  - non-specific neck pain
  - DJD of the cervical spine
  - upper crossed syndrome
  - mechanical/acquired torticollis
  - cervical disc syndrome
  - whiplash associated disorders.
- Assessment findings indicate the client's perception of injury and preferences for treatment.
- Consider Clinical Guidelines, available evidence, clinical efficacy and client preferences when planning treatment.
- Select the most appropriate remedial massage techniques for the affected tissue(s) (e.g. muscle-specific techniques like trigger point therapy for muscle strains; joint mobilisation for facet lesions). Be conservative in treatment: if in doubt, perform pain-free Swedish massage.
- Although serious conditions of the cervical region are rare, clients with such conditions will present for remedial massage from time to time. Caution is required when treating all clients with neck pain post trauma or associated with neurological signs.
- Educating clients about likely causal and predisposing factors is an essential part of remedial massage therapy.
- Over time, increase the client self-help component of treatment wherever possible to reduce likelihood of recurrence and/or to promote health maintenance and illness prevention.

Review questions

1. A client comes to your clinic with neck pain. She reports being unable to turn her head when she woke up. She is in her late twenties and has had some minor episodes of neck pain in the past but this one is by far the worst. She has had no previous accidents or falls and can't think of anything that could have brought this on. She is in a great deal of pain and is unable to go to work. This history is consistent with:
   a) cervical facet syndrome
   b) cervical disc syndrome
   c) acute torticollis
   d) cervical DJD
2. In general, traction tests are positive when:
   a) a facet joint is subluxated
   b) a ligament has been sprained
   c) an intervertebral disc has bulged
   d) a muscle has been strained
3. After a whiplash injury, a patient may be suffering with:
   a) a strained sternocleidomastoid muscle
   b) cervical facet syndrome
   c) cervical ligament sprain
   d) all of the above
4. The most common level for a cervical disc herniation to occur is:
   a) C1/C2 b) C3/C4
   c) C5/C6 d) C7/T1
5. Which muscles are usually weakened in upper crossed syndrome? Prescribe a home exercise program to help strengthen these muscles.
6. Draw or describe a home stretch for the following muscles:
   a) upper trapezius
   b) levator scapulae
   c) scalene muscles
7. List three red flags for acute neck pain.
8. The compression test is used to indicate the presence of:
   a) a space-occupying lesion such as a disc prolapse
   b) a muscle strain
   c) upper crossed syndrome
   d) DJD
9. Osteophytes, loss of disc height and endplate sclerosis may indicate:
   a) DJD
   b) acute torticollis
   c) a space-occupying lesion such as a disc prolapse
   d) upper crossed syndrome
10. Describe the typical presenting symptoms and signs associated with cervical DJD.

REFERENCES

1. WorkCover SA. Acute neck pain. Available: http://www.workcover.com/site/treat_home/guidelines_by_injury_type/acute_neck_pain.aspx; 2009.
2. Carnes M, Vizniak N. Quick reference evidence-based conditions manual. 3rd edn. Burnaby, BC: Professional Health Systems; 2009.
3. Australian Acute Musculoskeletal Pain Guidelines Group. Evidence-based management of acute musculoskeletal pain: a guide for clinicians. Bowen Hills, Qld: Australian Academic Press; 2004.
4. Swartz E, Floyd R, Cendoma M. Cervical spine functional anatomy and the biomechanics of injury due to compressive loading. J Athlet Train 2005;40(3):155–61.
5. Simons D, Travell J, Simons L. Myofascial pain and dysfunction: the trigger point manual. Vol 1: upper half of body. 2nd edn. Philadelphia: Williams and Wilkins; 1999.
6. Stiell I, Wells G, Vandemheen K, et al. The Canadian C-spine rule for radiography in alert and stable trauma patients. JAMA 2001;286:1841–8.
7. New Zealand Guidelines Group. New Zealand acute low back pain guide. Available: www.nzgg.org.nz/guidelines/0072/acc1038_col.pdf; 2004.
8. Reese N, Bandy W. Joint range of motion and muscle length testing. Philadelphia: WB Saunders; 2002.
9. Kendall McCreary E, Provance P, McIntyre Rodgers M, et al. Muscles, testing and function, with posture and pain. 5th edn. Philadelphia: Lippincott Williams and Wilkins; 2005.
10. Cleland J, Koppenhaver S. Netter's orthopaedic clinical examination: an evidence-based approach. 2nd edn. Philadelphia: Saunders; 2011.
11. Vernon H, Humphreys K, Hagino C. Chronic mechanical neck pain in adults treated by manual therapy: a systematic review of change scores in randomized clinical trials [erratum appears in J Manipulative Physiol Ther 2007;30(6):473–8]. J Manipulative Physiol Ther 2007;30(3):215–27.
12. Haraldsson BG, Gross AR, Myers CD, et al. Massage for mechanical neck disorders. Cochrane Database Syst Rev 006(3)CD004871.
13. Aker P, Gross A, Goldsmith C, et al. Conservative management of mechanical neck pain: systematic overview and meta-analysis. BMJ 1996;313:1291–6.
14. Yochum T, Rowe L. Essentials of skeletal radiology. 3rd edn. Baltimore: Lippincott Williams and Wilkins; 2005.
15. Towheed TE, Maxwell L, Anastassiades TP, et al. Glucosamine therapy for treating osteoarthritis. Cochrane Database Syst Rev [serial on the Internet] 2005;(2):CD0029.
16. Magee D. Orthopedic physical assessment. 5th edn. Philadelphia: Saunders; 2008.
17. Spitzer W, Skovron M, Salmi L, et al. Scientific monograph of the Quebec Task Force on whiplash associated disorders: redefining 'whiplash' and its management. Spine 1995;20(Suppl 8):1S–73S.
18. Rebbeck T, Sindhusake D, Cameron I, et al. A prospective cohort study of health outcomes following whiplash associated disorders in an Australian population. Inj Prev 2006;12:93–8.
19. Verhagen A, Scholten-Peeters G, van Wijngaarden S, et al. Conservative treatments for whiplash. Cochrane Database Syst Rev 2007;(2):CD003338.
20. Motor Accident Authority NSW. Guidelines for the management of acute whiplash-associated disorders for health professionals. Sydney: NSW Government; 2007.
21. Ettlin T, Schuster C, Stoffel R, et al. A distinct pattern of myofascial findings in patients after whiplash injury. Arch Phys Med Rehabil 2008;89(7):1290–3.

13 The head and face

The content of this chapter relates to the following Units of Competency:

HLTREM503C Plan remedial massage treatment strategy
HLTREM504C Apply remedial massage assessment framework
HLTREM502C Provide remedial massage treatment
HLTREM505C Perform remedial massage health assessment

Health Training Package HLT07

Learning Outcomes

- Assess clients with conditions of the head and face for remedial massage, including identification of red and yellow flags.
- Assess clients for signs and symptoms associated with common conditions of the head and face (including headache, sinusitis and temporomandibular joint disorders) and treat and/or manage these conditions with remedial massage therapy.
- Develop treatment plans for clients with conditions of the head and face, taking assessment findings, duration and severity of the condition, likely tissue types, clinical guidelines, the best available evidence and client preferences into account.
- Adapt remedial massage therapy to suit individual client needs based on duration and severity of injury, the client's age and gender, the presence of underlying conditions and co-morbidities and other consideration for special population groups.

INTRODUCTION

This chapter is divided into three sections. The first describes assessment and treatment of headache, which is the most common condition of the head and face for which clients seek remedial massage. Two further sections deal with sinusitis and temporomandibular joint (TMJ) disorders which are also commonly treated by remedial massage therapists. Some of the treatments introduced in this chapter have long been used in remedial massage but have rarely been the subject of scientific research. It is important for massage therapists to be acquainted with traditional treatments and to make their own judgments, through experience and research, about their efficacy.

HEADACHE

Headaches are common occurrences. A survey conducted by Headache Australia and Pfizer Australia in 2003 found that 84% of Australians reported having experienced a severe headache or migraine in the past 12 months and that nearly 40% of these people did not receive any treatment.[1, 2] There were up to seven million sufferers of tension-type headache.[3] The prevalence of cervicogenic headaches is estimated at about 18% of adults[4] and the use of manual therapy in the treatment of cervicogenic headache is supported by current evidence.[5, 6]

Headache is defined as pain in any part of the head, including the scalp, face and interior of the head.[7] Primary headaches (such as migraine, cluster headache and tension-type headache) are those for which no other causative factor can be found. Secondary headaches can have numerous causes including dental disorders, glaucoma, sinusitis, brain tumours, cerebral haemorrhages, viral infections, caffeine withdrawal and dehydration. Headaches arise from activation of pain-sensitive structures including skin and subcutaneous tissue, muscles, extracranial coverings and arteries, periosteum of the skull, intracranial venous sinuses, dura mater at the base of the brain, cranial nerves V, IX and X and the first three cervical nerves. However, the pathophysiology of many headache types is poorly understood. Migraine and tension headaches may be caused by electrical and chemical instability of key brain centres that regulate blood vessels around the head and neck, as well as the flow of pain messages into the brain. This instability may be inherited and appears to involve neurotransmitters like serotonin.

ASSESSMENT OF THE HEADACHE CLIENT

Assessment of the headache client provides essential information for development and negotiation of treatment plans, including:

- client's suitability for remedial massage therapy
- duration of the condition (i.e. acute or chronic)
- severity of the condition (i.e. mild, moderate or severe pain)
- type(s) of tissues involved and the most appropriate treatment for the condition[8]

Assessment of the headache client

1. Case history
2. Outcome measure
3. Postural analysis
4. Functional tests
   AROM cervical spine
   Flexion, extension, lateral flexion, rotation
   PROM cervical spine
   Flexion, extension, lateral flexion, rotation
   RROM cervical spine
   Flexion, extension, lateral flexion, rotation
   Resisted and length tests for specific muscles, including
   - Sub-occipital muscles
   - Posterior cervical muscles
   - Upper trapezius
   - Sternocleidomastoid

   Special tests as indicated
   Special tests for the cervical spine (see Chapter 10)
5. Palpation

- priorities for treatment if more than one injury or condition is present
- whether the signs and symptoms suggest one of the classifications of headache
- special considerations for individual clients (e.g. client's preference for treatment types and styles, special population considerations).

Although serious causes of headache are rare, headache clients require careful screening to identify those clients who require referral for further investigation.

Case history

A thorough case history with targeted questions is the most important assessment strategy for identifying potentially serious causes of headaches. Practitioners should be vigilant for red flags which suggest such disorders (see Table 13.1). Clients with one or more red flags should be referred for an immediate medical consultation and further investigation.[8]

Note:

- Headaches that have been present for more than 6 months are usually not life threatening.
- Recurring headaches in clients who appear well and have a normal examination are rarely serious. Recurring headaches that began in childhood or early adulthood in clients with a normal examination are usually benign. However, if the type or pattern of the headache changes in clients with a known primary headache disorder, investigation for secondary headache should be carried out.[9]
- Most single symptoms of primary headache disorders other than aura are non-specific. A combination of symptoms and signs is more characteristic. A retrospective study of 111 patients with headache in a hospital in Malaysia in 1999 found that paralysis, papilloedema, drowsiness, confusion, memory impairment and loss of consciousness were significant predictors of abnormal neuroimaging. Three or more red flags were found in clients with abnormal neuroimaging.[12]
- Questions are not only designed to identify red and yellow flags but also to suggest the type of headache. Ask about:

Table 13.1 Red flags for serious conditions associated with headache

Red flags for headache[9–11]	Possible condition
Thunderclap headache (severe headache that peaks within a few seconds)	Subarachnoid haemorrhage
New headache after the age of 50	Increased risk of serious cause (e.g. tumour, giant cell arteritis)
New onset headache with history of cancer or immunodeficiency	Brain infection, metastases
Headache with fever, neck stiffness and meningeal signs (Brudzinski's sign: lifting the head off the table in the supine position causes the legs to lift up; Kernig's sign: hip and knee flexed to 90°, knee extension from this position causes pain; nuchal rigidity)	Meningitis, subarachnoid haemorrhage, subdural empyema
Headache with neurological symptoms (e.g. altered mental state, confusion, neurogenic weakness, diplopia, papilloedema, focal neurological deficits) if not previously documented as a migraine with aura	Encephalitis, subdural haematoma, subarachnoid or intracerebral haemorrhage, tumour, other intracranial mass, increased intracranial pressure
Headache worsening with Valsalva manoeuvre or recumbency	Intracranial tumours
Progressively worsening headache	Mass lesion, subdural haematoma, medication overuse
Systemic symptoms (e.g. weight loss, fever)	Sepsis, thyrotoxicosis, cancer
Headache during pregnancy or post-partum	Cortical vein/cranial sinus thrombosis, carotid dissection, pituitary apoplexy

- Location of headache (e.g. headache in the occipital/suboccipital region could indicate cervicogenic headache or stress-induced headache; temporal pain may suggest temporal arteritis, tension-type headache, TMJ dysfunction; orbital headache may suggest eye strain, sinusitis or stress-induced headache; headaches preceded by aura may suggest migraine). Ask clients to point to the site of pain as they may have different understandings of anatomical terms.
- Character and intensity of pain (e.g. throbbing suggests vascular headache; dull aching could suggest cervicogenic headache). Is the pain incapacitating? Ask if the headache wakes the client from sleep. Clients with severe pain require referral.
- Onset and chronicity. Ask how long the client has been experiencing headaches and how quickly the headache

reaches a peak. Clients with abrupt onset headaches reaching a peak in 5 or 10 minutes require referral.
  - Precipitating and aggravating factors (e.g. headache aggravated by stooping, straining, coughing may suggest hypertension; headache precipitated by bright light, noise, stress or certain foods could be a migraine; headaches aggravated by a head-low position could be vascular or suggest sinusitis; headaches before menstrual periods could be related to hormonal change).
  - Frequency and duration (e.g. headache lasting from several hours to 1 or 2 days suggests migraine; intermittently persistent headache several times a days could suggest a brain tumour). It is important to ascertain if the headaches are becoming more frequent and severe over a period of months and if so refer for further investigation.
- Determine if the pain is likely to have a mechanical cause. Is the pain associated with rest or activity, certain postures or time of day? Cervicogenic headache is caused or aggravated by neck movements and sustained postures.[4] Ask clients to demonstrate movements and positions that aggravate or relieve their pain and to be specific with descriptions of aggravating or relieving activities. Cervicogenic headaches usually present as one-sided neck and occipital pain and may radiate to the forehead, eyes, temples or ears. Morning pain relieved with daily activity is often associated with arthritis.
- Determine if the headache is likely to be vascular. Migraine is the most common vascular headache. Clients are typically 10 to 40 years of age, are more likely to be female than male and describe episodes of throbbing pain that may last several hours, or up to 3 days.
- Enquire whether the clients' previous treatments for headache have included massage therapy and if so ask about their response to treatment.

TYPES OF HEADACHE

The following classifications have been adapted from the International Headache Society.[1] The most relevant classifications for remedial massage therapists are discussed here.

Classification of headache[1]

Primary (no other causative disorder)

1. Migraine – classic (with aura)
   – common (without aura)
2. Tension-type headache (psychogenic, stress, muscle contraction)
3. Cluster headache

Secondary (caused by another disorder)

Headache attributed to:

1. Head and/or neck trauma
2. Cranial or cervical vascular disorder
3. Non-vascular intracranial disorder
4. A substance or its withdrawal
5. Infection
6. Disorder of homeostasis (e.g. high-altitude headache, sleep apnoea headache, arterial hypertension headache)
7. Disorder of the cranium, neck, eyes, ears, nose, sinuses, teeth, mouth or other facial or cranial structures
8. Psychiatric disorder

Primary headache

1. Migraine

The term *migraine* is derived from the old French word *migraigne* meaning half head and reminds us that 60% of migraine sufferers experience pain unilaterally. One in five sufferers experience an aura (a group of neurological symptoms, including disturbances of vision that precede head pain). Migraines are often severe. They are episodic and can occur as often as once or twice a week but not daily. The International Headache Society has established the following diagnostic criteria for migraine.

Migraine without aura

A. At least two attacks fulfilling criteria B–D
B. Headache lasting 4–72 hours
C. Headache has at least two of the following characteristics:
   1. unilateral location
   2. pulsating quality
   3. moderate or severe pain intensity
   4. aggravated by or causing avoidance of routine physical activity (e.g. walking, climbing stairs)
D. During headache, at least one of the following:
   1. nausea ± vomiting
   2. photophobia and phonophobia
E. Not attributed to another disorder

Migraine with aura

A. At least two attacks fulfilling criterion B
B. Aura consisting of at least one of the following but no motor weakness:
   1. fully reversible visual symptoms including flickering lights, spots or lines, loss of vision
   2. fully reversible sensory symptoms including pins and needles and numbness
   3. fully reversible dysphasic speech disturbance
C. At least two of the following:
   1. homonymous visual symptoms and/or unilateral sensory symptoms
   2. at least one aura symptom develops gradually over ≥5 minutes and/or different aura symptoms occur in succession over ≥5 minutes
   3. each symptom lasts ≥5 minutes and ≤60 minutes
D. Not attributed to another disorder

2. Tension-type headache

Tension-type headaches typically are felt as a steady ache rather than throbbing and usually affect both sides of the head. They are often associated with a response to stressful events. Tension-type headaches may be chronic, occurring frequently or even daily. Clients may go to bed with a headache and wake up with it the next day. The International Headache Society has established the following diagnostic criteria.

A. Infrequent (at least 10 episodes occurring on <1 day/month on average), frequent (at least 10 episodes occurring on ≥1 but <15 days/month for ≥3 months) or chronic (occurring on ≥15 days/month on average for >3 months) and fulfilling criteria B–D
B. lasts from 30 minutes to 7 days
C. At least two of the following characteristics:
   1. bilateral location

2. pressing/tightening (non-pulsating) quality
3. mild to moderate intensity
4. not aggravated by physical activity such as walking or climbing stairs

D. Both of the following:
1. no nausea or vomiting
2. no more than one of photophobia and phonophobia

E. Not attributed to another disorder

3. Cluster headaches

Cluster headaches are a relatively rare form of migraine, affecting about 1% of the population. The headaches are typically unilateral, intense and brief (last no more than 1 or 2 hours). There may be many attacks in quick succession for a few hours or days, followed by a prolonged period of freedom. Clients describe severe and burning pain, primarily in the frontal region and one eye. The pain often spreads to the face and neck. The eye may be inflamed and watery. Cluster headaches may strike in the middle of the night and clients often describe pacing the floor holding their head. Many clients have a history of heavy smoking and drinking. Most sufferers (85%) are young males. Cluster headaches are thought to be due to histamine sensitivity related to heavy alcohol intake and cigarette smoking. The International Headache Society has established the following diagnostic criteria.

A. At least 5 attacks fulfilling criteria B–D

B. Severe or very severe unilateral orbital, supraorbital and/or temporal pain lasting 15–180 minutes if untreated

C. Headache is accompanied by at least one of the following:
1. ipsilateral conjunctival injection (red eye) and/or lacrimation
2. ipsilateral nasal congestion and/or rhinorrhoea
3. ipsilateral eyelid oedema
4. ipsilateral forehead and facial sweating
5. ipsilateral miosis and/or ptosis
6. a sense of restlessness or agitation

D. Attacks have a frequency from 1 every other day to 8/day

E. Not attributed to another disorder

Secondary headache

1. Headache attributable to head and/or neck trauma

Headache is the most common symptom following car accidents and falls. The headache can be dull, constant and aching. Other symptoms may accompany the headache, such as faintness, poor memory, inability to concentrate, anxiety, fatigue, insomnia, irritability, depression, tinnitus and vertigo. About 85% of chronic post-traumatic headache sufferers will recover completely but this can take many months or even years. The International Headache Society has established the following diagnostic criteria.

A. Headache, no typical characteristics known, fulfilling criteria C–D

B. Head trauma with at least 1 of the following:
1. Loss of consciousness for >30 minutes
2. Glasgow Coma Scale[a] > 13
3. Post-traumatic amnesia for >48 hours
4. Imaging demonstration of a traumatic brain lesion (cerebral haematoma, intracerebral/subarachnoid haemorrhage, brain contusion, skull fracture)

C. Headache develops within 7 days after head trauma or after regaining consciousness following head trauma

D. Headache persists for >3 months after head trauma

[a]The Glasgow Coma Scale rates levels of consciousness from 3 (deep unconsciousness) to 15 (normal).

2. Headache attributable to a substance or its withdrawal

One example of this type of headache arises from headache medication overuse including ergotamine intake. Headache is present on 15 or more days a month. Clients describe regular overuse for more than 3 months of one or more drugs that can be taken for acute and/or symptomatic treatment of headache. Other examples of this type of headache include oestrogen-withdrawal headache and analgesic overuse.

3. Headache or facial pain attributed to disorder of cranium, neck, eyes, ears, nose, sinuses, teeth, mouth or other facial or cranial structures

The most common headache in this category is cervicogenic headache which is estimated to account for 14–18% of all chronic headaches.[13] Cervicogenic headaches are also among the most responsive to remedial massage treatment.

Cervicogenic headache

Cervicogenic headaches may be related to a number of mechanisms including cervical facet dysfunction, cervical degenerative joint disease, musculotendinous lesions, entrapment neuropathy of the occipital nerves, and a connective tissue bridge between rectus capitis posterior minor and the dorsal spinal dura.[14] Pain is typically felt in the suboccipital region, unilaterally or bilaterally, and radiates to the head behind the eyes or into the face. The pain is usually dull and aching and is often worse on rising. The headache usually eases as the day goes on but may be aggravated by neck and head movements or by jolting (e.g. when riding in a bus). The International Headache Society has established the following diagnostic criteria:

A. Pain referred from a source in the neck and perceived in one or more regions of the head and/or face, fulfilling criteria C–D

B. Clinical, laboratory and/or imaging evidence of a disorder or lesion within the cervical spine or soft tissues of the neck known to be, or generally accepted as, a valid cause of headache

C. Evidence that the pain can be attributed to the neck disorder or lesion, based on at least one of the following:
1. demonstration of clinical signs that implicate a source of pain in the neck
2. abolition of headache following diagnostic blockage of a cervical structure or its nerve supply using placebo or other adequate controls

D. Pain resolves within 3 months after successful treatment of the causative disorder or lesion

Table 13.2 compares characteristics of common types of headache.

Table 13.2 Types of headache[1,15]

Features	Vascular headache (migraine)	Cervicogenic headache	Tension	Cluster
Age of onset	10–40 years	20–60 years	Any age	Common in adolescence and middle age
Gender	Three to four times more common in females than males	Four times more common in females than males	Slightly more common in females than males	80% males
Onset	Rapid	Slow	Slow	Rapid
Location	Temporal or frontal	Occipital, behind the eyes, temporal	Front, top and sides of the head	Frontal and one eye
Unilateral/bilateral	Unilateral or bilateral	Unilateral	Bilateral	Unilateral
Nature of pain	Throbbing/pulsing	Dull ache	Steady ache	Burning
Severity	Moderate to severe	Mild to moderate	Mild to moderate	Severe
Constancy	Episodic	Constant	Chronic, occur frequently, even daily	1 every other day to 8/day
Duration	4–72 hours (migraine)	Days	30 minutes to 7 days	Short (15 minutes to 3 hours)
Associated symptoms	Neurological symptoms common	Occasional neurological symptoms	None	Inflamed, watery eye
Triggers	Foods, drugs, stress	Trauma, posture	Stressful event	Allergic response, heavy drinking, smoking
Treatment	Avoid precipitating factors. Massage and other physical therapy, stress reduction, medication	Physical therapies including remedial massage therapy (e.g. muscle and joint-specific techniques, heat therapy, myofascial release, posture and exercise rehabilitation)	Physical therapies including remedial massage therapy (e.g. muscle and joint-specific techniques, heat therapy, myofascial release, posture and exercise rehabilitation), stress management including Swedish massage	Avoid precipitating factors. Massage and other physical therapy, medication

Outcome measures

Outcome measures are specifically designed questionnaires that are used to assess clients' level of impairment and to define benefits of treatment. Outcome measures for headache include the Migraine Disability Assessment Test (MIDAS). MIDAS is a simple five-question survey that measures days lost to headache disability during the last 3 months and headache pain on a 10-point scale (see Appendix 13.1).

Postural analysis

Postural analysis may reveal biomechanical compensations resulting from habitual postures or structural factors such as idiopathic scoliosis that can contribute to headache (see Chapter 2).

Functional tests

CERVICAL SPINE

a) Active range of motion

Flexion (50°)[16]

- Stand in front of the client and ask them to take their chin towards their chest as far as they comfortably can.
- The client should be able to touch their chin to their chest.

Extension (60°)

- Ask the client to look up to the ceiling as far as they comfortably can.
- The client should be able to extend their neck so that their face is parallel to the ceiling.

Lateral flexion (sidebend) (45°)

- Ask the client to take their ear toward their shoulder as far as they comfortably can.
- The client should be able to tilt their ear to their shoulder approximately 45°.

Rotation (80°)

- Ask the client to look over their shoulder as far as they comfortably can.
- The client should be able to rotate their neck so that their chin is almost in line with their shoulder.

b) Passive range of motion (see Chapter 12)

Lie the client supine to relax the neck muscles. Great care is needed when performing cervical passive range of motion tests. Perform all neck movements slowly and gently and only ever after you have observed the client's ability to perform active ranges of motion (the See-Move-Touch principle discussed in Chapter 2). Note the end-feel at the end of each range of motion. Stop the movement if neurological symptoms such as pain, paraesthesia or numbness are produced.

Flexion

- Cup the client's occiput with both hands and gently flex the client's neck.

Extension

- When the client is positioned with shoulders level with the top of the table, the neck can be gently extended. Alternatively, the neck can be passively extended by lifting the neck towards the ceiling.

Lateral flexion

- Place one hand on the client's shoulder and with the other, cup the occiput. Gently laterally flex the client's neck with the cupped hand.

Rotation

- Cup the client's occiput with both hands and gently rotate the neck to one side and then the other.

c) Resisted range of motion

Resisted range of motion (RROM) tests are designed to identify muscle groups that may be contributing to the client's condition. Resist the movement as the client flexes, extends, laterally flexes and rotates their head. The client may be seated or lying supine. These tests are usually carried out in conjunction with passive range of motion tests. For example, passive rotation of the neck can be followed immediately by resisted rotation before testing another movement in another plane. If any RROM tests are positive, resisted tests for specific muscle tests are required to identify individual muscles.

Tests for specific muscles associated with neck conditions

Muscle imbalances are commonly associated with headache. Resisted tests and length tests for specific muscles could include suboccipital muscles, posterior cervical muscles and upper trapezius.

d) Special tests

Special tests for headache clients include cervical special tests such as cervical compression, cervical distraction and Valsalva (see Chapter 12) and taking blood pressure. Clients over 50 years of age who present with a new or unaccustomed headache should be referred for blood pressure testing.

Palpation

Hypertonic muscles are commonly palpated in headache sufferers. Palpation should be gentle, as heavy palpation of affected tissues (e.g. trigger points in the upper trapezius, sub-occipital or temporalis muscles, or facet joints) may reproduce or aggravate headache. The following guide to palpation of the posterior cervical muscles is suggested by Simons et al:[17]

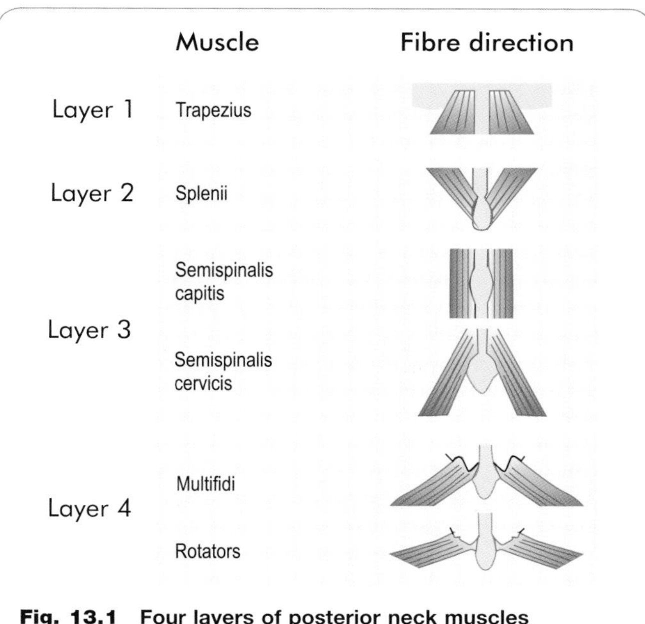

Fig. 13.1 Four layers of posterior neck muscles

Slight flexion of the head and neck makes the posterior neck muscles more distinguishable by palpation. Palpate posterior cervical muscles in four layers (see Figure 13.1).

- Most superficial layer: upper trapezius muscle converging to form a roof-top shape.
- Bilateral splenius fibres converge below to form a V shape.
- Semispinalis capitis fibres lie nearly vertical.
- Muscle fibres in the deepest layers converge to form a roof-top (e.g. semispinalis cervicis) and multifidi and rotators (the fourth layer).

Palpate the temporalis muscles. Spread fingertips across the superior aspects of the temporal fossae on either side of the head. Compare the left and right temporalis muscles as the fingertips move inferiorly through the muscle. Palpate the tendon of temporalis just above the zygomatic arch.

REMEDIAL MASSAGE TREATMENT FOR HEADACHE

Cervicogenic headaches are likely to respond well to spinal manipulation, remedial massage techniques for muscle contractures, trigger point therapy, cryotherapy, thermotherapy and ergonomic advice. However, such treatments may also be useful for other types of headache that are associated with cervical joint dysfunction and myospasm of the suboccipital and posterior neck muscles. Clients with headaches arising from non-mechanical causes should be referred for further investigation and treatment. Treatment can include conventional biomedicine, dietary modification, allergy assessment, herbal and nutritional supplements (e.g. vitamin B_2, vitamin A, calcium and magnesium, feverfew), homoeopathy, acupuncture and stress management.

Treatment options must always be considered in the context of the best available evidence for treatment effectiveness and clinical practice guidelines where they exist. Reviews investigating the effectiveness of non-invasive physical treatments

Table 13.3 Summary of evidence for the effectiveness of remedial massage therapy and other physical therapies for headache and mechanical neck disorders

Level of evidence	Research
Inconclusive	Fernandez-de-Las-Penas et al[19] conducted a systematic review on the effectiveness of manual therapies in reducing pain from tension-type headache. The authors concluded that there is an urgent need for further research to establish the efficacy beyond placebo of the different manual therapies currently provided to patients with tension-type headache.
	Haraldsson et al[20] conducted a review of the use of massage for mechanical neck disorders and were unable to make recommendations for practice because the effectiveness of massage for neck pain remains uncertain. The authors suggested that pilot studies are needed to characterise massage treatment (frequency, duration, number of sessions and massage technique) and establish the optimal treatment to be used in subsequent larger trials that examine the effect of massage as either a stand-alone treatment or part of a multimodal intervention.
	Biondi[18] conducted a structured review of physical treatments for headache which included massage, chiropractic, osteopathy and physical therapy. He concluded that further studies of improved quality are needed to more firmly establish the place of physical modalities in the treatment of primary neck disorder.

have so far not supported the use of manual therapy for long-term management of migraine or other tension-type headache.[6, 18, 19] However, remedial massage therapy for such headaches is often used as an adjunct to other treatments including pharmaceutical or dietary modification. Further research is also needed to investigate the effectiveness of manual therapies used in complex treatment combinations for non-biomechanical headaches. Findings of some current research are summarised in Table 13.3.

TREATMENT PROTOCOLS IN REMEDIAL MASSAGE PRACTICE

All remedial massage treatments are adapted to suit the needs of individual clients. Treatment protocols are templates from which individualised treatments can be developed. A typical remedial massage protocol for a cervicogenic headache includes:

- Swedish massage to the neck, upper back, head and face.
- Remedial massage therapy for muscle strains or imbalances, which includes:
  - deep gliding frictions along the muscle fibres
  - cross-fibre frictions
  - active and passive soft tissue releasing techniques
  - deep transverse friction
  - trigger point therapy
  - muscle stretches.

These techniques are described in Chapter 12 (Table 12.4).

- Apply myofascial releasing techniques for myofascial restrictions. The cranial base release is particularly useful for treating headaches (see Chapter 8).
- Cervical passive joint articulation may be beneficial for facet joint lesions (see Chapter 7). Techniques include:
  - cervical lateral flexion
  - cervical rotation
  - cervical extension
  - horizontal traction
  - stair-step technique
  - facet rotation
  - facet lateral flexion.
- Vascular headaches are usually treated with a cold compress to the head and sub-occipital area and heat to lower back, legs or feet. For non-vascular headaches, thermotherapy may be beneficial for hypertonic posterior cervical muscles and upper trapezius.
- Longer-term treatment addresses any underlying conditions or predisposing factors including scoliosis, hyperlordosis, hyperkyphosis or muscle imbalances.

Remedial massage treatments may also include aromatherapy, acupressure, reflexology and Bowen therapy. Although little scientific evidence is available to support their use, these techniques are often used in clinical practice. They are part of the range of techniques available to remedial massage therapists when negotiating treatment plans with clients. They can be integrated into the treatment plan in a number of ways. For example, an essential oil blend may be used as the lubricant in Swedish massage (5 drops in 10 mL of carrier oil) or vapourised in an oil-burner during the treatment. In its traditional form, Bowen is a stand-alone therapy, but a derivative form is presented here which may be integrated with other remedial techniques (although it usually follows Swedish massage). Acupressure is often integrated with Swedish massage.

Aromatherapy

Essential oils that may relieve headaches include lavender, basil, clary sage, eucalyptus, melissa, peppermint, rosemary, hypericum and chamomile.[21, 22]

Acupressure

Gentle pressure is applied on each acupuncture point for 10 seconds. Points for headache include (see Figure 13.2 on p 233):

- Colon 4 (midway along 2nd metacarpal, thumb side) for tension, headache, sinusitis
- Liver 3 (between first and second toes, 3 fingerbreadths proximal to web on dorsal aspect of foot) for tension, hypertension, urogenital problems
- Facial acupressure headache points (Bladder 1 and 2, Colon 20, Triple Heater 3)
- Suboccipital points (Gall Bladder 20).

Reflexology

Reflexologists use points associated with the head, neck and the underlying cause or predisposing factors of the headache if known (e.g. sinus points for sinusitis or adrenal glands for stress). Techniques include mild pressure directly on the reflex point using fingers, thumbs or knuckles, and *caterpillars*

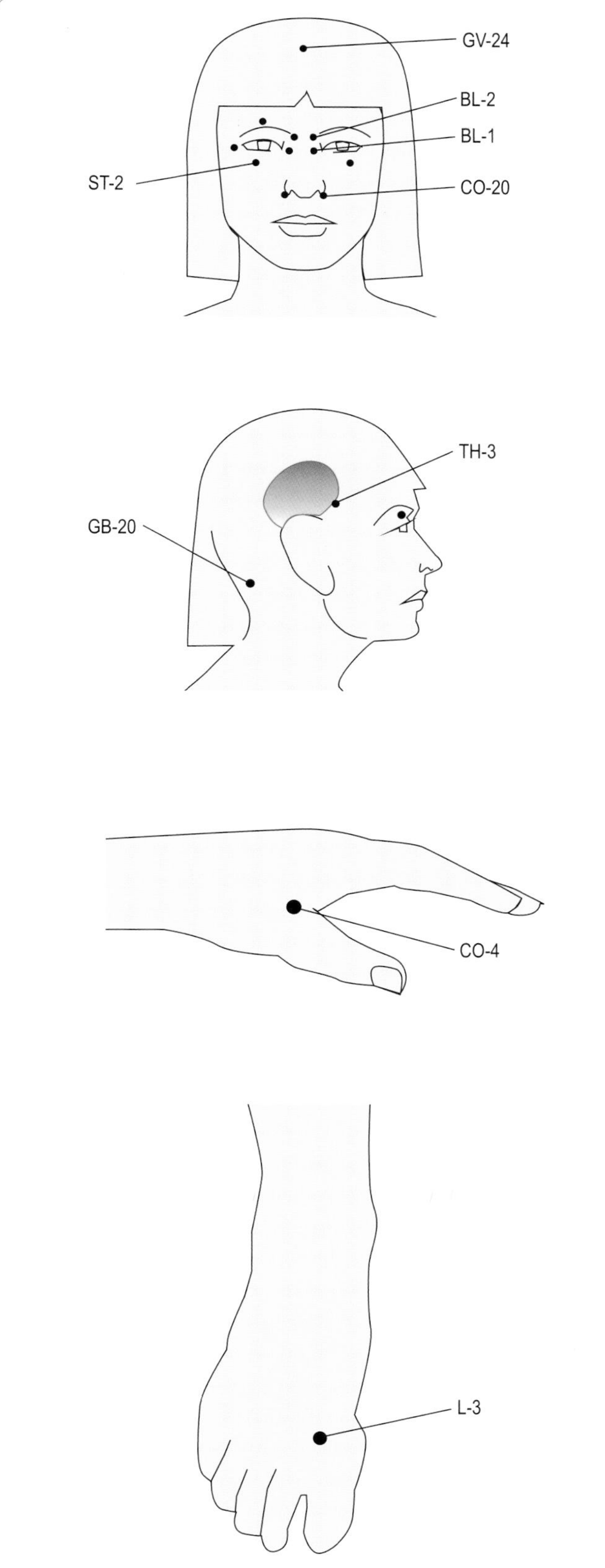

Fig. 13.2 **Acupressure points for headache and sinusitis**

(a stroke involving repeated flexion and extension of the interphalangeal joint of the thumb) (see Figure 13.3 on p 234).

The headache technique (derived from Bowen)

The client lies supine. Sit at the head of the table (see Figure 13.4 on p 234)

1. Using tips of middle fingers, apply light pressure to the inner corner of each eye (Position 1). Avoid any contact with the eye. Hold for 2 seconds. Take up Position 2 before releasing Position 1.
2. Using tips of index fingers, apply light pressure to the inner corner of the eyebrows (Position 2). Hold for 2 seconds. Take up Position 3 before releasing Position 2.
3. Use tips of thumbs, apply light pressure in the middle of the forehead at the hairline (Position 3). Hold for 2 seconds. Take up Position 4 before releasing Position 3.
4. Using the tips of the ring finger or little finger, apply light pressure over the temples (Position 4). Hold for 2 seconds. Take up Position 1 again before releasing Position 4.
   Repeat this procedure (applying light pressure from Position 1, 2, 3 to 4) four times.
5. Apply pressure to Position 4 for 5 seconds using the heels of both hands.

Client education

Client education includes recommendations for self-help such as stress management and avoidance of migraine triggers. Posture advice includes avoiding sustained neck flexion (e.g. when reading or working at a computer) and correcting ergonomics for desk work. The desk should be at elbow height. The top of the screen should be level with or slightly lower than the eyes (see Chapter 12, Figure 12.20).[23]

Home exercises

Lying supine with a rolled towel placed horizontally under the neck may help improve cervical biomechanics. Fold a towel in half lengthways and roll it up. Place the rolled towel behind the neck between the head and the shoulders. The height of the roll can be adjusted by unrolling the towel to the most comfortable height. The position should be painless and able to be maintained for 15–20 minutes. A cold compress (for vascular headache) or heat pack (for cervicogenic headache) can be placed over the towel if indicated.

Stretches and strengthening exercises should be prescribed for specific muscles and commenced as soon as possible. Isometric contractions usually begin when full range of motion has been restored. Strengthening exercises can progress to range of motion exercises performed with the chest and neck over the edge of a bench. Such exercises use resistance against gravity to build strong neck muscles that can support and protect the cervical spine in the same way that strong core muscles support the lumbar spine.

SINUSITIS

The paranasal sinuses are air-filled spaces in the bones of the face (frontal, maxillary, ethmoid and sphenoid) (see Figure 13.5 on p 234). They lighten the skull, produce mucus to moisten inspired air and provide a resonance chamber for

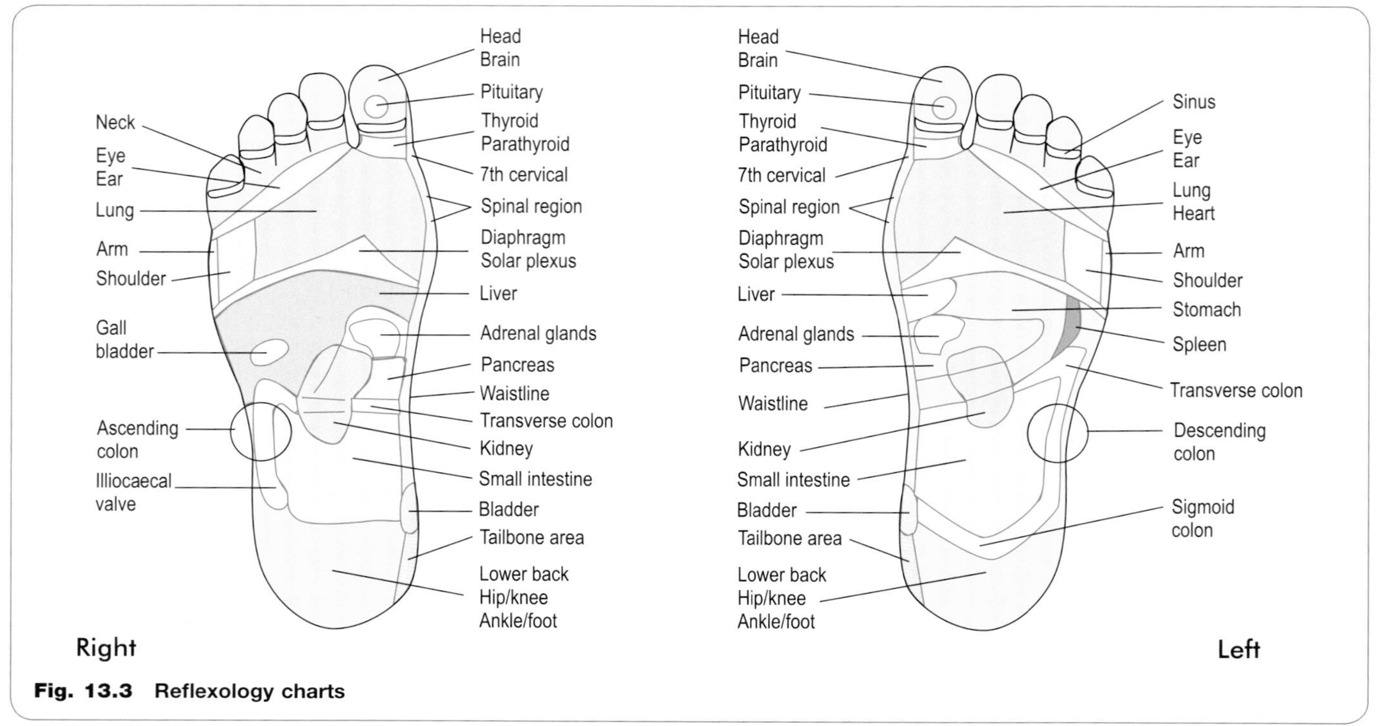

Fig. 13.3 Reflexology charts

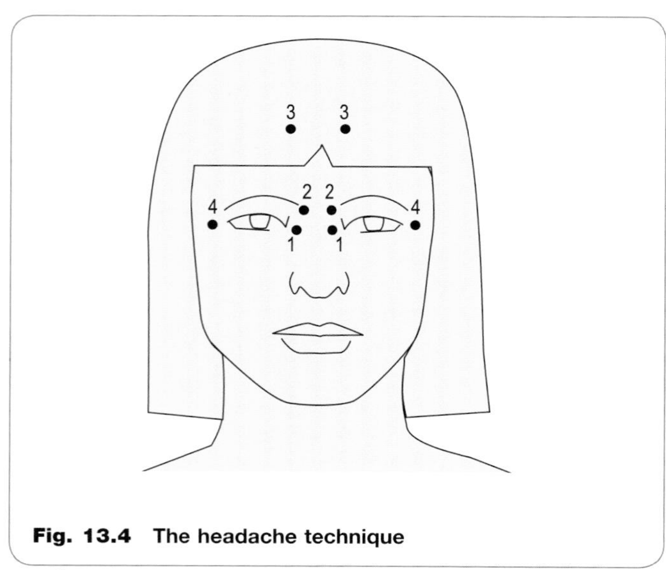

Fig. 13.4 The headache technique

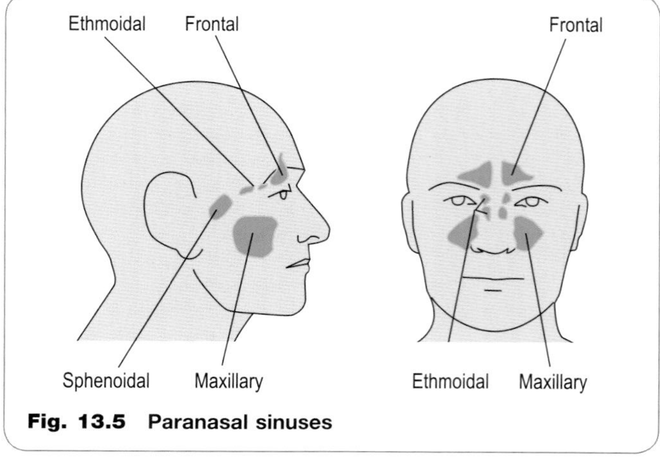

Fig. 13.5 Paranasal sinuses

voice production. Sinusitis refers to inflammation of the paranasal sinuses from over-production of mucus or a swelling of the lining of the sinuses and nose, which causes nasal obstruction and headache. It commonly accompanies a nasal infection but may also be an allergic response to such allergens as pollens or dairy products. It is also associated with cigarette smoking.

ASSESSMENT OF THE CLIENT WITH SINUS PAIN

Assessment of clients for sinusitis focuses on case history, observation and palpation.

Case history

Sinusitis is usually identified by case history. Infection of the frontal sinuses often produces headache that typically reaches a peak within 2 or 3 hours after rising and then subsides through the day. A purulent nasal or postnasal discharge is usually present. Clients describe a feeling of pressure in the head. Infection in the maxillary sinuses may be mistaken for toothache.[24] An allergic rather than microbial cause is suggested if the client reports sneezing and watery rhinorrhoea and has no systemic signs, such as fever or malaise.

The International Headache Society[1] describe the following diagnostic characteristics of sinus headache:

A. Frontal headache accompanied by pain in one or more regions of the face, ears or teeth and fulfilling criteria C and D.

B. Clinical, nasal endoscopic, CT and/or MRI imaging and/or laboratory evidence of acute or acute superimposed on chronic rhinosinusitis.
C. Headache and facial pain develop simultaneously with onset or acute exacerbation of rhinosinusitis.
D. Headache and/or facial pain resolve within 7 days after remission or successful treatment of acute or acute superimposed on chronic rhinosinusitis.

Observation

Nasal congestion is often apparent in the client's breathing and speech. Facial signs of allergic responses (atopic facies) such as dark circles under the eyes and watery eyes may be present.

Palpation

Tenderness is often reported on pressure over the affected sinuses. Press in a superior direction on the frontal and maxillary areas (avoid pressure on eyes) or tap directly over the frontal and maxillary sinuses.[25]

Nasal and sinus infection is often accompanied by swollen and tender lymph nodes in the neck. To palpate lymph nodes the client should be relaxed with their neck slightly flexed and rotated towards the side of the examination. Using the pads of the index and middle fingers palpate (see Figure 13.6):

- pre-auricular nodes – in front of the ear
- posterior auricular nodes – superficial to the mastoid process
- occipital nodes – at the base of the skull posteriorly
- tonsillar nodes – at the angle of the mandible
- submaxillary nodes – halfway between the angle and the tip of the mandible
- submental nodes – in the midline behind the tip of the mandible
- superficial cervical nodes – superficial to the sternocleidomastoid muscle
- posterior cervical chain – along the anterior edge of the trapezius
- deep cervical chain – deep to the sternocleidomastoid muscle (often inaccessible). Hook thumb and fingers around either side of the sternocleidomastoid muscle to find them (caution: the carotid artery and internal jugular vein are deep to the sternocleidomastoid muscle)
- supraclavicular – deep in the angle formed by the clavicle and the sternocleidomastoid muscle.

Note that non-tender nodes are frequently found in healthy people. Unexplained enlarged or tender nodes should be referred for further examination.

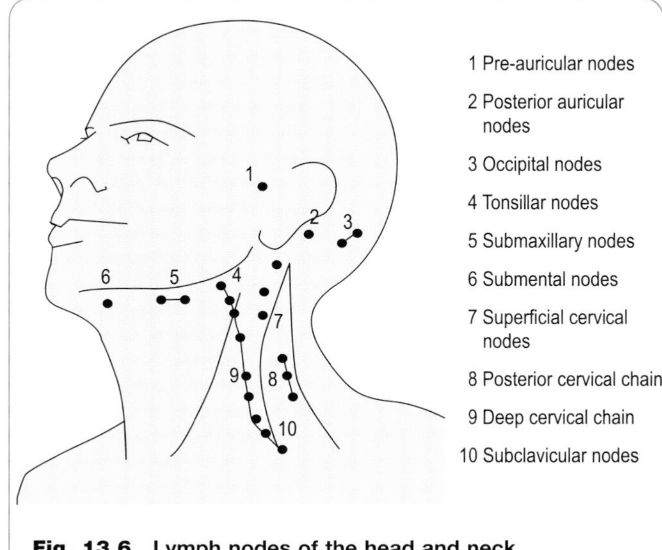

Fig. 13.6 Lymph nodes of the head and neck

REMEDIAL MASSAGE TREATMENT FOR SINUSITIS

Remedial massage therapy for sinusitis is designed to help reduce sinus congestion and thereby bring about symptom relief. Eliminating the infection or exposure to allergens is required for resolution of the cause of inflammation.

A typical remedial massage treatment for sinusitis includes:

- Swedish massage to the face, head and neck. Note that sinusitis sufferers often find lying prone very uncomfortable, not only because of the pressure exerted by the massage table on the affected sinuses, but also because Swedish massage therapy that focuses on relaxation and muscle techniques rather than lymph drainage tends to increase lymphatic congestion in the head. Prone neck and head massage should observe the direction of lymphatic drainage; that is, from cervical spinous processes *laterally* and *inferiorly* towards the posterior cervical chains and supraclavicular nodes.
- Remedial massage for sinusitis consists of lymphatic drainage to the neck and head and gentle pressures on the frontal bone and maxilla designed to open the frontal and maxillary sinuses.

Lymphatic drainage of the neck and head

Lymphatic drainage is described in detail in Chapter 9. A modified version of lymphatic drainage for the neck and head is described here. As with all lymphatic drainage the techniques are applied:

- slowly
- lightly
- monotonously (i.e. a high frequency of repetitions)
- with changes in pressure (i.e. pumping lymphatic fluid is achieved by alternating between pressure on and off with the fingers)
- in the direction of lymphatic flow (see Figure 13.7 on p 236).

1. LYMPHATIC PUMP OVER THE STERNUM

Begin and end all lymphatic drainage with a lymphatic pump. The client lies supine. Stand at the head of the table. With one hand on top of the other or side by side, place palms over the sternum or upper chest, fingers pointed inferiorly. Passively move hands up and down with the client's breathing. Ask the client to breathe deeply through the mouth. At the end of one full expiration by the client, maintain enough pressure on the sternum to prevent the rib cage rising as the client inhales. Towards the end of the inhalation, release the pressure as quickly as possible by jumping the hands off the sternum. The client usually makes an involuntary gasping sound as the

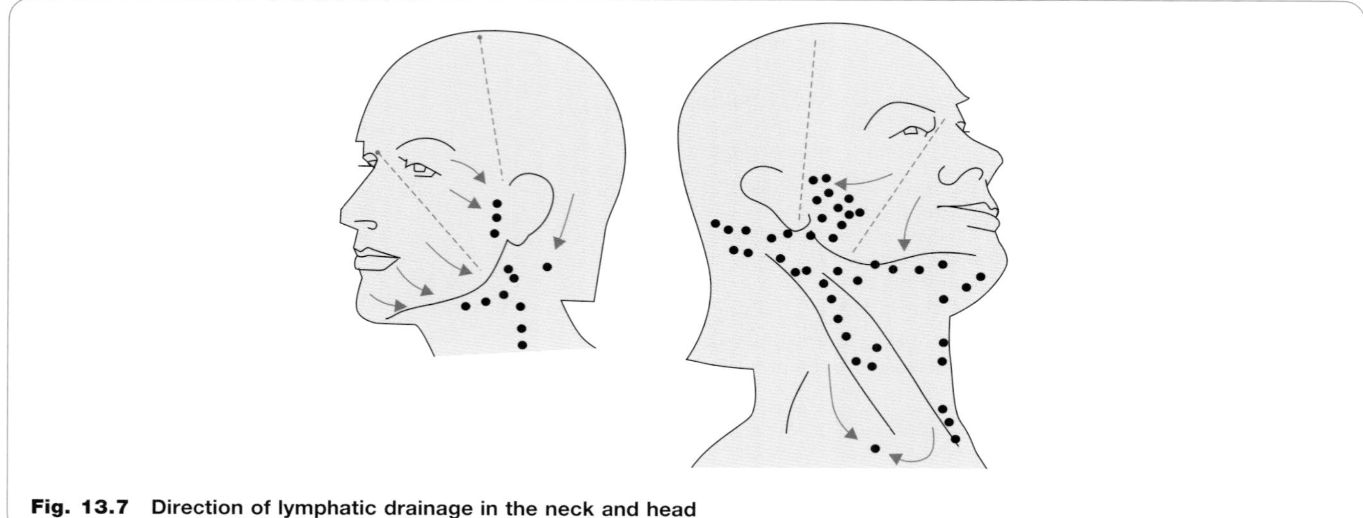

Fig. 13.7 Direction of lymphatic drainage in the neck and head

lungs suddenly expand. Note the difference between a lymphatic pump and the technique used in cardiopulmonary resuscitation: there is no attempt to depress the sternum beyond its natural level at the end of a forced expiration. This technique is contraindicated in clients with osteoporosis.

2. LYMPHATIC DRAINAGE OF THE HEAD AND NECK

The client is supine with slight elevation of the head (use a pillow or adjust the headpiece) to assist lymphatic drainage. Treatment begins with lymphatic drainage of the neck.

- Apply gentle pressure to the supraclavicular nodes for 10–15 seconds.
- Using fingertips, make spiral movements or stationary circles up the cervical chains (via the sternocleidomastoid muscle) towards the mastoid process, breaking contact to move in small increments along the muscle. At each point of contact, repeat the spiral/circular movement 5 to 7 times, making sure the pressure varies with each application (*pressure on–pressure off*).
- Drain the cervical chain towards the suprasternal nodes using a light pumping or stripping movement of the thumb or fingers. Pressure variation is achieved by slightly firmer stripping strokes draining inferiorly, followed by lighter return strokes. To pump the lymph, alternately apply gentle pressure with the fingers and release it moving progressively inferiorly along the sternocleidomastoid.

Repeat this procedure several times. Apply a similar procedure from the mastoid process along the base of the occiput to the midline and drain back towards the posterior auricular nodes.

3. LYMPHATIC DRAINAGE OF THE FACE

- Apply gentle pressure to the pre-auricular nodes for 10–15 seconds.
- Apply spirals or stationary circles away from the pre-auricular nodes in three sections:
  i) towards the midline of the mandible (include tonsillar, submaxillary and submental nodes)
  ii) towards the nose
  iii) towards the midline of the forehead.
- At each point of contact, repeat the spiral/circular movement 5 to 7 times, making sure pressure varies with each application (*pressure on–pressure off*). Break contact to move in small increments towards the midline of the face.
- Drain lymph towards pre-auricular glands using thumb or fingers to strip or pump towards the ears. Use a slightly firmer drainage stroke and a lighter return stroke to vary the pressure when using a stripping technique. To pump the lymph, alternately apply gentle pressure with the fingertips and release it, moving progressively towards the pre-auricular nodes.

Repeat this procedure several times. The technique can also be applied to submaxillary nodes halfway between the chin and angle of the mandible. Lymph is drained from the sides of the nose towards the submaxillary nodes.

4. REPEAT THE LYMPHATIC PUMP DESCRIBED IN 1.

Another useful lymphatic drainage technique for the neck is known as the *claw technique*. The client lies supine. Stand at the side of the table facing superiorly. With fingers spread so that the index finger is at C1–2 level and the little finger is at C6–C7 level just lateral to the spinous processes on the contralateral side, slowly draw the fingers anteriorly and inferiorly, flattening the fingers as they reach the sternocleidomastoid muscle and draining towards the supraclavicular nodes (see Figure 13.8 on p 237). Repeat several times.

Opening the frontal and maxillary sinuses

- Standing or sitting at the side of the table, place the lateral aspect of the cephalad thumb on the client's forehead (hook under the supraorbital ridges) and hold the bridge of the nose with the thumb and index finger of the other hand. Make sure your hand is not covering the client's nose or mouth. Apply superior pressure with the contact on the frontal bone for 5 seconds (Figure 13.9a on p 237).
- Stand or sit at the head of the table. Using either the lateral aspects of the thumbs or tips of the fingers, hook around the medial aspect of the zygomatic arches either side of the

nose. Apply lateral pressure for 5 seconds (Figure 13.9b on p 237).

- Stand or sit at the corner of the top of the table. Using either the lateral aspects of the thumbs or the tips of fingers, hook around the supraorbital ridge with one hand and the medial aspect of the opposite zygomatic arch with the other. Caution: do not contact eyes. Apply diagonal pressure for 5 seconds. Repeat on the other side (see Figures 13.9c).

Other remedial massage techniques for sinusitis include:

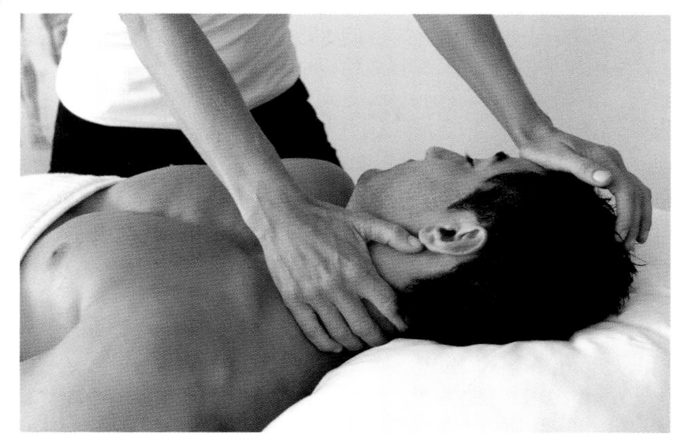

Fig. 13.8 Claw technique

Aromatherapy

Essential oils for sinusitis include eucalyptus, peppermint, pine, tea tree, French basil, cajeput and niaouli.[21] They can be vapourised in an oil burner during the massage, or recommended to the client for use in steam inhalations at home (5 drops of essential oil in a bowl containing 1 litre of steaming water, head covered with a towel, leaning over the bowl with eyes shut and inhaling). Alternatively, 5 drops of essential oil can be added to bath water just before turning off the taps.[21]

Acupressure

Acupressure can be integrated into the massage at any stage. Gently apply digital pressure for 10 seconds to the following acupressure points: Bladder 1, Bladder 2, Colon 20, Triple heater 3, Colon 4, Gall bladder 20 (see Figure 13.2 on p 233). Note that pressure over the sinuses may cause pain if the sinuses are acutely inflamed. Always work within the client's pain tolerance.

Reflexology

Reflexologists use reflex points associated with the head, neck and underlying cause or predisposing factors if known. Mild pressure can be applied directly on the reflex point using fingers, thumbs or knuckles (see Figure 13.3 on p 234).

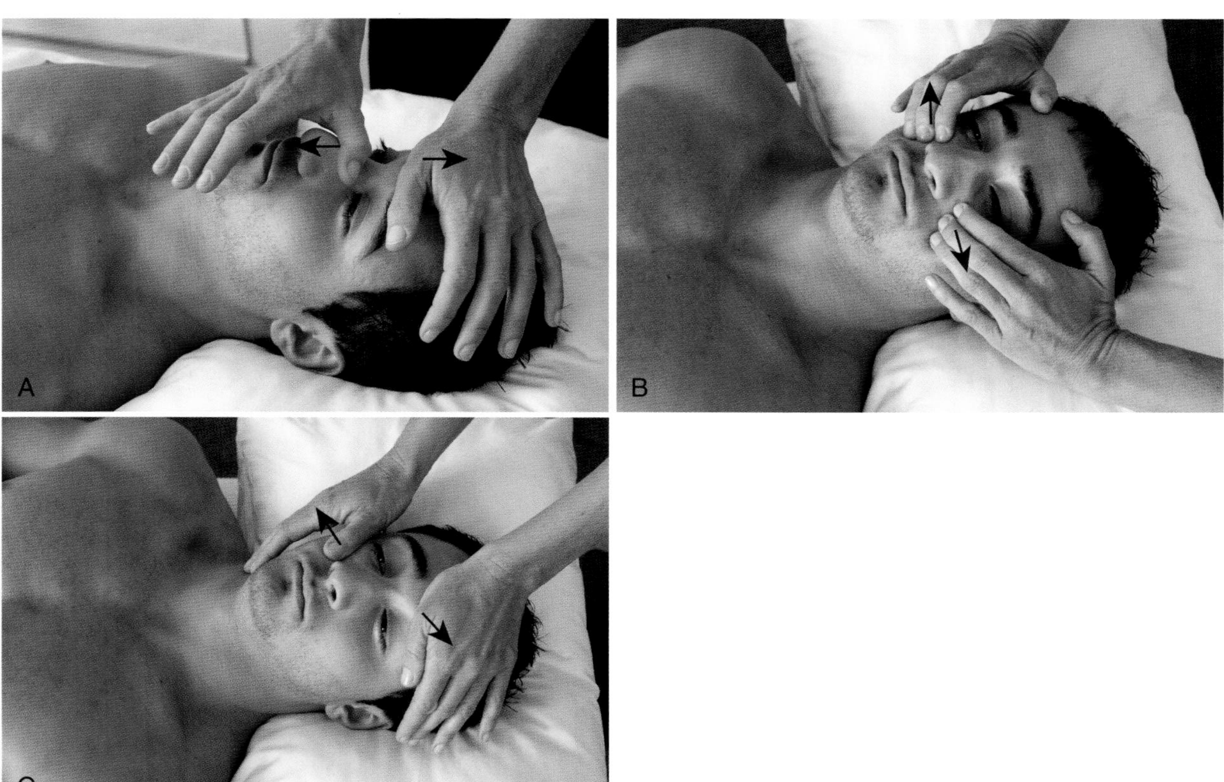

Fig. 13.9 Opening the frontal and maxillary sinuses

Client education

Advise clients to address the cause of the sinusitis if possible (e.g. pharmaceutical treatment for bacterial infection, allergy testing, avoiding allergens). Traditional treatments include increased daily water intake and steam inhalations. Where appropriate, refer clients to *Quit Smoking* programs.

HOME EXERCISES

Ocean swimming may help drain the sinuses.

TEMPOROMANDIBULAR JOINT DISORDERS

The temporomandibular joint (TMJ) is the most used joint in the body. It opens and closes approximately 1500–2000 times a day. It is a condylar joint formed between the mandibular fossa of the temporal bone and the condyle of the mandible and covered in white fibrocartilage. The TMJ is surrounded by fibrous capsule lined with synovial membrane. The capsular ligaments lie medially and laterally: the meniscotemporomandibular frenum (retrodiscal pad) lies posteriorly. Further posteriorly and medially are the stylomandibular and sphenomandibular ligaments (Figure 13.10). Three muscles (temporalis, masseter and medial pterygoid) close the mouth and provide the power to bite and chew; one muscle, lateral pterygoid, opens the mouth (see Table 13.4). Opening is achieved by a combination of rotation and gliding. A disc divides the joint into an upper part for rotation and a lower part for glide. The dual heads of the lateral pterygoid muscle act asynchronously, the upper head hinging the head of the mandible and the lower head pulling the mandible forward.

DISORDERS OF THE TEMPOROMANDIBULAR JOINT

It is estimated that up to 50% of the population have some symptoms of TMJ dysfunction. Clients are often young adults aged 20–40 years. Females with TMJ dysfunction outnumber males 4 to 1.[4] Causes of TMJ disorders include trauma, wear and tear, behavioural factors like grinding teeth and regularly chewing gum and malocclusion.

Temporomandibular joint disorders include three main groups:

1. Muscle disorders (the most common TMJ disorder).
2. Derangement disorders (e.g. dislocated jaw, displacement or distortion of the disc). *Clicking jaw* occurs when the condyle of the mandible overrides an anteromedially *displaced disc.* In some cases, the disc may become so distorted that it stops the condyle from translating forwards and locks the jaw closed (see Figure 13.11 on p 238).
3. Degenerative disorders such as arthritis which causes destruction of cartilage overlaying the TMJ.

ASSESSMENT OF THE CLIENT WITH TMJ DISORDER

Because the biomechanics of the TMJ, cervical spine and cranium are interconnected, assessment of the TMJ also involves assessment of the neck and head.

Case history

Clients almost always give the diagnosis in the history. Presenting symptoms include sharp unilateral facial pain on movement of the jaw, pain increasing as the mouth is opened, difficulty chewing, clicking jaw and sometimes ear symptoms (pain, impaired hearing, tinnitus), neuralgia and headache. The International Headache Society[1] describes the following characteristics of headache due to TMJ disorder:

A. Recurrent pain in one or more regions of the head and/or face, fulfilling criteria C and D.
B. X-ray, MRI and/or bone scintigraphy[b] demonstrate TMJ disorder.

[b]Scintigraphy is a diagnostic technique that involves the ingestion of radioisotopes to produce two-dimensional images.

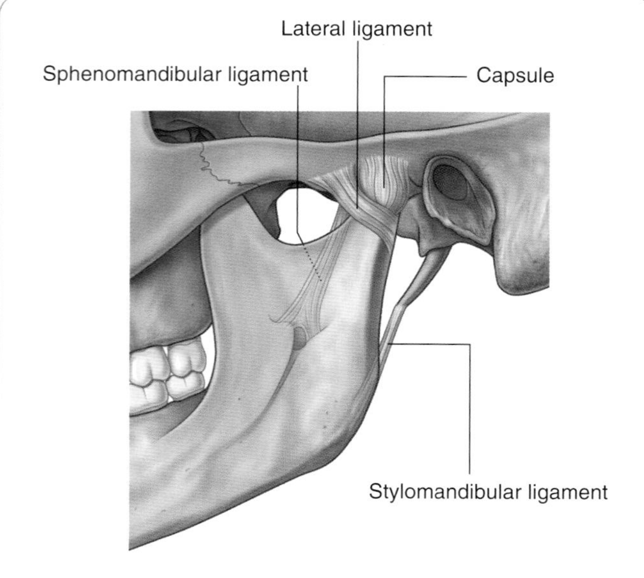

Fig. 13.10 The temporomandibular joint

Table 13.4 Muscles that move the jaw

Muscle	Origin	Insertion	Action
Temporalis	temporal bone	coronoid process of mandible	elevates and retracts mandible
Masseter	maxilla and zygomatic arch	angle and ramus of mandible	elevates mandible
Medial pterygoid	medial surface of lateral pterygoid plate of sphenoid	angle and ramus of mandible	elevates and protrudes mandible, moves mandible from side to side
Lateral pterygoid	greater wing and lateral surface of lateral plate of sphenoid bone	lower head: condyle of mandible Upper head: disc and fibrous capsule	protrudes mandible, opens mouth, moves mandible from side to side

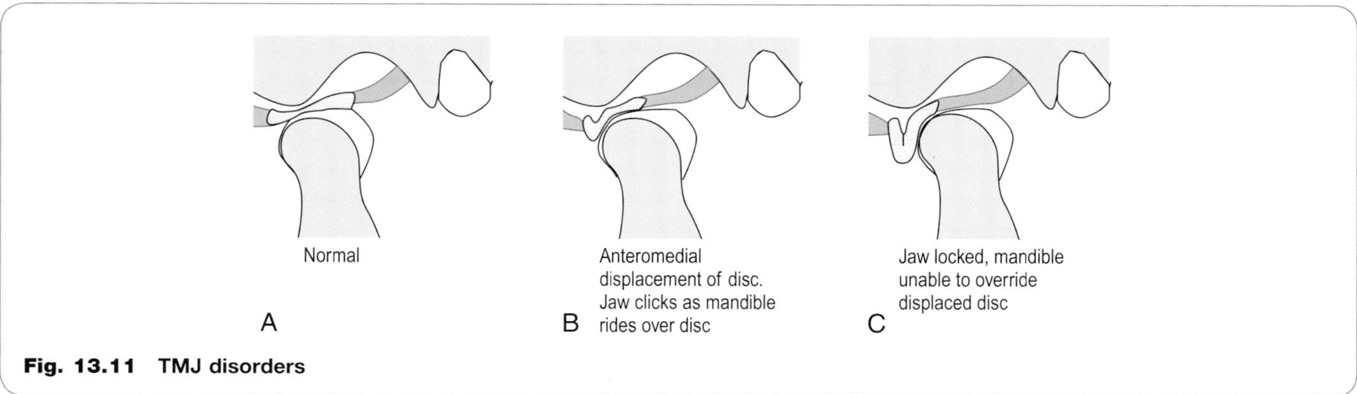

Fig. 13.11 TMJ disorders

C. Evidence that pain can be attributed to the TMJ disorder, based on at least one of the following:
   1. pain is precipitated by jaw movements and/or chewing of hard or tough food
   2. reduced range of or irregular jaw opening
   3. noise from one or both TMJs during jaw movements
   4. tenderness of the joint capsule(s) of one or both TMJs.

D. Headache resolves within 3 months, and does not recur, after successful treatment of the TMJ disorder.

Observation

Observe the mandible in motion and at rest. At rest the teeth are usually not in contact. On closure, teeth are in apposition with the spaces between the upper and lower central incisors aligned.

Postural analysis

TMJ dysfunction may be associated with forward head carriage and myofascial restrictions (e.g. restrictions of the deep front line, superficial back line and spiral line[26]) which may be detected during postural observation.

Functional tests

ACTIVE RANGE OF MOTION TESTS OF THE CERVICAL SPINE (FLEXION, EXTENSION, LATERAL FLEXION, ROTATION)

If any active range of motion tests of the cervical spine are positive, further assessment of the cervical spine is indicated (see Chapter 12).

ACTIVE RANGE OF MOTION OF THE TMJ

- Mandibular depression (opening): clients should be able to open their mouth wide enough for three fingers to be inserted vertically between the incisors.
- Mandibular elevation (closing): the upper and lower teeth should touch.
- Mandibular protrusion: the mandible should protrude far enough for the lower teeth to be placed in front of the upper teeth.
- Mandibular retraction.

RESISTED RANGE OF MOTION OF THE TMJ

It is difficult to isolate muscles of the TMJ because their actions overlap. Consequently, muscles are tested in groups (see Table 13.5).

Table 13.5 Resisted and length tests for muscles of the TMJ

	Resisted test	**Test for contracture**
Closing the mouth • medial pterygoid • temporalis • masseter	Ask the client to open their mouth. Place the web between your thumb and index finger on the mandible below the level of the teeth. Resist as the client tries to close their mouth.	Limited mouth opening (i.e. unable to place three fingers vertically between upper and lower teeth).
Opening the mouth • lateral pterygoid	Hold the client's mandible at the chin and resist mouth opening.	Inability to bring the teeth together.

Palpation

The masseter muscle is easily located in the cheeks when clients clench their teeth. With the muscle relaxed, palpate from the zygomatic arch to the angle of the mandible. Palpating bilaterally enables comparison of the muscles on either side.

Palpate the temporalis muscle in the temporal fossa. Palpate from its superior aspect inferiorly and feel the muscle as it gathers to pass beneath the zygomatic arch. Linear fibrotic tissue may be palpable superiorly to the zygomatic arch, and often anteriorly. To palpate the attachment of temporalis on the coronoid process, have the client open their mouth. Temporalis may be palpable at the coronoid process immediately beneath the zygomatic arch when the client's mouth is open.

Accessibility of lateral pterygoid for palpation is questioned by some authors, who maintain that the muscle is not palpable under the buccinator and medial pterygoid.[27] Traditionally the technique for palpating lateral pteryoid is to place a gloved index finger in the client's mouth between the buccal mucosa and the superior gum and point the tip of the finger posteriorly past the last molar to the neck of the mandible. As the client opens their mouth lateral pterygoid is thought to be palpable as it tightens against the practitioner's finger.

The following techniques may be used to palpate the TMJ:

i) Place index and middle fingers just anterior to the ears and ask the client to open and close their mouth. Observe the degree of opening, lateral deviation and synchronicity of movement of both temporomandibular joints.

ii) Place gloved index fingers into client's ears and palpate anteriorly as the client opens and closes their mouth.

REMEDIAL MASSAGE TREATMENTS FOR TMJ DISORDERS

If acute inflammation is present, treatment usually involves cryotherapy or anti-inflammatory medication. Introduce gentle range of motion exercises as soon as they can be tolerated by the client. A typical remedial massage treatment for a mild or moderate TMJ disorder includes:

- Swedish massage therapy to the upper back, neck, head and face.
- Remedial massage techniques for muscle imbalances and/or muscle strains, including (see Table 13.6):
  - deep gliding frictions along the muscle fibres
  - cross-fibre frictions
  - active and passive soft tissue releasing techniques
  - deep transverse frictions

Table 13.6 Remedial massage for muscles of the TMJ

Muscle	Soft-tissue releasing techniques	Trigger point	Client education	Stretch
Temporalis	Apply pressure to site of muscle lesion as client slowly opens and closes their mouth. 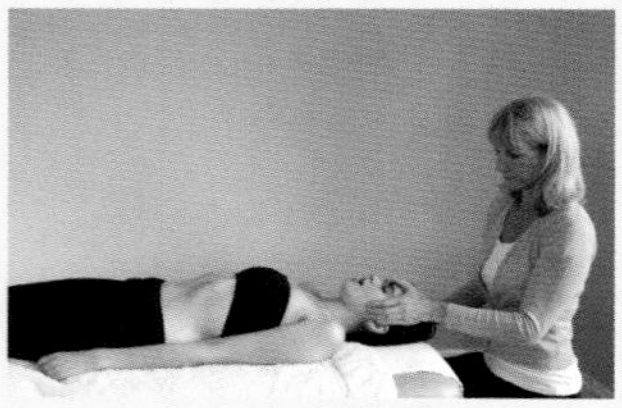	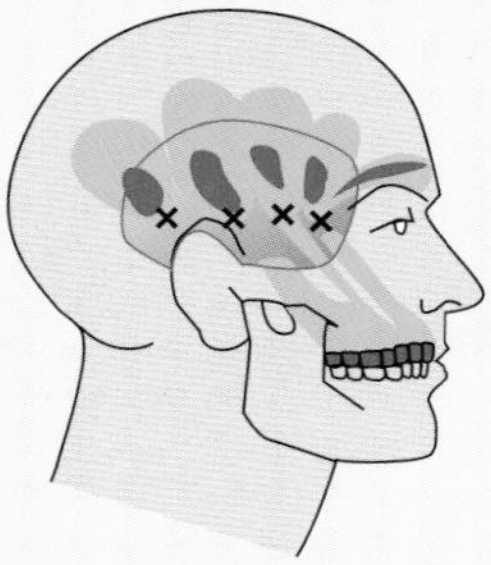	• Correct forward head posture. • Avoid excessive chewing, clenching and grinding teeth, chewing gum, biting hard food. • Reduce stress.	• Open mouth as far as possible; pull the jaw downward and to the opposite side.
Masseter	As above	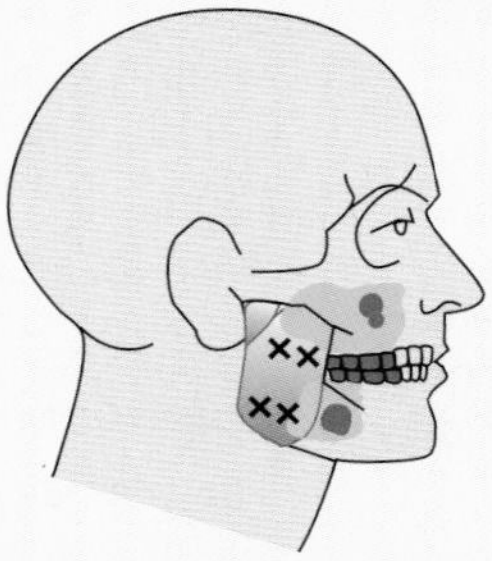	As above	As above
Medial pterygoid	As above	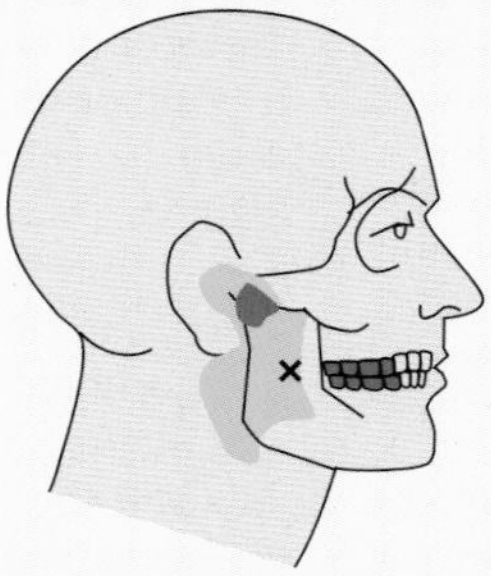	As above	• Open mouth as far as possible. • With the web between the thumb and index finger, gently push the chin posteriorly. • Move jaw to the side as far as possible.
Lateral pterygoid	As above	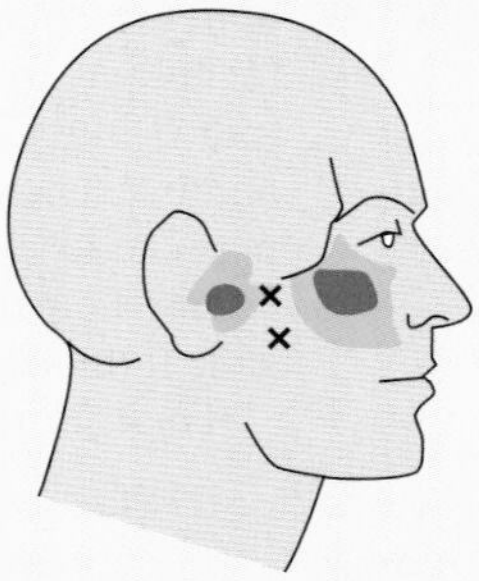	• Avoid excessive chewing, clenching and grinding teeth, chewing gum, biting hard food. • Reduce stress. • May need occlusal splint.	• With the web between the thumb and index finger, gently push the chin posteriorly. • Move jaw to the side as far as possible.

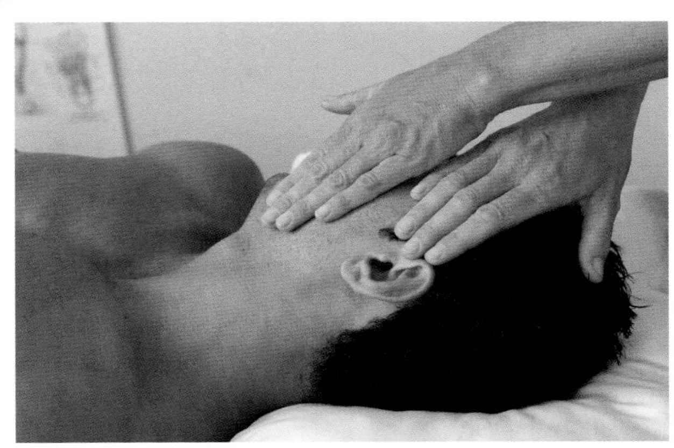

Fig. 13.12 Myofascial releasing techniques for the temporomandibular joint

- trigger point therapy
- muscle stretches.
- Myofascial releasing techniques may be beneficial for fascial restrictions (see Figure 13.12).

Client education

Advise clients that most TMJ disorders are temporary and resolve with simple conservative treatment. Avoid hard foods, cut food into small pieces, chew using molars on both sides and avoid chewing gum. Thermotherapy may relieve muscle spasm and pain. Correcting forward head carriage and other posture distortions will improve the biomechanics of the region. Refer to a chiropractor, osteopath or physiotherapist for osseous manipulation. Some clients may require dental splinting. Stress management may be indicated to eliminate teeth clenching and grinding.

HOME EXERCISE PROGRAM

Ask the client to stand in front of a mirror and slowly open and close their mouth making sure the jaw moves in a straight line. Within pain tolerance they should try to correct any deviations they observe. Specific stretching exercises (see Table 13.6) and strengthening exercises (resisting TMJ opening, closing or translating to the side) can be performed as required.

KEY MESSAGES

HEADACHE

- Remedial massage therapy has a key role to play in the treatment and management of headache: in cases of cervicogenic headache and tension-type headache remedial massage may be the primary treatment; in other types of headache remedial massage may be a useful adjunct to other treatments.
- Assessment of clients with headache involves history, outcome measures, postural analysis, functional tests (including resisted tests for specific muscles of the neck and face), special tests for the cervical spine and palpation.
- Case history is particularly important for identifying red flags. There are many different types of headaches, but only rarely are they the result of a serious pathology. Red flags include[1] sudden onset of a new severe headache;[2] a worsening pattern of a pre-existing headache in the absence of obvious predisposing factors;[3] more than three headaches per week;[4] headaches requiring pain-killers every day or almost daily;[5] headaches whose relief requires more than over-the-counter medication;[6] headache associated with fever, neck stiffness, skin rash and with a history of cancer, HIV or other systemic illness;[7] headache associated with focal neurological signs other than typical aura;[8] moderate or severe headache triggered by cough, exertion, or bearing down;[9] new onset of a headache during or following pregnancy;[10] headaches beginning after the age of 50.
- Consider Clinical Guidelines, available evidence and client preferences when planning therapy. Current evidence supports the use of manual therapy for cervicogenic headaches.
- Be conservative in treatment: if in doubt, refer for further investigation.
- Remedial massage treatment aims to address muscle imbalances, improve facet joint movement, release myofascial restrictions, provide relaxation therapy and educate clients about self-management of headaches.

SINUSITIS

- Remedial massage therapy may provide symptomatic relief for sinusitis sufferers but does not address causative factors (e.g. infections, allergies).
- Assessment of clients with sinusitis involves history, outcome measures, observation and palpation. Be vigilant for red flags, particularly if clients present with headache, although they are unlikely.
- Consider Clinical Guidelines, available evidence and client preferences when planning therapy.
- Remedial massage treatment aims to relieve sinus congestion and to educate clients about self-management of sinusitis.

TEMPOROMANDIBULAR JOINT

- Assessment of clients with TMJ disorders involves history, outcome measures, postural analysis, functional tests (including functional tests of the cervical region and the TMJ) and palpation.
- Consider Clinical Guidelines, available evidence and client preferences when planning therapy.
- Remedial massage may provide symptom relief for mild to moderate TMJ disorders by addressing imbalances in muscles that move the jaw, releasing myofascial restrictions, providing relaxation therapy and educating clients about self-management of TMJ disorders.

Review questions

Headache

1. List five red flags for serious causes of headache.
2. What are the main characteristics of migraine headaches (e.g. location, type of pain, chronicitiy, duration)?
3. What percentage of migraine sufferers experience an aura? What symptoms might they have?
4. How would you distinguish between a vascular and a cervicogenic headache?
5. How can remedial massage assist in the treatment of tension-type headache?
6. Indicate the correct answer by circling True or False:
   i) The most common type of headache is cervicogenic. True/False
   ii) Migraines often strike in the middle of the night. True/False
   iii) Tension-type headaches last no more than 1 or 2 days. True/False
   iv) Sinusitis headache is aggravated by bending forward. True/False
   v) Cervicogenic headaches typically start at the back of the neck and radiate over the head to the forehead. True/False
7. List three important questions that you would include in history taking to help eliminate the possibility of a pathological headache or other headache requiring referral.

Sinusitis

1. Where are the paranasal sinuses located?
2. Name two common causes of sinusitis.
3. What is the role of remedial massage in the treatment of sinusitis?
4. Swedish massage can increase lymphatic congestion in the head. How would you modify your Swedish massage treatment to minimise this effect?
5. What home advice would you give a client with sinusitis?

Temporomandibular joint disorder

1. Describe how lateral pterygoid acts to open the jaw.
2. List four symptoms that can be associated with TMJ dysfunction.
3. A client with normal range of motion of the TMJ should be able to:
   i) Open their mouth wide enough to ______________________________
   ii) Protrude their jaw far enough to ______________________________
4. Draw the pain referral patterns for the following trigger points.

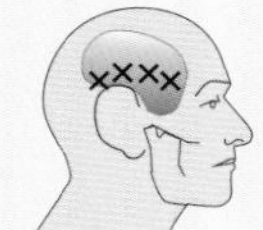
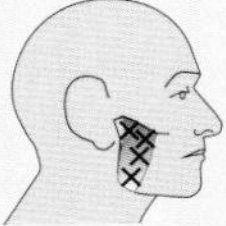
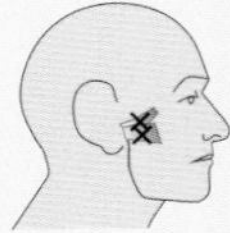
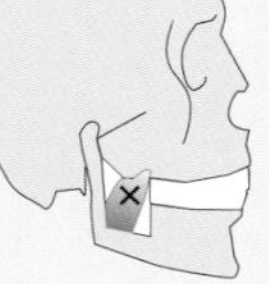

5. What home advice would you give a client with a clicking jaw?

APPENDIX 13.1

MIDAS (The Migraine Disability Assessment Test)

The MIDAS (migraine disability assessment) questionnaire was put together to help you measure the impact your headaches have had on your life over the last 3 months and to communicate this more effectively. The best way to do this is by counting the numbers of days of your life which are affected by headaches. You can do this for yourself as follows:

Please complete questions about ALL your headaches you have had over the last month. Leave the box set to zero if you did not do the activity in the last three months.

For questions 1 and 2, **work or school** means paid work or education if you are a student at school or college. For Questions 3 and 4, **household work** means activities such as housework, home repairs and maintenance, shopping as well as caring for children and relatives.

INSTRUCTIONS • Please answer the following questions about ALL your headaches you have had over the last 3 months. Select your answer in the box next to each question. If a single headache affects more than one area of your life (e.g. work and family life) it is counted more than once. Select zero if you did not have the activity in the last 3 months.

1. On how many days in the last 3 months did you miss work or school because of your headaches? [0]

2. How many days in the last 3 months was your productivity at work or school reduced by half or more because of your headaches?
(Do not include days you counted in question 1 where you missed work or school.) [0]

3. On how many days in the last 3 months did you not do household work because of your headaches? [0]

4. How many days in the last three months was your productivity in household work reduced by half or more because of your headaches?
(Do not include days you counted in question 3 where you did not do household work.) [0]

5. On how many days in the last 3 months did you miss family, social or leisure activities because of your headaches? [0]

What your doctor will need to know about your headache:

A. On how many days in the last 3 months did you have a headache?
(If a headache lasted more than 1 day, count each day.) [0]

B. On a scale of 0 to 10, on average how painful were these headaches?
(where 0 = no pain at all and 10 = pain as bad as it can be.) [0]

Please enter your e-mail address if you would also like an e-mail copy of the results.
(Leave this box blank if you do not need a copy.)

Calculate my Score

This survey was developed by Richard B. Lipton, MD, Professor of Neurology, Albert Einstein College of Medicine, New York, NY, and Walter F. Stewart, MPH, PhD, Associate Professor of Epidemiology, Johns Hopkins University, Baltimore, MD.

REFERENCES

1. International Headache Society. The International classification of headache disorders. 2nd edn. Cephalalgia 2005;25:460–5.
2. Pfizer Australia Pty Ltd. Pfizer Australia Health Report 2004; (15). Online. Available: www.healthreport.com.au/Reports/15.pdf.
3. Alexander L. Prevalance and cost of headache. Online. Available: http://www.headacheaustralia.org.au/what_is_headache/prevalence_and_cost_of_headache; 2003.
4. Carnes M, Vizniak N. Quick reference evidence-based conditions manual. 3rd edn. Burnaby, BC: Professional Health System; 2009.
5. Jull G, Trott P, Potter H. A randomized controlled trial of exercise and manipulative therapy for cervicogenic headache. Spine 2002;27:1835–43.
6. Bronfort G, Nilsson N, Haas M, et al. Non-invasive physical treatments for chronic/recurrent headache. Cochrane Database Syst Rev 2004;(3):CD001878.
7. Beers M, Porter R. The Merck Manual of Diagnosis and Therapy. 17th edn. West Point, PA: Merck; 1999.
8. Hall T, Briffa K, Hopper D. Clinical evaluation of cervicogenic headache: a clinical perspective. J Man Manip Ther 2008;16(2):73–80.
9. Siberstein S. Approach to the patient with headache. Online. Available from: http://www.merck.com/mmpe/sec16/ch216/ch216a.html; 2008.
10. Department of Health Western Australia. Adult patient with a headache. Online. Available: http://www.imagingpathways.health.wa.gov.au/includes/pdf/headache.pdf; 2005.
11. Bigal M, Lipton R. The differential diagnosis of chronic daily headaches: an algorithm-based approach. J Headache Pain 2007;8(5):263–72.
12. Sobri M, Lamont A, Alias N, et al. Red flags in patients presenting with headache: clinical indications for neuroimaging. Br J Radiol 2003;76:532–5.
13. Zito G, Jull G, Story I. Clinical tests of musculoskeletal dysfunction in the diagnosis of cervicogenic headache. Man Ther 2006;11(2):118–29.
14. Hack G, Koritzer R, Robinson W, et al. Anatomical relation between the rectus capitis posterior minor muscle and the dura mater. Spine 1997;22(8):924–6.
15. Brukner P, Khan K. Clinical Sports Medicine. 3rd edn. North Ryde, NSW: McGraw-Hill Book Company; 2010.
16. Reese N, Bandy W. Joint range of motion and muscle length testing. Philadelphia: W.B. Saunders; 2002.
17. Simons D, Travell J, Simons L. Myofascial pain and dysfunction: The trigger point manual. Vol 1: upper half of body. 2nd edn. Philadelphia: Williams and Wilkins; 1999.
18. Biondi D. Physical treatment for headache: a structured review. Headache 2005;45:738–46.
19. Fernandez-de-Las-Penas C, Alonso-Blanco C, Cuadrado M, et al. Are manual therapies effective in reducing pain from tension-type headache? A systematic review. Clin J Pain 2006;22:278–85.
20. Haraldsson BG, Gross AR, Myers CD, et al. Massage for mechanical neck disorders. Cochrane Database Syst Rev 2006;(3):CD004871.
21. Lawless J. The illustrated encyclopaedia of essential oils: the complete guide to the use of oils in aromatherapy and herbalism. Shaftesbury: Elements; 1995.
22. Battaglia S. The complete guide to aromatherapy. 2nd edn. Virginia, Qld: Perfect Potion; 2004.
23. Swinburne University of Technology. OH&S workstation assessment: Setting up your workstation. Online. Available: www.swinburne.edu.au/corporate/hr/ohs/ohs_ergonomics.htm; 2009.
24. Munro J, Campbell I, editors. Macleod's clinical examination. Edinburgh: Churchill Livingstone; 2000.
25. Bickley L, Szilagyi P, editors. Bates' guide to physical examination and history taking. 10th edn. Philadelphia: Lippincott-Raven; 2009.
26. Myers T. Anatomy trains. Edinburgh: Churchill Livingstone; 2001.
27. Stratmann U, Mokrys K, Meyer U, et al. Clinical anatomy and palpability of the inferior lateral pterygoid muscle. J Prosthet Dent 2000;83(5):548–54.

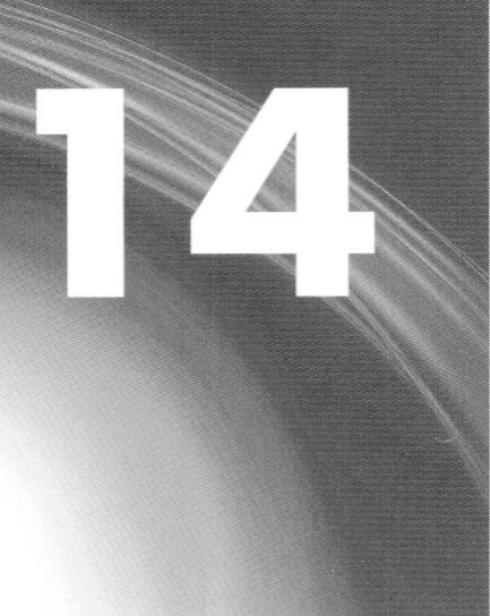

The chest

The content of this chapter relates to the following Units of Competency:

HLTREM503C Plan remedial massage treatment strategy
HLTREM504C Apply remedial massage assessment framework
HLTREM502C Provide remedial massage treatment
HLTREM505C Perform remedial massage health assessment

Health Training Package HLT07

Learning Outcomes

- Assess clients with chest conditions for remedial massage, including identification of red and yellow flags.
- Assess and treat clients with symptoms associated with muscle strains, rib subluxations and costochondritis.
- Provide supportive massage therapy to clients with chronic respiratory conditions.
- Develop treatment plans for clients with chest conditions, taking into account assessment findings, duration and severity of the condition, likely tissue types, clinical guidelines, the best available evidence and client preferences.
- Develop short- and long-term treatment plans to address presenting symptoms, underlying conditions and predisposing factors, and to progressively increase the self-help component of therapy.
- Adapt remedial massage therapy to suit the needs of individual clients based on duration and severity of injury, the client's age and gender, the presence of underlying conditions and other considerations for special population groups.

INTRODUCTION

Musculoskeletal chest pain has been defined as chest pain that is aggravated by movement.[1] Although chest complaints are an uncommon presenting condition in remedial massage clinics, tight chest muscles are frequently treated in upper crossed syndrome and in any presentation that involves a rounded shoulder posture. Remedial massage therapists are also called upon to assist in management of chronic respiratory conditions like chronic bronchitis and asthma. However, it is important to rule out serious and potentially life-threatening conditions of the cardiac, respiratory and gastrointestinal systems. As a general rule, no complaint of chest pain should ever be assumed to be musculoskeletal until other causes have been excluded.[2]

FUNCTIONAL ANATOMY REVIEW

The configuration of the rib cage gives it the flexibility it needs for smooth inspiration and expiration. The sternum is made up of three bony parts: the manubrium, body and xiphoid process to which the diaphragm attaches. Ribs 1 to 10 have both bony and cartilaginous components. The cartilages are located anteriorly and extend approximately 5 to 8 cm from the sternum. The costal cartilages of the first seven pairs (the true ribs) attach directly to the sternum at the sternocostal joints. Ribs 8 to 12 are called false ribs because their costal cartilages attach to the sternum indirectly or not at all. The 11th and 12th ribs are also called floating ribs because they do not attach anteriorly to the sternum (see Figure 14.1 on p 245).

The biomechanics of the sternum and ribs are intimately related to the thoracic vertebrae. All 12 pairs of ribs attach posteriorly to the thoracic vertebrae. The upper ribs 1 to 8 attach to the correspondingly numbered vertebral body and its transverse process and to the vertebral body below. Ribs 9 to 12 attach to the correspondingly numbered vertebrae and transverse processes only.

At each level of the thoracic column, a pair of ribs is connected at two joints (see Figure 14.2 on p 245):

a) costovertebral joint, which is a synovial joint between the head of the rib, the intervertebral disc and the vertebral bodies. The facet on the rib head articulates with a facet of a single vertebra or demifacets of two adjacent vertebrae. An interosseous ligament attaches to the head of the rib between the two articular facets and to the intervertebral disc.
b) costotransverse joint, which is a synovial joint between the rib tubercle and the transverse process of the vertebra below. It is strengthened by three costotransverse ligaments (interosseous, posterior and anterior).

The vertebral bodies are joined by the anterior and posterior longitudinal ligaments. The anterior longitudinal ligament extends along the anterior surfaces of the bodies of the vertebrae; the posterior longitudinal ligament lies within the vertebral canal on the posterior surface of the vertebral bodies.

The ligamenta flava connect the laminae of adjacent vertebrae. These ligaments are thicker in the thoracic spine than in the cervical, and thickest of all in the lumbar spine. The supraspinous ligament connects the spines of C7 to the sacrum. It is thinner and narrower in the thoracic region than in the lumbar. In the cervical region it is replaced by ligamentum nuchae. The intertransverse ligaments are rounded cords that are intimately connected with the deep muscles of the back (see Figure 14.3).

Major muscles of the chest are illustrated in Table 14.1.

When the external intercostal muscles contract, the ribs move in a similar way to a bucket handle, thereby increasing the lateral and anterior dimensions of the rib cage. The vertical dimension of the rib cage increases as the diaphragm

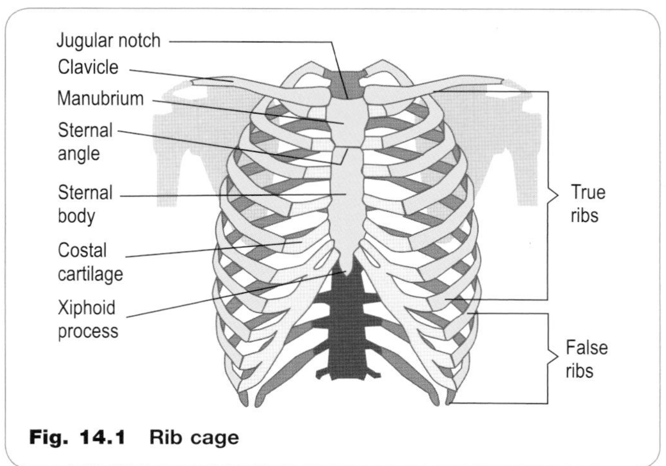

Fig. 14.1 Rib cage

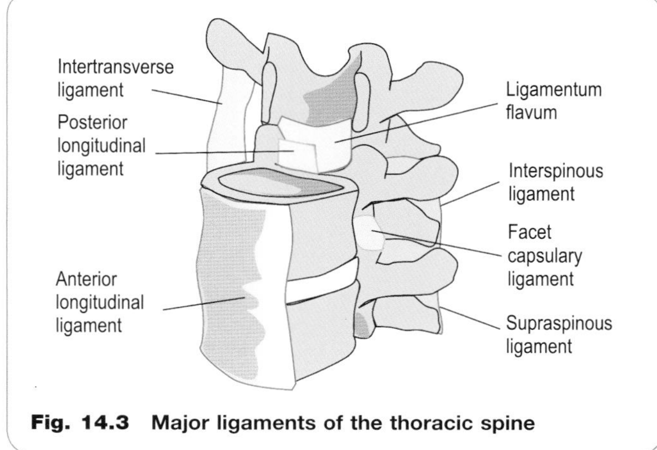

Fig. 14.3 Major ligaments of the thoracic spine

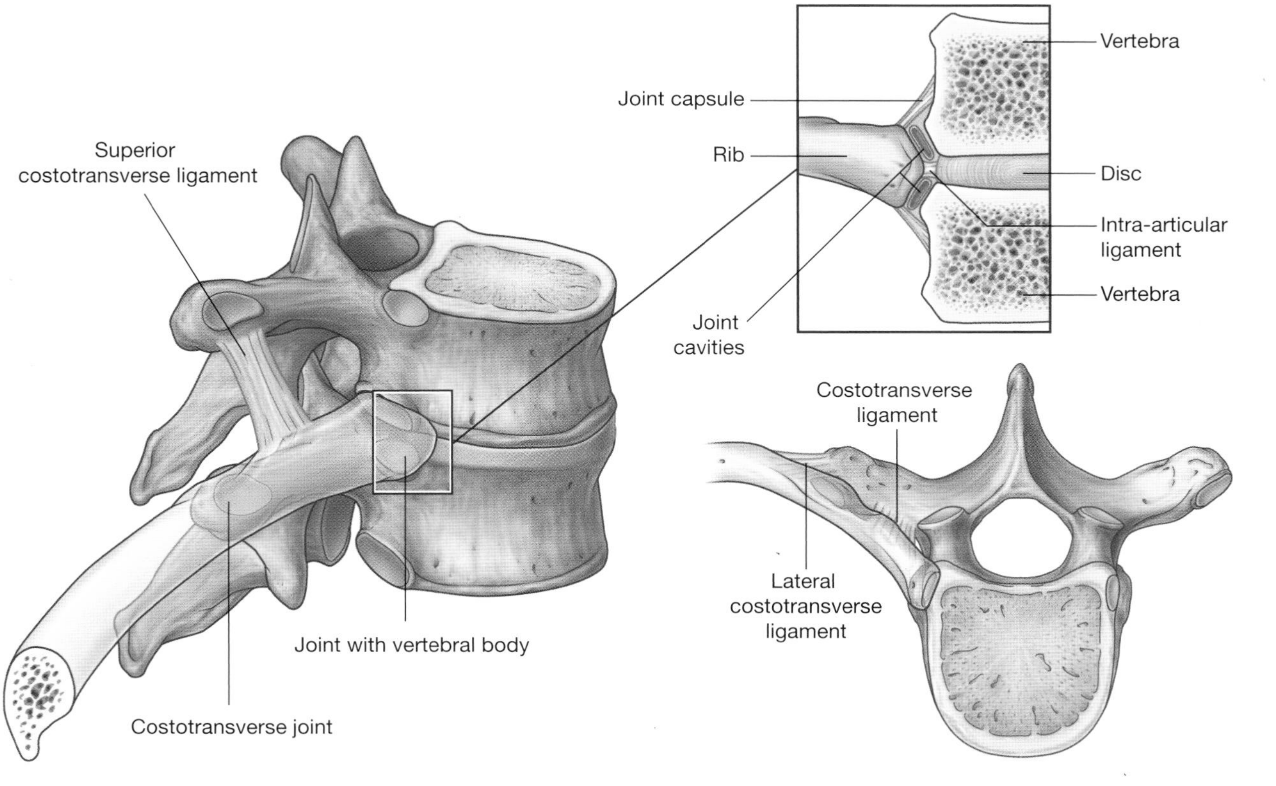

Fig. 14.2 Costovertebral and costotransverse joints

Table 14.1 Muscles of the chest

Muscle	Origin	Insertion	Action
Pectoralis major	Clavicular head: clavicle Sternal head: sternum and costal cartilages of ribs 2 to 6	Greater tubercle and intertubercular sulcus of the humerus	Together both parts flex and anteriorly adduct the humerus at the shoulder joint, The sternal part also internally rotates the humerus at the shoulder joint
Pectoralis minor	Ribs 2 to 5 (sometimes ribs 2 to 4 or ribs 3 to 5)	Coracoid process of the scapula	Protracts and abducts the scapula, elevates the ribs to which it attaches when the scapula is fixed as in forced inspiration
Intercostal muscles			
External intercostal	Inferior border of rib	Superior border of rib below	Elevates ribs at the sternocostal and costovertebral joints
Internal intercostal	Inner surface of rib	Inferior border of rib above	Depresses ribs at the sternocostal and costovertebral joints
Diaphragm	Sternal part: two muscular slips from dorsum of xiphoid process Costal part: inner surface of lower 6 costal cartilages and lower 6 ribs Lumbar part: by two muscular crura from bodies of upper lumbar vertebrae, and by arcuate ligaments	Central tendon	Increases volume and decreases pressure of the thoracic cavity

contracts and flattens its dome. These muscle contractions, and the increase in chest size that follows, cause a fall in intrapleural pressure and the lungs are forced to expand. Intrapulmonary pressure drops below atmospheric pressure and air moves into the lungs. When the diaphragm and external intercostal muscles relax, the thoracic cavity decreases and the lungs recoil creating an increase in intrapulmonary pressure (above atmospheric pressure), and air leaves the lungs.

ASSESSMENT

The aim of remedial massage assessment of the chest region includes:

- determining the suitability of clients for massage (red flags)
- determining duration (acute or subacute) and severity of injury, types of tissues involved
- determining if symptoms fit patterns of common conditions.

Assessment procedures for remedial massage clients are discussed in Chapter 2. Any client presenting with chest pain must be assessed for the presence of visceral disease including cardiac disease, peptic ulceration, reflux or malignancies.

The most common finding in people with musculoskeletal chest pain who presented to hospital with suspected myocardial infarction was tenderness and pain reproduced by anterior pressure over the costochondral junctions.[3] Thoracic spinal pain reproduced on movement or on compression was also evident.

Assessment of the chest

1. Case history
2. Outcome measures
3. Postural analysis
4. Functional tests
   Thoracic spine
   AROM
   flexion, extension, lateral flexion, rotation
   PROM
   flexion, extension, lateral flexion, rotation
   RROM
   flexion, extension, lateral flexion, rotation
   Resisted and length tests for specific muscles including
   Pectoralis major
   Pectoralis minor
   Special tests including
   Deep breathing
5. Palpation

CASE HISTORY

- Identify any red flags that require referral for further investigation (see Table 14.2 on p 247).
- Ask clients to point to the site of pain as they may have different understandings of anatomical terms.
- Determine if the pain is likely to have a mechanical cause. (Is the pain associated with rest or activity, certain postures or time of day?) Ask clients to demonstrate movements and positions that aggravate or relieve their pain and be specific

Table 14.2 Red flags for serious conditions associated with acute chest pain[6]

Red flags for acute chest pain	Possible condition
Presence of risk factors (e.g. previous history of heart disease, hypertension, smoking, diabetes, men >40 years, women >50 years), pallor, sweating, dyspnoea, nausea, palpitations	Myocardial infarction
Sharp or stabbing chest pain which may refer to lateral neck or shoulder, increased pain sidelying, relieved by sitting and bending forward	Pericarditis
History of trauma, osteoporosis, prolonged steroid use, age >70, loss of mobility, local tenderness/pain, increased thoracic kyphosis	Fracture
Recent bout of coughing, strenuous exercise or trauma, sudden sharp chest pain aggravated by inspiration, dyspnoea	Pneumothorax
Pleuritic pain associated with productive cough, pain may refer to shoulder, fever, chills, headaches, malaise, nausea	Pneumonia
Severe sharp stabbing pain with inspiration, history of recent respiratory disorder (e.g. infection, pneumonia, tumour, tuberculosis), dyspnoea	Pleurisy
Chest, shoulder, or upper abdominal pain aggravated by deep breathing, dyspnoea, haemoptysis, history of risk factors for developing deep venous thrombosis (recent surgery, recent long plane or bus trip, female smoker taking contraceptive pill)	Pulmonary embolism

with descriptions of aggravating or relieving activities. Any acute trauma must be treated as a medical emergency.
  - Mechanical pain is usually highly reactive to changes in posture, positions or activity.
  - The most common cause of chest pain in the young athlete is referred pain from the thoracic spine.[4]
  - History of trauma suggests rib injury.
- Determine if the pain is likely to be associated with visceral function. Pain of cardiac origin, peptic ulceration, gastro-esophageal reflux, pneumothorax and pulmonary embolism must be excluded. Look for associated symptoms like palpitations, shortness of breath, sweating, productive cough or pain relieved with antacid medication.
- Determine if the pain is likely to be associated with herpes zoster (shingles). Shingles is a unilaterally painful, blistering skin rash that is caused by the varicella-zoster virus, the virus that causes chickenpox. It usually affects adults over 60 years who had chickenpox in their first year of life. A weakened immune system predisposes. The pain and burning sensation can be severe and usually precede the rash which commonly occurs around the trunk from the spine to the front of the chest or abdomen in skin areas supplied by sensory nerves of one or more dorsal root ganglia.[5]
- Determine if the pain is likely to be associated with psychosocial causes (yellow flags).

A summary of serious symptoms that could require referral includes:[6]

- abnormal vital signs (bradycardia, tachycardia, tachypnoea, hypertension, hypotension)
- pallor, sweating, dyspnoea, palpitations
- fever, chills, headache, malaise, productive cough
- wheezing, accessory muscle retractions
- pain intensified with inspiration
- asymmetric pulses (pulsus paradoxus[a] over 10 mmHg)
- pain relieved by leaning forward
- increased pain by lying on the left side
- symptoms lasting more than 20–30 minutes.

OUTCOME MEASURES

Outcome measures are specifically designed questionnaires that are used to assess clients' level of impairment and to define benefits of treatment. The benefit is assessed in terms of client-perceived changes to health status. The Patient Specific Scale is an example of an outcome measure that could be used to assess conditions affecting the chest.

POSTURAL ANALYSIS[7]

Observe the shape and symmetry of the chest (see Figure 14.4 on p 247). Funnel chest (pectus excavatum) is a congenital chest deformity characterised by a depression in the lower sternum. If severe, it can impair cardiac and respiratory function. In pigeon chest (pectus carinatum), which is associated with longstanding early life obstructive airways disease such as chronic bronchitis or asthma, the sternum is displaced anteriorly. Barrel chest is associated with pulmonary emphysema and normal ageing. Normally the ratio of the anterior/posterior to lateral diameter of the adult chest is approximately 1 : 2. With emphysema and normal ageing the ratio approximates 1 : 1. The presence of thoracic kyphosis or scoliosis will affect the shape and symmetry of the chest.

Observe the rate and rhythm of breathing and any abnormal retraction of the supraclavicular fossae or the interspaces between the ribs during breathing (severe asthma, emphysema, tracheal obstruction) or abnormal bulging of the interspaces during expiration (asthma, emphysema). Note the use of accessory muscles including sternocleidomastoid, scalenes and upper trapezius on inspiration and abdominals on expiration during normal breathing.

FUNCTIONAL TESTS

The costovertebral joints transmit movements of the thoracic spine to the rib cage. Begin functional examination of the chest with range of motion testing of the thoracic spine (see Chapter 11).

[a]Blood pressure normally declines with inhalation and increases with exhalation. Pulsus paradoxus refers to an exaggeration of the normal blood pressure variation during the inspiration phase. It can suggest a number of conditions including cardiac tamponade, pericarditis, obstructive lung disease or chronic sleep apnoea.

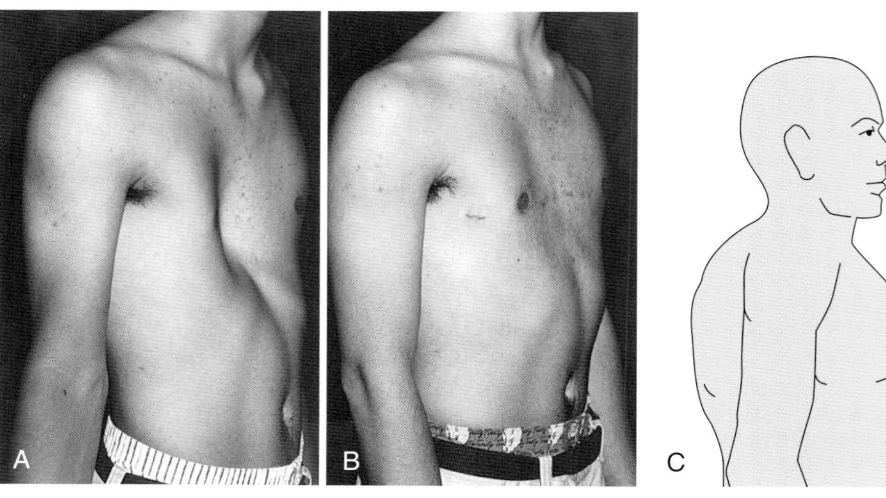

Fig. 14.4 Common rib cage distortions (A funnel chest; B pigeon chest; C barrel chest)

Thoracic spine

ACTIVE RANGE OF MOTION (AROM)

Flexion

- Stand behind the client.
- Instruct the client to bend forward slowly as far as they can without pain.

Extension

- Stand at the side of the client and place hand on the spine at T12 level. Ask client to bend backwards from the contact point as far as they comfortably can.

Lateral flexion (sidebend)

- Ask the client to take their shoulder towards the hip on the same side. Stabilise the iliac crest with one hand and gently guide the client with the other hand on their shoulder as they laterally flex the trunk.
- Compare both sides and observe the coupling of the thoracic spine facet joints and posterior ribs.

Rotation

- Ask the client to turn their shoulders to the left and then the right as far as they are comfortably able.

PASSIVE RANGE OF MOTION (PROM)

Passive range of motion of the thoracic spine can be performed with the client seated. Place your forearm across the top of the client's shoulders to guide the movements. Rest your other hand on the middle thoracic spine as the client's trunk is flexed, extended, laterally flexed and rotated. Next your spinal contact is moved to the upper thoracic spine and the movements are repeated (see Chapter 11).

RESISTED RANGE OF MOTION (RROM)

The six ranges of motion of the thoracic spine tested in AROM can also be tested against resistance. Resisted range of motion tests are best performed with the client sitting on the treatment table to minimise extraneous muscle recruitment (see Chapter 11).

Resisted and length test for specific muscles[9, 10]

Muscle imbalances arise from muscle contractures and muscle weaknesses. Mobilisers (e.g. upper trapezius) tend to tighten and shorten; stabilisers (e.g. lower trapezius and serratus anterior) tend to weaken and lengthen.[8] Length tests and resisted tests can be performed for the major muscles of the thoracic spine and chest. Resisted tests provide information about muscle strength and location of muscle strains. As with all clinical examination procedures findings from any test should be interpreted with caution and correlated with findings from other assessment procedures.[11]

1. Pectoralis major

Resisted test: Pectoralis major upper fibres (clavicular part) The client lies supine, shoulder flexed to 90°, elbow straight and palm facing towards the feet. Stand at the head of the table. Place one hand over the client's elevated forearm and resist as the client attempts to move their arm across their chest towards the opposite shoulder (see Figure 14.5 on p 249).

Resisted test: Pectoralis major lower fibres (sternal part) Use the same position as above but this time apply resistance as the client tries to move their arm towards their opposite hip (see Figure 14.5 on p 249).

Length test With the client supine, shoulder level with the edge of the table, the client abducts their arm to 90° and lets their arm drop down towards the floor. Shortness of the pectoralis major (clavicular part) prevents the arm dropping to the table level. Upper fibres (sternal part) are tested as above except that the arm is abducted to 135° (see Figure 14.6 on p 249).

Clinical significance Shortness is commonly observed in upper crossed and rounded shoulder postures.

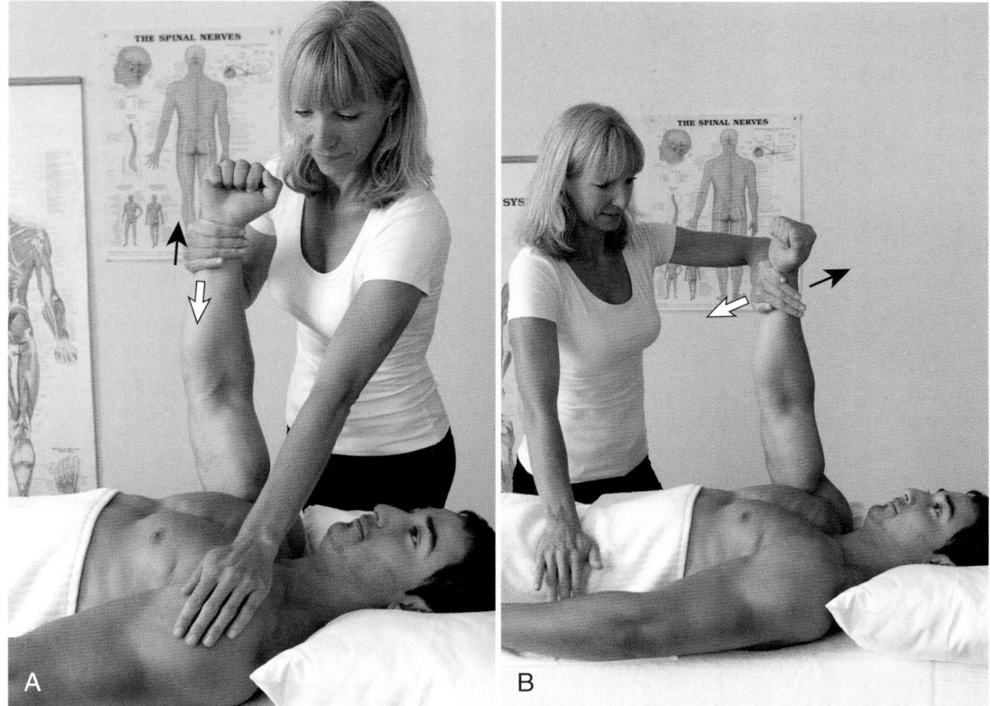

Fig. 14.5 Resisted test for pectoralis major (A clavicular and B sternal divisions)

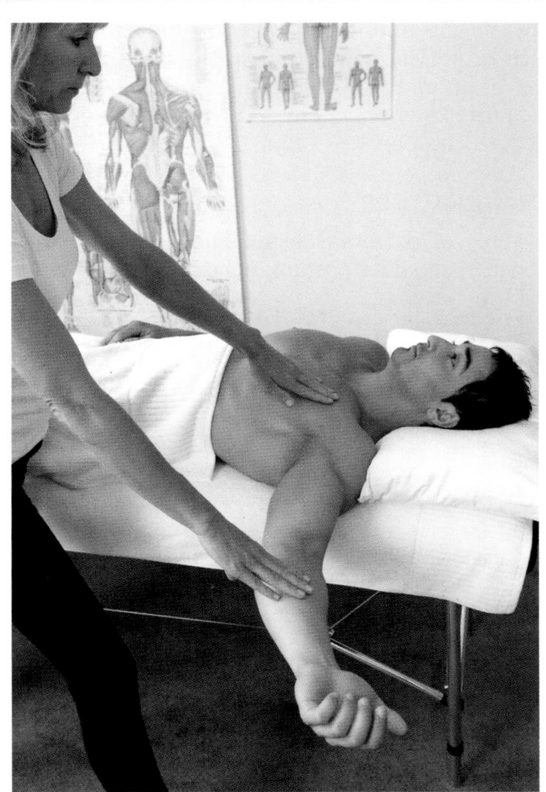

Fig. 14.6 Length test for pectoralis major

2. Pectoralis minor

Resisted test The client lies supine and thrusts their shoulder forward against resistance (see Figure 14.7 on p 250).

Length test The client lies supine with their arms alongside their body, elbows extended. Normally both shoulders lie flat against the table. A short pectoralis minor holds the shoulder off the table (see Figure 14.8 on p 250).

Clinical significance Short pectoralis minor muscles are often associated with forward head carriage.[9] Pectoralis minor contracture can pull the coracoid process of the scapula downward and compress cords of the brachial plexus and axillary blood vessels causing arm pain. Weakness of pectoralis minor may reduce the strength of arm extension and could add to respiratory distress when using accessory muscles to breathe.[10]

SPECIAL TESTS

If clients experience pain while performing special tests, ask the client to indicate the exact location of the pain.

Deep breathing

Pain aggravated by deep breathing or coughing could be related to a musculoskeletal or respiratory condition. Listen for audible rhonchi (e.g. snoring sound in chronic bronchitis and emphysema), wheezing (e.g. in asthma) or rales (e.g. crackles in acute bronchitis and pneumonia).

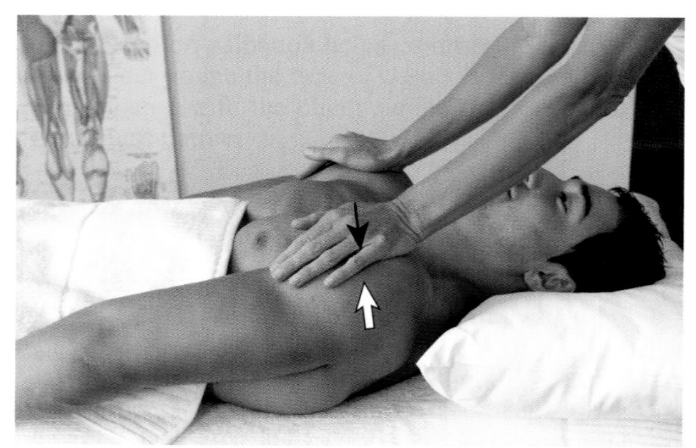

Fig. 14.7 Resisted test for pectoralis minor

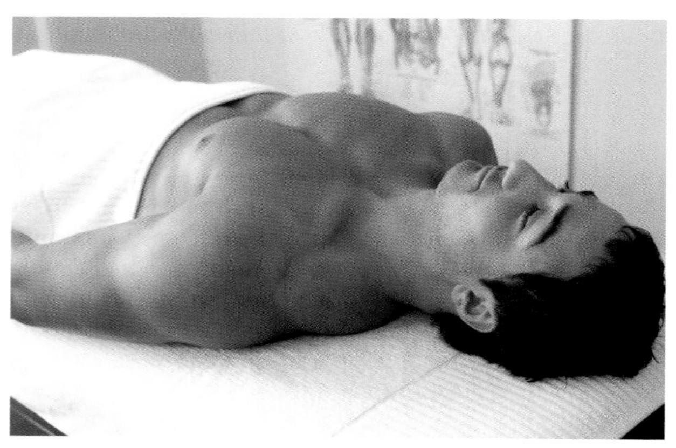

Fig. 14.8 Length test for pectoralis minor

PALPATION

Apply direct compression/pressure over the costochondral junctions, sternocostal joints, pectoral muscles and costal cartilages. Tender points and/or pain suggests musculoskeletal causes of chest pain.

With the client prone, palpate rib alignment by placing four fingertips in four consecutive intercostal spaces and sliding them laterally from the spine. Start at the floating ribs and work up the rib cage. If the space between two consecutive ribs narrows considerably the intercostal muscles at that location may be contracted and the ribs misaligned.

Respiratory excursion

To assess respiratory excursion, the client must be seated. Change in circumference of a client's chest can be measured with a tape measure at the level of the 4th intercostal space as the client inhales and exhales as far as possible. Expansion of less than 2.5 cm suggests decreased costovertebral movement, ankylosing spondylitis or respiratory pathology.[7, 12]

REMEDIAL MASSAGE TREATMENT

Assessment of the chest provides essential information for development and negotiation of treatment plans, including:

- client's suitability for remedial massage therapy
- duration of the condition (i.e. acute or chronic)
- severity of the condition (i.e. grade of injury; mild, moderate or severe pain)
- type(s) of tissues involved
- priorities for treatment if more than one injury or condition is present
- whether the signs and symptoms suggest a common condition of the chest region
- special considerations for individual clients (e.g. client's preference for treatment types and styles, special population considerations).

MUSCLE STRAIN

Muscle strains may occur as a result of sudden trauma, repetitive overuse or from coughing episodes. Chronic contractures of the pectoralis major and minor which are associated with prolonged hours of desk work, upper crossed syndrome and rounded shoulder postures may predispose the client to muscle strain.

Assessment

HISTORY

The client complains of localised chest pain associated with trauma (e.g. pectoralis major strain from performing bench press exercises) or repetitive overuse. Pain is usually aggravated by movement or by inspiration, although these features may also be present with intrathoracic disease. Chronic contractures of pectoralis major and minor (as may occur in head forward postures or upper crossed syndrome) may predispose the client to chest muscle strain.

POSTURAL ANALYSIS

Contractures of pectoralis major and minor are associated with rounded shoulder posture, upper crossed syndrome and forward head carriage.

Assessment findings for muscle strain

- History of trauma or repetitive overuse
- Postural analysis: rounded shoulder posture or upper crossed syndrome may be associated with longstanding contractures
- Functional tests:
  Thoracic range of motion
  - AROM: positive
  - PROM: may be positive at end of range as muscle is passively stretched
  - Resisted and length tests positive for specific muscles
  - Special test usually negative
- Palpation positive for tenderness/pain and/or spasm

FUNCTIONAL TESTS

Thoracic spine

AROM positive.
PROM positive as the muscle is passively stretched.
RROM positive.
Resisted and length tests positive for specific muscle.
Special test: usually negative.

PALPATION

Palpation at the site of lesion elicits tenderness or pain. Muscle spasm may be palpable.

Treatment

Acute injuries are treated with RICE. Gentle stretching exercises are introduced as soon as pain permits.

Remedial massage techniques for subacute or chronic grade 1 or 2 muscle strains include:

- Swedish massage to the chest, upper limb, neck, upper and mid back.
- A range of specific muscle techniques including (see Table 14.3):
  - deep gliding frictions along the muscle fibres
  - cross-fibre frictions
  - soft tissue releasing techniques
  - deep transverse friction
  - trigger point therapy
  - muscle stretching.
- Myofascial release (see Chapter 8).

Address any underlying or predisposing conditions (e.g. scoliosis, post Scheuermann's disease).

CLIENT EDUCATION

Advise clients to avoid aggravating activities. Correction of weight-lifting techniques may be required. Posture advice is essential and includes avoidance of all postures and activities that cause the head to be held forward. Advise clients about lumbar supports, correct sitting posture and improving the ergonomics of the work area (see Figure 12.20). Clients often respond well to a corrective exercise program, but referral for osseous manipulation may be required.

Home exercise program

Begin with gentle stretches and isometric exercises as soon as pain permits (see Table 14.3). Progressively introduce shoulder range of motion exercises and functional exercises. In clients with upper crossed syndrome, a program to strengthen weak middle and lower trapezius, rhomboids and serratus anterior should be progressively introduced for long-term biomechanical improvements.

RIB SUBLUXATION/FRACTURE

Rib subluxations or misalignments may occur at any age. Rib fractures are typically caused by impacts to the chest. However, even inconsequential traumas can fracture a rib in the presence of pre-existing weakness (e.g. osteopenia, tumour or bone infection). Onset can also be related to repetitive strain (e.g. twisting action in boxing or severe bouts of coughing).

Key assessment findings for rib subluxation/fracture

- History of impact or blow to the chest, presence of underlying pathology or repetitive strain; sharp localised rib pain, referring laterally along the rib. Severe pain if fracture present
- Functional tests:
  Thoracic spine:
  - AROM: limited especially rotation to the injured side
  - PROM: limited especially rotation to injured side
  - RROM: may be positive for associated intercostal strain
  - Resisted and length tests: may be positive for associated intercostals strain
  - Special tests: positive if fracture present
- Palpation: tenderness/pain is elicited at the injury site: severe pain and muscle guarding if fracture present

Assessment

HISTORY

Clients with rib subluxations complain of intense sharp localised pain at the site of lesion. Subluxations can occur at the insertion of the rib into the thoracic spine posteriorly or at the sternal cartilaginous attachment anteriorly. The pain often refers laterally along the rib. Both the anterior and the posterior attachment sites may be painful simultaneously. The client will often report a recent episode of twisting, for example boxing, paddling or repetitive twisting in the workplace such as moving items through a supermarket checkout or along a production line. If fracture has occurred, the client reports severe pain in the ribs. Coughing, laughing and deep breathing are painful and make normal breathing difficult. Usually a significant traumatic event is described (e.g. a football game or car accident). If traumatic event is absent, there is usually a history of underlying pathology or symptoms suggestive of one (e.g. osteopenia, bone tumour, bone infection).

FUNCTIONAL TESTS

Thoracic spine

AROM: positive, particularly on rotation to the side of lesion. If fracture is present, range of motion on most movements is greatly limited due to pain.
PROM: positive, particularly on rotation to the side of lesion. If fracture is present, range of motion on most movements is greatly limited due to pain.
RROM: may be positive for associated muscle strains.
Resisted and length tests for specific muscles may be positive for involved muscles.
Special tests: deep breathing, coughing, sneezing and laughing are positive if fracture is present.

PALPATION

Anteriorly the rib attaches to the sternum via costocartilage. Posteriorly the tubercle of the rib articulates with the transverse process and the rib head with either two adjacent vertebral bodies (ribs 1 to 8) or one vertebral body (ribs 9 to 12). Palpation at the site of lesion (anteriorly or posteriorly) elicits acute pain. The region may be boggy and inflamed. Associated

Table 14.3 Remedial massage techniques for muscles of the chest

Muscle	Soft tissue release	Trigger point	Stretch	Client education[13]	Home stretch
Pectoralis major	Stand at the head of the table, slightly to the involved side and place knuckles or fingers of the medial hand over the lateral aspect of pectoralis major. The client's straight arm is flexed to 90°. Hold the client's wrist with your other hand. Glide along the fibres of pectoralis major as the client's arm is passively horizontally abducted. Alternatively the client can actively perform the arm movement. 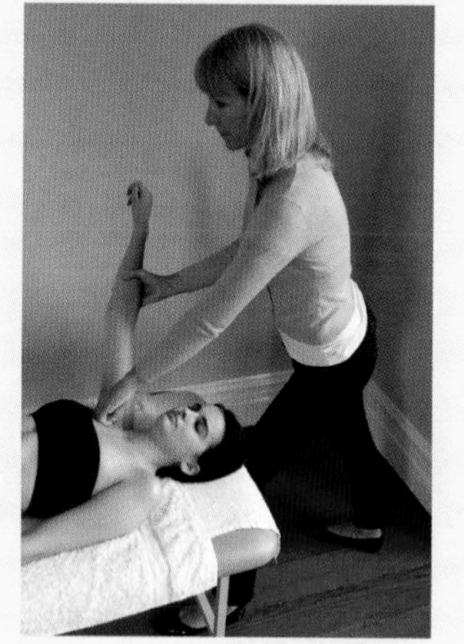	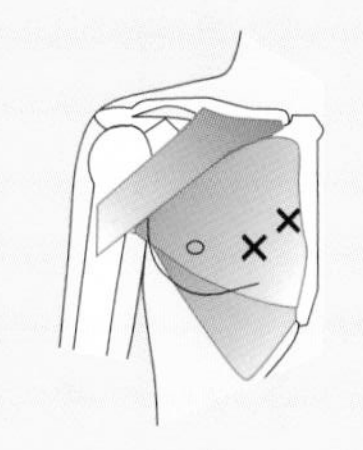	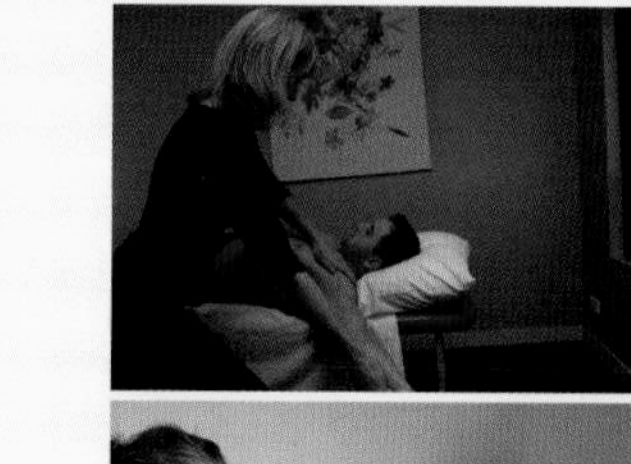 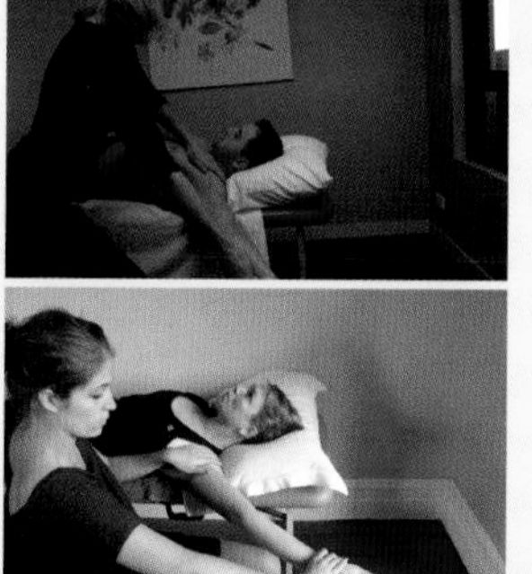 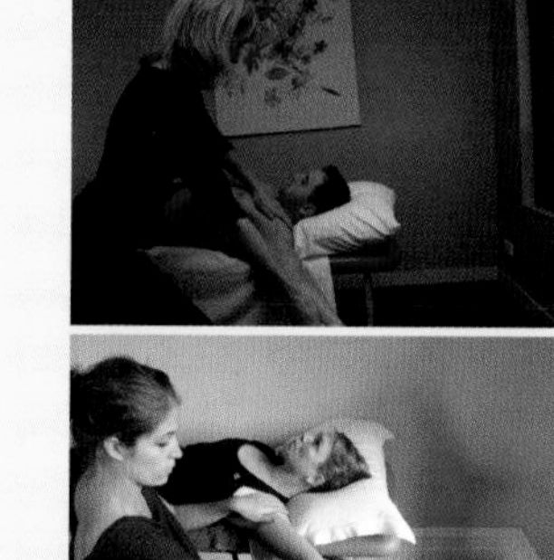	Correct standing and sitting posture, avoid mechanical overload.	In doorway stretch

Table 14.3 Remedial massage techniques for muscles of the chest—cont'd

Muscle	Soft tissue release	Trigger point	Stretch	Client education[13]	Home stretch
Pectoralis minor	Stand at the head of the table slightly to the involved side. Pressure is gently applied to the pectoralis minor with fingers, knuckles or thumbs maintained as the client protracts and retracts their shoulder. Note: clients often find this technique beyond their comfortable pain tolerance. Do not use this technique if the client reports pain of more than 7 out of 10 on a pain scale.	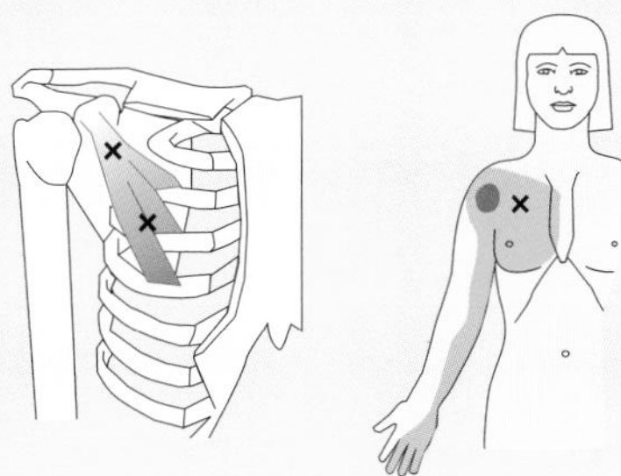	The client lies supine. Stand at the head of the table and gently apply downward (posterior) pressure to the shoulders with the palms of the hands. 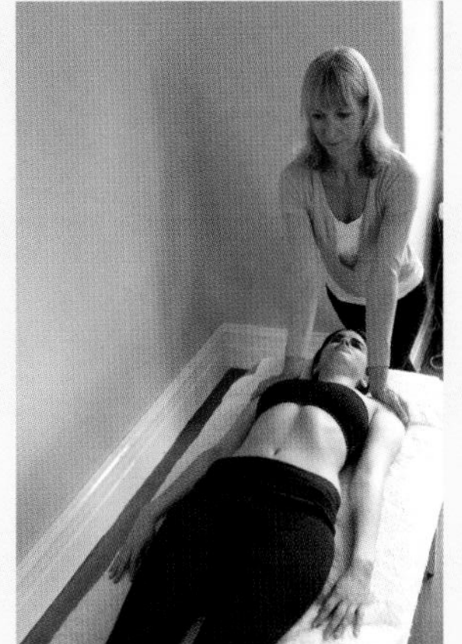 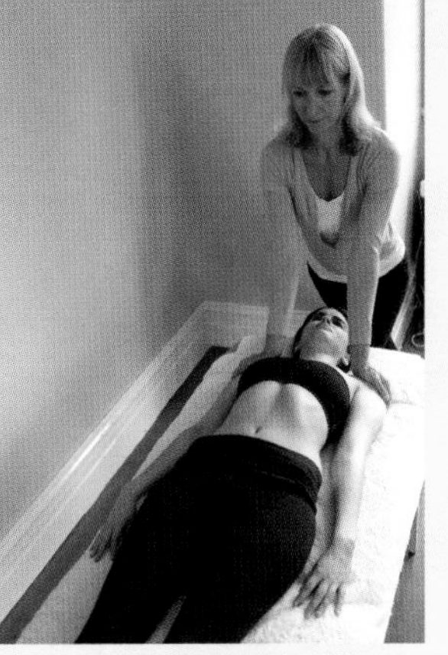	Correct standing and sitting posture, avoid mechanical overload	The client lies supine with arms alongside body and tries to take their shoulders to the floor.
Intercostal muscles and diaphragm	Stand to one side of the client facing the client's head. Place palms on either side of the lower ribs, fingers pointing towards the floor. With elbows almost horizontal, apply pressure to the rib cage as the client exhales. Instruct the client to breathe in deeply. As the client inhales the practitioner resists the expansion of the rib cage. (Note: contraindicated in osteoporosis.) 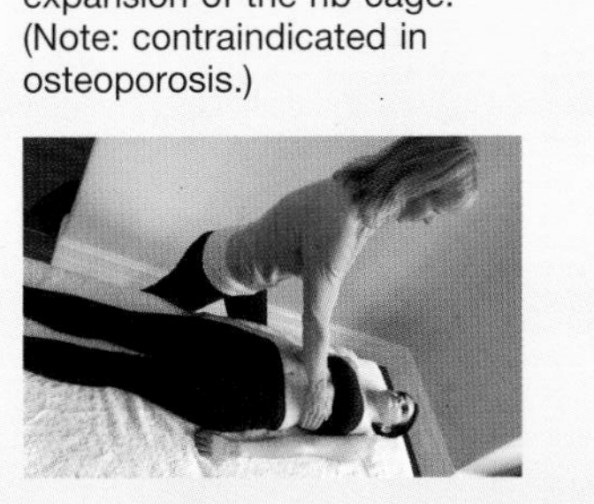	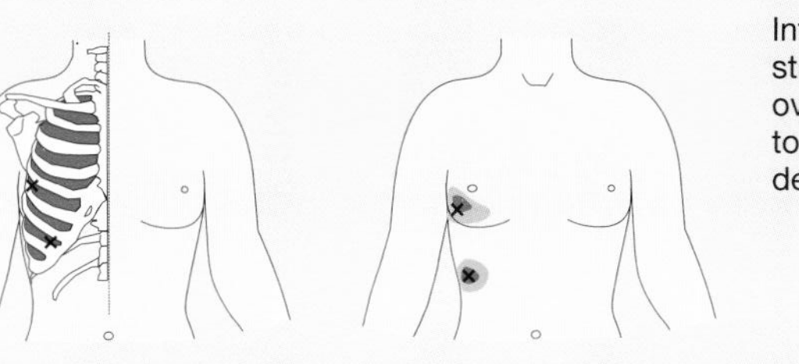	Intercostal muscles can be stretched by raising the arms overhead, trunk lateral flexion to the opposite side and deep breathing.	Correct paradoxical breathing, correct head forward and slumped posture	Breathing exercises (e.g. Buteyko, yoga)

intercostal muscles are typically contracted and sore and the ribs unevenly spaced. Palpating a fracture site may invoke involuntary muscle guarding.

DIFFERENTIAL DIAGNOSIS

Rib subluxations may be difficult to distinguish from fractures. The rib cage is highly innervated to enable normal coordinated breathing. Consequently rib subluxations are initially intensely painful. The severity of the trauma or the presence of underlying pathology suggest fracture. Severe pain that does not decrease over days and the presence of involuntary muscle guarding also suggest fracture. An X-ray of the region is required in order to make a definitive diagnosis.

Costochondritis

Costochondritis refers to inflammation of one or more rib cartilages usually on one side of the sternum. It is associated with pain related to activity and localised tenderness at the costochondral joint. Tietze's syndrome is a severe form of costrochondritis characterised by swelling of the affected costal cartilages. The cause is poorly understood. It is thought to arise from minor trauma or bouts of coughing, sneezing or vomiting. The condition usually resolves within 3 months but can become chronic. It may be associated with other conditions like fibromyalgia, inflammatory bowel disease, psoriatic arthritis and ankylosing spondylitis.

Sternocostal joint sprain

Clients with sternocostal joint sprain report a history of trauma and localised sharp pain that is aggravated by movement and relieved by rest. AROM and PROM of the thoracic spine aggravate symptoms. Pain and/or tenderness elicited by palpation of the affected sternocostal joints suggests sternocostal joint sprain.

Overview of treatment and management of rib subluxation

If fracture is suspected, referral is required. Remedial massage is contraindicated until the bone has healed (a minimum of 6 weeks). Initially, Swedish massage helps to reduce muscle spasm and pain. As tolerated, deep remedial techniques may be introduced.

Rib subluxation often involves ligamentous sprain, which may take 8 weeks to heal. Acute pain and inflammation usually subside in a few days. Cryotherapy may speed the process. Residual intercostal protective muscle spasm will be relieved with massage therapy. The client needs to avoid excessive rotation movements in order to prevent relapse within the first 8 weeks post injury.

A typical remedial massage treatment for rib subluxation includes:

- Swedish massage to the thoracic spine and chest.
- Remedial massage techniques, which include:
  - for ligamentous sprain: cross-fibre frictions and deep transverse friction
  - for muscle strain (see Table 14.3)
    - deep gliding frictions along the muscle fibres
    - cross-fibre frictions
    - soft tissue releasing techniques
    - deep transverse friction
    - trigger point therapy
    - muscle stretching.

  Adjacent rib spaces can be treated simultaneously using fingers in the intercostal spaces to gently separate the ribs.
- Gentle thoracic and rib mobilisation help restore normal movement patterns (see Chapter 7) including:
  - thoracic longitudinal mobilisation
  - thoracic diagonal mobilisation
  - arm overhead rib mobilisation
  - rib rotation.

  (Note that mobilisations are contraindicated in clients with osteoporosis.)
- Thermotherapy may provide pain relief.
- Myofascial releasing techniques may be beneficial (see Chapter 8) (see Figure 14.9).

CLIENT EDUCATION

Advise clients to take several deep breaths each day within their pain tolerance. Heat packs may provide pain relief after the acute phase.

Home exercise program

Introduce gentle stretches as soon as they can be tolerated. For example, standing upright with hands on hips, the client raises the arm overhead on the side of rib lesion. The client slowly bends to the opposite side to open the rib cage and stretches the intercostal muscles on the side of injury. Predisposing biomechanical factors may include weak or contracted erector spinae muscles and weak core muscles. Progressively introduce a strengthening program as required.

RESPIRATORY CONDITIONS

Remedial massage therapists can assist in the management of respiratory conditions, particularly asthma and chronic bronchitis. A Cochrane review was conducted on the use of manual therapy (including chiropractic and osteopathic techniques, tapotement and massage) for asthma.[14] The authors found that there was not enough evidence from trials to show whether

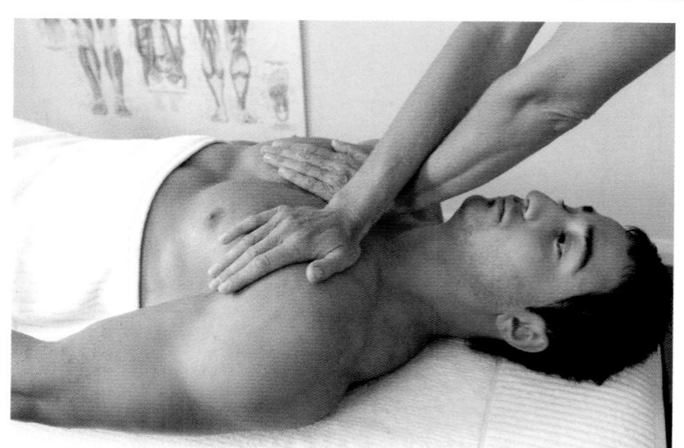

Fig. 14.9 Myofascial release: rib subluxation

these therapies can improve asthma symptoms and recommended that further research be carried out. Reviews have also been conducted for the effect of acupuncture, breathing exercises and physical training on asthma. There was insufficient evidence to make recommendations about the value of acupuncture as a treatment for asthma.[15] However, trends towards improvement, particularly in quality of life measurements, were found in studies on breathing exercises for asthma and further research is encouraged.[16] Physical training was found to have no effect on resting lung function or the number of days of wheeze. However, cardiopulmonary fitness was improved.[17] In one study by Field et al[18] 32 children with asthma received daily massage by their parents for 30 days. The younger children (aged between 6 and 8 years) showed reduced behavioural anxiety and cortisol levels directly after massage but not after the series of treatments. Lung function tests significantly improved after 30 days of massage. The older children (aged between 9 and 16 years) showed considerably less benefit.

Symptoms of cough, shortness of breath and chest pain require referral for assessment by a medical practitioner (see red flags). Some conditions affecting the respiratory system are presented in Table 14.4.

For those clients for whom remedial massage is suitable, observe the shape of the chest and any use of accessory muscles of breathing, especially sternocleidomastoid, scalenes and upper trapezius muscles on inspiration, and abdominals on expiration. Note the breathing rate and character. Observe the client's general colour (pink colour may suggest emphysema, blue colour may suggest chronic bronchitis). Is there any clubbing of the fingers?[b]

Listen to the client's breathing. Is there any wheezing, crackles or laboured breathing? Table 14.5 contains some of the physical signs of bronchitis, bronchial asthma and emphysema.

Table 14.4 Conditions of the respiratory system

Bronchial asthma	Chronic airway inflammation and narrowing of airways from smooth muscle spasm in small bronchi and bronchioles, oedema of the airway and excessive mucus. This results in dyspnoea, wheezing, chest tightness and coughing.
Chronic bronchitis	Excessive secretion of bronchial mucus and productive cough. Lasts for at least 3 months of the year for 2 consecutive years.
Coryza	Common cold caused by viruses.
Emphysema	Loss of elasticity of alveolar walls. Lungs become permanently inflated with reduced surface area for gas exchange. Inspiration is forced to obtain more oxygen. Barrel-chested.
Influenza	Chills, fever, headache, muscle aches, and cough due to infection with the influenza virus.
Pertussis (whooping cough)	Contagious disease caused by bacterium Bordetella pertussis. Dry, harassing cough developing into paroxysms followed by a long, drawn inspiration with a 'whoop' sound.
Pleurisy	Inflammation of the pleural linings of the lungs, usually accompanied by viral infection. Sharp pain on inhalation (pleuritic chest pain).
Pneumonia	Acute inflammation of the alveoli of the lungs which fill up with fluid. Decreased ventilation and gas exchange. Most commonly caused by Streptococcus pneumonia.
Pneumothorax	Lung collapse due to air in the pleural space in people with chronic lung disease or spontaneous collapse from penetrating wound.
Sinusitis	Infection and inflammation of the mucous membranes of the paranasal sinuses (maxillary, frontal, ethmoid, sphenoid). Chronic sinusitis may result in the formation of the tumour-like processes called polyps (see Chapter 13).
Tuberculosis	Infection caused by Mycobacterium tuberculosis which causes inflammation of the pleura and lungs. Symptoms include fatigue, weight loss, anorexia, low-grade fever, night sweats, dyspnoea, cough and chest pain. Contagious through inhalation.

Overview of treatment and management of respiratory conditions

Remedial massage treatment of asthma or chronic bronchitis includes the following:

- Swedish massage to the back, including T3 (nerve supply to lungs, bronchial tubes, pleura, chest), neck (the phrenic nerve, which supplies the diaphragm, originates mainly from C4) and chest (focus on intercostal muscles). Tapotement is useful in loosening mucus.
- Remedial massage techniques include:
  - specific muscle techniques, particularly for muscles of respiration (pectoralis minor, external intercostal, subclavius, scalene and sternocleidomastoid muscles). Techniques include (see Tables 14.3 and 12.4):
    - deep gliding frictions
    - cross-fibre frictions
    - soft tissue releasing techniques
    - trigger point therapy
    - muscle stretching.
- Deep gliding and cross-fibre frictions of the subclavius are useful when treating respiratory conditions. The muscle is an accessory respiratory muscle and is often overworked in asthmatics and in people with chest infections (see Figure 14.10 on p 256).
- Acupressure points can be incorporated into Swedish massage. Apply digital pressure to specific respiratory points along acupuncture meridians or energy lines of the

[b]Clubbing refers to swelling in the subcutaneous tissues over the terminal phalanges. The angle at the base of the nail is decreased (the nail turns downwards like the rounded part of an upside-down spoon). Clubbing occurs in patients with heart and lung disease, lung cancer or liver and gastrointestinal disease.

Table 14.5 Physical signs of bronchitis, bronchial asthma and emphysema[19]

Pathological process	Movement of chest wall	Breath sounds	Added sounds
Bronchitis	Normal or symmetrically diminished	Vesicular with prolonged expiration	Rhonchi, usually with some coarse crepitations
Bronchial asthma	Symmetrically diminished	Vesicular with prolonged expiration	Rhonchi, mainly expiratory and high-pitched
Diffuse pulmonary emphysema	Symmetrically diminished	Diminished vesicular with prolonged expiration	Expiratory rhonchi

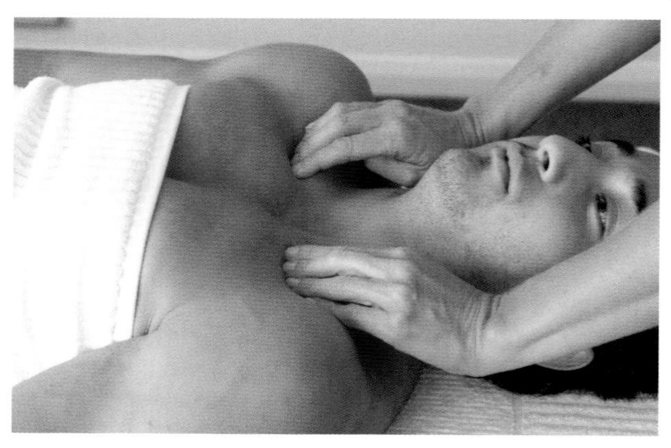

Fig. 14.10 Subclavius: deep gliding and cross-fibre frictions

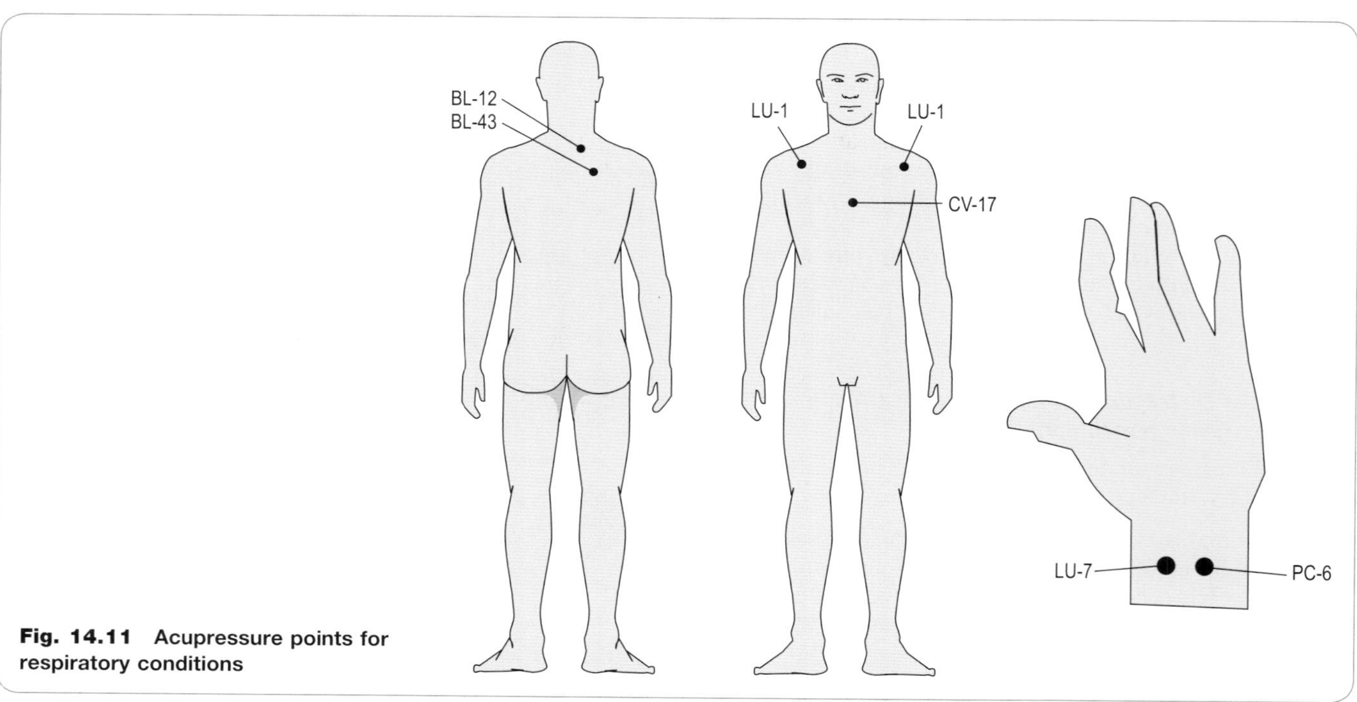

Fig. 14.11 Acupressure points for respiratory conditions

body. Apply thumb or knuckle pressure on points for approximately 10 seconds. Points commonly used to treat asthma and chronic bronchitis include (see Figure 14.11):

- Lung 1 (L1): In the interspace between the first and second ribs, 8 fingerbreadths lateral to the midline.
- Lung 7 (L7): Proximal to styloid process of the radius, 2 fingerbreadths above the transverse crease of the wrist.
- Conception vessel 17 (CV17): Centre of the chest, between the nipples.
- Pericardium 6 (P6): 2 thumb widths above the transverse crease of the wrist between the tendons of palmaris longus and flexor carpi radialis.
- Bladder 12 (BL12): 2 fingerbreadths either side of the spinous process of T2.
- Bladder 43 (BL43): 4 fingerbreadths either side of the spinous process of T4.

Note that the distances refer to the client's own finger and thumb size.

Note: Lung 1 is located in the delto-pectoral groove or triangle. It is generally regarded as a forbidden point for needling although pressure and/or heat (moxibustion) may be applied. Pectoralis minor and the coracoid process also lie in this region. Circular frictions at this point may be useful for treating lung conditions.

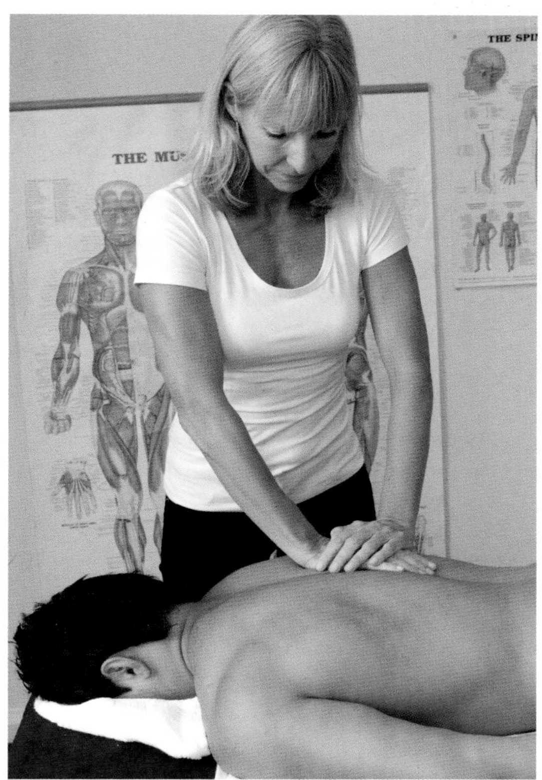

Fig. 14.12 Compressions

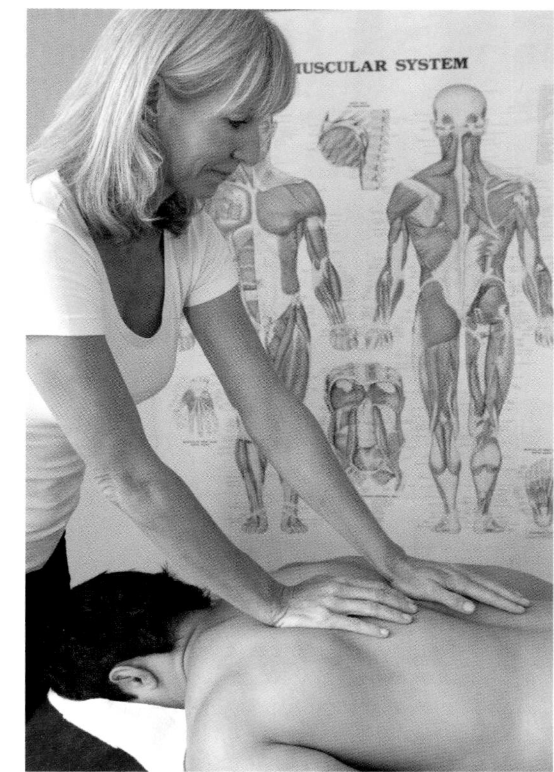

Fig. 14.13 Cat walk

- Gentle mobilisations of the thoracic spine including (see Chapter 7):
  - thoracic longitudinal mobilisation
  - thoracic diagonal mobilisation
  - arm overhead rib mobilisation
  - rib rotation.

  (Note: mobilisation techniques are contraindicated in clients with osteoporosis.)
- Further mobilisations include:
  - Prone
    1. i) Compressions. Remove oil or cover the client with a towel and stand facing transversely across the client. Apply slow rhythmic compressions making brief contact and releasing the hand to allow the rib cage to recoil, first on one side of the rib cage and then to the other (see Figure 14.12).
    2. ii) Cat walk. Stand at the head of the table. Remove oil or cover the client with a towel. Place the heels of both hands on the upper thoracic paravertebral muscles, fingers pointing inferiorly. Apply pressure downward with one hand, release, and transfer weight to the other hand. Repeat this transfer of pressure on one side of the spine and then on the other as the hands 'walk' down the rib cage. Apply pressure slowly as the client exhales (see Figure 14.13).
  - Sidelying
    1. i) Assisted breathing: sidelying, arm overhead. The client lies on their side with their uppermost arm overhead. Face caudally and gently traction the fully abducted arm with the cephalad hand. Apply gentle pressure with your caudal palm to the lower ribs as the client exhales (see Figure 14.14).

       (Note: all assisted breathing techniques are contraindicated in osteoporosis.)

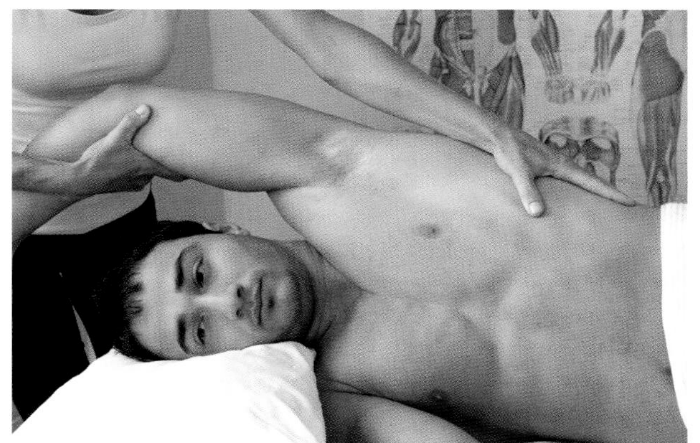
Fig. 14.14 Assisted breathing: sidelying, arm overhead

  - Supine: Stand at client's head. Work in two sections: upper ribs and lower ribs above and below a towel folded horizontally across the breasts. (It is beyond the scope of remedial massage therapy to massage breast tissue.)

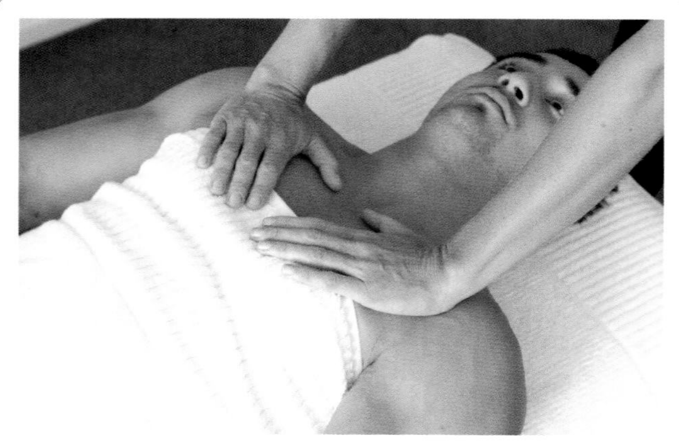
Fig. 14.15 **Assisted breathing: supine, upper ribs**

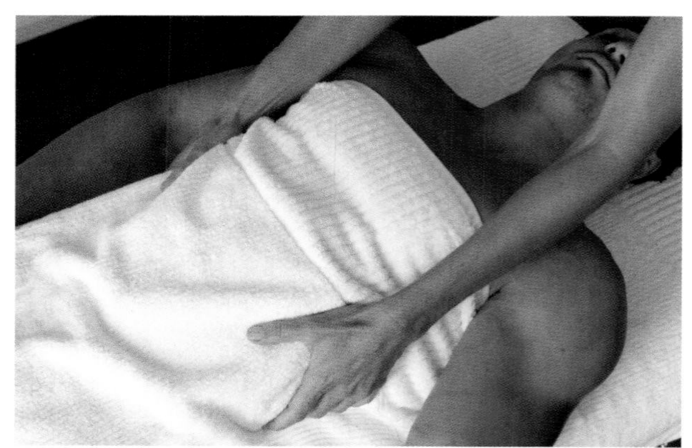
Fig. 14.16 **Assisted breathing: supine, lower ribs**

i) Assisted breathing: supine, upper and lower ribs
Stand at the head of the table. Apply gentle pressure on the anterior upper chest with both palms (heels of hands laterally and fingers pointing medially) as the client exhales, and then quickly change hand position to the posterolateral aspect of the lower ribs and lift the lower ribs as the client inhales. Repeat for several breaths (see Figures 14.15 and 14.16).
ii) Assisted breathing: supine, upper ribs
Stand at the head of the table. Cover the client's chest with a towel. Place the palm of one hand over the sternum. Alternatively, place palms on either side of the upper chest, fingers pointing medially. Apply downward pressure as the client exhales, then instruct the client to inhale deeply. At about half inspiration, suddenly release your palm pressure by lifting the hands rapidly off the chest. This will often cause the client to gasp. Repeat up to 3 times.
iii) Assisted breathing supine, lower ribs
Stand to one side of the client facing the client's head. Place palms on either side of the lower ribs, fingers pointing towards the floor. With elbows almost horizontal, apply pressure to the rib cage as the client exhales. Instruct the client to breathe in deeply and at about half inspiration, release the pressure.
iv) Diaphragm release
Face the client's head. Place thumb tips under the client's costal margin. Try to contract the underside of the costal margin with the thumbs. Begin lateral to the xiphoid process and, as the client exhales, slowly slide the thumbs under the costal margin from medial to lateral (see Figure 14.17).

- Remedial massage treatments may also include aromatherapy, reflexology and Bowen therapy. Although little scientific evidence is available to support their use, these techniques are often used in clinical practice. They are part of the range of techniques available to remedial massage therapists when they negotiate treatment plans with clients.
  - Reflexology
  Reflexologists use reflex points that are associated with the lungs and bronchi (see Figure 14.18). Techniques include mild pressure directly on the reflex points on the

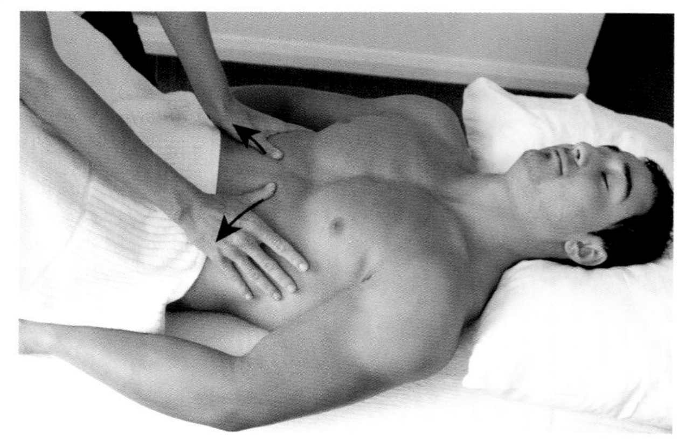
Fig. 14.17 **Diaphragm release**

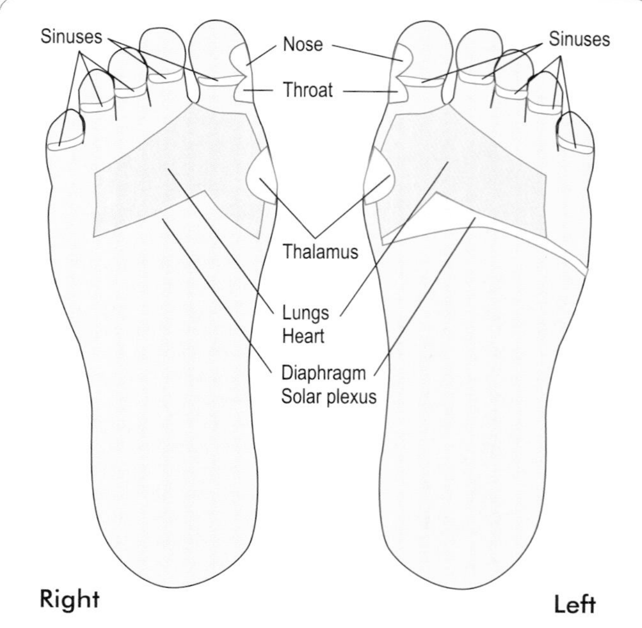

Fig. 14.18 **Reflexology for lungs and bronchi**

feet using fingers, thumbs or knuckles and *caterpillars* (a stroke involving repeated flexion and extension of the interphalangeal joint of the thumb).

- Aromatherapy
  An essential oil blend may be used as the lubricant in Swedish massage (5 drops in 10 mL carrier oil) or vapourised in an oil-burner during the treatment. Useful oils for asthma include aniseed, atlas cedarwood, cajeput, clary sage, Roman chamomile, cypress, fennel, frankincense, everlasting, eucalyptus radiate, hyssop var. decumbens, lavender, pinus sylvestris, spike lavender, lemon, mandarin, myrtle, peppermint, petitgrain, rosemary. (Caution: always check the client's sensitivity/allergic response before using essential oils.)

CLIENT EDUCATION

Steam inhalations and humidifiers using essential oils (e.g. eucalyptus and pine) have traditionally been used. Breathing exercises, swimming, yoga, Buteyko[c] and hydrotherapy may be recommended.

The Victorian government Better Health channel recommends the following simple breathing exercises.[20]

Relaxed deep breathing

Sit down, relax your shoulders and breathe in through your nose and out through your mouth. Your abdomen should move in and out as you breathe. This shows you are using your diaphragm.

Prolonged breathing out

Breathe in for two counts and breathe out for three or four counts. This helps to expel any trapped air.

Simons et al[13] identified paradoxical breathing (i.e. the rib cage deflating as the client inhales and inflating as they exhale) as a common perpetuating factor for trigger points in chest muscles. If there is no underlying pathology, clients can correct paradoxical breathing by placing one hand on the upper ribs and one on the abdomen and practising breathing in such a way that the hand on the rib cage rises as they inhale and falls as they exhale.

It is imperative that clients continue their usual medication. Clients can be referred to a naturopath, homoeopath, acupuncturist and/or manipulative therapist for further treatment. Allergy testing may also be required.

[c]The Buteyko breathing method is a series of exercises involving nasal breathing, relaxation and holding the breath. It is used in the treatment of asthma.

KEY MESSAGES

- Assessment of clients with chest conditions involves case history, outcome measures, postural observation, functional tests (including resisted tests and length tests for specific muscles) and deep breathing.
- No chest pain should ever be assumed to be musculoskeletal until other causes have been eliminated. Be vigilant for red flags for serious conditions associated with chest pain (e.g. cardiac, respiratory or gastrointestinal causes).
- Assessment findings may indicate the type of tissue involved (contractile or inert), duration of condition (acute or subacute) and severity.
- Consider Clinical Guidelines, available evidence and client preferences when planning therapy.
- Remedial massage therapy for chest conditions commonly involves treatment of chronic contractures of chest muscles (e.g. when treating clients with upper crossed syndrome or forward head carriage). Remedial massage therapists also treat chest muscle strains and rib subluxations, and provide supportive treatment for clients with chronic respiratory conditions.
- Educating clients about likely causal and predisposing factors is an essential part of remedial massage therapy. Over time, increase the client self-help component of treatment wherever possible to reduce likelihood of recurrence and/or to promote health maintenance and illness prevention.

Review questions

1. A 70-year-old client presents with pain in the chest. She has recently recovered from a chest infection and cough. The pain is sharp, localised and continuing to be very painful. She is unable to take a deep breath without pain. Palpation of the injury site is very tender and there is evidence of reflex muscle guarding. This history suggests:
   a) bronchitis
   b) a fractured rib
   c) a herniated thoracic disc
   d) intercostal muscle strain
2. Describe a test for:
   i) the length of pectoralis minor
   ii) the length of pectoralis major sternal division
   iii) differentiating a musculoskeletal chest pain from a visceral one.
3. A 48-year-old man is suffering from chest pain. He has high blood pressure, is overweight and smokes about 20 cigarettes a day. He looks pale, is having difficulty breathing and appears to be in some distress. This history suggests:
   a) cardiovascular disease
   b) pectoralis major strain
   c) pericarditis
   d) shingles
4. Costochondritis may be associated with:
   a) cardiovascular disease
   b) pericarditis
   c) inflammatory bowel disease
   d) a fractured rib
5. The most common cause of chest pain in a 25-year-old athlete is:
   a) referral from the thoracic spine
   b) rib subluxation
   c) rib stress fracture
   d) pectoralis major trigger point
6. A pigeon chest is associated with:
   a) normal ageing
   b) childhood asthma
   c) emphysema
   d) pertussis
7. What symptoms and signs differentiate a rib fracture and a rib subluxation?
8. List five red flags associated with chest pain.
9. Give three characteristics of musculoskeletal chest pain that differentiate it from pain of visceral or other origin.
10. What role can remedial massage play in the treatment and management of asthma?
11. List the primary and accessory muscles of respiration.
12. a) What is *paradoxical* breathing?
    b) How can it be corrected?

REFERENCES

1. Eslick G, Jones M, Talley N. Non-cardiac chest pain: prevalence, risk factors, impact and consulting – a population-based study. Aliment Pharmacol Ther 2003;17:1115–24.
2. Birnbaum J. The musculoskeletal manual. 2nd rev edn. Philadelphia: Grune and Stratton; 1986.
3. How J, Volz G, Doe S, et al. The causes of musculoskeletal chest pain in patients admitted to hospital with suspected myocardial infarction. Eur J Intern Med 2005;16(6):432–6.
4. Brukner P, Khan K. Clinical sports medicine. 3rd edn. North Ryde, NSW: McGraw-Hill; 2010.
5. Beirman R. Handbook of clinical diagnosis. Sydney: R. Beirman; 2003.
6. Zitkus B. Take chest pain to heart. Nurse Pract 2010;35(9):41–7.
7. Bickley L, Szilagyi P, editors. Bates' guide to physical examination and history taking. 10th edn. Philadelphia: Lippincott-Raven; 2009.
8. Chaitow L. Muscle energy techniques. 2nd edn. Edinburgh: Churchill Livingstone; 2001.
9. Kendall McCreary E, Provance P, McIntyre Rodgers M, et al. Muscles, testing and function, with posture and pain. 5th edn. Philadelphia: Lippincott Williams and Wilkins; 2005.
10. Hislop H, Montgomery J. Daniels and Worthingham's muscle testing: techniques of manual examination. 8th edn. Oxford: Saunders Elsevier; 2007.
11. Lewis JS, Valentine RE. The pectoralis minor length test: a study of the intra-rater reliability and diagnostic accuracy in subjects with and without shoulder symptoms. BMC Musculoskelet Disord [serial on the Internet] 2007;8:64. Online. Available: www.biomedcentral.com/content/pdf/1471-2474-8-64.pdf.
12. Vizniak N. Physical assessment. Burnaby, BC: Professional Health Systems; 2008.
13. Simons D, Travell J, Simons L. Myofascial pain and dysfunction: the trigger point manual. Vol 1: upper half of body. 2nd edn. Philadelphia: Williams and Wilkins; 1999.
14. Hondras M, Linde K, Jones A. Manual therapy for asthma; (2). Online. Available: www.cochrane.org/reviews/en/ab001002.html; 2005.
15. McCarney RW, Brinkhaus B, Lasserson TJ, et al. Acupuncture for chronic asthma. Cochrane Database Syst Rev 1999;(1)CD000008.
16. Holloway E, Ram FSF. Breathing exercises for asthma. Cochrane Database Syst Rev 2004;(1)CD001277.
17. Ram F, Robinson S, Black P, et al. Physical training for asthma. Cochrane Database Syst Rev 2005;(4):CD001116.
18. Field T, Henteleff T, Hernandez-Reif M, et al. Children with asthma have improved pulmonary functions after massage therapy. J Pediatr 1998;132:854–8.
19. Bates B. Bates' guide to physical examination and history taking. 10th edn. Philadelphia: Lippincott Williams and Wilkins; 2008.
20. State Government of Victoria, Australia. Department of health: breathing problems and exercise. Online. Available: http://www.betterhealth.vic.gov.au/bhcv2/bhcarticles.nsf/pages/Breathing_problems_and_excercise; 2010.

The shoulder region 15

The content of this chapter relates to the following Units of Competency:

HLTREM503C Plan remedial massage treatment strategy
HLTREM504C Apply remedial massage assessment framework
HLTREM502C Provide remedial massage treatment
HLTREM505C Perform remedial massage health assessment

Health Training Package HLT07

Learning Outcomes

- Assess clients with conditions of the shoulder region for remedial massage, including identification of red and yellow flags.
- Assess clients for signs and symptoms associated with common conditions of the shoulder region (including muscle strains, impingement syndrome, glenohumeral degenerative joint disease and adhesive capulitis), and treat and/or manage these conditions with remedial massage therapy.
- Develop treatment plans for clients with conditions of the shoulder region, taking assessment findings, duration and severity of the condition, likely tissue types, clinical guidelines, the best available evidence and client preferences into account.
- Develop short- and long-term treatment plans to address presenting symptoms, underlying conditions and predisposing factors, and to progressively increase the self-help component of therapy.
- Adapt remedial massage therapy to suit individual client needs based on duration and severity of injury, the client's age and gender, the presence of underlying conditions and other considerations for special population groups.

INTRODUCTION

Prevalence figures for shoulder complaints differ according to the various ways these complaints are defined,[1] although anecdotal evidence about the number of shoulder complaints treated in remedial massage clinics suggests that they are the third most common after low back and neck. It is estimated that about 10% of the adult population experience an episode of shoulder pain at some stage in their lives and that most cases of acute shoulder pain (e.g. from sprains and strains, rotator cuff pathologies, impingement syndrome, adhesive capsulitis, instability disorders, bruises and contusions) arise from mechanical causes.[2]

FUNCTIONAL ANATOMY

The shoulder joint comprises a relatively shallow ball and socket joint which enables the extensive mobility required for manual dexterity. Its stability relies on overlying muscles and tendons, particularly the rotator cuff muscles, the glenohumeral ligaments, glenoid labrum, joint capsule and fascia. Normal shoulder function requires coordination of stabilising and movement forces of the glenohumeral joint, the scapula, and the acromioclavicular (AC) and sternoclavicular (SC) joints. The subacromial bursa sits on top of the supraspinatus tendon and is designed to reduce friction between the supraspinatus tendon and the acromion. This bursa extends over the superior region of the humerus and out from under the acromion process deep to the deltoid muscle (see Figure 15.1 on p 262).

Major muscles of the shoulder region are shown in Figure 15.2 on page 262 and summarised in Table 15.1. The rotator cuff muscles (see Figure 15.3 on p 263) and the coracobrachialis control the position of the head of the humerus in the glenoid fossa. The supraspinatus in particular counteracts the upward pull of the deltoid muscle on the head of the humerus when the shoulder is abducted. Smooth scapulohumeral rhythm requires strong scapular stabilisers (lower trapezius, serratus anterior, rhomboids, levator scapulae and pectoralis minor muscles) and normal length of scapulohumeral muscles (infraspinatus, teres minor and subscapularis). Most shoulder pathologies are associated with disturbances of these integrated movement and stabilising forces.

ASSESSMENT

The purpose of remedial massage assessment includes:

- determining the suitability of clients for massage (contraindications and red flags, see Table 15.2)

- determining the duration (acute or subacute), severity and types of tissues involved in the injury/condition
- determining whether symptoms fit patterns of common conditions.

Clinical assessment alone cannot produce an accurate diagnosis of the causes of shoulder pain but positive outcomes can be achieved from treatment of many shoulder conditions without identifying the exact cause.[4]

Principles of remedial massage assessment are discussed in Chapter 2. This section presents specific considerations for assessment of the shoulder region.

CASE HISTORY

Information from case histories can alert practitioners to the presence of serious conditions requiring referral. However, individual features in case histories may have low significance for diagnosis and should always be interpreted in the context of information from other assessments.[4] Use targeted questioning to collect the most useful and relevant information, including:

- Identifying red and yellow flags that require referral for further investigation.
- Identifying the exact location of the symptoms by asking clients to point to the site of pain.
- Determining if the pain is likely to have a mechanical cause. (Is the pain associated with rest or activity, certain postures or time of day?) Obtain descriptions of the specific

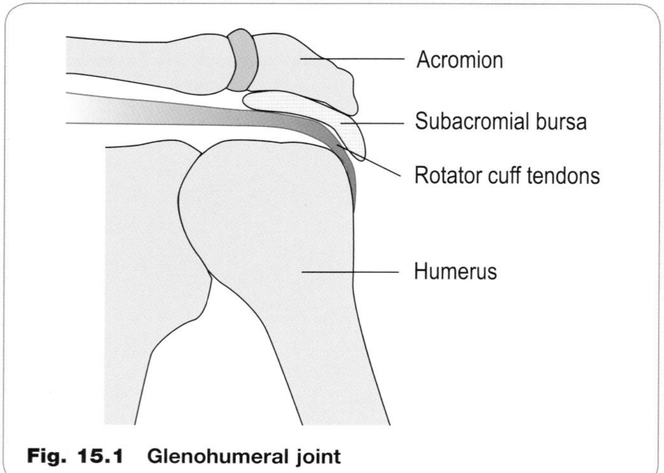

Fig. 15.1 Glenohumeral joint

Assessment of the shoulder region

1. Case history
2. Outcome measures, e.g. The Shoulder Pain and Disability Index (see Appendix 15.1) and The Patient Specific Scale
3. Postural analysis
4. Functional tests
   Cervical spine
   Active range of motion tests
   Flexion, extension, lateral flexion, rotation
   Shoulder joint
   Active range of motion tests
   Flexion, extension, abduction, horizontal adduction, internal rotation, external rotation
   Passive range of motion tests
   Flexion, extension, abduction, horizontal adduction, internal rotation, external rotation
   Resisted range of motion tests
   Flexion, extension, abduction, horizontal adduction, internal rotation, external rotation
   Resisted and length tests for specific muscles, including
   supraspinatus, infraspinatus, subscapularis, teres major, teres minor, deltoid, pectoralis major
   Special tests
   Apley's scratch test
   Drop arm test
   Impingement test
   Apprehension test
   Yergason's test
   Empty can test
5. Palpation

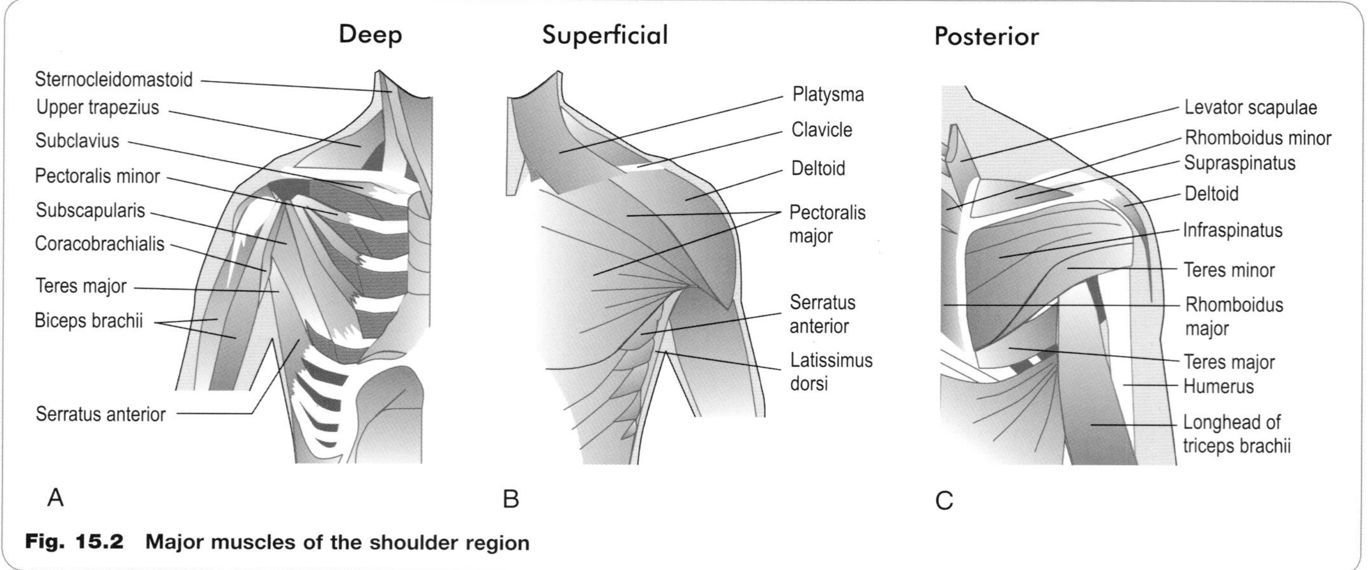

Fig. 15.2 Major muscles of the shoulder region

Table 15.1 Muscles of the shoulder region[3]

Muscles that move the humerus	Origin	Insertion	Action
Deltoid	acromial extremity of clavicle (anterior fibres), acromion of scapula (lateral fibres) and spine of scapula (posterior fibres)	deltoid tuberosity of humerus	lateral fibres abduct humerus; anterior fibres flex and medially rotate arm at shoulder joint; posterior fibres extend and laterally rotate arm at shoulder joint
Supraspinatus	supraspinatus fossa of scapula	greater tubercle of humerus	assists deltoid muscle in abducting humerus
Infraspinatus	infraspinous fossa of scapula	greater tubercle of humerus	externally rotates and adducts humerus
Teres major	inferior angle of scapula	intertubercular sulcus of humerus	extends humerus and assists in adduction and internal rotation of humerus
Teres minor	inferior lateral border of scapula	greater tubercle of humerus	externally rotates, extends and adducts the humerus
Subscapularis	subscapular fossa of scapula	lesser tubercle of humerus	internally rotates humerus
Biceps brachii	long head originates from the supraglenoid tubercle; short head originates from coracoid process of scapula	radial tuberosity and bicipital aponeurosis	flexes humerus at shoulder joint, flexes forearm at elbow joint, supinates forearm at radioulnar joints
Coracobrachialis	coracoid process of scapula	middle of medial surface of shaft of humerus	flexes and adducts humerus
Triceps brachii	long head: infraglenoid tubercle lateral head: lateral and posterior surface of humerus superior to radial groove medial head: entire posterior surface of humerus inferior to a groove for the radial nerve	olecranon of ulna	extends humerus at shoulder joint and extends forearm at elbow joint

Note: latissimus dorsi, rhomboid muscles and serratus anterior are described in Chapter 11; pectoralis major and minor are described in Chapter 14.

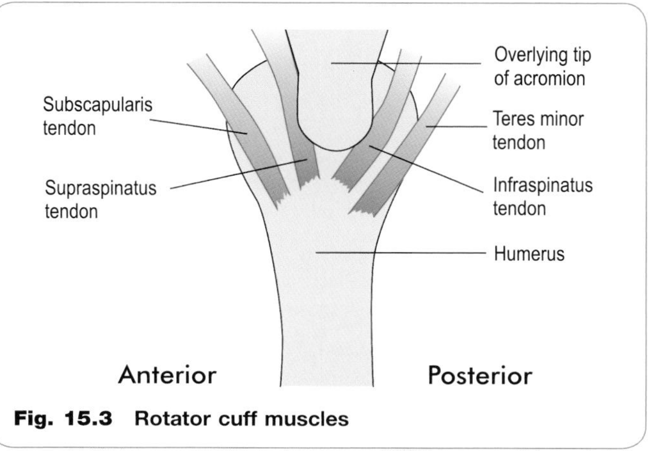

Fig. 15.3 Rotator cuff muscles

Table 15.2 Red flags for serious conditions associated with acute shoulder pain[4]

Feature or risk factor	Condition
Symptoms and signs of infection (e.g. fever) Risk factors for infection (e.g. underlying disease process, immunosuppression, penetrating wound)	Infection
History of trauma Sudden onset of pain	Fracture/dislocation
Past history of malignancy Age >50 years Failure to improve with treatment Unexplained weight loss Pain at multiple sites Pain at rest	Tumour

mechanism of the injury and the forces involved. For example, falls onto the outstretched hand may be associated with AC injuries, wrenching the arm backwards may suggest anterior dislocation, and morning pain relieved with daily activity is often associated with arthritis. Enquire about the onset of symptoms, nature of the pain, disability and functional impairment, previous injuries to the area, type of work, typical postures, sleeping posture, overuse and overhead work. Ask clients to demonstrate movements and positions that aggravate or relieve their pain and to be specific with descriptions of aggravating or relieving activities.

- Determining if pain is likely to be associated with visceral function or is neurogenic or psychosocial (yellow flags). Pain can be referred to the shoulder from diseases of the heart, gall bladder, liver, lung and diaphragm.[5, 6] Clients with numbness, pins and needles and muscle weakness associated with their shoulder condition may have brachial plexus injuries or cervical radiculopathy. Refer clients with sensory symptoms or muscle weakness for further investigation. Psychosocial factors (e.g. job dissatisfaction and work demands) along with biological factors (e.g. age, female gender, past history and response to repetitive physical task) may contribute to the onset and development of acute shoulder pain.[4]

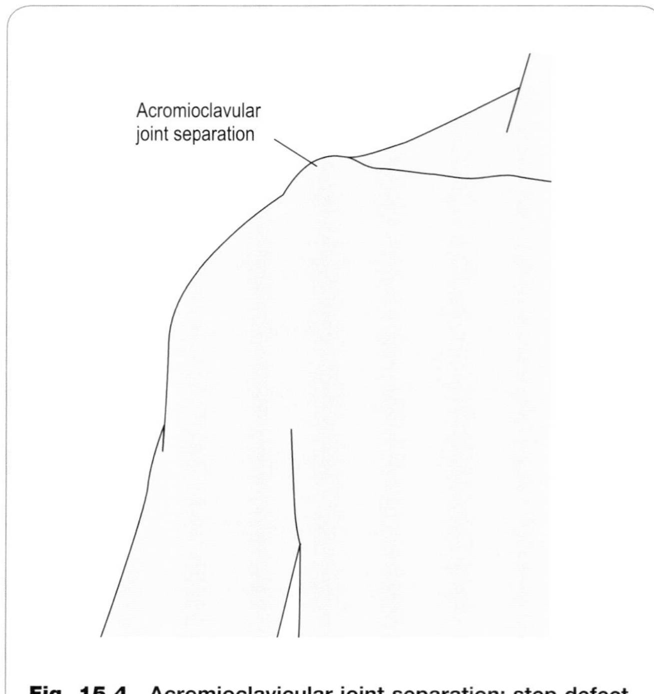

Fig. 15.4 Acromioclavicular joint separation: step defect

OUTCOME MEASURES

Outcome measures are questionnaires that are specifically designed to assess clients' level of impairment and to define benefits of treatment. The Shoulder Pain and Disability Index can be used to assess pain and routine functional skills (see Appendix 15.1).[7] The Patient Specific Scale can be used to measure progress of treatment of clients with any musculoskeletal condition, including shoulder conditions.

POSTURAL ANALYSIS

Postural analysis enables observation of the whole client and facilitates identification of important features through bilateral comparison. It also facilitates detection of possible predisposing or contributing factors by observing the position of the cervical and thoracic spines, glenohumeral joints and scapula. Observe and compare the shoulders anteriorly and posteriorly noting their symmetry. The shoulder muscles normally appear full and round. Observe any bruising, colour changes, swelling, surgical incisions and scars. Differences in bony contour may be apparent in AC joint separation (the step defect, see Figure 15.4), SC separation and clavicle fractures. The level of the shoulders is often distorted in clients with scoliosis. Observe winging of the scapula and muscle hypertonicity or atrophy.

FUNCTIONAL TESTS

For any tests involving joint movements it is important to compare both sides and take into account any underlying pathology and the age and lifestyle of the client. Findings from physical examinations should be interpreted in the light of evidence for their diagnostic accuracy. 'No clinical test is both reliable and valid for any specific diagnostic entity.'[4] However, despite their limitations, functional tests help alert practitioners to the presence of potentially serious conditions and suggest types of tissues that are likely to be involved. Range of motion tests have been shown to be reliable but their diagnostic utility is unknown. Manual muscle strength testing also appears to be reliable.[8]

Active range of motion of the cervical spine (flexion, extension, lateral flexion and rotation)

Examination of the shoulder complex begins with functional tests of the cervical spine to help rule out brachial plexus and cervical radiculopathy which refer pain to the shoulder region (see Figure 15.5). If active range of motion tests of the cervical spine reproduce the shoulder symptoms, further examination of the cervical spine is indicated (see Chapter 12).

Active range of motion of the glenohumeral joint

The client may be standing or sitting, elbow bent or straight as convenient. Face the client and demonstrate the movements. Examine the following ranges of motion:

- Flexion/extension (165°/60°)[9]
- Internal/external rotation (70°/90°)
  Instruct the client to bend their elbows and keep their elbows close to their body as they move their forearms outwards from the body and inwards across the body.
- Abduction/adduction (165°)
  Painful arc: Look for a painful arc (i.e. pain that comes on after the arm has been abducted to the middle of the arc (40°–120°) and dissipates with further abduction). The presence of a painful arc suggests rotator cuff, AC joint pathology or impingement syndrome.

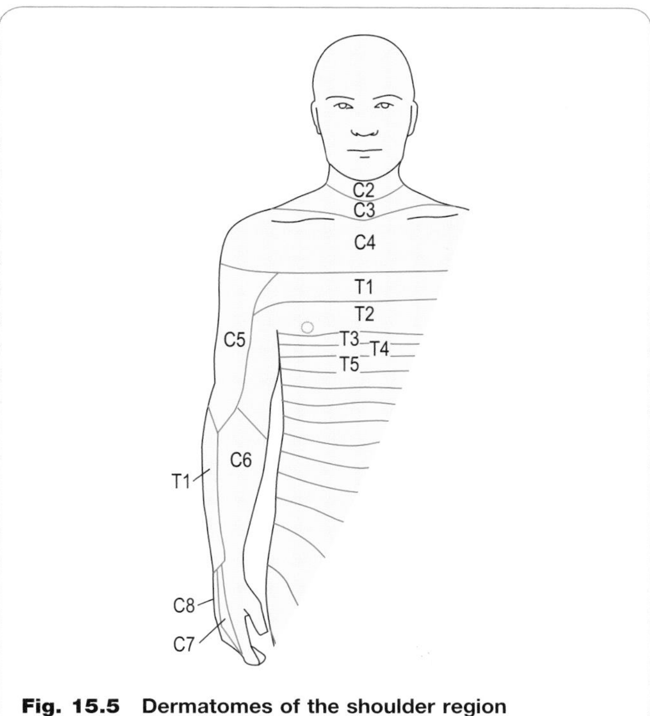

Fig. 15.5 Dermatomes of the shoulder region

Table 15.3 Shoulder joint: end-feel[10]

Normal end feel	Flexion	Elastic, firm, capsular
	Extension	Firm
	Internal/external rotation	Firm
	Horizontal adduction	Soft tissue
	Horizontal abduction	Elastic, firm
Abnormal end feel	Empty	Severe instability
	Hard, capsular	Frozen shoulder
	Late myospasm	Instability

- **Scapulohumeral rhythm:** Glenohumeral abduction and scapulothoracic abduction occur in the ratio 2 to 1 (beginning after the upper limb has reached 20° of abduction); that is, when the humerus is abducted 120°, the scapula abducts 60°. Disturbances to the smooth scapulohumeral rhythm may be due to weak scapula stabilisers and/or tightness of the scapulohumeral muscles (infraspinatus, teres minor, subscapularis).
- Horizontal adduction (130°).

Passive range of motion

If the client is unable to perform normal AROM in any direction, further investigation is required. PROM testing should be performed with one hand stabilising and palpating the shoulder joint while the other hand moves the upper limb. Note that PROM shoulder tests may be performed with the elbow flexed. Palpate for crepitus, capsular pattern and end-feel (see Table 15.3). The capsular pattern of restriction for the glenohumeral joint is external rotation more limited than abduction; abduction more limited than internal rotation.[10]

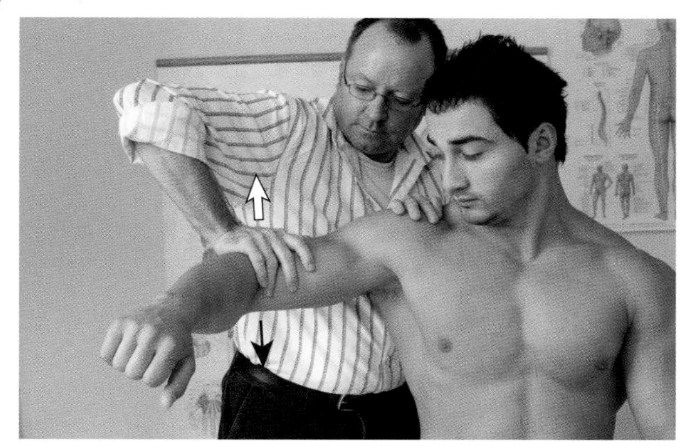
Fig. 15.6 Resisted test for middle deltoid

Resisted range of motion

RROM tests should also be performed if AROM testing indicates the likelihood of a shoulder problem. RROM tests include:

- flexion: anterior deltoid, biceps brachii, coracobrachialis, pectoralis major
- extension: posterior deltoid, latissimus dorsi, triceps brachii, teres major
- abduction: middle deltoid, supraspinatus
- adduction: latissimus dorsi, teres major, pectoralis major
- horizontal adduction: pectoralis major, coracobrachialis, anterior deltoid
- internal rotation: subscapularis, teres major, latissimus dorsi, pectoralis major
- external rotation: infraspinatus, teres minor
- scapular elevation: upper trapezius, levator scapulae, rhomboid major, rhomboid minor
- scapular retraction: rhomboid major, rhomboid minor, middle trapezius
- scapular protraction: serratus anterior

Resisted tests and length tests for specific muscles[11, 12]

If RROM tests reproduce symptoms, then further tests may be used to help identify specific muscles involved.

1. DELTOID MUSCLE

Middle deltoid

Resisted test

The client abducts their arm to 90° with their elbow flexed at 90°. Place one hand on the client's shoulder and the other on the elbow. Ask the client to hold their arm in this position against your downward pressure (see Figure 15.6).

Anterior deltoid

Resisted test

Position as above. One of your palms contacts the anterior aspect of the upper arm, the other is placed over the shoulder

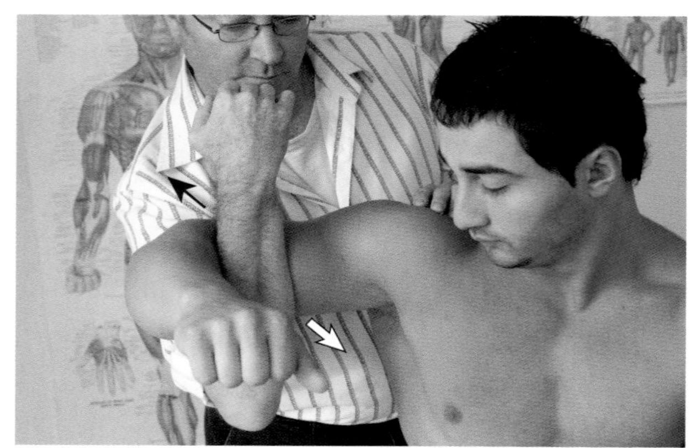

Fig. 15.7 Resisted test for anterior deltoid

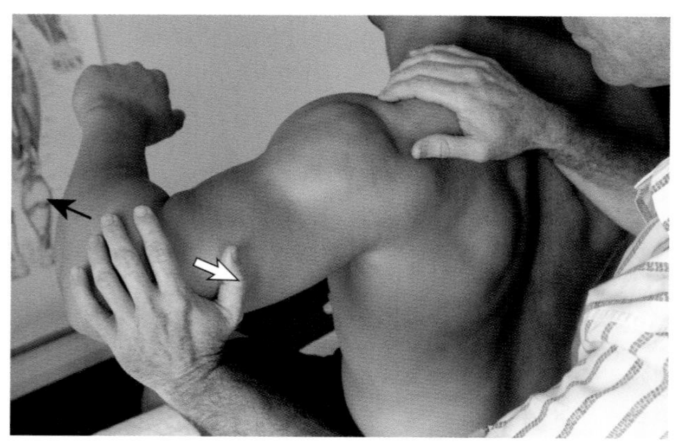

Fig. 15.8 Resisted test for posterior deltoid

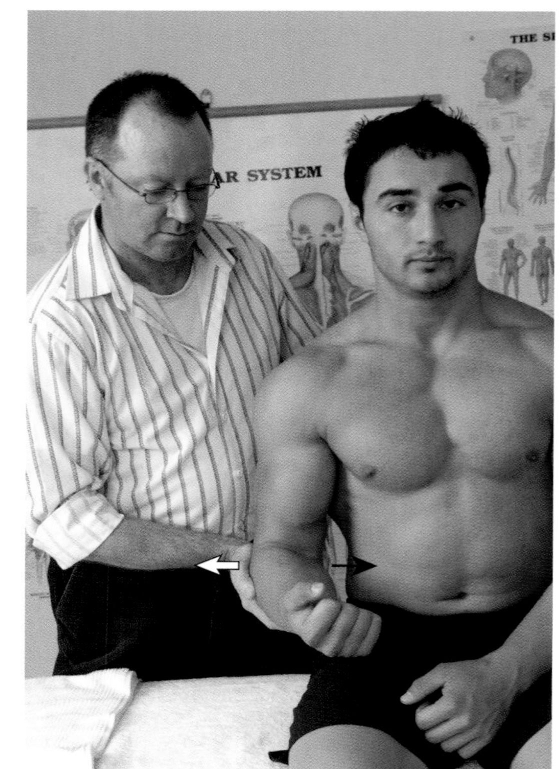

Fig. 15.9 Resisted test for supraspinatus

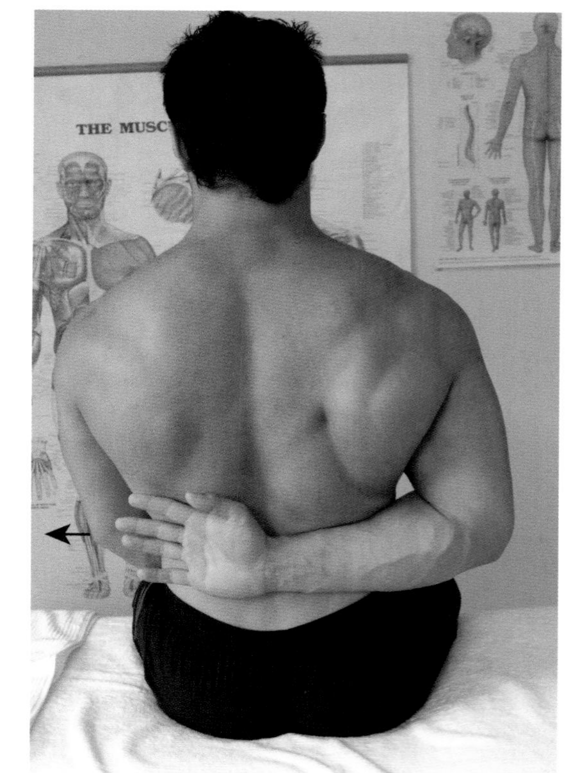

Fig. 15.10 Length test for supraspinatus

joint. The client tries to bring their forearm forwards against your resistance (see Figure 15.7).

Posterior deltoid

Resisted test

Position as above. One of your palms contacts the posterior aspect of the client's upper arm. The client tries to move their upper arm backwards against your resistance.

Length test

The length of middle deltoid is tested with supraspinatus (see Figure 15.10).

2. SUPRASPINATUS

Resisted test

Place one hand on the client's forearm or elbow, the other hand contacts the shoulder joint. The client abducts their arm up to 30° against your resistance (see Figure 15.9).

Length test

Supraspinatus and middle deltoid are tested together. The client adducts their arm by reaching across their back as far as possible. The client should be able to reach the elbow if their other arm. (see Figure 15.10).

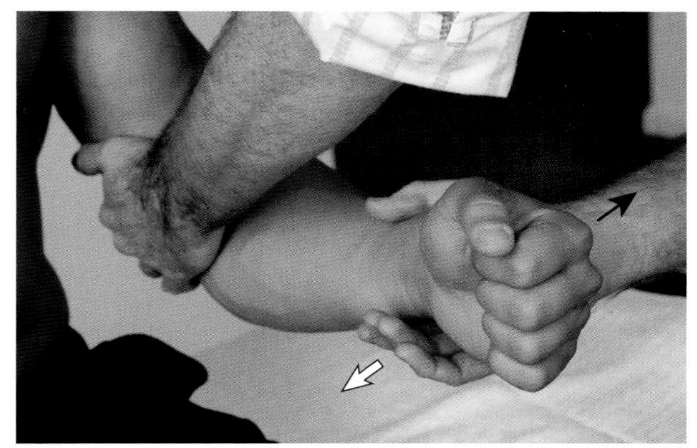

Fig. 15.11 Resisted test for infraspinatus/teres minor

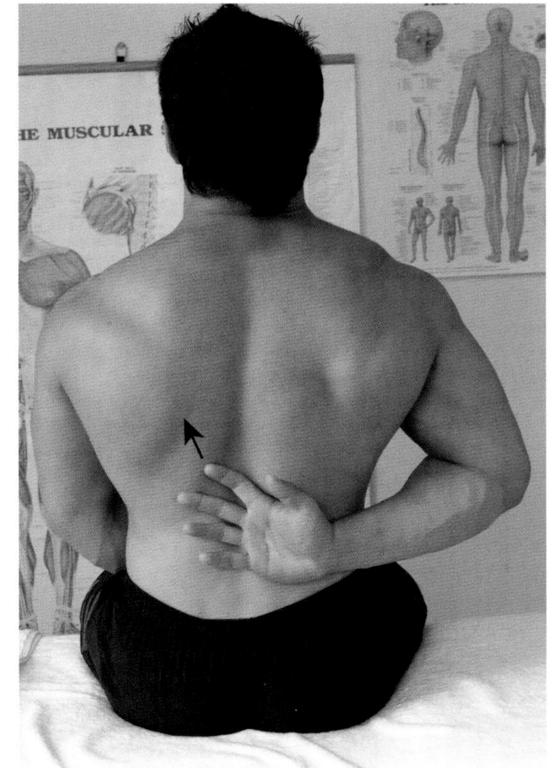

Fig. 15.12 Length test for infraspinatus/teres minor

3. INFRASPINATUS/TERES MINOR

Resisted test

The client places their arm against their side with their elbow flexed to 90°, their forearm is semi-supinated. Place one hand on the patient's elbow to prevent abduction and the other hand on the dorsum of the wrist. The client tries to laterally rotate their forearm against your resistance (see Figure 15.11).

Length test

The client should be able to touch the inferior tip of the opposite shoulder blade with their fingers (see Figure 15.12).

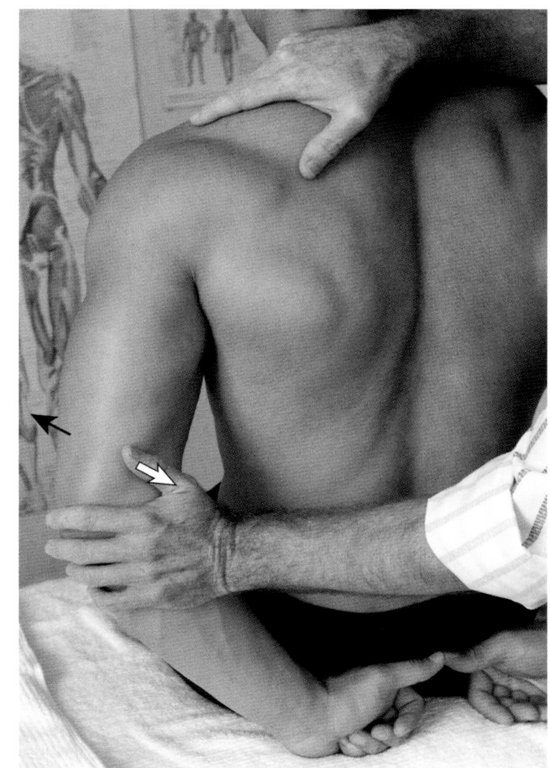

Fig. 15.13 Resisted test for teres major

4. TERES MAJOR

Resisted test

The client places the dorsum of one hand on the posterior aspect of their iliac crest. Place one hand on the shoulder; the other hand contacts the posterior aspect of the elbow. The client tries to hold this position as you apply pressure to the elbow in the direction of abduction and flexion (see Figure 15.13).

Length test

The length of the external rotator muscles is tested with the client supine and one hand placed behind their neck. The client's elbow should touch the table (see Figure 15.14 on p 268).

5. SUBSCAPULARIS

Resisted test

The client places their arm against their side with their elbow flexed to 90°, their forearm is semi-supinated. The practitioner places one hand on the patient's elbow to prevent abduction and the other hand on the dorsum of the wrist. The client tries to internally rotate their forearm against resistance. (Note: This test recruits all shoulder internal rotator muscles. Latissimus dorsi (see Chapter 11) and teres major (see above) may be distinguished from subscapularis with further resisted tests.)

Length test

The shoulder internal rotators are tested together (see Figure 15.14 on p 268).

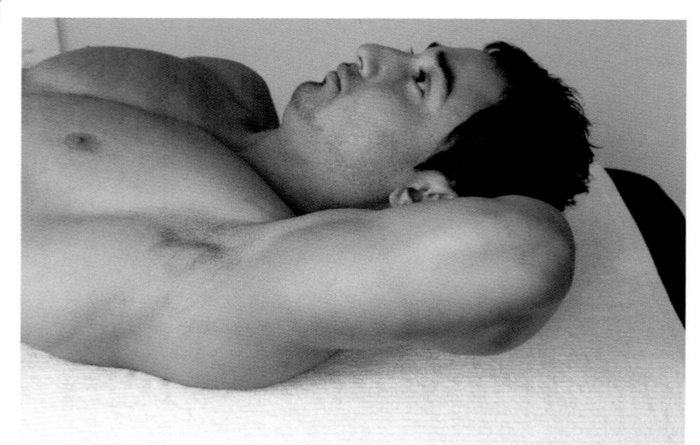

Fig. 15.14 Length test for shoulder internal rotators

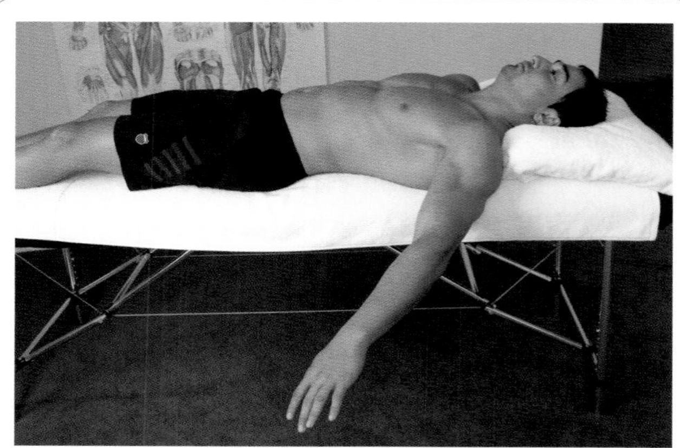

Fig. 15.17 Length test for biceps brachii

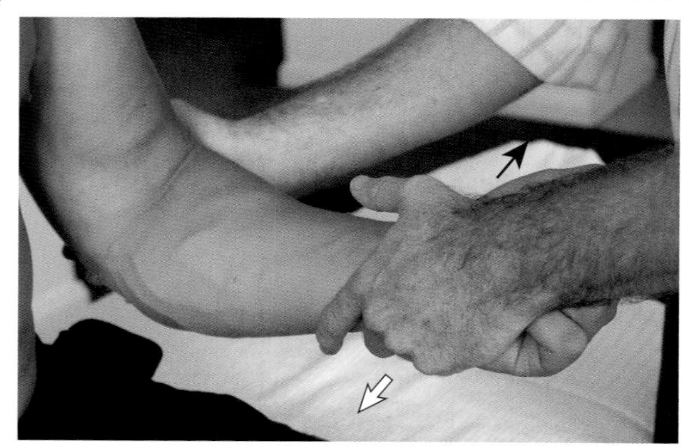

Fig. 15.15 Resisted test for subscapularis

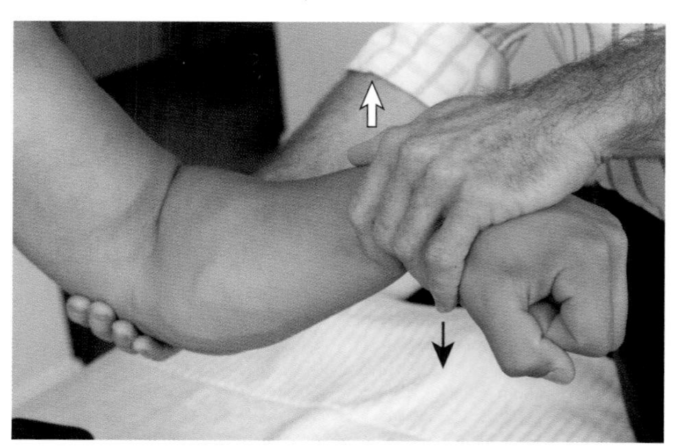

Fig. 15.18 Resisted test for coracobrachialis

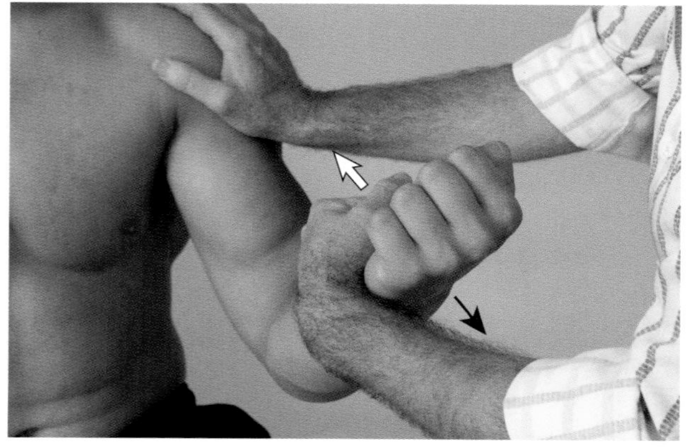

Fig. 15.16 Resisted test for biceps brachii

6. BICEPS BRACHII

Resisted test

The client flexes their elbow to 90°. One of your hands supports the elbow, the other contacts the client's supinated wrist. Apply resistance as the client tries to flex their elbow (see Figure 15.16).

Length test

The client lies supine with their shoulder level with the edge of the table, elbow extended and forearm pronated. The client extends their shoulder, keeping their elbow fully extended (see Figure 15.17). There are no know normative data for this flexibility test.[13]

7. CORACOBRACHIALIS

Resisted test

The client flexes their shoulder to 90° and tries to hold this position as the practitioner applies downward pressure (see Figure 15.18). (Note: This procedure tests all shoulder flexor muscles. Biceps brachii and anterior deltoid can be distinguished with further resisted tests described above.)

Length test

See biceps brachii length test (Figure 15.17).

8. TRICEPS BRACHII

Resisted test

Contact the client's elbow with one hand and wrist with the other and resist as the client tries to extend their elbow.

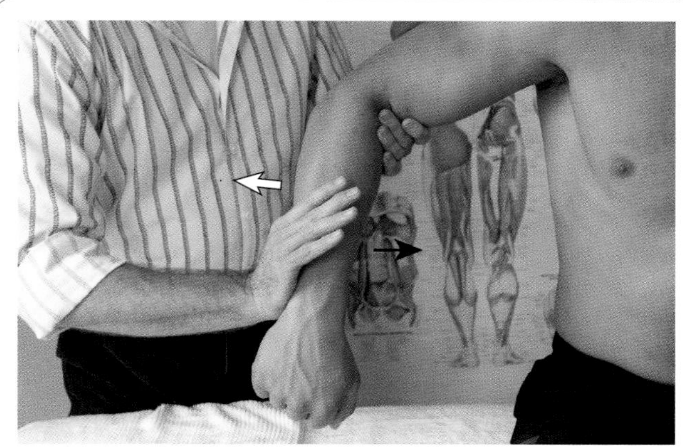

Fig. 15.19 Resisted test for triceps brachii

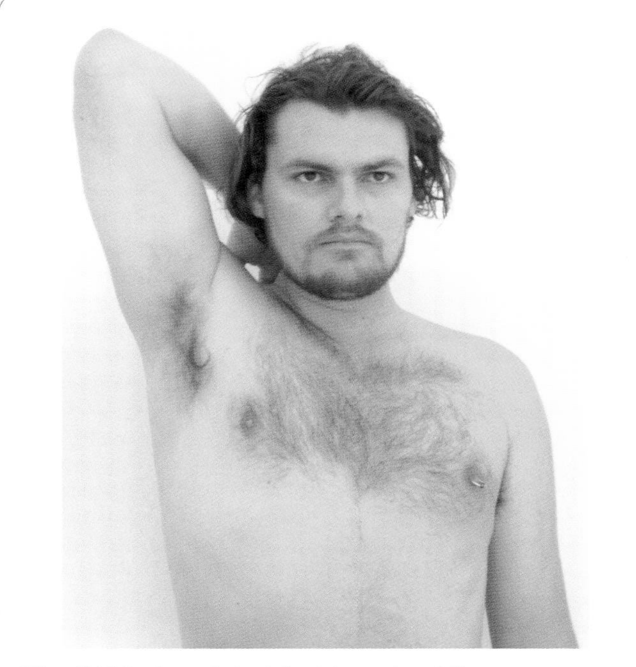

Fig. 15.20 Length test for triceps brachii

Length test

The client tries to touch the back of the shoulder on the same side with the shoulder flexed to 180°. There are no known normative data for this flexibility test (see Figure 15.20).[13]

Special tests

Special tests are designed to reproduce the client's symptoms. If pain is reported when performing a special test, ask the client to identify the exact location of the pain and confirm that it is the same pain as the pain described in the case history. Positive special test results should always be interpreted cautiously and in the context of other clinical findings (see Chapter 2).

APLEY'S SCRATCH TEST

The client tries to touch the opposite scapula approaching from above and from below. Pain when performing these movements or inability to perform the movements normally suggests rotator cuff pathology, labral pathology, AC arthritis or capsular/muscle contracture (see Figure 15.21 on p 270).

DROP ARM TEST

The drop arm test is designed to identify tears of the supraspinatus muscle. Stand behind the client and abduct their arms to 90° supporting their arm at the elbow. Suddenly release the elbow support and ask the client to stop their arms from dropping. Pain or weakness may indicate rotator cuff strain or tear, bursitis or impingement (see Figure 15.22 on p 270).

IMPINGEMENT TEST

The client raises their arm to 90° flexion with the palm facing up (externally rotated) and then returns their arm to the starting position. Next, the client raises their arm to 90° with the thumbs down (internally rotated). Pain during flexion with external rotation may suggest supraspinatus impingement; pain during flexion with internal rotation may suggest long head of biceps impingement (see Figure 15.23 on p 270).

APPREHENSION TEST

Stand behind the client and abduct their humerus to 90° with the elbow bent (the stop sign position). Observe the client for distress or anxiety while slow and gentle anterior pressure is applied to the shoulder joint. Apprehension on the client's part suggests anterior glenohumeral instability (see Figure 15.24 on p 271).

YERGASON'S TEST

Begin with the client's elbow flexed to 90° and wrist pronated. Demonstrate the hitchhiker movement (i.e. supinating, flexing and externally rotating their forearm). Next, palpate the long head of the biceps with one hand and hold the client's forearm with the other. The client performs the hitchhiker movement against your resistance. Pain in the region of the bicipital groove suggests biceps brachii tendinosis or strain. Pain in the shoulder suggests glenoid labrum pathology. If the transverse humeral ligament is torn, the tendon will snap out of the groove (bicipital tendinopathy) (see Figure 15.25 on p 271).

EMPTY CAN TEST

The client abducts both arms to 120° with their palms facing upwards. Next, the client internally rotates their arm by turning their thumbs downwards towards the floor (empty can position) and, maintaining the internal rotation, slowly lowers their arms to their sides. Pain or weakness may indicate a supraspatus muscle injury (see Figure 15.26 on p 271).

PALPATION

Palpatory findings, along with findings from other assessments, are used to guide treatment plans. From the suprasternal notch, palpate the sternoclavicular joints immediately laterally. Clavicular dislocations are usually easily palpated, the medial end of the clavicle displacing medially and superiorly. The tip of the coracoid process can be palpated 2.5 cm

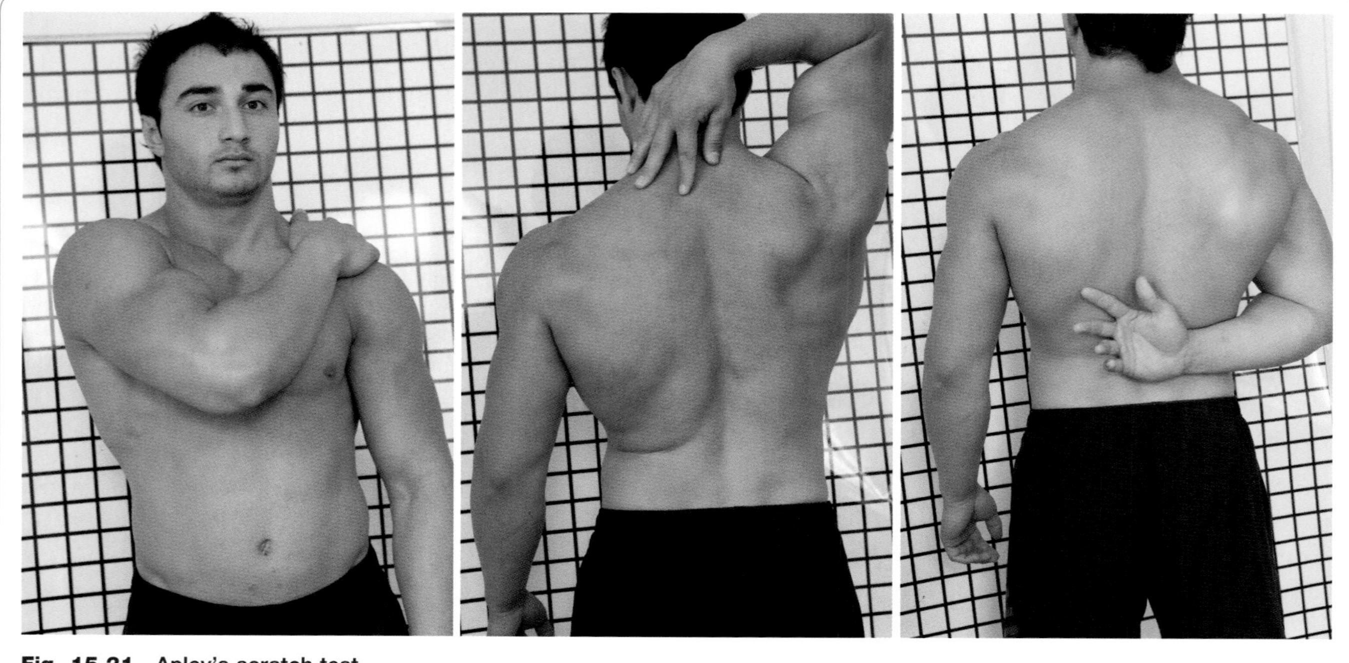

Fig. 15.21 Apley's scratch test

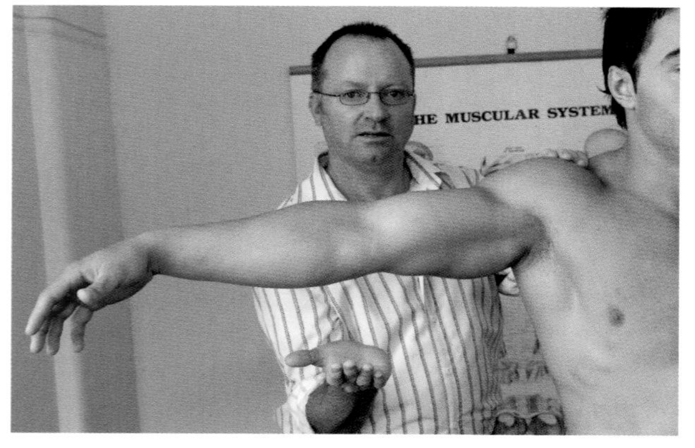

Fig. 15.22 Drop arm test

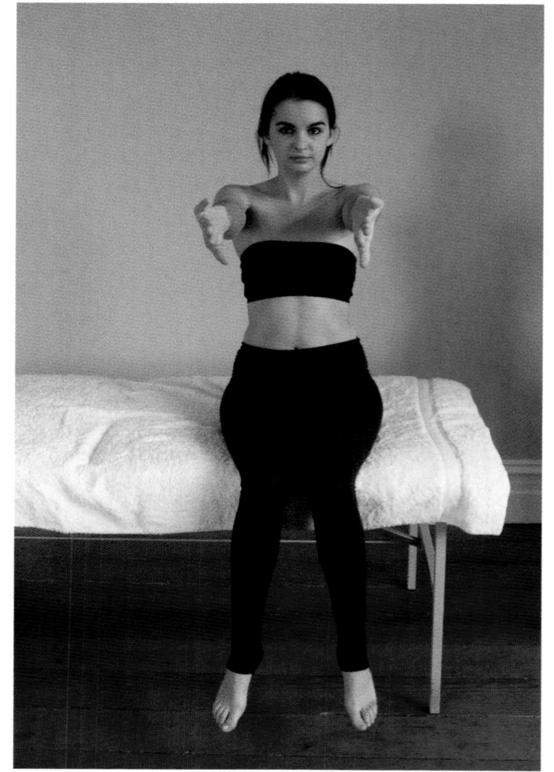

Fig. 15.23 Shoulder impingement test

below the clavicle through the pectoralis major muscle. Palpate the AC joint and the acromion. The greater tuberosity of the humerus can be palpated lateral and inferior to the acromion. Externally rotate the client's shoulder to palpate the intertubercular groove which is anterior and medial to the greater tuberosity, and the lesser tuberosity medial to the groove. Palpate the tendon of the long head of biceps brachii in the bicipital groove (see Figure 15.27 on p 271).

The deltoid attaches to the acromion and inserts into the deltoid tuberosity. It overlays the greater tuberosity of the humerus and gives the shoulder its full and rounded appearance. Three of the rotator cuff muscles (the supraspinatus, infraspinatus and the teres minor, commonly referred to by the acronym SIT muscles[14]) insert into the greater tuberosity. The fourth muscle of the rotator cuff, the subscapularis,

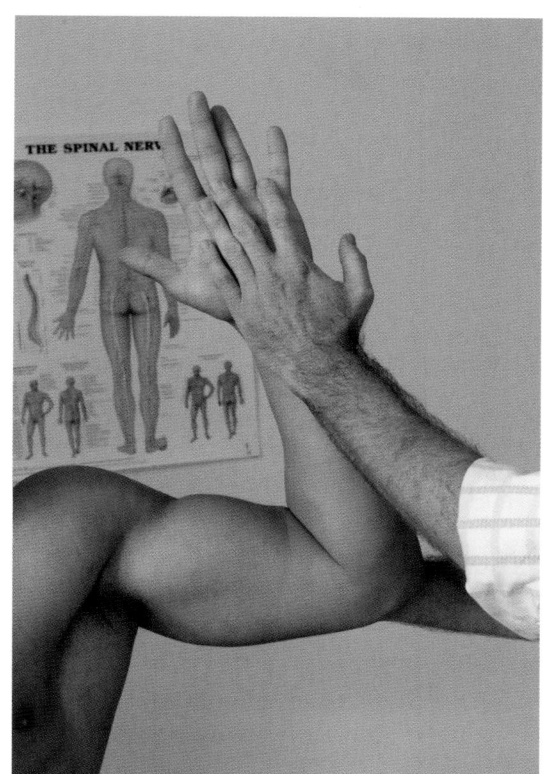

Fig. 15.24 Shoulder apprehension test

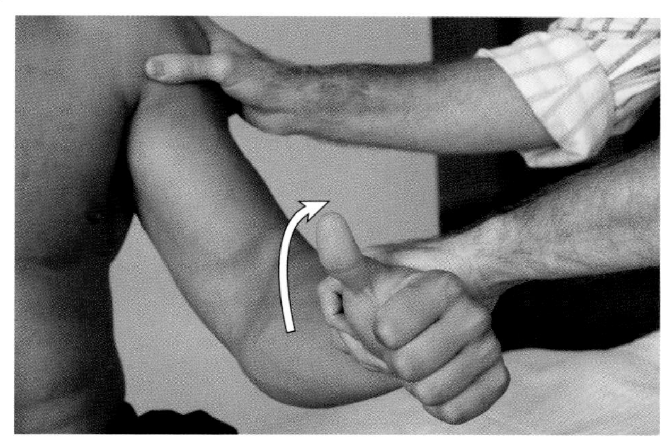

Fig. 15.25 Yergason's test

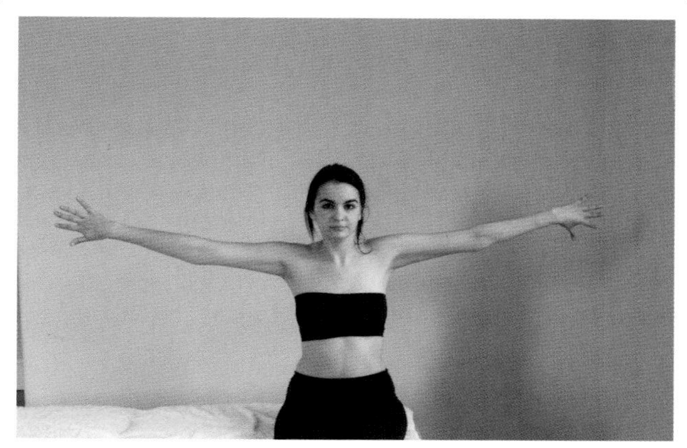

Fig. 15.26 Empty can test

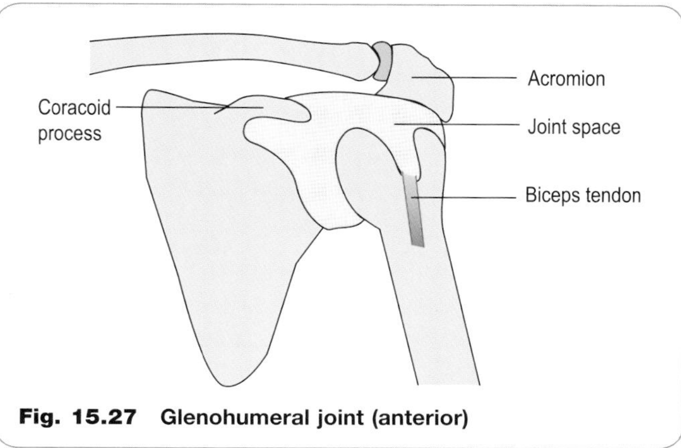

Fig. 15.27 Glenohumeral joint (anterior)

attaches to the lesser tuberosity and is not easily palpated. When the client's arm is by their side, the supraspinatus attachment lies under the acromion, the subscapularis attachment is anterior, and the infraspinatus and teres minor attachments are posterior. Passively extending the client's shoulder moves the SIT muscles into a more easily palpable position. Tenderness elicited during palpation of the muscle attachments suggests tear or strain. Note that the supraspinatus tendon is the most commonly injured muscle of the shoulder joint.[15] The subacromial and subdeltoid bursa may be palpable immediately below the anterior and lateral aspects of the acromion when the arm is in the neutral position by the side.

Palpate the spine of the scapula posteriorly. The superior angle of the scapula and the insertion of the levator scapulae muscle are palpated through the trapezius muscle. Palpate the medial border of the scapula, inferior angle, lateral border and overlying latissimus dorsi, teres major and teres minor muscles. The latissimus dorsi muscle forms the posterior border of the axilla and the subscapularis muscle may be palpated deep to latissimus dorsi. Pectoralis major makes up the anterior border of the axilla. Ribs 2–6 and the overlying serratus anterior muscle are palpated in the medial axilla. Lymph node enlargements may be palpated at the apex of the axilla.

REMEDIAL MASSAGE TREATMENT

Many conditions with acute shoulder pain will resolve spontaneously. A prospective study of clients reporting new episodes of shoulder pain in general practice found that 23% of all new episodes of shoulder pain resolved fully within one month and 44% resolved within three months of onset.[16] With conservative treatment approximately 50% of people with acute shoulder pain recovered within 6 months and approximately 60% within 12 months. Persistent symptoms at 6 months after initial consultation have been consistently associated with long duration of symptoms, gradual onset of pain and high pain severity at presentation.[17] The risk that uncomplicated shoulder pain will persist beyond the acute phase appears to be also related to personality traits, coping style and occupational factors.[18, 19] Shoulder pain may recur even when a full recovery appears to have been made in the short term.

Assessment of the shoulder region provides essential information for development of treatment plans, including:

- clients' suitability for remedial massage therapy
- duration of the condition (i.e. acute or chronic)
- severity of the condition (i.e. grade of injury; mild, moderate or severe pain)
- type(s) of tissues involved
- priorities for treatment if more than one injury or condition are present
- whether the signs and symptoms suggest a common condition of the shoulder region
- special considerations for individual clients (e.g. client's preference for treatment types and styles, special population considerations).

Treatment options must always be considered in the context of the best available evidence for treatment effectiveness and clinical practice guidelines where they exist. One systematic review found that manual therapy appears to increase either active or passive mobility of the shoulder joint and that there appears to be a trend favouring manual therapy for decreasing pain, but its effect on function and quality of life is inconclusive.[20] Further research is required to prove effectiveness of many shoulder treatments. Findings of current research are summarised in Table 15.4.

Most shoulder pathology is related to either impingement or instability.[21] Common mechanisms of injury include throwing overhead, falling on the outstretched arm or shoulder tip and forcing the shoulder into external or internal rotation while the arm is abducted.

OVERVIEW

Develop a short- and a long-term plan for each client. The short-term plan directs treatment to the highest priority (usually determined by symptoms). The long-term plan can be introduced when presenting symptoms have subsided. Long-term treatment focuses on contributing or predisposing factors such as underlying structural features and lifestyle factors. A significant part of both short-term and long-term treatment involves educating clients about likely causal or aggravating factors and guiding their management of these factors. If massage therapy is being used in conjunction with other treatments such as corticosteroid injections, it is important to communicate with other treating practitioners.

MUSCLE STRAIN

The most common sites of pathology in the shoulder are the rotator cuff muscles (particularly supraspinatus), the subacromial bursa and the tendon of the long head of biceps brachii.[22]

Rotator cuff tendinosis

Rotator cuff tendinosis refers to strain of the supraspinatus, infraspinatus, teres minor or subscapularis tendons. Most rotator cuff strains are partial tears. They are the result of progressive collagen breakdown and develop from prolonged repetitive strain, especially from overhead activities, throwing or lifting, shovelling, spiking in volleyball, bowling in cricket and racquet sports.[10, 23] Strains may also arise from sudden trauma or excessive force applied to the shoulder. Full thickness tears of the tendon tend to result from serious acute injuries with high force loads.

Supraspinatus is the most commonly strained rotator cuff muscle. Repeated compression under the acromion eventually leads to tissue degeneration and fibre tearing. Decreased

Table 15.4 Summary of evidence for the effectiveness of treatments for acute shoulder pain[4]

Evidence of effectiveness	• Subacromial corticosteroid injection for acute shoulder pain may improve pain at four weeks compared to placebo but this benefit is not maintained at 12 weeks. • Exercises may improve shoulder pain compared to placebo in people with rotator cuff disease in both the short and longer term. • Topical and oral non-steroidal anti-inflammatory drugs (NSAIDs) improve acute shoulder pain by a small to moderate degree for up to four weeks compared to placebo. Serious adverse effects of NSAIDs include gastrointestinal complications (e.g. bleeding, perforation). • Therapeutic ultrasound may provide short-term pain relief in calcific tendinitis compared to placebo.
Insufficient evidence	• There are no randomised controlled trials investigating the use of analgesics (paracetamol or compound analgesics) for acute or chronic shoulder pain. • Shoulder joint mobilisation with combined treatments (hot packs, active exercise, stretching, soft tissue mobilisation and education) may improve acute shoulder pain in the short term compared to combined treatments alone. • There are no randomised controlled trials investigating the use of oral corticosteroids compared with placebo or no treatment for adhesive capsulitis. • There are no published randomised controlled trials investigating the effectiveness of surgery for acute shoulder pain, although studies exist for chronic populations. • There is insufficient evidence for the use of TENS for acute shoulder pain.
Conflicting evidence	• There is conflicting evidence about the effectiveness of acupuncture compared to placebo ultrasound for shoulder pain and function.

vascularity near the supraspinatus insertion can also lead to slower healing and calcification of the tendon.[24] The infraspinatus and teres minor muscles laterally rotate the humerus (concentric contraction) and also decelerate medial rotation of the humerus as in the eccentric contraction phase (follow through) of throwing. The subscapularis is rarely strained as other stronger accessory muscles, such as pectoralis major, latissimus dorsi and teres major provide mechanical support. Subscapularis strains are more likely in clients over 40 and are often associated with glenohumeral dislocation.

Biceps brachii tendinosis[10]

Biceps brachii tendinosis is a result of progressive degeneration of the long head of the biceps brachii tendon as it passes from the superior aspect of the glenoid fossa through the joint capsule to the bicipital groove of the humerus. The tendon is surrounded by a synovial sheath. Tendinosis is usually the result of overuse, especially with excessive weight training (e.g. excessive bench press and dips). The tendon is stabilised in the bicipital groove by the transverse humeral ligament and may pop out of the groove if the transverse ligament is impaired. The tendon may also pull away from the glenoid labrum if excessive force is applied. Refer all severe injuries for further investigation.

Assessment

HISTORY

The client complains of shoulder pain after prolonged or repetitive overuse, especially after overhand throwing, shovelling, racquet sports or a single blow, fall onto an outstretched hand or sports injury. Pain can be experienced immediately or within the next 24–48 hours. Pain is associated with activities and generally relieved with rest.

FUNCTIONAL TESTS

AROM: limited in one or more directions.
PROM: mild to no pain except at end of range when muscle is stretched.
RROM: painful.
Resisted and length tests painful for involved muscles.
Special tests for specific muscle strains positive (e.g. Apley's scratch test, drop arm test, empty can test, Yergason's test).

Key assessment findings for muscle strain

- History of trauma or repetitive overuse
- Functional tests
  - AROM limited in one or more directions
  - PROM usually negative except at end of range if muscle is passively stretched
  - RROM painful in one or more directions
  - Resisted test and length test positive for specific muscle
  - Special tests may be positive for specific muscles (e.g. Apley's scratch for rotator cuff pathology, empty can test for supraspinatus, Yergason's test for long head of biceps brachii)
- Palpation positive for tenderness/pain, spasm, myofibril tears/scar tissue

PALPATION

Muscle spasm is usually evident. The client reports tenderness or pain on palpation of the affected muscle.

Overview of treatment of muscle strains

A typical remedial massage treatment for mild to moderate muscle strains of the shoulder includes:

- Swedish massage to the shoulder, upper back, neck, upper limb and chest.
- Remedial techniques including:
  - deep gliding frictions along the muscle fibres
  - cross-fibre frictions
  - soft tissue releasing techniques
  - deep transverse friction
  - trigger point therapy.

  Remedial massage techniques for muscles of the shoulder region are illustrated in Table 15.5.
- Myofascial release including cross-arm techniques and the arm pull (see Chapter 8). (Fig 15.28 on p 274).
- Thermotherapy might be useful for pain relief.

Other remedial techniques for muscle strains/imbalances include:

- **Horizontal fibre release (derived from Bowen)**
  In its traditional form Bowen is a stand-alone therapy. A derivative form is described here which may be integrated with other remedial techniques.
  The client is seated. Stand behind the client and place your foot on the table next to the client (hip and knee flexed). For hygiene purposes, place foot on paper towel. Instruct the client to raise their arm into the stop sign position (shoulder abducted to 90°, elbow flexed to 90°). The client's elbow is placed on your knee. Place both hands together over the client's shoulder joint and deltoid, with fingers anteriorly and thumbs posteriorly. Instruct the client to slowly move their hand as far forward as they can (internal rotation) and then as far back again (external rotation). As the client moves, grip the shoulder muscles to separate the myofibrils horizontally (see Figure 15.29 on p 274).
- Shoulder passive joint articulation may be a useful supplement to the muscle-specific techniques described above (see Chapter 7):
  - shoulder rotation
  - shoulder traction
  - shoulder progressive cylindrical articulation
  - shoulder progressive external rotation
  - shoulder progressive internal rotation
  - shoulder figure-8.

Address any underlying conditions or predisposing factors (e.g scoliosis or thoracic hyperkyphosis).

CLIENT EDUCATION

Where possible, clients should take an increasingly active role in their treatment through rehabilitation and health promotion activities. Shoulders are particularly susceptible to injury from activities and sports which place sustained demands on the arms and shoulders or where there is a risk of sudden trauma. The importance of a general and sport-specific physical conditioning program in the prevention of shoulder injuries

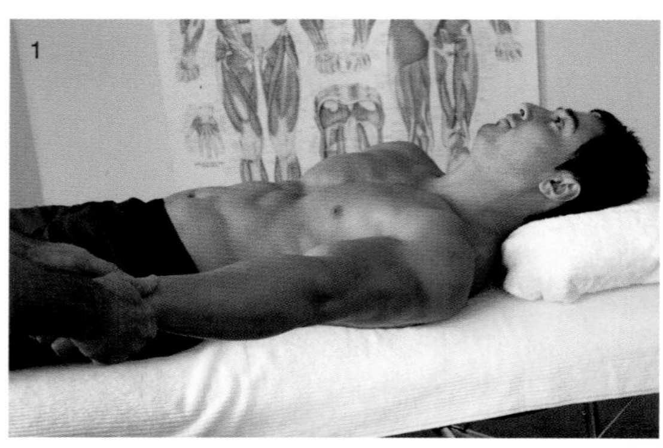

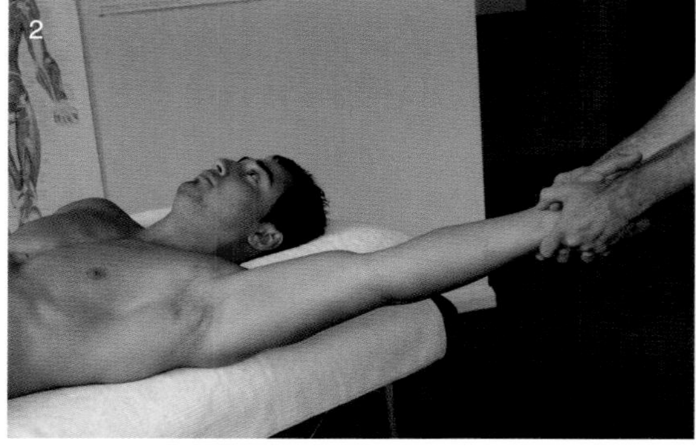

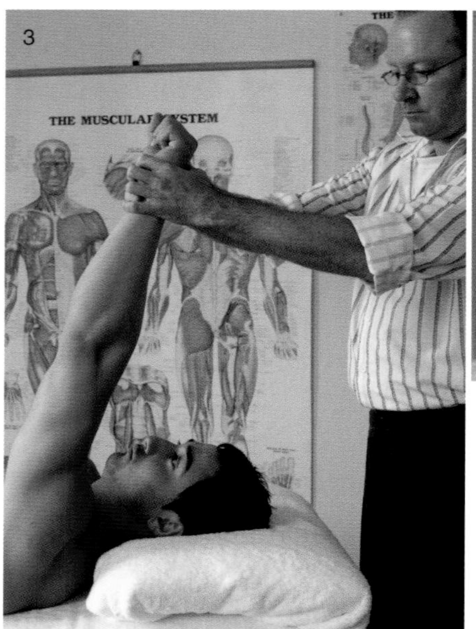

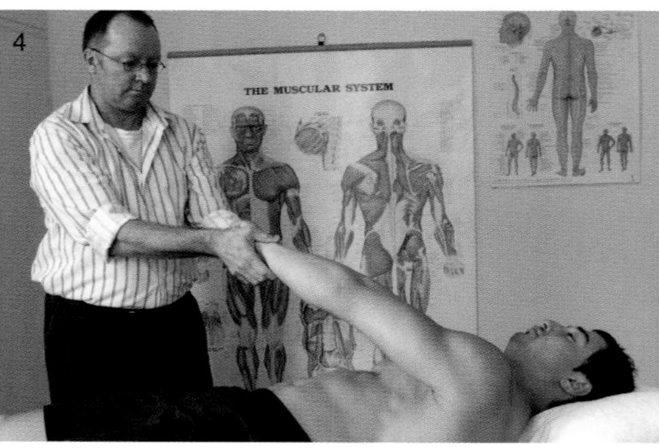

Fig. 15.28 Myofascial release: Arm pull

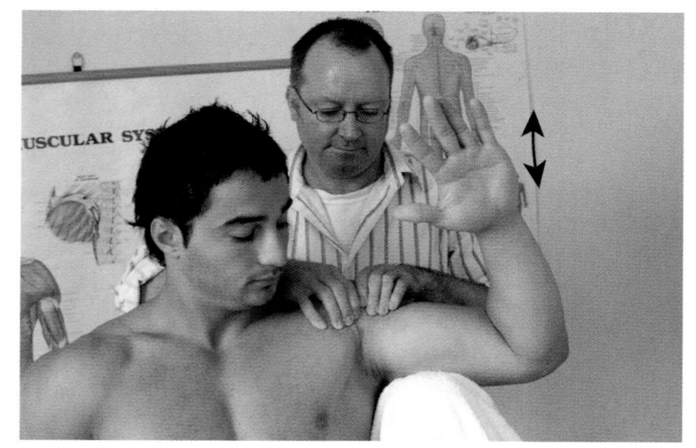

Fig. 15.29 Horizontal fibre release (derived from Bowen)

cannot be overstated. To prevent overuse injuries technique correction (e.g. for throwing, spiking, overhead smashing, overhand serving, crawl and butterfly swimming, and tackling) may be required.

Home exercise program

A program of progressive rehabilitation should accompany remedial massage treatment. Aim for maximum strength and full length of all major muscles. Unresolved strains lead ultimately to faulty biomechanics and other conditions such as adhesive capsulitis and degenerative joint disease may follow.

Introduce stretching exercises as soon as possible after injury (depending on severity and pain tolerance). Introduce non-resistive pendulum exercises gradually progressing to active resistive isometric, isotonic and isokinetic exercises after most ROM has been regained. Apply ice after exercises if pain or swelling returns (exercises should be performed at less than 90° flexion and abduction). Focus on glenohumeral rotation (aim for a strength ratio of 2 : 3 of external rotators to internal rotators).[10] Strengthening programs should progress towards functional exercises (e.g. wall push ups, overhead

Table 15.5 Remedial massage techniques for muscles of the shoulder region

Muscle	Soft tissue release	Trigger point	Deep transverse friction	Stretch	Corrective action[25, 26]	Home exercise
Middle deltoid	Horizontal fibre release (derived from Bowen). Practitioner: stands behind the seated client with their foot on the table (on a paper towel). Client: raises arm into stop sign position (shoulder abducted to 90°, elbow flexed to 90°) and rests flexed elbow on practitioner's knee. The practitioner places both hands together over the deltoid, with fingers anterior and thumbs posterior. The client slowly moves their hand as far forward as they can (shoulder internal rotation) and then as far back (shoulder external rotation). As the client moves, the practitioner grips the deltoid muscle to spread the fibres. 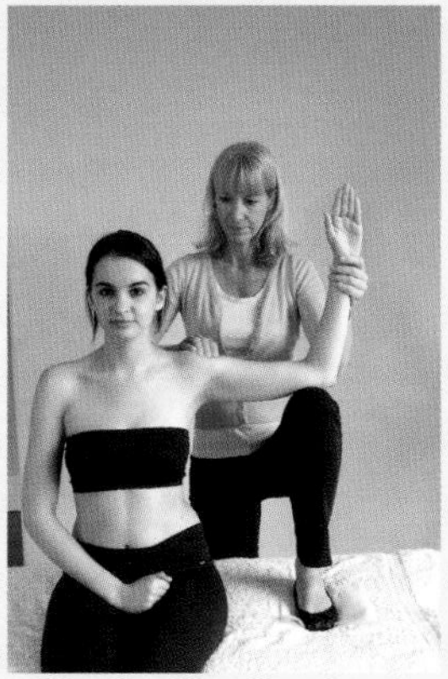	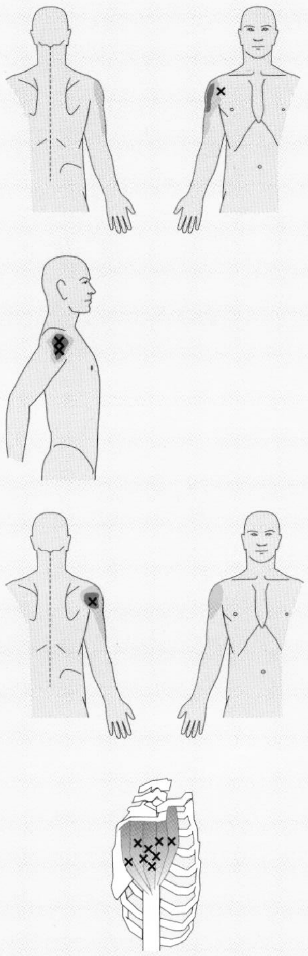	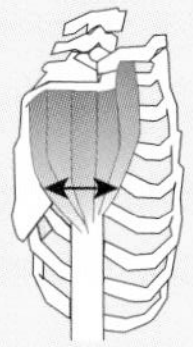	Middle deltoid: As for supraspinatus.	Eliminate perpetuating mechanical stresses (e.g. drive with two hands on steering wheel). Technique correction with overhead sports.	Stretch: Reach behind back as far as possible within pain tolerance towards opposite side of body. (Other hand can assist by pulling flexed elbow further medially.) 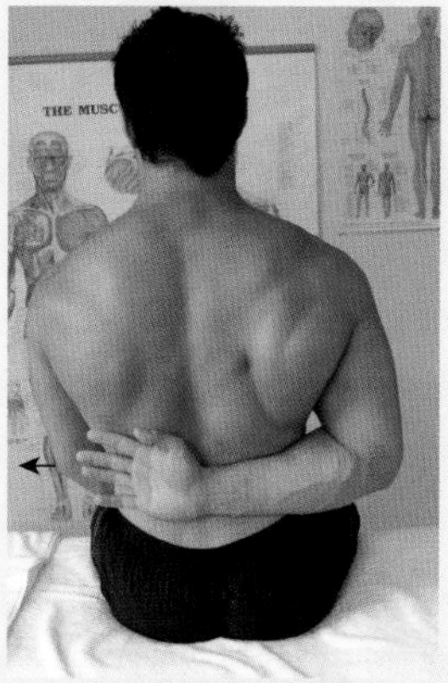

Continued

Table 15.5 Remedial massage techniques for muscles of the shoulder region—cont'd

Muscle	Soft tissue release	Trigger point	Deep transverse friction	Stretch	Corrective action[25, 26]	Home exercise
Supraspinatus	Client: sitting or supine with elbow bent to 90°. Practitioner: applies gentle sustained pressure to the belly of the supraspinatus using thumbs or knuckles as client slowly abducts and adducts their arm as far as possible within pain tolerance. Repeat several times. In the dynamic variation, the practitioner glides their contact along the supraspinatus belly while the client adducts the arm (i.e. lengthening supraspinatus).			CRAC stretch: Client: seated, adducts arm by reaching behind their back across their body towards their other arm as far as possible within pain tolerance. Practitioner: applies resistance at the client's flexed elbow as they try to abduct their arm for 6–8 seconds. After the resistance, the client returns their arm to their side and then adducts their arm again as far as possible within pain tolerance. Repeat the whole procedure three times.	Avoid overloading the muscle (e.g. avoid carrying heavy loads). Do not sleep with hands above head.	Stretch:

Table 15.5 Remedial massage techniques for muscles of the shoulder region—cont'd

Muscle	Soft tissue release	Trigger point	Deep transverse friction	Stretch	Corrective action[25, 26]	Home exercise
Infraspinatus/ teres minor	Client: seated, elbow flexed to 90°. Practitioner: maintains pressure on taut band/ lesion of the muscle using thumbs or knuckles, as the forearm is actively or passively taken inwards across the body (shoulder internal rotation) and outwards (shoulder external rotation), keeping elbow at side of body. Dynamic variation: practitioner slowly glides along the muscle fibres as the muscle is lengthened (i.e. the humerus internally rotates) Can be performed prone, beginning with client's shoulder abducted to 90°	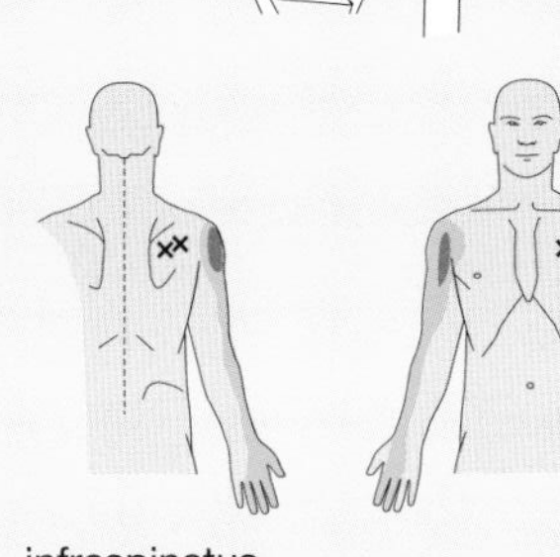 infraspinatus 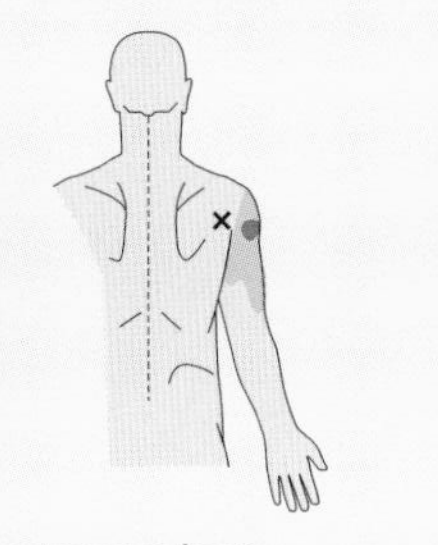 teres minor		CRAC stretch: Client: reaches behind their back towards inferior angle of opposite scapula within pain tolerance. Practitioner: holding client's wrist and elbow, resists the client's attempt to return arm to their side for 6–8 seconds. Client returns arm to their side. Next, client reaches behind their back towards inferior angle of scapula again within pain tolerance. Repeat the whole procedure three times. 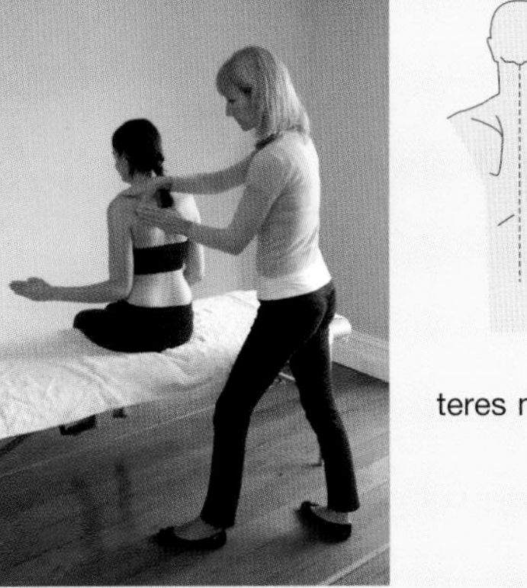	Avoid overloading the muscle (e.g. reaching into back seat of car). Support arm on a pillow for pain relief when sleeping. Avoid rounded shoulder posture.	Stretch: Try to touch hands behind back with one arm overhead and the other behind the back. Can hold a small towel between hands if required. Hold for up to 30 seconds. Repeat three times. 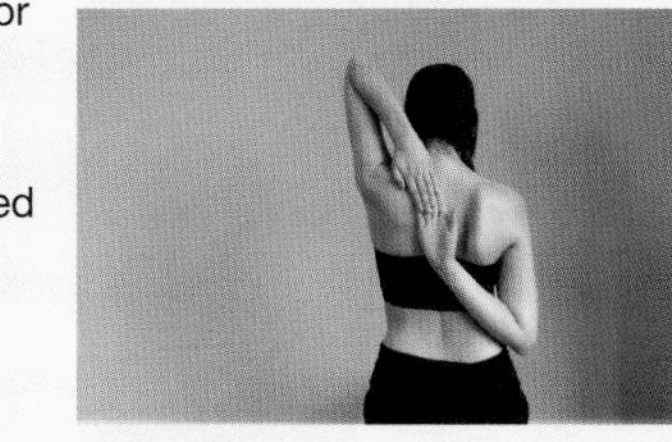 Strengthen: Resisted shoulder external rotation 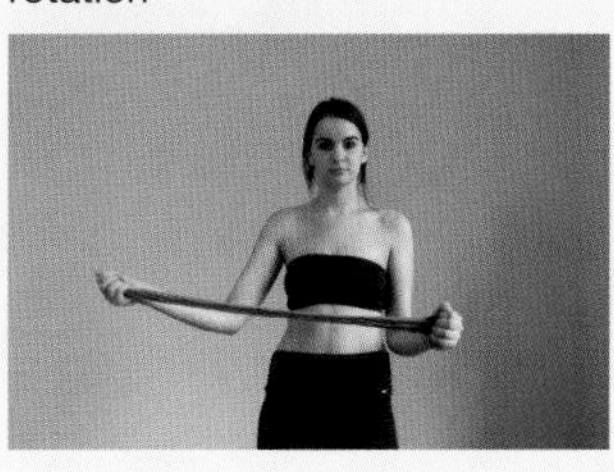

Continued

Table 15.5 Remedial massage techniques for muscles of the shoulder region—cont'd

Muscle	Soft tissue release	Trigger point	Deep transverse friction	Stretch	Corrective action[25, 26]	Home exercise
Teres major	Client: seated, elbow flexed to 90°. Practitioner: maintains pressure on taut band/lesion of the muscle using thumbs or knuckles as the forearm is actively or passively taken inwards across the body (shoulder internal rotation) and outwards (shoulder external rotation), keeping elbow at side of body. Can be performed prone, beginning with client's shoulder abducted to 90°.			CRAC stretch: Client lies supine, elbow flexed to 90° and externally rotates forearm as far as possible within pain tolerance, keeping elbow alongside body. The practitioner applies resistance for 6–8 seconds as the client tries to bring their forearm across their body (internally rotate shoulder). When the resistance is released, the client tries to externally rotate their forearm as far as possible again. The whole procedure is repeated three times. Progress to different starting positions (e.g. humerus abducted to 30°, 60° or 90°, practitioner supporting abducted elbow), making sure the client's scapula remains flat on the treatment table throughout the stretch.	Avoid overloading the muscle (e.g. drive with two hands on the steering wheel). To sleep, lie on the affected side and place a pillow between the elbow and the front of the body. Check gym activities.	Lie supine, place both hands behind the neck and let elbows fall towards the floor as far as possible. Strengthen: Resisted internal rotation

Table 15.5 Remedial massage techniques for muscles of the shoulder region—cont'd

Muscle	Soft tissue release	Trigger point	Deep transverse friction	Stretch	Corrective action[25, 26]	Home exercise
Subscapularis	Client: supine, humerus abducted to 90° and elbow flexed to 90°. Practitioner: contacts the lateral aspect of the subscapularis using a flat finger contact and moves medially into the posterior axilla. The practitioner contacts the client's forearm at the wrist and slowly externally and internally rotates the arm while applying pressure to the subscapularis.		The distal musculotendinous junction where most tears occur is accessible. The practitioner grasps either side of the posterior axilla between thumb and index finger and applies deep friction to the fibres by dragging the contacts laterally.	CRAC stretch: Client: supine or seated, elbow flexed to 90° and externally rotates the arm as far as possible within pain tolerance. Practitioner: applies resistance for 6–8 seconds as the client tries to internally rotate their arm. After the resistance, the client tries to externally rotate their arm to their comfortable limit. Repeat the whole procedure three times.	Correct rounded shoulder posture.	Stretch: Lie supine, humerus abducted to 90° or as far as possible, elbow flexed to 90°. Let the forearm fall backwards towards the floor as far as possible within pain tolerance. Hold for 30 seconds. Make sure that the scapula remains flat on the floor throughout the stretch. Alternatively, the doorway stretch (see Chapter 14) can also be used to stretch subscapularis. Strengthen: Resisted internal rotation.

Continued

Table 15.5 Remedial massage techniques for muscles of the shoulder region—cont'd

Muscle	Soft tissue release	Trigger point	Deep transverse friction	Stretch	Corrective action[25, 26]	Home exercise
Biceps brachii	Client: supine or seated, elbow fully flexed at the beginning of this technique to shorten the biceps. Practitioner: maintains pressure with thumbs, fingers or knuckles, or performs a deep glide along the muscle fibres as the client's forearm is actively or passively extended and flexed. The client can hold a weight in their hand to recruit more fibres.		At the humeral insertion, deep friction techniques are applied in a longitudinal rather than transverse direction to prevent dislocation of the tendon from the groove.	Passive stretch: Biceps brachii is stretched by extending the shoulder, extending the elbow and then pronating the forearm.	Lift objects with forearms in pronation. Decrease load when carrying with flexed elbows. Strengthen triceps brachii. Correct sleeping posture. Check work ergonomics.	Extend the shoulder, extend the elbow and point thumb downwards. Hold for 30 seconds. A variant of the doorway stretch can be used: stand in front of the doorway, hold the door jamb with thumbs pointing downward, elbows extended and lean forward.

Table 15.5 Remedial massage techniques for muscles of the shoulder region—cont'd

Muscle	Soft tissue release	Trigger point	Deep transverse friction	Stretch	Corrective action[25, 26]	Home exercise
Triceps brachii	Client: prone or seated (or supine with arm extended overhead). Practitioner: maintains pressure with thumbs, fingers or knuckles or performs a deep glide along the muscle fibres as the client slowly flexes and extends their elbow.			CRAC stretch: Client: seated, elbow fully flexed, and humerus flexed to comfortable limit. Practitioner: stands behind the client, holds the elbow and resists as the client tries to extend their humerus (i.e. bring their elbow forward) for 6–8 seconds. After the resistance, the client tries to flex the humerus again to their comfortable limit. Repeat the whole procedure three times.	Avoid overload. Modify chairs with inadequate elbow support. Review arm position in repetitive manual work. Use tennis racquet with a large grip. Avoid overhead activities.	Fully flex the elbow and flex the humerus as far as possible. Use the other hand to try to pull the flexed elbow towards a vertical position within a comfortable limit. Hold the stretch for up to 30 seconds. Repeat three times.

work, ball throwing) which should be maintained long term. Include proprioceptive exercises (e.g. gymball).

Clients may be referred for manipulation of the neck, upper back and shoulders. Refer any client who worsens or fails to improve within 2 weeks or shows only slight improvement within 4 weeks.

SHOULDER IMPINGEMENT SYNDROME

Shoulder impingement syndrome (sometimes called swimmer's shoulder) describes the compression of several soft tissue structures between the coracoacromial arch (made up of the coracoid process, the acromion and the coracoacromial ligament) and the greater tuberosity of the humerus. Soft tissues that may be compressed include the supraspinatus muscle or tendon, the tendon of the long head of biceps brachii, the upper glenohumeral joint capsule and the subacromial bursa. When the subacromial bursa becomes inflamed it can swell to the size of a golf ball. Subacromial bursitis often occurs from repetitive compression underneath the coracoacromial arch as can occur in overhead movements (e.g. tennis serve, bowling in cricket, or freestyle swimming). Other causes of bursitis include autoimmune disease, crystal deposition, or infection.

Impingement is classified as primary or secondary. Primary impingement may be caused by reduced space under the acromion due to a flattened or tilted acromion, or osteophytes which have developed under the acromion. Secondary impingement may be caused by repeated overhead movements as occur in throwing, overhead strokes in swimming, cricket, weight lifting, water polo and tennis, decreased vascularity to the rotator cuff or biceps brachii tendons, or a raised humeral head due to a previous dislocation.

Shoulder impingement tends to initiate a cycle of degeneration. Once the shoulder muscles are impinged, they are less effective at maintaining the humeral head in the glenoid fossa, which in turn leads to further impingement. Treatment outcomes depend on how quickly treatment is commenced. Three progressive stages of impingement have been described.[27] Stage 1 is characterised by acute inflammation, oedema and haemorrhage in the rotator cuff muscles. Stage 2 progresses to fibrosis and tendinosis of the rotator cuff muscles. In Stage 3 mechanical disruption of the rotator cuff tendons and changes to the coracoacromial arch occur. As with most musculoskeletal conditions, early intervention is likely to produce the best outcomes.

Assessment

Key assessment findings for shoulder impingement syndrome

- History of repetitive overhead activity; painful abduction and flexion
- Functional tests
  - AROM positive (painful arc)
  - PROM ± painful
  - RROM positive in some directions
  - Resisted and length tests positive for affected muscles
  - Special tests: shoulder impingement test positive
- Palpation positive for pain/tenderness, spasm, myofibril tears/scar tissue

HISTORY

The client complains of pain during active flexion and abduction of the shoulder, usually between 70° and 120° (painful arc). The client may describe recurring or constant shoulder pain, often worse at night. There is often a history of several previous episodes of shoulder pain that are associated with repetitive overhead activity. Pain may refer to the lateral and posterolateral upper arm.

FUNCTIONAL TESTS

Cervical AROM negative.

Shoulder:
AROM: positive flexion and abduction (painful arc).
PROM: may be positive in flexion and abduction.
RROM: Weakness and pain depending on muscle(s) involved (e.g. if supraspinatus involved, pain ± weakness on resisted shoulder abduction; if biceps brachii tendon is involved, pain on resisted shoulder flexion).
Resisted tests and length tests are positive for affected muscles.
Special tests: Impingement test positive, empty can test and Apley's scratch test positive if supraspinatus is affected.

PALPATION

Tenderness may be elicited during palpation over the greater tuberosity and anterior acromion. (Note: tenderness may also be present in glenohumeral or AC arthrosis). Muscle atrophy may follow long-standing impingement. Crepitus/snapping may be present. (Note: crepitus/snapping is also associated with glenohumeral and AC arthrosis and labral tears.[10])

Overview of treatment and management

One of the challenges of treating impingement is that the tissues that have been compressed are often fibrotic. They are also difficult to access under the acromion. Effective techniques to accessible tissues include friction to the supraspinatus tendon, deep longitudinal stripping to the supraspinatus belly, and deep friction to the infraspinatus and teres minor muscles. Attention should be focused on tissues that contribute to biomechanical imbalance, such as tightness in the deltoid or weakness of the lateral and internal rotators which could raise the humeral head in the glenoid fossa predisposing to impingement during overhead movements.

A typical remedial massage treatment for mild or moderate impingement syndrome includes:

- Swedish massage therapy to the shoulder and upper arm, neck, upper back (and chest).
- Remedial massage techniques, including (see Table 15.5):
  - deep gliding frictions along the muscle fibres
  - cross-fibre frictions
  - soft tissue releasing techniques
  - deep transverse friction
  - trigger point therapy
  - muscle stretching.

  If assessment results suggest inert structures then myofascial releasing techniques (see Chapter 8) and passive joint articulations (see Chapter 7) may be appropriate. Passive joint articulation for the shoulder includes:
  - shoulder rotation
  - shoulder traction

- shoulder progressive cylindrical articulation
- shoulder progressive external rotation
- shoulder progressive internal rotation
- shoulder figure-8.

CLIENT EDUCATION

Advise clients to avoid all overhead or painful activities. Posture correction especially for the cervical spine and pectoral girdle may be required. Review aggravating sporting techniques or work activities and correct if possible. A rehabilitation exercise program should be started as soon as tolerated by the client. The goal of the program is to restore normal shoulder biomechanics. This usually involves strengthening the shoulder stabilisers and rotator cuff muscles. Restoration of normal scapular rotation about a medial to lateral axis and serratus anterior muscle function are particularly important in the rehabilitation of clients whose symptoms are related to occupational overhead work.[28] Refer for spinal and shoulder manipulation.

Care must be taken to ensure that strength-training programs do not aggravate the condition. Exercises should progress from pain-free stretches (e.g. pendulum exercises) and isometric exercises to increasingly loaded muscle strength training and functional exercises (e.g. wall push ups, overhead work, ball throwing) which should be maintained long term. Flexibility exercises should be continued through all phases of rehabilitation.

Note: Oral anti-inflammatory medication or subacromial corticosteroid injections are sometimes used to decrease inflammation. There are concerns about injecting corticosteroids into the connective tissue because of the long-term detrimental effects. Surgical techniques to create space under the acromion are considered when conservative approaches fail. Acromioplasty involves shaving off the underside of the acromion in order to reshape it or remove bone spurs.

DEGENERATIVE JOINT DISEASE (DEGENERATIVE ARTHRITIS, OSTEOARTHRITIS)

Degenerative joint disease (DJD) of the shoulder is uncommon unless there is a history of previous significant trauma or overuse, or DJD in other joints. DJD is more commonly found in the AC joint than the glenohumeral joint. It is characterised by progressive degeneration of articular cartilage, subchondral sclerosis and osteophyte formation[10] (see Figure 15.30). The client is usually middle-aged or elderly or has a history of previous significant trauma, or work or sport that involves repetitive shoulder activity.

Assessment

Key assessment findings for DJD of the glenohumeral joint

- History of chronic shoulder pain and limitation aggravated by use; client usually over 50 years old
- Functional tests:
  - AROM limited ± painful in some directions
  - PROM limited ± painful (capsular pattern)
  - RROM usually negative
  - Special tests negative
- Palpation positive for crepitus and hard or capsular end-feel

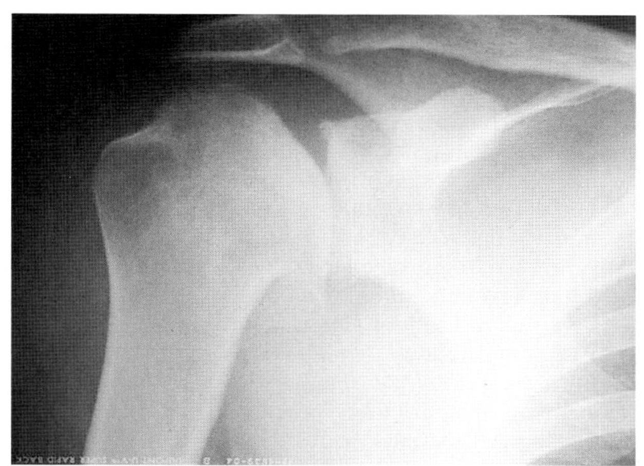

Fig. 15.30 Radiograph of glenohumeral DJD

HISTORY

The client complains of chronic shoulder pain and stiffness that is aggravated by use. The client is usually over 50 years old or has a history of significant previous injury or overuse. DJD of the glenohumeral joint is not a common presenting condition although it is more common when other joints are also affected.

FUNCTIONAL TESTS

Cervical AROM does not reproduce shoulder symptoms.

Shoulder:
AROM positive (limited external rotation, abduction and medial rotation).
PROM positive (capsular pattern: limited external rotation, abduction and medial rotation), crepitus often present.
RROM negative.
Resisted and length tests for specific muscles: DJD is often accompanied by capsule tightening and muscle contractures. In such cases, muscle length tests reveal shortening of affected muscles.
Special tests usually negative.

PALPATION

Crepitus and abnormal hard or capsular end-feel are usually palpated.

Treatment of DJD of the glenohumeral joint

Although DJD is a chronic degenerative condition, acute episodes can occur from time to time, usually after overactivity. If acute inflammation is present, treatment could include cryotherapy for analgesia, acupressure, Reiki, reflexology or anti-inflammatory medication. The client should be advised to modify activities to avoid aggravating the condition.

A typical remedial massage treatment for mild or moderate subacute or chronic DJD includes:

- Swedish massage therapy to the shoulder and upper arm, neck, upper back and chest.

- Remedial massage therapy, which includes heat therapy, myofascial releasing techniques (see Chapter 8) and passive joint articulation (see Chapter 7), including:
  - shoulder rotation
  - shoulder traction
  - shoulder progressive cylindrical articulation
  - shoulder progressive external rotation
  - shoulder progressive internal rotation
  - shoulder figure-8.
- Apply remedial massage techniques to address any associated muscle contractures (see Table 15.5):
  - deep gliding frictions along the muscle fibres
  - cross-fibre frictions
  - soft tissue releasing techniques
  - deep transverse friction
  - trigger point therapy
  - muscle stretching.

CLIENT EDUCATION

The client should be advised to continue to use heat therapy for pain relief and to modify or avoid all aggravating activities. Home exercises should be commenced as soon as pain permits. Stretching and strengthening exercises can be introduced as indicated by assessment findings and should progress towards functional exercises (e.g. wall push-ups and overhead work) that mimic activities required for daily living. Educate clients about the importance of finding the right balance between too little activity (which can lead to capsule and muscle contractures and movement compensations) and too much activity (which can inflame the joint). Non-weight-bearing activities such as water aerobics are often beneficial.

Many clients with DJD of the shoulder joint will also have DJD in other areas of the body including the lower cervical spine. For such clients, massage and posture advice for the neck and upper back will be beneficial.

Nutritional supplements such as glucosamine may be beneficial.[29] Clients may be referred for other supportive therapies including specialist nutritional advice and acupuncture.

ADHESIVE CAPSULITIS (FROZEN SHOULDER)

Adhesive capsulitis is characterised by significantly limited movement caused when the normally loose capsule on the underside of the shoulder joint adheres to itself. Adhesive capsulitis develops over months beginning with painful early synovitis and progressing to an acute inflammatory phase with adhesion formation in the axillary fold. Stiffness and decreased range of motion ensue along with muscle atrophy and a reduction in the size of the synovial cavity and the glenohumeral space. In many cases prolonged immobility of the glenohumeral joint is related to inadequate rehabilitation of a previous shoulder injury (e.g. rotator cuff tears, bicipital tendinosis, shoulder trauma, trigger points of the subscapularis). In such cases the condition may be prevented by adequate rehabilitation of shoulder injuries, including continued shoulder movement within reasonable pain limits. The condition may also be secondary to cardiac disease or surgery, pulmonary disease, diabetes mellitus or thyroid disease. It can also be idiopathic and can subside in one shoulder only to reappear in the other. The condition tends to be self-perpetuating as clients avoid painful movements and this lack of movement further increases adhesions, immobility and pain. Symptoms generally resolve within 18 months to 2 years.[30, 31]

Key assessment findings for adhesive capsulitis of the glenohumeral joint

- History of significant functional limitation and pain; history of previous significant injury; the client is usually 40–60 years old
- Functional tests:
  - AROM limited and painful (external rotation > abduction > internal rotation)
  - PROM limited and painful (external rotation > abduction > internal rotation)
  - RROM positive in some directions
  - Resisted and length tests positive for affected muscles
  - Special tests: Apley's test positive
- Palpation positive for capsular end-feel, pain, ± muscle atrophy or contractures

Assessment

HISTORY

The client is usually 40 to 60 years old and complains of significantly limited functional movement of the entire upper limb. They are often unable to lift their arms above 90° and movement is often accompanied by significant pain. They may complain of being unable to reach into their back pocket, comb their hair or hang clothes on the line. There is usually a history of previous significant trauma. There may be a history of previous adhesive capsulitis in the other shoulder.

FUNCTIONAL TESTS

Cervical AROM does not usually reproduce the shoulder symptoms.

Shoulder tests:
AROM: positive for limitation and pain (capsular pattern: motion is limited in external rotation > abduction > internal rotation). The client shrugs their shoulder when trying to abduct their arm.
PROM: limited and painful (capsular pattern). Note that muscle contractures will follow immobility further restricting passive stretching of muscles.
RROM: Muscle contractures and atrophy are common accompaniments of adhesive capsulitis.
Resisted and length tests: Adhesive capsulitis is associated with capsule tightening and muscle contractures. Length tests reveal contractures of affected muscles.
Special tests: Apley's test positive.

Note: both adhesive capsulitis and subacromial impingement syndrome will limit abduction. However, adhesive capsulitis limits external rotation and impingement syndromes generally do not.

Treatment

A typical remedial massage treatment for adhesive capsulitis includes:

- Swedish massage therapy to the shoulder and upper arm, neck, upper back and chest.

- Remedial massage therapy, which includes heat therapy, myofascial releasing techniques (see Chapter 8) and passive joint articulation (see Chapter 7). Passive joint articulation initially focuses on restoring scapulothoracic/scapulohumeral rhythm and then progresses to restoring glenohumeral movement. Passive stretching, especially in external rotation, abduction and internal rotation, is beneficial. Joint articulations include:
  - shoulder rotation
  - shoulder traction
  - shoulder progressive cylindrical articulation
  - shoulder progressive external rotation
  - shoulder progressive internal rotation
  - shoulder figure-8.

  Select appropriate remedial massage techniques to address muscle contractures, particularly subscapularis. Techniques include (see Table 15.5):
  - deep gliding along the muscle fibre
  - cross-fibre frictions
  - soft tissue releasing techniques
  - deep transverse friction
  - trigger point therapy
  - muscle stretching.

CLIENT EDUCATION

The client should be advised to use ice/heat therapy for pain relief. Home exercises (pendulum exercises, wall climbing exercise, manoeuvring with a cord to reach their hands behind the back) and a gentle strengthening program should be commenced immediately and the client advised to work within their pain tolerance. Encourage clients to find the right balance between too little activity, which leads to further capsule adhesions and muscle contractures, and too much activity which can inflame the area. Support and encourage the client (e.g. recognise even small gains in ranges of motion). Progressively introduce strengthening exercises within the client's pain-free range. Strengthening programs usually begin with isometric exercises and progress towards functional exercises (e.g. wall push-ups, overhead work, ball throwing) which should be maintained long term.

Clients may also require treatment of the upper back, neck and pectoral girdle. Some clients may benefit from referral for spinal and shoulder manipulation and acupuncture.

ACROMIOCLAVICULAR SPRAINS, CLAVICLE FRACTURES AND GLENOHUMERAL DISLOCATIONS

Clients with acute traumatic shoulder injuries such as acromioclavicular sprains, clavicle fractures and glenohumeral dislocations require assessment and treatment by medical practitioners. The rehabilitation of such injuries can be drawn out and many clients experience symptoms or dysfunction for many years after the initial injury. Remedial massage techniques, particularly those that address muscle imbalance and myofascial restrictions, may improve shoulder biomechanics and provide symptom relief.

AC sprains (shoulder separation)

The AC ligaments (superior and inferior acromioclavicular ligaments and coracoacromial ligament) provide anterior/posterior and medial/lateral stability of the AC joint; the coracoclavicular ligaments are designed to provide stability against vertical forces. Injury usually occurs from a direct blow on the anterolateral shoulder from falling on the shoulder or outstretched arm or severe distraction of an abducted arm.

GRADES OF AC SPRAINS

Grade 1: No visible separation, mild injury to the AC ligaments
Grade 2: Elevation of the clavicle, moderate disruption of the AC and coracoclavicular ligaments
Grade 3: Marked elevation of the clavicle, severe disruption of the AC and coracoclavicular ligaments

Presenting symptoms depend on the severity of the initial trauma and subsequent treatment. Clients with Grade 3 injuries are often left with a cosmetic deformity (see Figure 15.4 on p 264). Fibrotic tissue may be evident in affected ligaments.

Clavicle fractures

Clavicle fractures are one of the most common fractures arising from sporting activities. They are usually caused by falls onto the point of the shoulder. In rare cases a bone fragment may cause arterial or nerve damage.

Glenohumeral dislocations

Most glenohumeral dislocations are anterior. They occur from the combined movements of abduction and external rotation and damage the inferior glenohumeral ligament and the glenoid labrum. Many clients will be left with ligamentous laxity and return positive apprehension tests.

Treatment

A typical treatment for a client with a history of chronic symptoms related to previous traumatic injury includes:

- Swedish massage to the shoulder, upper back, neck, upper limb and chest.
- Remedial massage techniques to restore muscle balance including:
  - deep gliding along the muscle fibre
  - cross-fibre frictions
  - soft tissue releasing techniques
  - deep transverse friction
  - trigger point therapy
  - muscle stretching.
- Passive joint articulation may be helpful (see Chapter 7) but any technique that stretches already overstretched ligaments must be avoided.
- Provide myofascial releasing techniques for myofascial restrictions. Thermotherapy may be beneficial.

CLIENT EDUCATION

Progressively introduce stretching and strengthening exercises as required. Advise clients about good posture, especially about avoiding rounded shoulders and head forward posture when sitting. Clients may require referral for osseous manipulation. For clients with a history of glenohumeral dislocation, strengthening rotator cuff, trapezius and serratus anterior may be beneficial. Avoid strengthening pectoralis major as it pulls the humeral head anteriorly.

KEY MESSAGES

- Assessment of clients with conditions of the shoulder region involves history, outcome measures, postural analysis, functional tests and palpation.
- Assessment findings may indicate the type of tissue involved (contractile or inert, muscle, joint, fascia, ligament), duration of condition (acute or subacute) and severity (grade).
- Assessment findings may indicate common presenting conditions such as muscle strain, shoulder impingement syndrome, subacromial bursitis, DJD or adhesive capsulitis.
- Assessment findings also indicate client perception of injury and preferences for treatment.
- Consider Clinical Guidelines, available evidence and client preferences when planning therapy.
- Be conservative in treatment: if in doubt, perform pain-free Swedish massage.
- Although serious conditions of the shoulder region are rare, all clients with symptoms of neurological or vascular impairment in the upper limb should be referred for further assessment.
- The selection of remedial massage techniques depends on assessment results. Swedish massage to the shoulder, upper back, neck, upper limb and chest may be followed by muscle techniques (e.g. deep gliding, cross-fibre frictions, soft tissue releasing techniques, trigger point therapy and deep transverse friction), passive joint articulation, myofascial release and thermotherapy as indicated.
- Educating clients about likely causal and predisposing factors and exercise rehabilitation are essential parts of remedial massage therapy.
- Over time, increase the client self-help component of treatment wherever possible (to reduce likelihood of recurrence and/or to promote health maintenance and illness prevention).

Review questions

1. Match the end-feels in Column A with the shoulder range of motion or condition in Column B

Column A	Column B
Elastic and firm	Horizontal adduction
Empty	Adhesive capsulitis
Hard and capsular	Horizontal abduction
Soft tissue	Severe instability

2. A test that would most likely be positive for a subscapularis muscle strain is:
   a) resisted shoulder adduction
   b) resisted shoulder external rotation
   c) resisted shoulder abduction
   d) resisted shoulder internal rotation
3. A client with shoulder pain has the following assessment results:
   - Positive active abduction (painful arc)
   - Positive passive abduction
   - Negative resisted abduction

   What is/are the most likely soft tissue structure(s) indicated by the assessment findings?
   a) muscle belly
   b) ligament
   c) tendon
   d) bursa
4. The apprehension test of the shoulder may help identify:
   a) grade 3 supraspinatus tear
   b) subacromial bursitis
   c) history of anterior glenohumeral dislocation
   d) impingement of structures between the acromion and the humerus
5. The capsular pattern for DJD describes limitations of ranges of motion that are specific to each joint. The capsular pattern for DJD of the glenohumeral joint suggests that its most restricted movement will be:
   a) abduction
   b) lateral rotation
   c) medial rotation
   d) flexion
6. A step deformity may be observed in a client with:
   a) adhesive capsulitis
   b) impingement syndrome
   c) AC joint separation
   d) a grade 3 supraspinatus tear
7. Describe a home stretch for:
   i) supraspinatus
   ii) teres major
   iii) biceps brachii
8. Home exercises for shoulder impingement syndrome usually include:
   i) stretching for
   ii) strengthening for
9. The following questions refer to the diagram below:

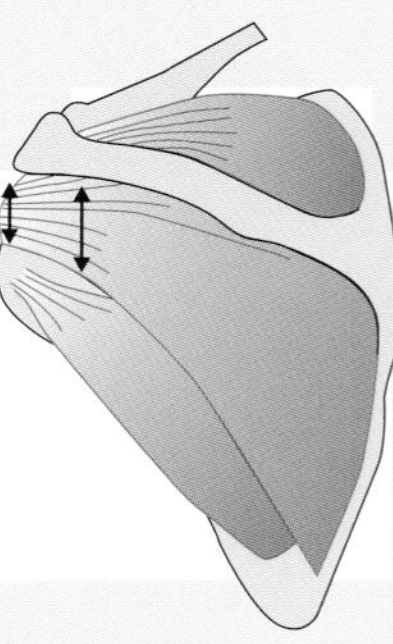

   i) Name the muscle that the arrows cross.
   ii) The arrows represent the direction of deep transverse friction. What are the specific indications for this technique? (For further information see Chapter 4.)
10. A 19-year-old female swimmer has recently increased her training program. She has developed pain in the left shoulder during the pull stroke. The pain seems to be getting worse. Postural analysis reveals a mild scoliosis. The results of her functional tests are as follows:
   Cervical spine:
   AROM: Negative
   Shoulder tests:

Review questions—cont'd

AROM: Painful in flexion, abduction (painful arc)
PROM: Negative
RROM: Painful shoulder flexion
Resisted tests: Positive for flexion
Special tests: Impingement test positive
What structure(s) could be involved?

11. Name five remedial massage techniques that would be suitable for a client with mild to moderate supraspinatus tendinosis.
12. Client education is an essential part of remedial massage therapy. List three recommendations for a client with chronic glenohumeral DJD.

APPENDIX 15.1

Shoulder pain and disability index[a]

The Shoulder Pain and Disability Index (SPADI) is a self-administered questionnaire that consists of two dimensions, one for pain and the other for functional activities. The pain dimension consists of five questions regarding the severity of an individual's pain. Functional activities are assessed with eight questions designed to measure the degree of difficulty an individual has with various activities of daily living that require upper-extremity use. The SPADI takes 5 to 10 minutes for a patient to complete and is the only reliable and valid region-specific measure for the shoulder.

SCORING INSTRUCTIONS

To answer the questions, patients place a mark on a 10 cm visual analogue scale for each question. Verbal anchors for the pain dimension are 'no pain at all' and 'worst pain imaginable', and those for the functional activities are 'no difficulty' and 'so difficult it required help'. The scores from both dimensions are averaged to derive a total score.

INTERPRETATION OF SCORES

Total pain score: / 50 × 100 = %
Note: If a person does not answer all questions divide by the total possible score (e.g. if 1 question missed divide by 40)
Total disability score: / 80 × 100 = %
Note: If a person does not answer all questions divide by the total possible score (e.g. if 1 question missed divide by 70)
Total Spadi score: / 130 × 100 = %
Note: If a person does not answer all questions divide by the total possible score (e.g. if 1 question missed divide by 120)
The means of the two subscales are averaged to produce a total score ranging from 0 (best) to 100 (worst).
Minimum Detectable Change (90% confidence) = 13 points (change less than this may be attributable to measurement error)

SHOULDER PAIN AND DISABILITY INDEX (SPADI)

Please place a mark on the line that best represents your experience during the last week attributable to your shoulder problem.

Pain scale

How severe is your pain?	
Circle the number that best describes your pain where: 0 = no pain and 10 = the worst pain imaginable. At its worst?	0 1 2 3 4 5 6 7 8 9 10
When lying on the involved side?	0 1 2 3 4 5 6 7 8 9 10
Reaching for something on a high shelf?	0 1 2 3 4 5 6 7 8 9 10
Touching the back of your neck?	0 1 2 3 4 5 6 7 8 9 10
Pushing with the involved arm?	0 1 2 3 4 5 6 7 8 9 10

Disability scale

How much difficulty do you have?	
Circle the number that best describes your experience where: 0 = no difficulty and 10 = so difficult it requires help. Washing your hair?	0 1 2 3 4 5 6 7 8 9 10
Washing your back?	0 1 2 3 4 5 6 7 8 9 10
Putting on an undershirt or jumper?	0 1 2 3 4 5 6 7 8 9 10
Putting on a shirt that buttons down the front?	0 1 2 3 4 5 6 7 8 9 10
Putting on your pants?	0 1 2 3 4 5 6 7 8 9 10
Placing an object on a high shelf?	0 1 2 3 4 5 6 7 8 9 10
Carrying a heavy object of 10 pounds (4.5 kilograms)?	0 1 2 3 4 5 6 7 8 9 10
Removing something from your back pocket?	0 1 2 3 4 5 6 7 8 9 10

[a] Roach K, Budiman-Mak E, Songsiridej N, Lertratanakul Y. Development of a shoulder pain and disability index. Arthritis Care and Research 1991;4(4):143–9.

REFERENCES

1. Luime J, Koes B, Hendriksen I, et al. Prevalence and incidence of shoulder pain in the general population: a systemic review. Scand J Rheumatol 2004;33(2):73–81.
2. WorkCover SA. Acute shoulder injuries. Online. Available: http://www.workcover.com/site/treat_home/guidelines_by_injury_type/acute_shoulder_injuries.aspx; 2010
3. Tortora G, Grabowski S. Principles of anatomy and physiology. Stafford, Qld: John Wiley; 2002.
4. Australian Acute Musculoskeletal Pain Guidelines Group. Evidence-based management of acute musculoskeletal pain: a guide for clinicians. Bowen Hills, Qld: Australian Academic Press; 2004.
5. Beirman R. Handbook of clinical diagnosis. Sydney: R. Beirman et al.; 2003.
6. Stevenson J, Trojian T. Evaluation of shoulder pain: applied evidence. J Fam Pract 2002;51(7):605–11.
7. Williams J, Holleman D, Simel D. Measuring shoulder function with the Shoulder Pain and Disability Index. J Rheumatol 1995;22:727–32.
8. Cleland J, Koppenhaver S. Netter's orthopaedic clinical examination: an evidence-based approach. 2nd edn. Philadelphia: Saunders; 2011.
9. Reese N, Bandy W. Joint range of motion and muscle length testing. Philadelphia: W.B. Saunders; 2002.
10. Carnes M, Vizniak N. Quick reference evidence-based conditions manual. 3rd edn. Burnaby, BC: Professional Health Systems; 2009.
11. Kendall McCreary E, Provance P, McIntyre Rodgers M, et al. Muscles, testing and function, with posture and pain. 5th edn. Philadelphia: Lippincott Williams and Wilkins; 2005.
12. Hislop H, Montgomery J. Daniels and Worthingham's muscle testing: techniques of manual examination. 8th edn. Oxford: Saunders Elsevier; 2007.
13. Reiman M, Manske R. Functional testing in human performance. Champaign, IL: Human Kinetics; 2009.
14. Hoppenfeld S. Physical examination of the spine and extremities. 2nd edn. Upper Saddle River, NJ: Prentice Hall; 2010.
15. Williams G, Rockwood C, Bigliani L, et al. Rotator cuff tears: why do we repair them? J Bone Joint Surg – American Volume 2004;86-A(12):1264–76.
16. van der Windt D, Koes B, Boeke A. Shoulder disorders in general practice: Prognostic indicators of outcome. Br J Gen Pract 1996;46:519–23.
17. Kuijpers T, van der Windt D, Boeke A, et al. Clinical prediction rules for the prognosis of shoulder pain in general practice. Pain 2006;120(3):276–85.
18. van der Heijden GJ. Shoulder disorders: a state of the art review. In: Croft P, Brooks P, editors. Ballière's Clinical Rheumatology; 1999. pp. 287–309.
19. Descatha A, Roquelaure Y, Chastang J, et al. Work, a prognosis factor for upper extremity musculoskeletal disorders? Occup Environ Med 2009;66(5):351–2.
20. Camarinos J, Marinko L. Effectiveness of manual physical therapy for painful shoulder conditions: a systematic review. J Manipulative Physiol Ther 2009;17(4):206–15.
21. Brukner P, Khan K. Clinical Sports Medicine. 3rd edn. North Ryde, NSW: McGraw-Hill; 2010.
22. Munro J, Campbell I, editors. Macleod's clinical examination. Edinburgh: Churchill Livingstone; 2000.
23. Wang H, Cochrane T. A descriptive epidemiological study of shoulder injury in top level English male volleyball players. Int J Sports Med 2001;22(2):159–63.
24. Lohr J, Uhthoff H. The microvascular pattern of the supraspinatus tendon. Clin Orthop Relat Res 1990;254:35–8.
25. Simons D, Travell J, Simons L. Myofascial pain and dysfunction: The trigger point manual. Volume 1 Upper half of body. 2nd edn. Philadelphia: Williams & Wilkins; 1999.
26. Niel-Asher S. Concise book of trigger points. Berkeley, CA: North Atlantic Books; 2005.
27. Wing K, Chang M. Shoulder impingement syndrome. Phys Med Rehabil Clin N Am 2004;15:493–510.
28. Ludewig P, Cook T. Alternations in shoulder kinematics and associated muscle atrophy in people with symptoms of shoulder impingement. Phys Ther 2000;80(3):276–91.
29. McAlindon TE, LaValley MP, Gulin JP, et al. Glucosamine and chondroitin for treatment of osteoarthritis: a systematic quality assessment and meta-analysis. JAMA 2000;283(11):1469–75.
30. Tauro J, Paulson M. Shoulder stiffness. Arthroscopy 2008;24:949–55.
31. Tasto J, Elias D. Adhesive capsulitis. Sports Med Athrosc 2007;15:216–21.

The elbow region

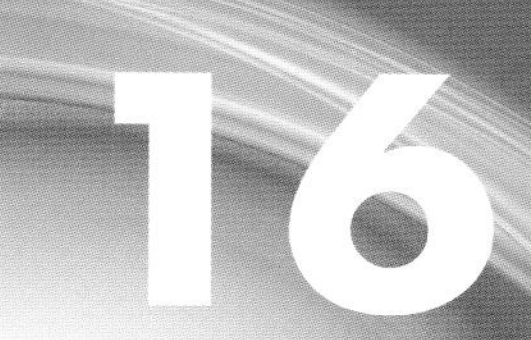

The content of this chapter relates to the following Units of Competency:

HLTREM503C Plan remedial massage treatment strategy
HLTREM504C Apply remedial massage assessment framework
HLTREM502C Provide remedial massage treatment
HLTREM505C Perform remedial massage health assessment

Health Training Package HLT07

Learning Outcomes

- Assess clients with conditions of the elbow region for remedial massage, including identification of red and yellow flags.
- Assess clients for signs and symptoms associated with common conditions of the elbow region (including muscle strains, olecranon bursitis and elbow sprains) and treat and/or manage these conditions with remedial massage therapy.
- Develop treatment plans for clients with conditions of the elbow region, taking assessment findings, duration and severity of the condition, likely tissue types, clinical guidelines, the best available evidence and client preferences into account.
- Develop short- and long-term treatment plans to address presenting symptoms, underlying conditions and predisposing factors, and to progressively increase the self-help component of therapy.
- Adapt remedial massage therapy to suit individual client needs based on duration and severity of injury, the client's age and gender, the presence of underlying conditions and other consideration for special population groups.

INTRODUCTION

Repetitive overuse, especially of wrist extension, is the most common mechanism of elbow injury. In the US, elbow disorders are among the most common causes of reported occupational injuries and workers' compensation claims.[1] Other elbow injuries arise from traumas such as falling on the outstretched arm. Conditions of the elbow often occur concurrently with conditions of the neck, shoulder and wrist. However, regardless of whether the elbow region is the primary or secondary lesion, treatment should be directed to the whole kinetic chain. Wherever possible, the practitioner should identify both the cause of the condition and aggravating factors so that treatment can be directed not only to normalising structural integrity of the region but also to underlying contributing factors.

FUNCTIONAL ANATOMY

The elbow is a combination hinge and pivot joint made up of three joints: the humeroulnar, the humeroradial and the radioulnar joints which are formed by the articulation of the distal humerus and proximal radius and ulna. The radius is on the lateral side of the joint; the ulna is on the medial side and its large olecranon process forms the posterior point of the elbow.

The humeroulnar and humeroradial joints are responsible for the hinge action. The trochlea of the humerus articulates with the semilunar notch of the ulna to form the humeroulnar joint (Figure 16.1 on p 290). The capitulum of the humerus articulates with the fovea on the head of the radius to form the humeroradial joint. The radial head also articulates with the radial notch of the ulna to form the pivot component of the joint which enable pronation and supination. The radius and ulna are connected by the interosseous membrane, a broad sheet of connective tissue which extends along their shafts and forms an attachment for tendons of some of the deep muscles of the forearm.

The medial and lateral epicondyles are prominent projections on either side of the humerus just above the elbow joint. They are the major attachment points for muscles of the forearm: the wrist flexors attach to the medial epicondyle and the wrist extensors to the lateral epicondyle. The ulna nerve (funny bone) lies on the posterior surface of the medial epicondyle.

The articular surfaces of the elbow are connected by an articular capsule which thickens either side to form the medial and lateral collateral ligaments. The radial annular ligament circles the head of the radius and attaches it to the radial notch of the ulna (Figure 16.2 on p 290).

Flexion of the forearm is largely due to the action of the brachialis muscle of the upper arm. It is assisted by biceps brachii and brachioradialis, and to a lesser extent by wrist flexors which attach to the medial epicondyle. Triceps brachii and anconeus are the main muscles responsible for elbow

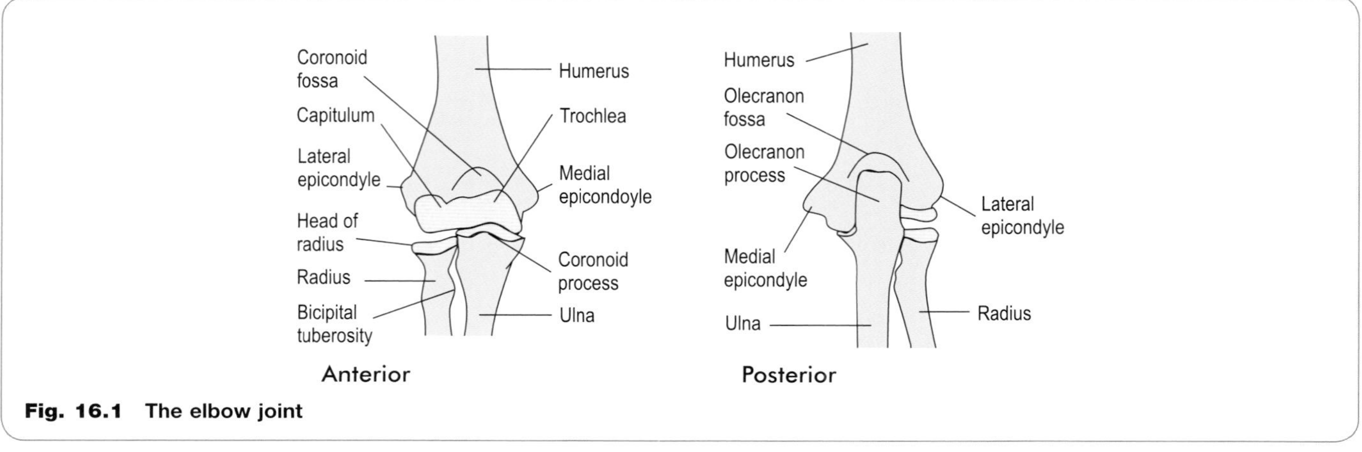

Fig. 16.1 The elbow joint

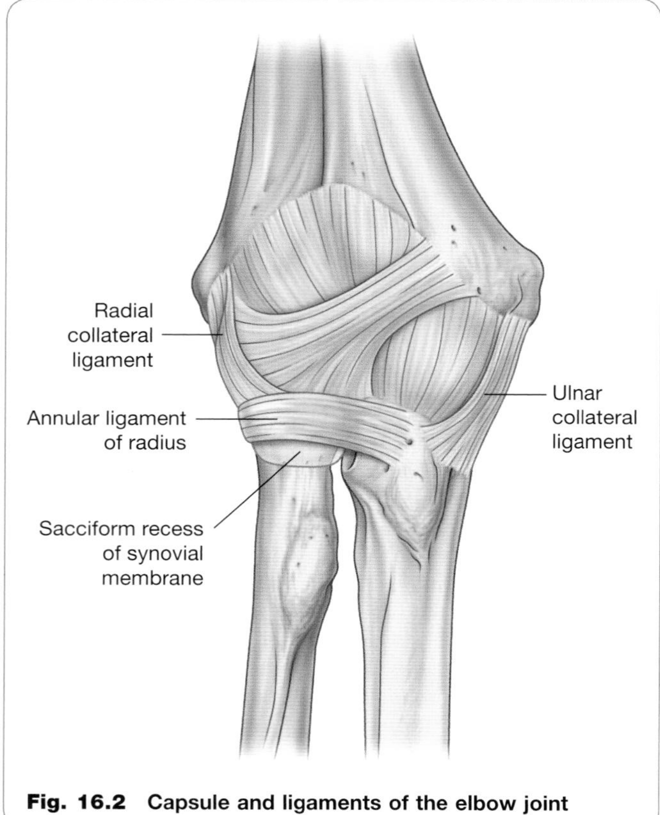

Fig. 16.2 Capsule and ligaments of the elbow joint

Assessment of the elbow region

1. Case history
2. Outcome measures, e.g. The Patient Specific Scale
3. Postural analysis
4. Functional tests
   Cervical spine
   Active range of motion tests
   Flexion, extension, lateral flexion, rotation
   Shoulder joint
   Active range of motion tests
   Flexion, extension, abduction, horizontal adduction, internal rotation, external rotation
   Elbow joint
   Active range of motion tests
   Flexion, extension, supination, pronation
   Passive range of motion tests
   Flexion, extension, supination, pronation
   Resisted range of motion tests
   Flexion, extension, supination, pronation
   Resisted and length tests for specific muscles, including:
   wrist flexor muscles, wrist extensor muscles, supinator, pronator quadratus, pronator teres
   Special tests including:
   Valgus stress test
   Varus stress test
   Elbow extension test
   Resisted wrist flexion
   Resisted wrist extension
5. Palpation

extension with assistance from wrist extensors attaching to the lateral epicondyle.

Supination is controlled by supinator, biceps brachii and brachioradialis (see Figure 16.3 on p 291, Figure 16.4 on p 292): pronation by pronator teres at the elbow joint and pronator quadratus at the wrist. Brachioradialis helps bring the forearm into mid-range pronation or supination depending on its starting position.

The common flexor tendon attaches to the medial epicondyle. It is shared by a number of superficial flexor muscles (flexor carpi radialis, flexor carpi ulnaris, palmaris longus, flexor digitorum superficialis) and pronator teres which is also a weak elbow flexor.

At the lateral epicondyle extensor carpi radialis brevis, extensor carpi radialis longus, extensor digitorum, extensor digiti minimi and extensor carpi ulnari attach via a common extensor tendon (see Figure 16.4 on p 292).

Major muscles of the elbow region are summarised in Table 16.1 on p 294.

ASSESSING THE ELBOW AND FOREARM

The purpose of remedial massage assessment includes:

- determining the suitability of clients for massage (contra-indications and red flags)

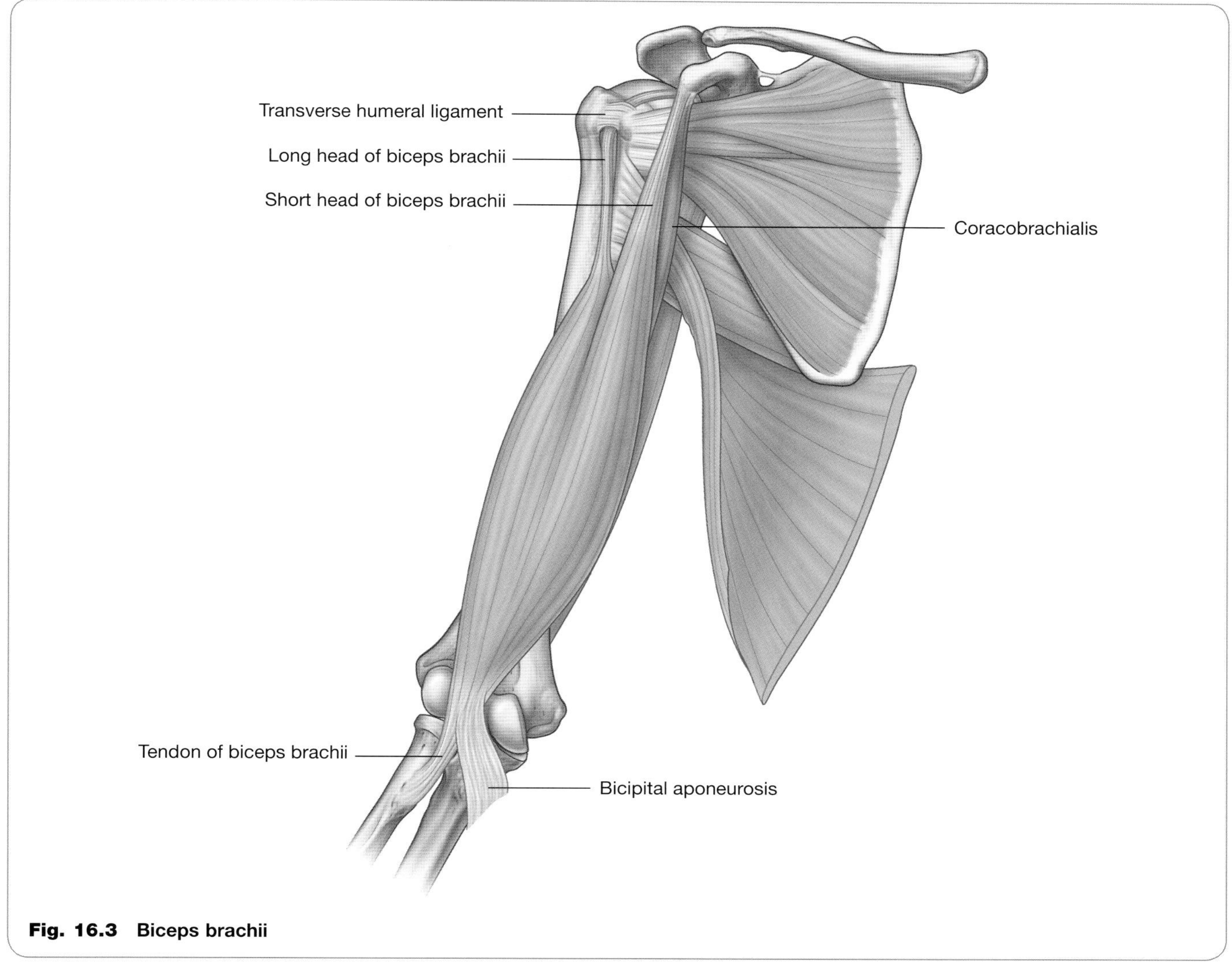

Fig. 16.3 Biceps brachii

- determining the duration (acute or subacute), severity of injury and types of tissues involved in the injury/condition
- determining whether symptoms fit patterns of common conditions.

Principles of remedial massage assessment are discussed in Chapter 2. This section presents specific considerations for assessment of the elbow and forearm.

CASE HISTORY

Information from case histories can alert practitioners to the presence of serious conditions requiring referral. However, little is known about the usefulness of subjective complaints with elbow pain.[3] Questioning should be targeted to include:

- Descriptions of the specific mechanism of the injury and the forces involved. Enquire about the onset of symptoms, nature of the pain, disability and functional impairment, previous injuries to the area, type of work, typical postures, overuse and overhead work. Ask clients to demonstrate movements and positions that aggravate or relieve their pain and to be specific with descriptions of aggravating or relieving activities. Identify whether the pain is located at the lateral, medial or posterior aspect of the elbow, or the forearm.
- Identifying red and yellow flags that require referral for further investigation. Red flags for serious causes of elbow pain are summarised in Table 16.2.
- Identifying the exact location of the symptoms by asking clients to point to the site of pain.
- Determining if the pain is local or referred. Local pain tends to be sharp and well-localised; referred pain tends to be dull and poorly localised. Is there any numbness, tingling or weakness? The presence of nerve impingement symptoms suggests referral from lower cervical nerves or local ulnar or radial nerve entrapment.

OUTCOME MEASURES

Outcome measures are questionnaires that are specifically designed to assess clients' level of impairment and to define benefits of treatment. The Patient Specific Scale can be used to measure progress of treatment of clients with any musculoskeletal condition, including elbow conditions.

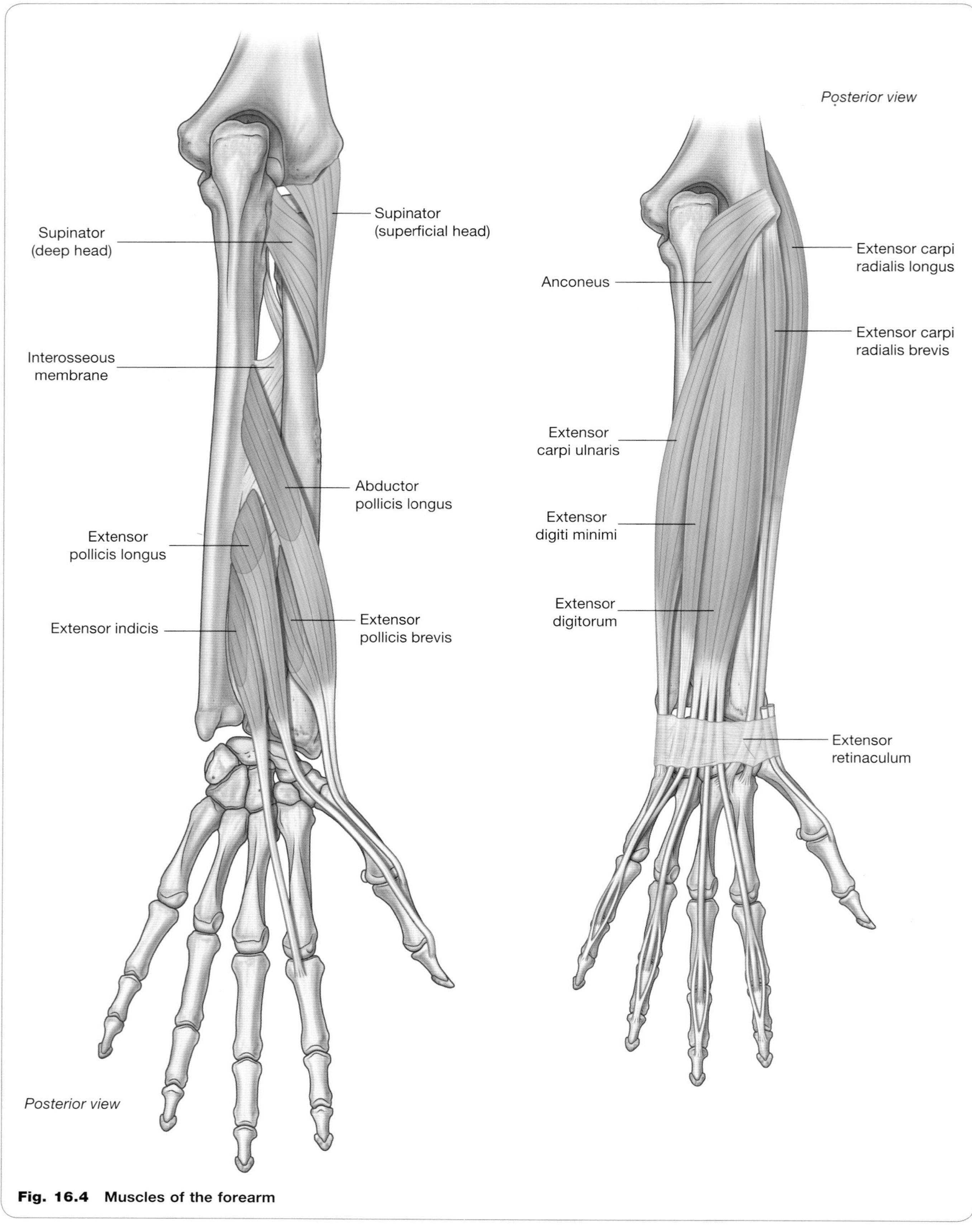

Fig. 16.4 Muscles of the forearm

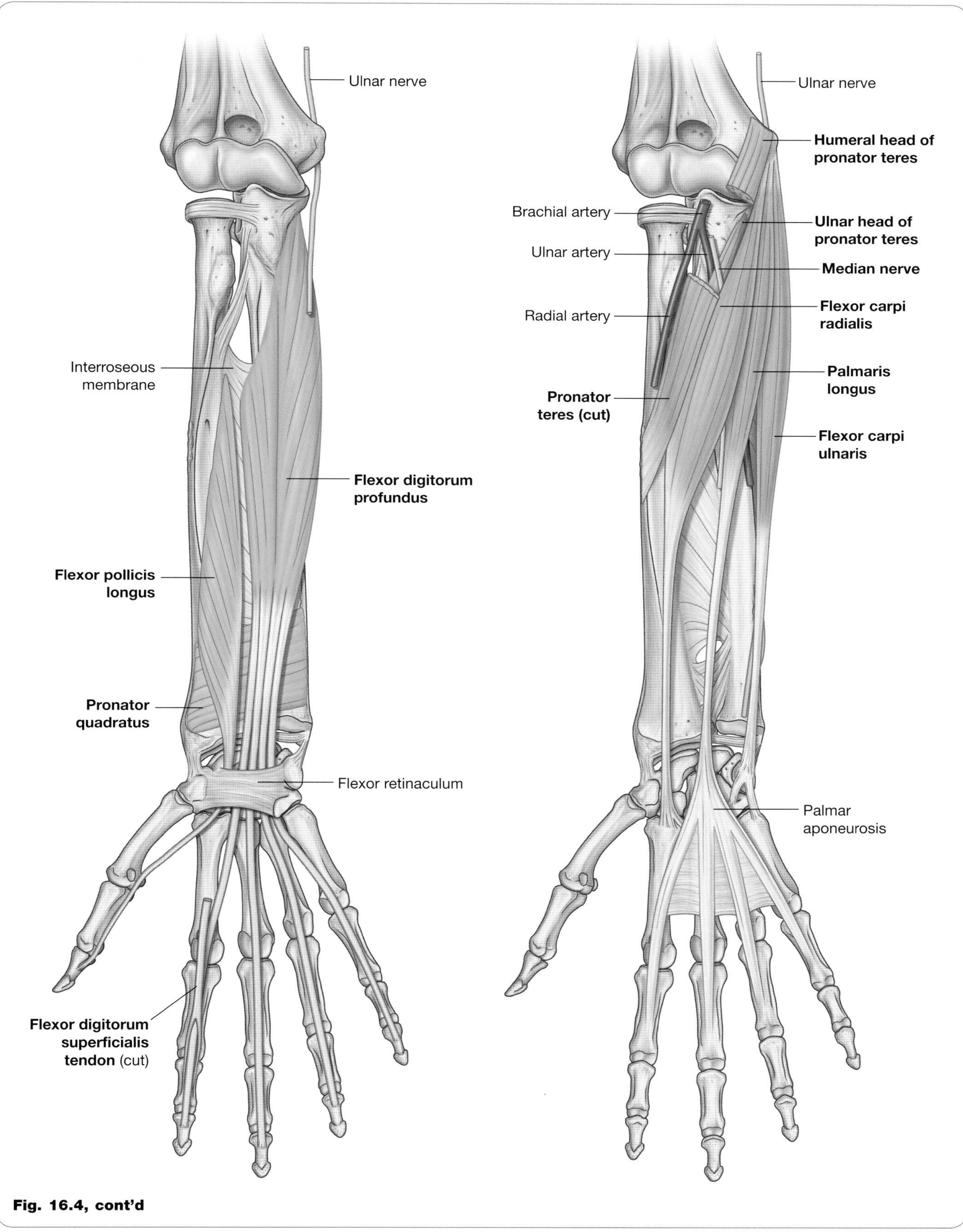

Fig. 16.4, cont'd

Table 16.1 Muscles of the elbow region[2]

Muscle	Origin	Insertion	Action
Forearm Flexors • Biceps brachii	Long head: supraglenoid tubercle Short head: coracoid process of scapula	Radial tuberosity of radius and bicipital aponeurosis	Flexes forearm at elbow joint, supinates forearm at radioulnar joints, and flexes humerus at shoulder joint
• Brachialis	Distal anterior surface of humerus	Ulnar tuberosity and coronoid process of ulna	Flexes forearm at elbow joint
• Brachioradialis	Lateral border of distal end of humerus	Superior to styloid process of radius	Flexes forearm at elbow joint, supinates and pronates forearm at radioulnar joints to neutral position
Forearm Extensors • Triceps brachii	Long head: infraglenoid tubercle Lateral head: lateral and posterior surface of humerus superior to radial groove Medial head: entire posterior surface of humerus inferior to radial groove	Olecranon of ulna	Extends forearm at elbow joint and extends humerus at shoulder joint
• Anconeus	Lateral epicondyle of humerus	Olecranon of ulna	Extends forearm at elbow joint
Forearm Pronators • Pronator teres	Medial epicondyle of humerus and coronoid process of ulna	Middle of lateral surface of radius	Pronates forearm at radioulnar joint and weakly flexes forearm at elbow
• Pronator quadratus	Distal portion of shaft of ulna	Distal portion of shaft of radius	Pronates forearm at radioulnar joints
Forearm Supinator • Supinator	Lateral epicondyle of humerus and supinator crest	Lateral surface of proximal one-third of radius	Supinates forearm at radioulnar joints
Superficial flexor compartment of the forearm • Flexor carpi radialis	Medial epicondyle of humerus	Second and third metacarpals	Flexes and abducts hand (radial deviation) at wrist joint
• Palmaris longus	Medial epicondyle of humerus	Flexor retinaculum and palmar aponeurosis	Weakly flexes hand at wrist joint
• Flexor carpi ulnaris	Medial epicondyle of humerus and superior posterior border of ulna	Pisiform, hamate and base of fifth metacarpal	Flexes and adducts hand (ulnar deviation) at wrist joint
• Flexor digitorum superficialis	Medial epicondyle of humerus, coronoid process of ulna, anterior oblique line of radius	Middle phalanx of each finger	Flexes middle phalanx of each finger at proximal interphalangeal joint, flexes proximal phalanx of each finger at metacarpophalangeal joint, and flexes hand at wrist joint
Superficial extensor compartment of the forearm • Extensor carpi radialis longus	Lateral supracondylar ridge of humerus	Second metacarpal	Extends and abducts hand at wrist joint
• Extensor carpi radialis brevis	Lateral epicondyle of humerus	Third metacarpal	Extends and abducts hand at wrist joint

Table 16.1 Muscles of the elbow region—cont'd

Muscle	Origin	Insertion	Action
• Extensor digitorum	Lateral epicondyle of humerus	Distal and middle phalanges of each finger	Extends distal and middle phalanges of each finger at interphalangeal joints, proximal phalanx of each finger at metacarpophalangeal joint, and hand at wrist joint
• Extensor digiti minimi	Lateral epicondyle of humerus	Tendon of extensor digitorum on fifth phalanx	Extends proximal phalanx of little finger at metacarpophalangeal joint and hand at wrist joint
• Extensor carpi ulnaris	Lateral epicondyle of humerus and posterior border of ulna	Ulnar side of fifth metacarpal	Extends and adducts hand at wrist joint

Table 16.2 Red flags for potentially serious elbow disorders[4]

Disorder	Symptoms	Signs
Fracture	History of significant trauma Fall on outstretched hand Fall onto lateral elbow	Deformity consistent with fracture Reduced range(s) of motion Pain with range of motion Disturbance in the triangular relationship between the olecranon and the epicondyles Significant bruising, if subacute (unusual)
Dislocation	History of fall/trauma as above History of deformity with or without spontaneous reduction	Deformity consistent with dislocation Haemarthrosis
Infection	Pain, swelling, redness Diabetes mellitus History of immunosuppression (e.g. transplant, chemotherapy, HIV) History of systemic symptoms	Localised heat, swelling, erythema Purulence Erythematous streaks, especially from a portal of entry Systemic signs of infection
Tumour	History of cancer Unintentional weight loss Continuous pain, especially at night and not improved with rest	Palpable mass not consistent with usual diagnoses
Inflammation	History of gout or pseudogout History of rheumatoid arthritis History of other inflammatory arthritides	Effusion Localised heat, swelling, erythema, tenderness
Rapidly Progressive Neurologic Deficit	History of neurologic disease Trauma	Abnormal neurologic examination Focal or global motor weakness distal to the elbow Weakness may be limited to one nerve, such as hand intrinsic muscles
Vascular Compromise	History of diabetes mellitus Tobacco use History of fracture or dislocation History of vascular disease of any kind	Decreased or absent peripheral pulses and delayed capillary refill Oedema
Compartment Syndrome	History of trauma, surgery or extreme unaccustomed forceful activity Persistent forearm pain and 'tightness' Tingling, burning or numbness	Palpable tenderness and tension of involved compartment Pain intensified with stretch to involved muscles Paraesthesia, paresis and sensory deficits Diminished pulse and prolonged capillary refill

POSTURAL ANALYSIS

Postural analysis enables observation of the whole client and facilitates identification of important features through bilateral comparison. It also facilitates detection of possible predisposing or contributing factors that may be implicated by observing the position of the head, cervical and thoracic spines, glenohumeral joints and scapula. Observe and compare the upper limbs anteriorly and posteriorly, noting symmetry, colour, swelling, lumps, bruising and carrying angle. (When the arm is extended in anatomical position, the longitudinal

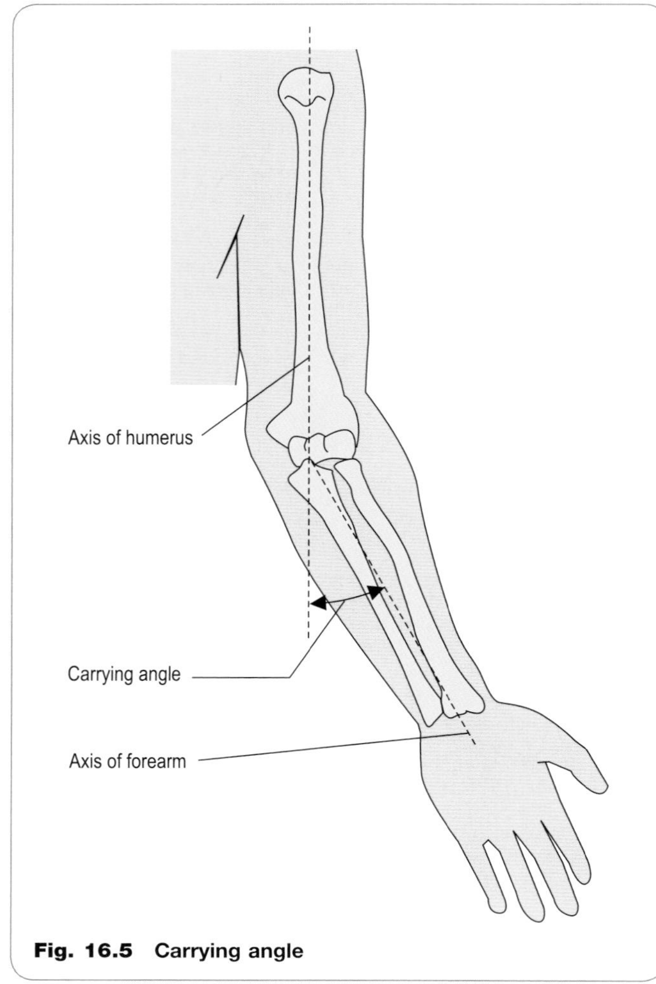

Fig. 16.5 Carrying angle

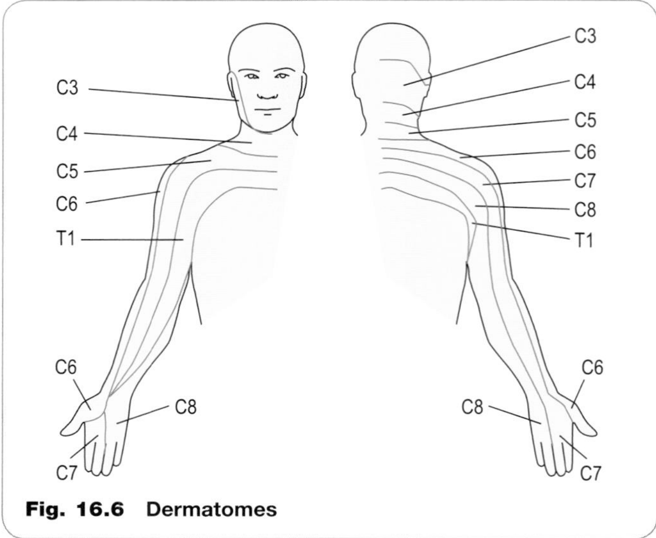

Fig. 16.6 Dermatomes

axes of the upper arm and forearm form a lateral (valgus) angle at the elbow joint known as the carrying angle (see Figure 16.5). A normal carrying angle measures approximately 5° in males and 10–15° in females. The carrying angle often increases with greater elasticity of the ligaments, especially in females and is associated with extension greater than 0°. The carrying angle may increase when the lateral epicondyle is fractured or decrease as a result of trauma. A reversed carrying angle (a gunstock deformity) may result from a supracondylar fracture in a child.

Observe the elbow region for swelling. Swelling may be local (e.g. olecranon bursitis) or diffuse (e.g. fracture or crush injury). Diffuse swelling involves the entire elbow region. The client often carries their elbow flexed at 45° to accommodate the swelling with minimal pain. Look for scars (e.g. surgical scars, burns, drug addiction) and muscle hypertonicity or atrophy.

FUNCTIONAL TESTS

For any tests involving joint movements it is important to compare both sides and take into account any underlying pathology and the age and lifestyle of the client. Measuring elbow range of motion has good to high reliability.[3]

Active range of motion of the cervical spine (flexion, extension, lateral flexion and rotation)

Examination of the elbow and forearm begins with active range of motion tests of the cervical spine to help rule out cervical radiculopathy or brachial plexus neuropathy which may refer pain to the elbow region. Dermatomes which cover the elbow region are shown in Figure 16.6. If active range of motion tests of the cervical spine reproduce elbow symptoms, further examination of the cervical spine is indicated (see Chapter 12).

Active range of motion (AROM) of the glenohumeral joint (flexion, extension, abduction, horizontal adduction, external and internal rotation)

Examination of the glenohumeral joint helps identify or eliminate elbow pain referred from the glenohumeral joint or associated structures (e.g. trigger points in shoulder muscles). If AROM tests of the glenohumeral joint produce elbow or other symptoms, a full examination of the glenohumeral joint is indicated.

Active range of motion of the elbow joint

The client may stand or sit as convenient. Face the client and demonstrate the movements for the client to follow. Examine the following ranges of motion:

- Flexion/extension (140°/0°[5])
- Pronation/supination (80°/80°).

Passive range of motion (PROM)

If the client is unable to perform normal AROM in any direction, further investigation is required. PROM testing should be performed with one hand stabilising and palpating the elbow joint while the other hand moves the forearm. Palpate for crepitus, capsular pattern and end-feel (see Table 16.3 on p 297). The capsular pattern of restriction for the humeroulnar joint is flexion more limited than extension.

Table 16.3 Elbow joint: end-feel[6]

	End-feel	Range of motion
Normal end-feel	Soft tissue approximation	Flexion
	Bony approximation	Extension
	Bony approximation or ligamentous	Pronation
	Ligamentous	Supination
	End-feel	**Suggested condition**
Abnormal end-feel	Boggy	Joint effusion
	Early myospasm	Acute injury
	Late myospasm	Instability
	Hard (mid range of motion)	Bony abnormality or loose body (bone fragment)
	Springy block	Loose body

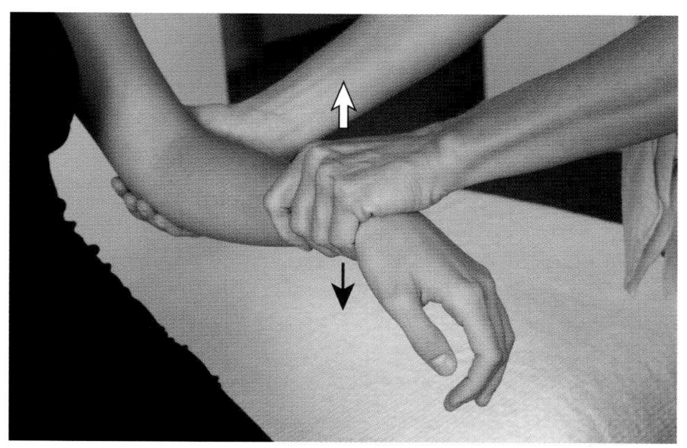

Fig. 16.7 Resisted test for brachialis

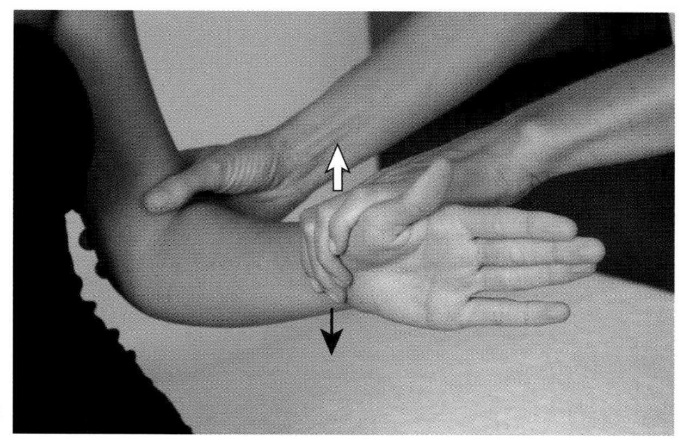

Fig. 16.8 Resisted test for brachioradialis

Resisted range of motion (RROM)

RROM tests should also be performed if AROM testing indicates the likelihood of an elbow problem. RROM tests include:

- flexion: biceps brachii, brachialis, brachioradialis
- extension: triceps brachii, anconeus
- pronation: pronator teres, pronator quadratus
- supination: biceps brachii, supinator.

Resisted tests and length tests for specific muscles[7, 8]

If RROM tests reproduce symptoms, further tests may be used to help identify specific muscles.

1. BRACHIALIS

Resisted test

This test is similar to the resisted test for biceps brachii except that it is performed with the wrist pronated. The client flexes their elbow to 90° and pronates their wrist. One of your hands supports the elbow. Your other hand applies resistance as the client tries to flex their elbow (see Figure 16.7).

Length test

The client should be able to fully extend their elbow with the wrist supinated.

2. BRACHIORADIALIS

Resisted test

This test is similar to the resisted test for biceps brachii and brachialis except that the wrist is semi-supinated (in the handshake position). The client flexes their elbow to 90° and semi-supinates their wrist. One of your hands supports the elbow while the other applies resistance as the client tries to flex their elbow (see Figure 16.8).

Length test

The client should be able to fully extend the elbow.

3. PRONATOR TERES

Resisted test

Stabilise the elbow to avoid shoulder movement. The client pronates the forearm with the elbow partially flexed and holds this position as you try to supinate the forearm above the wrist (see Figure 16.9 on p 298).

Length test

Shortening of the pronator muscles of the forearm is observed as limited supination which can interfere with many normal functions of the hand and forearm.

4. PRONATOR QUADRATUS

Resisted test

The test is similar to the resisted test for pronator teres except that the test is performed with the elbow fully flexed (see Figure 16.10 on p 298).

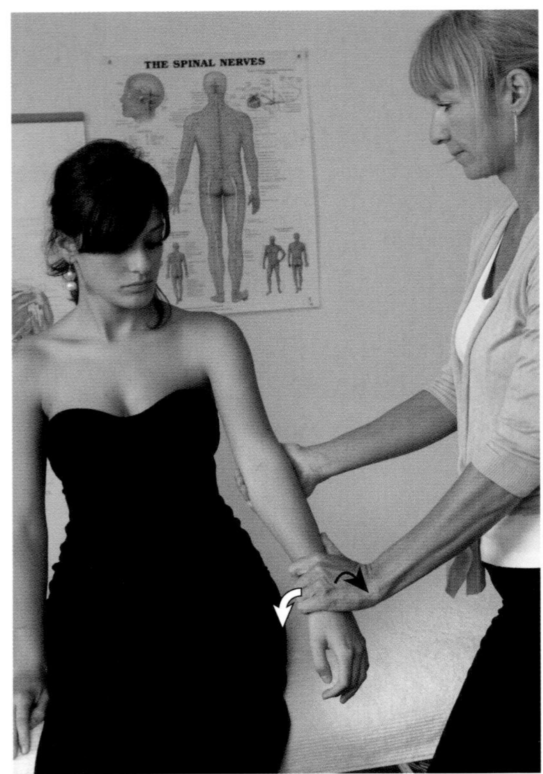

Fig. 16.9 Resisted test for pronator teres

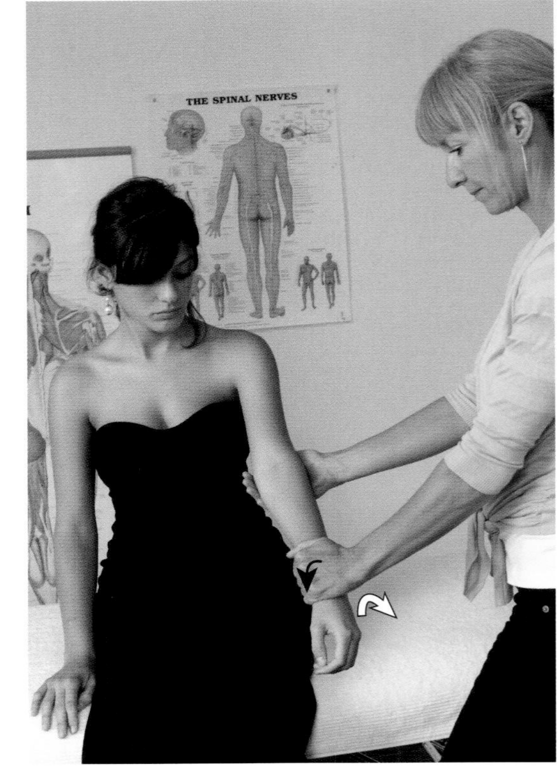

Fig. 16.11 Resisted test for supinator

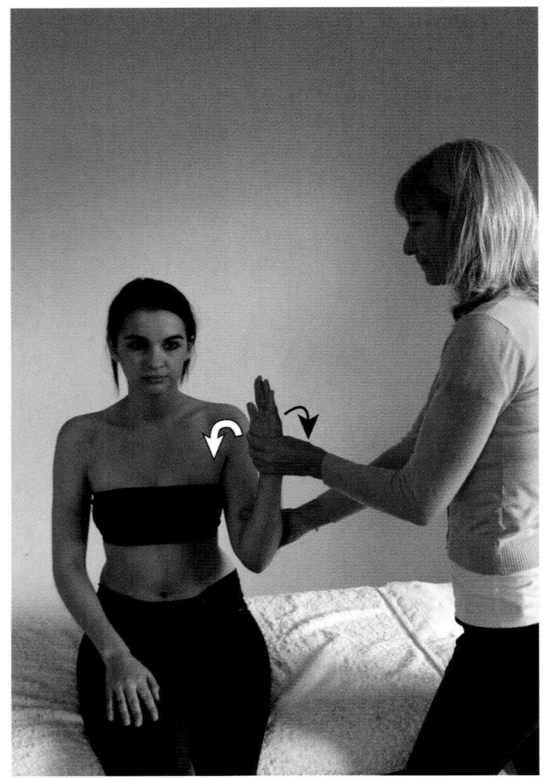

Fig. 16.10 Resisted test for pronator quadratus

Length test

Shortening of the pronator muscles of the forearm is observed as limited supination, which can interfere with many normal functions of the hand and forearm.

5. SUPINATOR

Resisted test

The client sits with the forearm supinated and the elbow either fully flexed or fully extended to shorten or elongate biceps brachii. In such positions the procedure is more likely to test the action of supinator. Stabilise the elbow. The client holds the supinated position as you try to pronate the client's forearm (see Figure 16.11). (To test the biceps brachii, the test is performed with the elbow partially flexed.)

Length test

Shortening of the supinator muscles is observed as limited pronation which can interfere with many normal functions of the hand and forearm.

6. WRIST EXTENSOR MUSCLES

The wrist extensor muscles can be tested as a group. The client makes a loose fist and pronates the forearm. Apply resistance to the client's hand as the client tries to extend the wrist (see Figure 16.12 on p 299). (Tests for individual wrist extensor muscles are described in Chapter 17.)

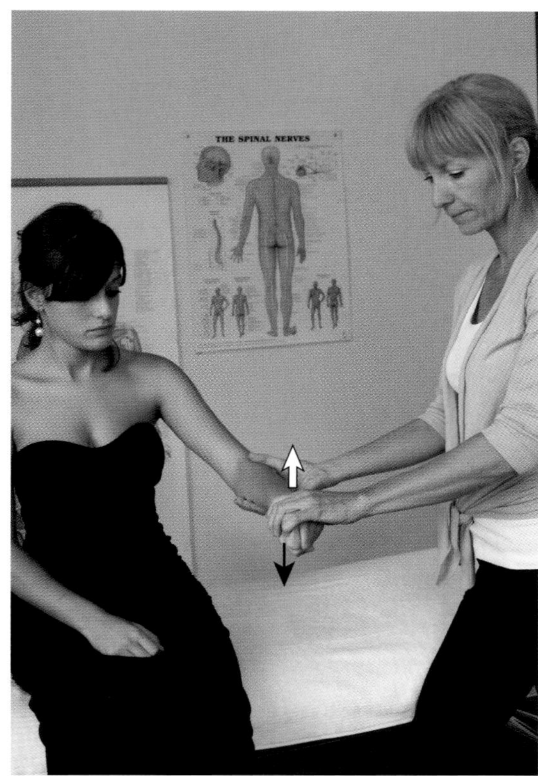

Fig. 16.12 Resisted test for wrist extensor muscles

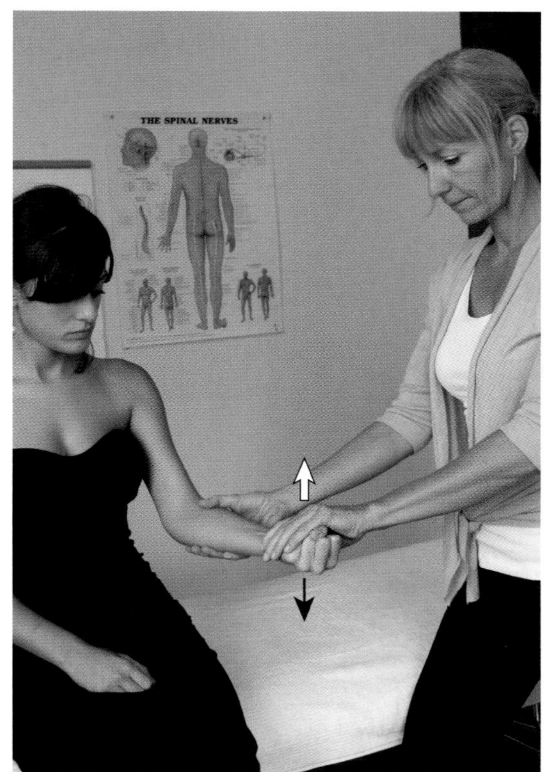

Fig. 16.13 Resisted test for wrist flexor muscles

7. WRIST FLEXOR MUSCLES

The wrist flexor muscles can be tested as a group. The client makes a loose fist and supinates the forearm. Apply resistance to the client's palm as the client tries to flex the wrist (see Figure 16.13). (Tests for individual wrist flexor muscles are described in Chapter 17.)

Special tests

If symptoms are reported when performing a special test, ask the client to identify their exact location and confirm that they are the same as those described in the case history. Positive special test results should always be interpreted cautiously and in the context of other clinical findings (see Chapter 2).

VALGUS STRESS TEST

The client is seated with the forearm supinated. Apply valgus stress to the elbow at full extension and at 30°, 60° and 90° of elbow flexion. Pain or excessive joint movement suggests medial collateral ligament sprain or instability (see Figure 16.14).

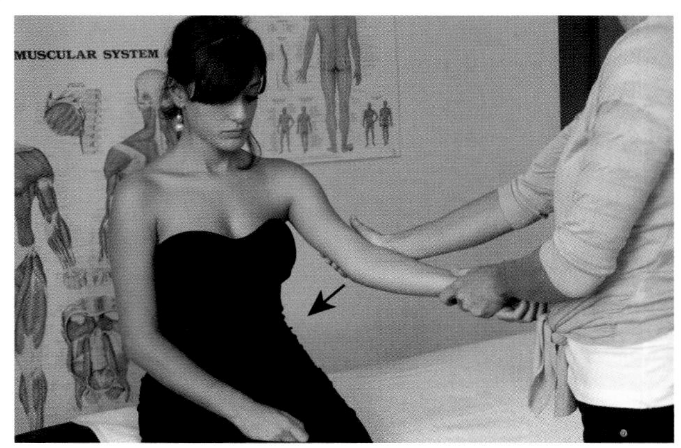

Fig. 16.14 Valgus stress test

VARUS STRESS TEST

The client is seated with the forearm supinated. Apply varus stress to the elbow at full extension and at 30°, 60° and 90° of elbow flexion. Pain or excessive joint movement suggests lateral collateral ligament sprain or instability (see Figure 16.15 on p 300). To date no studies have examined the usefulness of the varus stress test for identifying the presence of lateral collateral ligament tears.[3]

ELBOW EXTENSION TEST

The client sits with arms supinated and humerus flexed to 90° at the shoulder joint. The client then extends both elbows. Limited extension in one elbow compared with the other suggests bone or joint injury. This test has been consistently

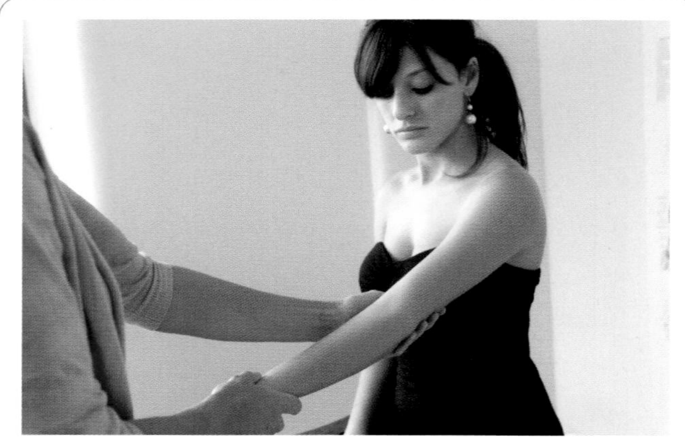
Fig. 16.15 Varus stress test

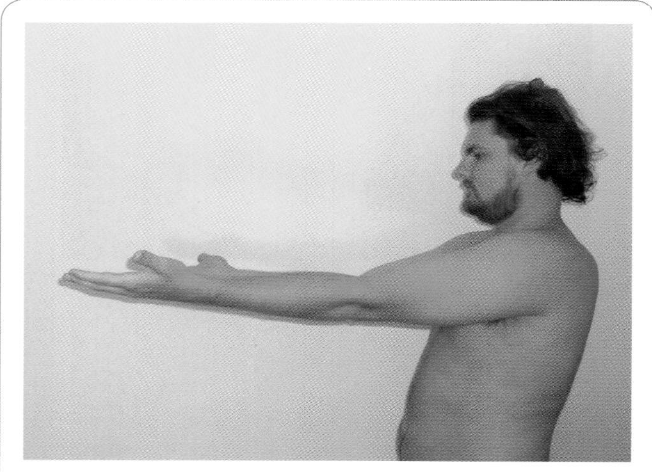
Fig. 16.16 Elbow extension test

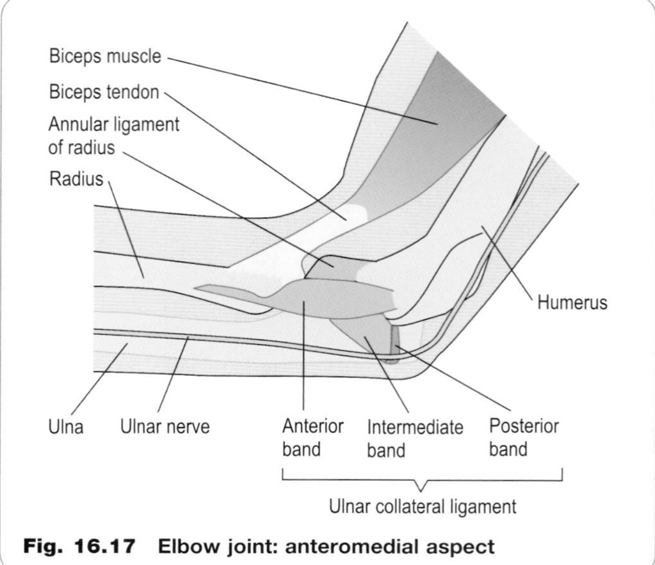

Fig. 16.17 Elbow joint: anteromedial aspect

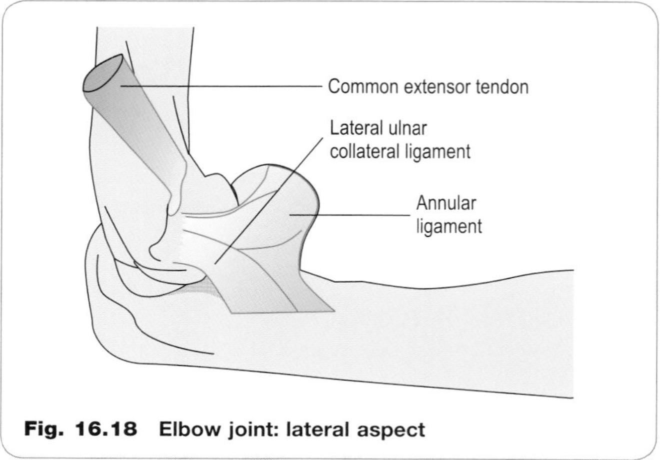

Fig. 16.18 Elbow joint: lateral aspect

shown to accurately rule out the presence of bone or joint injury[3] (see Figure 16.16).

RESISTED WRIST FLEXION/EXTENSION

Although resisted wrist flexion and extension are not special orthopaedic tests, they are included here so that the elbow-testing procedure captures the conditions that most commonly produce elbow pain, namely flexor/extensor tendinosis. The client makes a fist and extends and flexes their wrist against the practitioner's resistance (see Figures 16.12 and 16.13 on p 299). Pain at the lateral or medial epicondyle suggests flexor/extensor tendinosis respectively.

PALPATION

Locate the olecranon process on the posterior aspect of the elbow. Move to the medial epicondyle to locate the ulnar nerve which feels soft and tubular. Avoid compressing the nerve which may cause paraesthesia in the forearm, ring and little fingers. Trace the border of the ulna to the wrist.

Palpate the epicondyles on either side of the distal humerus. On the anterior aspect of the forearm locate the medial epicondyle and just inferiorly palpate the attachment of the wrist and finger flexors and pronator quadratus. The medial collateral ligament extends from the medial epicondyle of the humerus to the coronoid process and olecranon of the ulna. Supracondylar lymph nodes may be palpable when there is an infection in the arm or hand. Palpate the wrist flexor muscles on the anteromedial medial aspect of the forearm and trace their tendons as they cross the anterior aspect of the wrist.

Palpate the cubital fossa, the brachioradialis laterally and pronator teres medially. Locate the brachial artery (a pulse medial to the biceps tendon). The median nerve is directly medial to the brachial artery.

Palpate the lateral epicondyle, the attachment site for some of the wrist and finger extensors which form the bulk of the posterolateral forearm. Brachioradialis is medial to the wrist extensor muscles. To make brachioradialis more prominent, instruct the client to make a fist with the thumb up and push the fist upwards under the table. Palpate the lateral collateral ligament of the elbow which extends from the lateral epicondyle to the annular ligament of the radius and the radial notch of the ulna. Palpate the radial head and the radial annular ligament (see Figure 16.19).

REMEDIAL MASSAGE TREATMENT

Assessment of the elbow and forearm provides essential information for development of treatment plans, including:

- client's suitability for remedial massage therapy
- duration of the condition (i.e. acute or chronic)
- severity of the condition (i.e. grade of injury; mild, moderate or severe pain)
- type(s) of tissues involved
- priorities for treatment if more than one injury or condition are present
- whether the signs and symptoms suggest a common condition of the elbow region
- special considerations for individual clients (e.g. client's preference for treatment types and styles, special population considerations).

Clients who present to remedial massage clinics with elbow pain almost invariably have extensor tendinosis or flexor tendinosis and occasionally olecranon bursitis. Treatment options must always be considered in the context of the best available evidence for treatment effectiveness and clinical practice guidelines where they exist. Over 40 different treatment methods for lateral epicondylitis have been reported in the literature.[9] The American College of Occupational and Environmental Medicine reviewed the available research on the effectiveness of a range of mainstream and complementary and alternative medical treatments for elbow conditions and were unable to make recommendations for or against the use of massage for lateral or medial epicondylitis or olecranon bursitis because of insufficient evidence (see Table 16.4).[4] A Cochrane Review on the effectiveness of deep friction massage for the treatment of tendinitis reviewed two randomised controlled trials and concluded that deep transverse friction massage combined with other physiotherapy modalities did not show consistent benefit for pain or improvement of grip strength and functional status for patients with iliotibial band friction syndrome or extensor carpi radialis tendinosis. These conclusions are limited by the small sample size of the randomised controlled trials in the review. No conclusions can be drawn concerning the use or non-use of deep transverse friction massage for the treatment of tendinitis.[10]

The most common mechanism of elbow injury is repetitive overuse, especially of wrist extension. Other causes include throwing overhead, falling on the outstretched arm, hyperextension and valgus or varus stress.

OVERVIEW

Develop a short- and a long-term plan for each client. The short-term plan directs treatment to the highest priority (usually determined by symptoms). The long-term plan can be introduced when presenting symptoms have subsided. Long-term treatment focuses on contributing or predisposing factors such as underlying structural features and lifestyle factors. A significant part of both short-term and long-term treatment involves educating clients about likely causal or aggravating factors and guiding their management of these factors. If massage therapy is being used in conjunction with other treatments such as corticosteroid injections, it is important to communicate with other treating practitioners.

Table 16.4 Evidence for some recommendations for common elbow conditions[4]

Condition	Recommendation	Evidence
Lateral epicondylitis	Avoid aggravating activity	Insufficient evidence
	Topical non-steroidal anti-inflammatory drugs (NSAIDs) for acute, subacute and chronic lateral epicondylitis	Moderately strong evidence
	Tennis elbow bands	Insufficient evidence
	Home exercises	Insufficient evidence
	Self-application of heat/ice	Insufficient evidence
	Glucocorticoid injections for subacute or chronic lateral epicondylitis	Moderate evidence
	Surgical release for chronic lesions	Insufficient evidence
Medial epicondylitis	No quality literature available	
Olecranon bursitis	Soft padding, supports	Insufficient evidence
	Modify activity	Insufficient evidence
	Aspiration or surgical drainage	Insufficient evidence
Elbow sprains	Slings	Insufficient evidence

MUSCLE STRAIN

The most common sites of pathology in the elbow are the tendinous attachments of the wrist extensors and flexors.

Extensor tendinitis/tendinosis (tennis elbow/ lateral epicondylitis)

Extensor tendinosis is one of the most common repetitive strain or overuse injuries. This condition is also known as tennis elbow because it can affect tennis players, but the overall percentage of clients who develop this condition from tennis is actually small. Clients more typically develop extensor tendinosis from repetitive tasks that involve wrist extension such as typing. It is thought that repeated microtrauma of the tendons from repeated stretching and contraction of the extensors of the forearm and hand causes disruption of the internal structure and degeneration of the cells and matrix.[11] The condition is also referred to as lateral epicondylitis; however, extensor tendinosis is the currently preferred term as it more accurately represents the pathology, which is often degenerative rather than inflammatory. It appears that dense populations of fibroblasts, vascular hyperplasia and disorganised collagen contribute to degenerative processes.

Key assessment findings for extensor tendinosis

- History of repetitive overuse
- Functional tests:
  - AROM painful during wrist extension and flexion with the elbow extended
  - PROM painful at end of wrist flexion with elbow extended
  - RROM may be negative for muscles that move the elbow joint, but positive for muscles that extend the wrist
  - Special tests: positive for resisted wrist extension
- Palpation: local tenderness or pain. Fibrotic tissue is usually palpable.

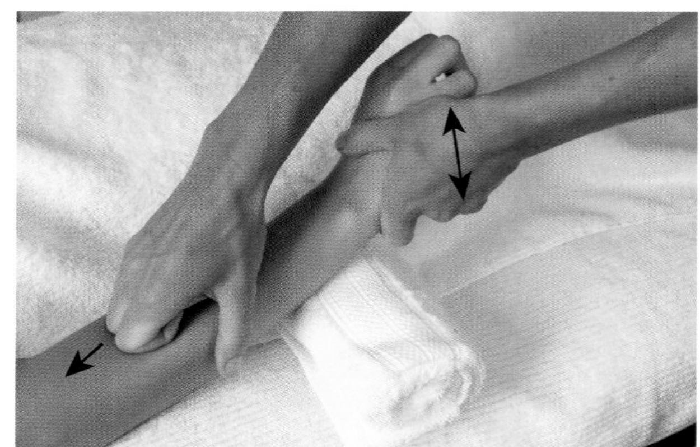

Fig. 16.19 Soft-tissue release for extensor tendinosis

The site of injury is usually the common extensor tendon of the wrist, in particular the fibres of extensor carpi radialis brevis just inferior to its attachment at the lateral epicondyle. Most cases develop from excessive amounts of eccentric wrist flexion (e.g. from racket sports or using a hammer) or concentric wrist extension and supination (e.g. using a screwdriver) which cause microtears in the tendon and ultimately lead to fibrosis, adhesions and necrosis.[6] Excessive or repetitive eccentric loads on the wrist extensor muscles can also occur during typing (repetitive finger flexion and extension), scanning groceries at a checkout (repetitive ulnar and radial deviation) or from performing massage therapy.[12] Sustained contraction of wrist muscles may lead to myofascial trigger points which will also require treatment.

ASSESSMENT

History

The client may present with intermittent lateral elbow pain. The pain usually develops gradually and may begin with morning stiffness or stiffness after rest. There is usually a history of repetitive overuse (e.g. racket sports, typing). Grasping objects may be associated with pain and weakness. Note: radial neuropathy may cause elbow pain. However, it is more commonly associated with sensory changes in the dorsum of the first web space and wrist and finger extensor weakness.

Functional tests

Cervical AROM tests do not reproduce elbow symptoms.
Shoulder AROM tests do not reproduce elbow symptoms.

Elbow tests

AROM may be painful during wrist extension (± flexion) when the elbow is extended.
PROM may be painful at the end of wrist flexion when the elbow is extended.
RROM is usually negative for muscles that move the elbow joint but positive for muscles that extend the wrist.
Special tests: Resisted wrist extension is painful. Wrist supination may also cause pain.

Palpation

There is local tenderness around the lateral epicondyle. Fibrotic tissue is often palpable in the extensor tendon.

OVERVIEW OF TREATMENT AND MANAGEMENT

Lengthy recovery times are sometimes associated with extensor tendinosis. Acute presentations may require cryotherapy. Advise clients to avoid aggravating conditions. Tennis elbow splints which usually comprise a Velcro strap worn around the forearm below the elbow joint have traditionally been recommended although their efficacy is currently being questioned.[13] One study found that wrist extensor splints provided greater pain relief than forearm straps for clients with lateral epicondylitis.[14]

A typical remedial massage treatment for subacute or chronic extensor tendinosis includes:

- Swedish massage therapy to the elbow, upper limb, neck and upper back.
- Remedial massage techniques including (see Table 16.5):
  - deep gliding frictions along the muscle fibres (including extensor carpi ulnaris, extensor digiti minimi, extensor digitorum, extensor carpi radialis brevis, anconeus, brachioradialis)
  - cross-fibre frictions
  - soft tissue releasing techniques
    The client is supine with the palm down and the hand over the edge of the table. Alternatively, a rolled towel or bolster may be placed under the client's wrist to allow full wrist flexion. Static pressure is applied to a point of hypertonicity in the wrist extensors using fingers, thumbs or knuckles. The wrist is then slowly passively or actively flexed and extended. You may also perform deep longitudinal stripping while the wrist is moving (see Figure 16.19).
  - deep transverse friction applied directly to the damaged tendon may help stimulate collagen production. A review of the use of deep transverse friction (Cyriax frictions) in the treatment of tennis elbow concluded that more research was needed to assess the effectiveness and effects of the technique.[15]
  - trigger point therapy for wrist extensor muscles
  - muscle stretches

Table 16.5 Remedial massage techniques for muscles of the elbow region

Muscle	Soft tissue release	Trigger point	Deep transverse friction	Stretch	Corrective action[16, 17]	Home exercise
Wrist extensors	Client: supine, wrist pronated over the edge of the table or over a bolster. Practitioner: applies static pressure or deep gliding to a taut band/lesion in the muscle using fingers, thumbs or knuckles as wrist is slowly passively or actively flexed and extended.	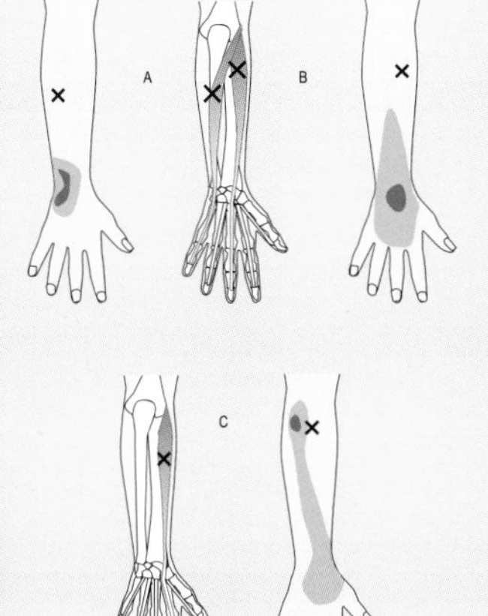	Common wrist extensor tendon insertion at the lateral epicondyle, distal to common extensor tendon (up to several cms) along line of tendon. 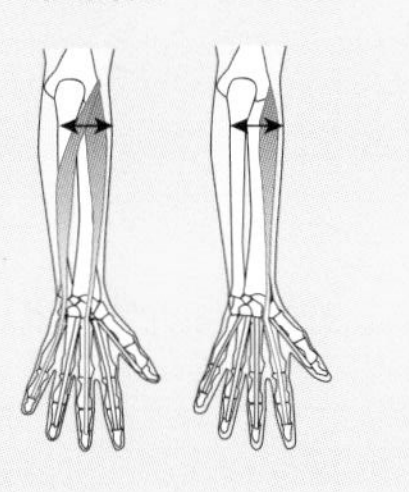	CRAC: Client: wrist flexion with elbow extension within pain tolerance. Practitioner: resists as client tries to extend wrist for 6–8 seconds. Release pressure. Client flexes wrist with elbow extension as far as possible within pain tolerance. Repeat whole procedure 3 times.	Eliminate or avoid muscle overload (e.g. avoid sustained or excessive gripping in sport). Tennis elbow splint. Check work ergonomics, especially keyboard and mouse. Change grip in tennis and golf.	Stretch: Extend elbow and flex the wrist. Use the other hand to further flex the wrist within pain tolerance. Hold 30 seconds. Repeat 3 times. 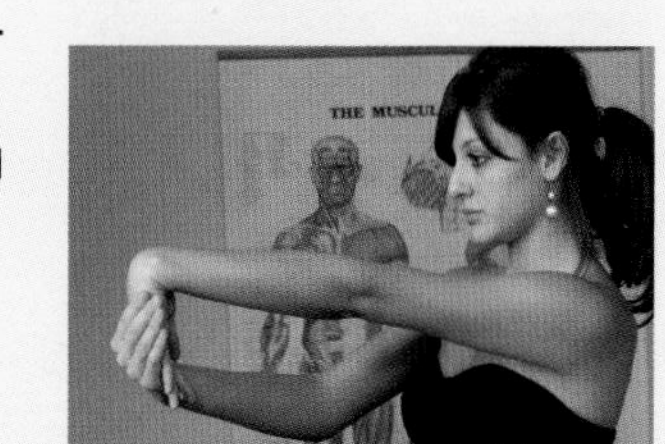
Wrist flexors	Client: supine, wrist supinated over the edge of the table or over a bolster. Practitioner: applies static pressure or deep gliding to a taut band/lesion using fingers, thumbs or knuckles as wrist is slowly passively or actively flexed and extended. 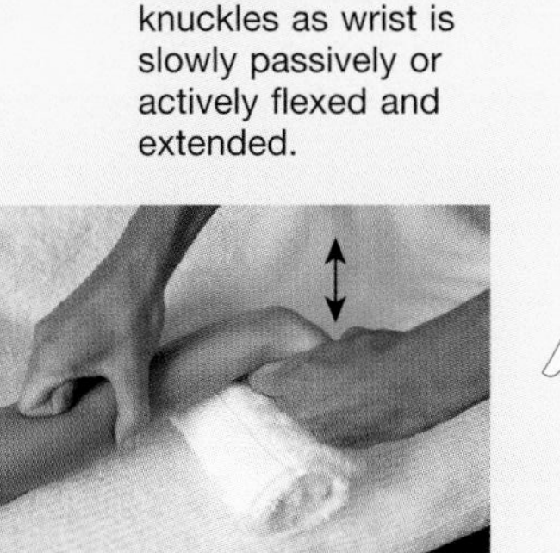	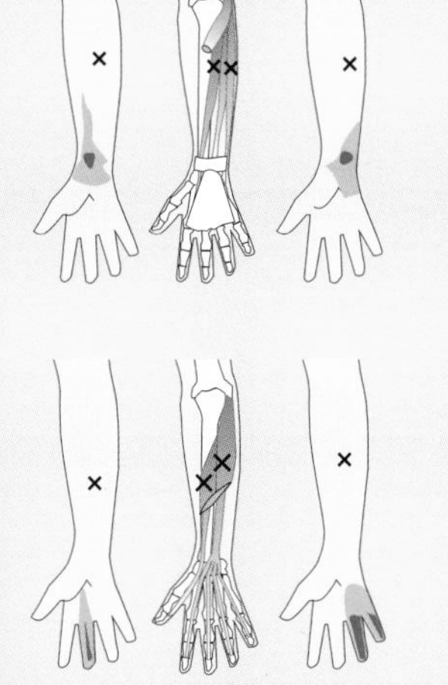	2.5 cm below medial epicondyle, common wrist flexor tendon insertion at the medial epicondyle.	CRAC: Client: wrist extension with elbow extension within pain tolerance. Practitioner: resists as client tries to flex wrist for 6–8 seconds. Release pressure. Client extends wrist with elbow extension as far as possible within pain tolerance. Repeat whole procedure 3 times.	Avoid prolonged tight gripping (e.g. power tools). Palmaris longus: avoid palmar cupping. Change golf grip.	Stretch: Extend elbow and extend the wrist. Use the other hand to further extend the wrist within pain tolerance. Hold 30 seconds. Repeat 3 times. 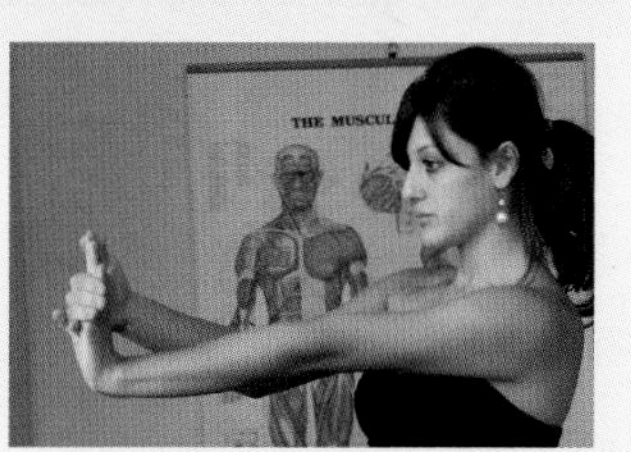

Continued

Table 16.5 Remedial massage techniques for muscles of the elbow region—cont'd

Muscle	Soft tissue release	Trigger point	Deep transverse friction	Stretch	Corrective action[16, 17]	Home exercise
Pronator teres/ pronator quadratus	For pronator teres: Client: supine, wrist supinated, elbow extended. Practitioner: applies static pressure or deep gliding using fingers, thumbs or knuckles as wrist is slowly passively or actively supinated or pronated.			Passive stretch: Practitioner stabilises the client's elbow and supinates their forearm to pain tolerance/muscle stretch end-feel and holds the stretch for up to 30 seconds.	Avoid overloading muscle (e.g. driving with two hands on the steering wheel). Change grip and technique in tennis and golf.	Stretch: Sit at a table, forearms flat on table. Keeping elbows on table, supinate wrists as far as possible, hold 30 seconds. Repeat 3 times. Strengthen: Sit or stand, arms by sides, elbows flexed to 90°. Begin holding light weight, pronate the wrist. Relax and return to starting position. Repeat to fatigue. Progress to increased weight and number of repetitions.

Table 16.5 Remedial massage techniques for muscles of the elbow region—cont'd

Muscle	Soft tissue release	Trigger point	Deep transverse friction	Stretch	Corrective action[16, 17]	Home exercise
Supinator	Palpate in space between biceps tendon, pronator teres and brachioradialis. Client: supine, forearm supinated. Practitioner: applies static pressure to supinator as the forearm is slowly actively or passively pronated and supinated.			Passive stretch: Practitioner stabilises the client's elbow and pronates their forearm to pain tolerance/muscle stretch end-feel.	Avoid overloading muscle (e.g. prolonged gripping or carrying – use backpack). Correct tennis technique and grip size. Carry loads with forearms supinated.	Stretch: Sit at a table, forearms flat on table. Keeping elbows on table, pronate wrists as far as possible, hold 30 seconds. Repeat 3 times.

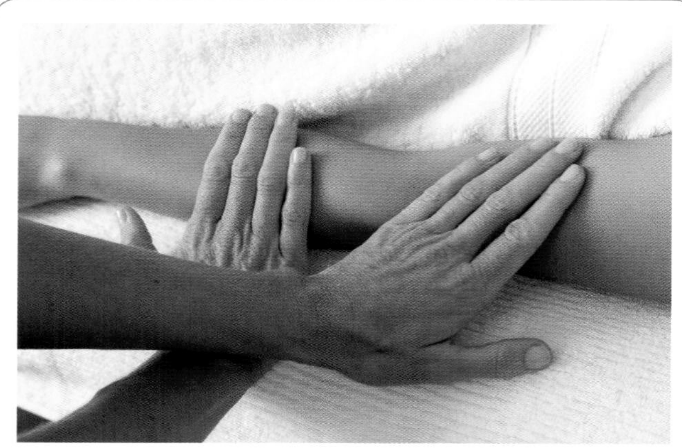

Fig. 16.20 Myofascial release: cross-hand technique

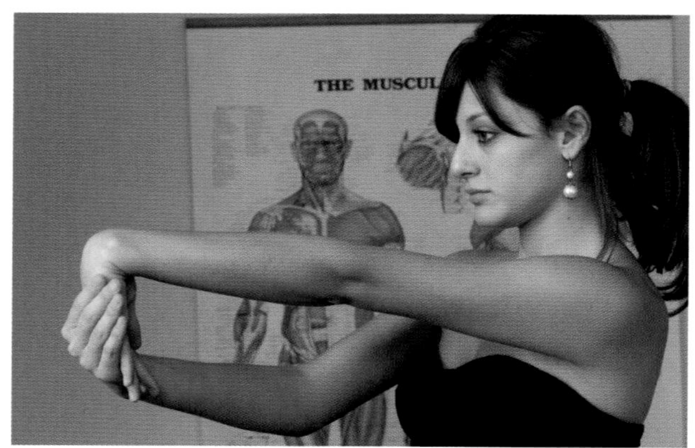

Fig. 16.21 Home stretch for extensor tendinosis

- Myofascial release including cross-arm techniques (see Figure 16.20) and the arm pull (see Chapter 8).
- Cryotherapy or thermotherapy may be indicated.
- Other remedial techniques such as elbow joint articulation (see Chapter 7) may be introduced as required.

Client education

Advise the client to rest from aggravating activities to reduce the stress on the damaged tendons. Rehabilitation exercises are designed to improve overall strength, endurance and flexibility in the muscles of the entire upper limb kinetic chain. This includes the muscles of the neck, shoulder, elbow and wrist. Initially wrist extensor stretches (flexing the wrist and extending and pronating the forearm) are recommended (see Figure 16.21). Isometric exercises for muscles of the shoulder including biceps brachii, triceps brachii and rotator cuff may be introduced. When full range of wrist flexion and extension can be performed within pain tolerance, strengthening exercises for the wrist extensors, flexors, pronators and supinators are introduced. Tennis players should review their technique (e.g. a two-handed backstroke, adequate warm-up, changing racquet, avoiding high string tension). For carpenters or others regularly using a hammer, use a larger shock-absorbing handle and/or padded gloves.

Refer for osseous manipulation and for physical therapy modalities such as ultrasound, phonophoresis or electrical stimulation. Most cases of tennis elbow respond to nonsurgical management. However, if conservative methods fail, surgical treatment is sometimes considered. Surgical approaches include arthroscopic debridement of the extensor carpi radialis brevis,[9] laser and injection with botulinum toxin.

Flexor tendinosis (golfer's elbow, medial epicondylitis)

The common flexor tendons of the wrist that attach at the medial epicondyle are also susceptible to overuse trauma, especially flexor carpi radialis. The condition is commonly called golfer's elbow although it is also associated with repetitive overhead throwing, tennis serving and using a hammer. In golf, the problem occurs when the ball is struck at the low point of the swing. At the point of impact the wrist flexors concentrically contract to swing the club towards the ground. When the ball is hit there is a sudden eccentric load on the flexor group which is exaggerated by the length of the golf club. Medial epicondylitis rarely involves inflammation of the tendon. Rather it is a problem of collagen degeneration in the tendon fibres from chronic tensile loads. The most common site of pathology occurs 2.5 cm distal to the medial epicondyle at the interface between pronator teres and flexor carpi radialis origins.[6] Early stages of the condition, referred to as flexor tendinitis, often require cryotherapy. The wrist flexor tendons travel through the carpal tunnel and it is not uncommon to find flexor tendinosis occurring concurrently with carpal tunnel syndrome.

ASSESSMENT

History

The client complains of aching pain over the medial elbow. In the early stages the pain is brought on by activities such as overhead throwing, tennis serving or swinging a golf club and relieved by rest. Left unchecked, the condition can progress to constant pain and weakness in grip strength.

Functional tests

Cervical AROM tests do not reproduce elbow symptoms.
Shoulder AROM tests do not reproduce elbow symptoms.

Key assessment findings for flexor tendinosis

- History of repetitive overuse
- Functional tests:
  - AROM painful during wrist flexion ± extension with elbow extended
  - PROM painful at end of wrist extension with elbow extended
  - RROM negative for muscles that move the elbow; positive for muscles that flex the wrist
  - Special tests: positive for resisted wrist flexion
- Palpation: local tenderness or pain. Fibrotic tissue is often palpable.

Elbow tests

AROM painful during wrist flexion (± extension) when elbow is extended.

PROM painful at the end of wrist extension when elbow is extended.

RROM negative for muscles that move the elbow but positive for muscles that flex the wrist.

Special tests: Resisted wrist flexion painful. Resisted wrist pronation may also cause pain.

Palpation

There is local tenderness around the medial epicondyle. Fibrotic tissue is often palpable in the flexor tendon.

OVERVIEW OF TREATMENT AND MANAGEMENT

The approach to remedial massage treatment is similar to that for extensor tendinosis. In the acute phase, advise the client to eliminate or avoid the aggravating condition. Traditionally ice and forearm splints are prescribed.

A typical remedial massage treatment for subacute or chronic flexor tendinosis includes:

- Swedish massage therapy to the elbow, upper limb, neck and upper back.
- Remedial massage techniques for muscles including (see Table 16.5):
  - deep gliding frictions along the muscle fibres (including flexor carpi radialis, palmaris longus, flexor carpi ulnaris, flexor digitorum superficialis, pronator teres, supinator, pronator quadrates)
  - cross-fibre frictions (see Figure 16.23)
  - soft tissue releasing techniques
  The client is supine with the palm supinated and the hand over the edge of the table. Alternatively, a rolled towel or bolster can be placed under the wrist to allow for full range of wrist extension. Static pressure is applied to a point of hypertonicity/lesion in the wrist flexors using fingers, thumbs or knuckles while the wrist is slowly passively or actively flexed and extended. Alternatively, you may perform deep longitudinal stripping while the wrist is moving (see Figure 16.22).
- Deep transverse friction applied directly to the damaged tendon may help stimulate collagen production.
- Trigger point therapy, including wrist flexors and extensors and rotator cuff muscles.
- Muscle stretching, including wrist flexors, elbow flexors, pronators and supinators.
- Myofascial release including cross-arm techniques (see Figure 16.20).
- Other remedial techniques such as elbow joint articulation (see Chapter 7) may be introduced as required.

Client education

Advise the client to reduce or eliminate aggravating activities. The use of anti-inflammatory medication and corticosteroid injection is controversial.[4] Most cases respond to conservative management and exercise rehabilitation, although recovery can take time. Refer clients for osseous manipulation. In some instances, surgery to remove damaged tissue may be performed.

Home exercises

Stretching the wrist flexor muscles (extend the wrist and elbow and use the other hand to further extend the wrist – see Figure 16.24) and elbow flexors and forearm pronators. Progressively introduce isometric exercises and weights to strengthen the elbow and wrist flexors and extensors, forearm

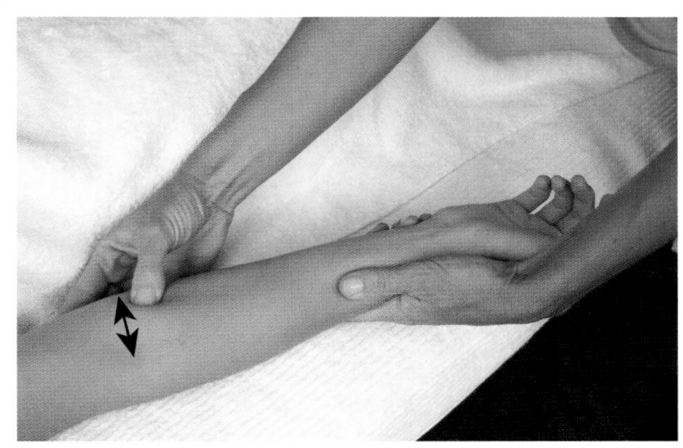

Fig. 16.23 **Cross-fibre frictions at the common flexor tendon**

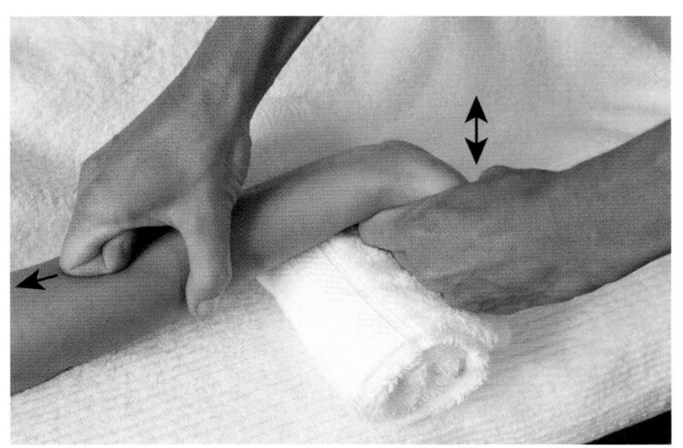

Fig. 16.22 **Soft tissue release for flexor tendinosis**

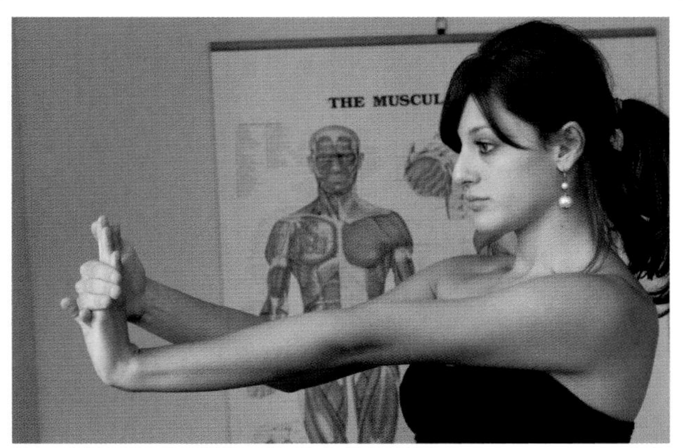

Fig. 16.24 **Home stretch for flexor tendinosis**

pronators and rotator cuff muscles. Later introduce sports-specific activities.

OLECRANON BURSITIS

Olecranon bursitis is painful inflammation of the bursa which overlies the olecranon at the back of the elbow and lubricates movement of the olecranon under the skin. Its usual cause is either a direct blow or sustained irritation exerted by pressure, rubbing or bumping. It is commonly referred to as student's elbow. The history of its development is important since there are occasions where bleeding into the bursa may occur after direct trauma or the bursa ruptures through excessively forced flexion at the elbow. Slow onset with no apparent cause suggests infection and should be referred for medical examination.

Treatment

Apply ice and firm compression. Advise clients to eliminate the responsible activity. This may involve avoiding resting the elbow on a hard surface, modifying the work environment or wearing an elbow pad. If the aetiology is associated with a tight triceps brachii or forearm extensor muscles, include specific remedial massage techniques (including deep gliding, cross-fibre frictions, soft tissue release, trigger point therapy and muscle stretches – see Table 16.5) to restore full muscle length in the subacute or chronic phase. Myofascial release may be beneficial. Refer clients for osseous manipulation if required.

Note: Joint infection or gout can occur at the elbow. Refer any client with systemic signs such as raised temperature and inflamed lymph nodes associated with olecranon bursitis.

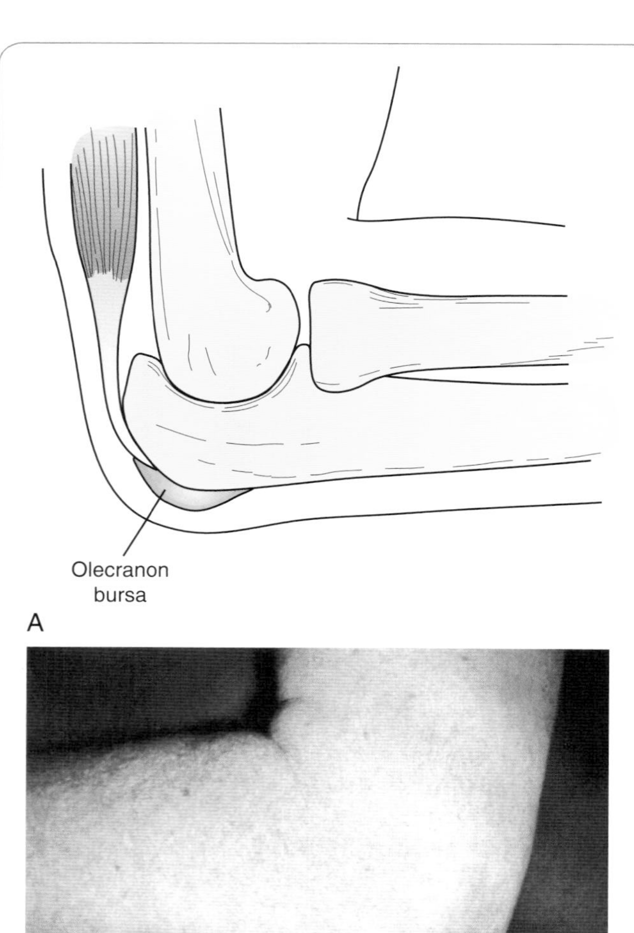

Fig. 16.25 Olecranon bursitis

ELBOW SPRAIN

Elbow sprains are uncommon. Sprains of the medial and lateral collateral ligaments may occur as a result of trauma (e.g. falls on the outstretched arm and direct blows to the elbow) or repeated excessive varus and valgus stress (e.g. from throwing). Clients complain of pain, swelling around the elbow and limited movement. Severe sprains should be referred to a physiotherapist, osteopath or chiropractor. Remedial massage therapists may be called upon to assist in the rehabilitation of mild and moderate strains. Treatment includes RICE for acute injuries and then deep transverse friction to the injury site within pain tolerance. Address muscle imbalances, encourage full range of motion in the joint through gentle joint articulation in the pain-free range and eliminate myofascial adhesions using myofascial release techniques. Rehabilitation exercises should be commenced when pain tolerance allows.

FRACTURES AND DISLOCATIONS

Fractures are extremely disabling and may leave permanently restricted movement. Heavy falls on the outstretched arm can crush the head of the radius or chip the joint with similar damage to the end of the humerus. Bone chips may also break from the medial epicondyle of the humerus and the tip of the olecranon. In children the head of the radius may be dislocated through wrenching movements (pulled elbow). Dislocations are usually reduced by medical or paramedical staff by forearm rotation in flexion. Remedial massage therapists may be called upon to treat clients after fractures and dislocations have healed. At this stage the purpose of treatment is usually to address muscle imbalances, to encourage full range of motion in the joint through gentle joint articulation, and to eliminate myofascial adhesions using myofascial release techniques.

KEY MESSAGES

- Assessment of clients with conditions of the elbow region involves case history, outcome measures, postural analysis, functional tests and palpation.
- Assessment findings may indicate the type of tissue involved (contractile or inert; muscle, joint, fascia, ligament), duration of condition (acute or subacute) and severity (grade).
- Assessment findings may indicate a common presenting condition such as wrist extensor/flexor tendinosis or olecranon bursitis.
- Assessment findings also indicate client perception of injury and preferences for treatment.

- Consider Clinical Guidelines, available evidence and client preferences when planning therapy.
- Be conservative in treatment: if in doubt, perform pain-free Swedish massage.
- Although serious conditions of the elbow region are rare, be vigilant for red flags during assessment (including history of significant trauma, constant pain, systemic signs accompanying joint pain, symptoms of neurological or vascular compromise).
- The selection of remedial massage techniques depends on assessment results. Swedish massage to the elbow, upper limb, neck and upper back may be followed by muscle techniques (e.g. deep gliding, cross-fibre frictions, soft tissue releasing techniques, trigger point therapy, deep transverse friction and muscle stretching), passive joint articulation, myofascial release and thermotherapy as indicated.
- Educating clients about likely causal and predisposing factors and exercise rehabilitation are essential parts of remedial massage therapy.
- Over time, increase the client self-help component of treatment wherever possible (to reduce likelihood of recurrence and/or to promote health maintenance and illness prevention).

Review questions

1. The carrying angle in an adult female is approximately:
   a) 5°
   b) 5–10°
   c) 10–15°
   d) 15–20°
2. Name four wrist flexor muscles that attach to the medial epicondyle via the common flexor tendon.
3. When performing resisted tests for forearm pronation, how can pronator teres be differentiated from pronator quadratus?
4. Which dermatomes cross the posterior aspect of the wrist?
   a) C5
   b) T1
   c) C7
   d) C8
5. Boggy end-feel during elbow range of motion testing suggests:
   a) joint effusion
   b) instability
   c) loose body
   d) capsular tightening
6. A client has pain on resisted elbow flexion. Biceps brachii, brachialis and brachioradialis all flex the elbow joint. How can resisted wrist flexion tests be modified to isolate each of the elbow flexors?
7. Massage therapists are prone to develop wrist extensor tendinosis. What recommendations would you make to a beginning therapist to help them avoid injury?
8. Extensor tendinosis most commonly involves:
   a) extensor carpi ulnaris
   b) extensor digitorim
   c) extensor carpi radialis brevis
   d) extensor carpi radialis longus
9. Name two common presentations of elbow injury to remedial massage clinics.
10. Describe your treatment for olecranon bursitis:
    i) in the acute phase
    ii) in the subacute phase
11. Name four remedial massage techniques that could be used to treat subacute extensor tendinosis.
12. A resisted test of the wrist flexors reproduces pain at the medial epicondyle. What condition does this suggest?
    a) sprained ligament
    b) tennis elbow
    c) golfer's elbow
    d) olecranon bursitis

REFERENCES

1. American College of Occupational and Environmental Medicine (ACOEM). Elbow disorders. Elk Grove Village, IL: American College of Occupational and Environmental Medicine; 2010. Online. Available: www.acoem.org/guidelines_elbow.aspx.
2. Tortora GJ, Grabowski SR. Principles of anatomy and physiology. 10th edn. John Wiley; 2002.
3. Cleland J, Koppenhaver S. Netter's orthopaedic clinical examination: an evidence-based approach. 2nd edn. Philadelphia: Saunders; 2011.
4. American College of Occupational and Environmental Medicine (ACOEM). Elbow disorders. Elk Grove Village (IL): American College of Occupational and Environmental Medicine (ACOEM); 2007.
5. Reese N, Bandy W. Joint range of motion and muscle length testing. Philadelphia: WB Saunders; 2002.
6. Carnes M, Vizniak N. Quick reference evidence-based conditions manual. 3rd edn. Burnaby, BC: Professional Health Systems; 2009.
7. Hislop H, Montgomery J. Daniels and Worthingham's muscle testing: techniques of manual examination. 8th edn. Oxford: Saunders Elsevier; 2007.
8. Kendall F, McCreary E, Provance P, et al. Muscles, testing and function, with posture and pain. 5th edn. Philadelphia: Lippincott Williams and Wilkins; 2005.
9. Lattermann C, Romeo AA, Meininger AK, et al. Arthroscopic debridement of the extensor carpi radialis brevis for recalcitrant lateral epicondylitis. J Shoulder Elbow Surg 2010;19(5):651–6.
10. Brosseau L, Casimiro L, Milne S, et al. Deep transverse friction massage for treating tendinitis. Cochrane Database Syst Rev 2002;(4):CD003528.
11. Kraushaar B, Nirschl R. Current concepts review: tendinosis of the elbow (tennis elbow). J Bone Joint Surg (Am) 1999;81(2):259–78.
12. Jang Y, Chi C, Tsauo J, et al. Prevalence and risk factors of work-related musculoskeletal disorders in massage practitioners. J Occup Rehabil 2006;16(3):425–38.
13. Luginbuhl R, Brunner F, Schneeberger AG. No effect of forearm band and extensor strengthening exercises for the treatment of tennis elbow: a prospective randomised study. Chir Organi Mov 2008;91:35–40.
14. Garg R, Adamson GJ, Dawson PA, et al. A prospective randomized study comparing a forearm strap brace versus a wrist splint for the treatment of lateral epicondylitis. J Shoulder Elbow Surg 2010;19(4):508–12.
15. Stasinopoulos D, Johnson M. Cyriax physiotherapy for tennis elbow/lateral epicondylitis. Brit J Sport Med 2004;38(6):675–7.
16. Simons D, Travell J, Simons L. Myofascial pain and dysfunction: The trigger point manual. Volume 1 Upper half of body. 2nd edn. Philadelphia: Williams & Wilkins; 1999.
17. Niel-Asher S. Concise book of trigger points. Berkeley, CA: North Atlantic Books; 2005.

17 The wrist and hand

The content of this chapter relates to the following Units of Competency:

HLTREM503C Plan remedial massage treatment strategy
HLTREM504C Apply remedial massage assessment framework
HLTREM502C Provide remedial massage treatment
HLTREM505C Perform remedial massage health assessment

Health Training Package HLT07

Learning Outcomes

- Assess clients with conditions of the wrist and hand for remedial massage, including identification of red and yellow flags.
- Assess clients for signs and symptoms associated with common conditions of the wrist and hand (including muscle strains, carpal tunnel syndrome, repetitive strain injury, de Quervain's tenosynovitis, degenerative joint disease and wrist sprains) and treat and/or manage these conditions with remedial massage therapy.
- Develop treatment plans for clients with conditions of the wrist and hand, taking into account assessment findings, duration and severity of the condition, likely tissue types, clinical guidelines, the best available evidence and client preferences.
- Develop short- and long-term treatment plans to address presenting symptoms, underlying conditions and predisposing factors, and to progressively increase the self-help component of therapy.
- Adapt remedial massage therapy to suit the individual client's needs based on duration and severity of injury, the client's age and gender, the presence of underlying conditions and other consideration for special population groups.

INTRODUCTION

The wrist and hand are frequently injured as a result of repetitive work-related tasks, falls on the outstretched hand and playing sport. Remedial massage therapists commonly encounter repetition strains of the wrist such as carpal tunnel syndrome and de Quervain's tenosynovitis, and first- and second-degree sprains. It is of concern that a number of studies have reported a high incidence of work-related musculoskeletal disorders among massage and other physical therapists. A survey of 667 physical therapists and physical therapist assistants reported that 32% and 35% respectively had sustained a musculoskeletal injury.[1] Injuries of the upper back, wrist and hand had the second highest prevalence (23%) after injures of the low back (56%). A survey of musculoskeletal injuries amongst 502 Canadian massage therapists found that there was a high prevalence of pain to all areas of the upper extremity, especially the wrist and thumb.[2] Jang et al[3] conducted a study on 161 visually impaired massage therapists and found that 71.4% had experienced at least one work-related musculoskeletal injury in the past 12 months, 50.3% reporting injuries of the fingers or thumb.[4]

FUNCTIONAL ANATOMY

The wrist and hand are made up of eight carpal bones in two rows (proximal row: scaphoid, lunate, triquetrum and pisiform; distal row: trapezium, trapezoid, capitate and hamate), five metacarpal bones, five proximal phalanges, four middle phalanges and five distal phalanges. The distal end of the radius articulates with the scaphoid and lunate to form the wrist or radiocarpal joint. There is no direct articulation between the distal ulna and the carpal bones. Instead, the distal ulna joins the wrist via the fibrocartilaginous disc of the distal radioulnar joint (see Figure 17.1 on p 311).

The wrist joint is enclosed by a fibrous capsule which extends from the distal radius and ulna to the proximal carpal row. The capsule is strengthened by dorsal and palmar radiocarpal ligaments and also by radial and ulnar collateral ligaments. The flexor retinaculum, a thickening of the deep fascia of the forearm, is a strong transverse band that forms the roof of the carpal tunnel. Nine flexor tendons and the median nerve pass under the flexor retinaculum as they pass through the carpal tunnel.

The metacarpals and phalanges form hinge joints for flexion and extension. The five metacarpal bones each have a base, shaft and head. The heads of the metacarpal bones articulate with proximal phalanges to form the metacarpophalangeal joints (knuckles of the hand). Each finger has three phalanges (proximal, middle and distal); the thumb only has two. The opposable thumb is formed by the rotation of the first metacarpophalangeal joint. The movements of the thumb

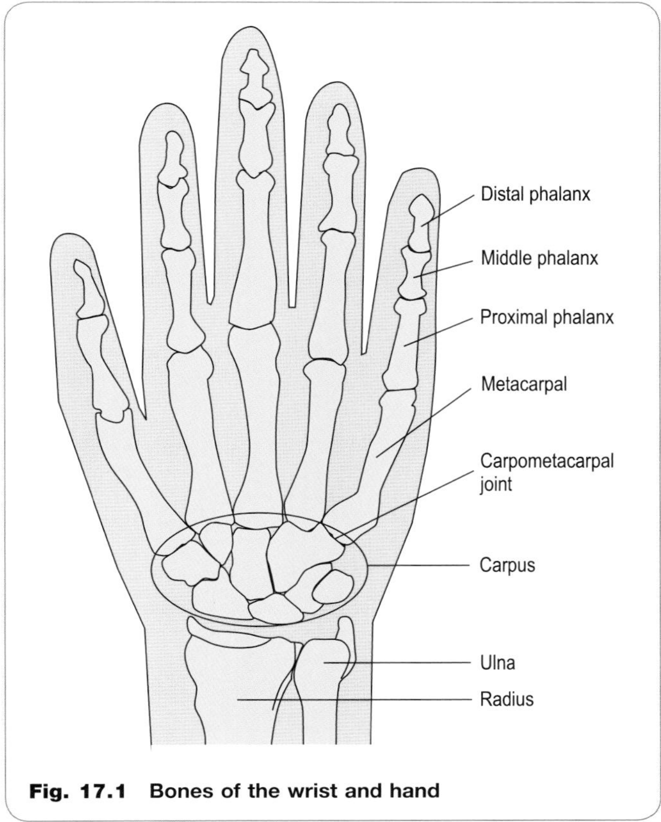

Fig. 17.1 Bones of the wrist and hand

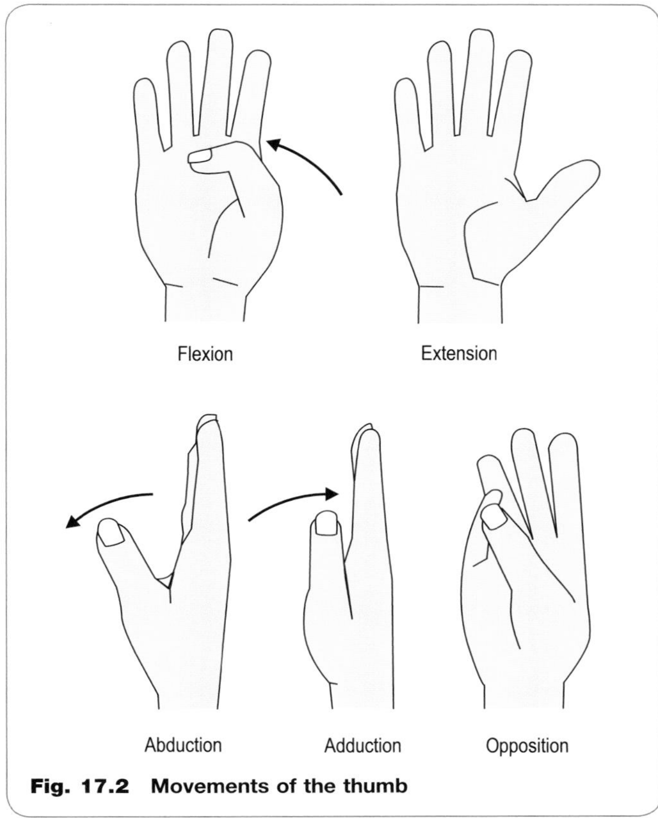

Fig. 17.2 Movements of the thumb

are described as if the thumb were in line with the row of fingers (see Figure 17.2).

Normal hand function requires complex coordination and control of muscles, many of which begin at the elbow or forearm. Muscles of the forearm often help maintain the position of the wrist and hand when the thumb and fingers perform fine motor movements or grip an object (see Figure 17.3 on p 312 and 313). Muscles of the thenar eminence (abductor pollicis brevis, opponens pollicis, flexor pollicis brevis) and the hypothenar eminence (abductor digiti minimi, flexor digiti minimi brevis, opponens digiti minimi and palmaris brevis) usually run from the carpal bones to the thumb and fingers. They enable the hand to grip and hold (see Figure 17.4 on p 314).

Nerve supply to the hand and fingers originates from the brachial plexus (C4 to T2). Three major nerves supply the hand:

1 ulnar nerve is responsible for sensation to the medial side of the hand, the medial half of the ring finger and the little finger, and motor activity of flexor carpi ulnaris, part of flexor digitorum profundus and some of the muscles of the hand
2 median nerve is responsible for sensation to the palmar surface of the thumb, index, middle and half of the ring finger, and motor activity of thenar muscles and the rest of the muscles on the front of the forearm and hand
3 radial nerve is responsible for sensation to the radial side of the forearm, dorsum of the hand, thumb, 2nd and 3rd digits, and motor activity of triceps and muscles of the back of the forearm

Table 17.1 summarises the major muscles of the wrist and hand.

ASSESSMENT

The purpose of remedial massage assessment includes:

- determining the suitability of clients for massage (contraindications and red flags)
- determining the duration (acute or subacute), severity of injury and types of tissues involved in the injury/condition
- determining whether symptoms fit patterns of common conditions.

Principles of remedial massage assessment are discussed in Chapter 2. This section presents specific considerations for assessment of the wrist and hand.

CASE HISTORY

Information from case histories can alert you to the presence of serious conditions requiring referral.[5] However, information from case histories should always be interpreted with findings from other assessments. For example, subjective complaints do not appear to be useful in identifying carpal tunnel syndrome. Reports of dropping objects and shaking hands to improve symptoms were shown to minimally alter the probability of diagnosis (+LR = 1.7–1.9, –LR = 0.34–0.47).[6]

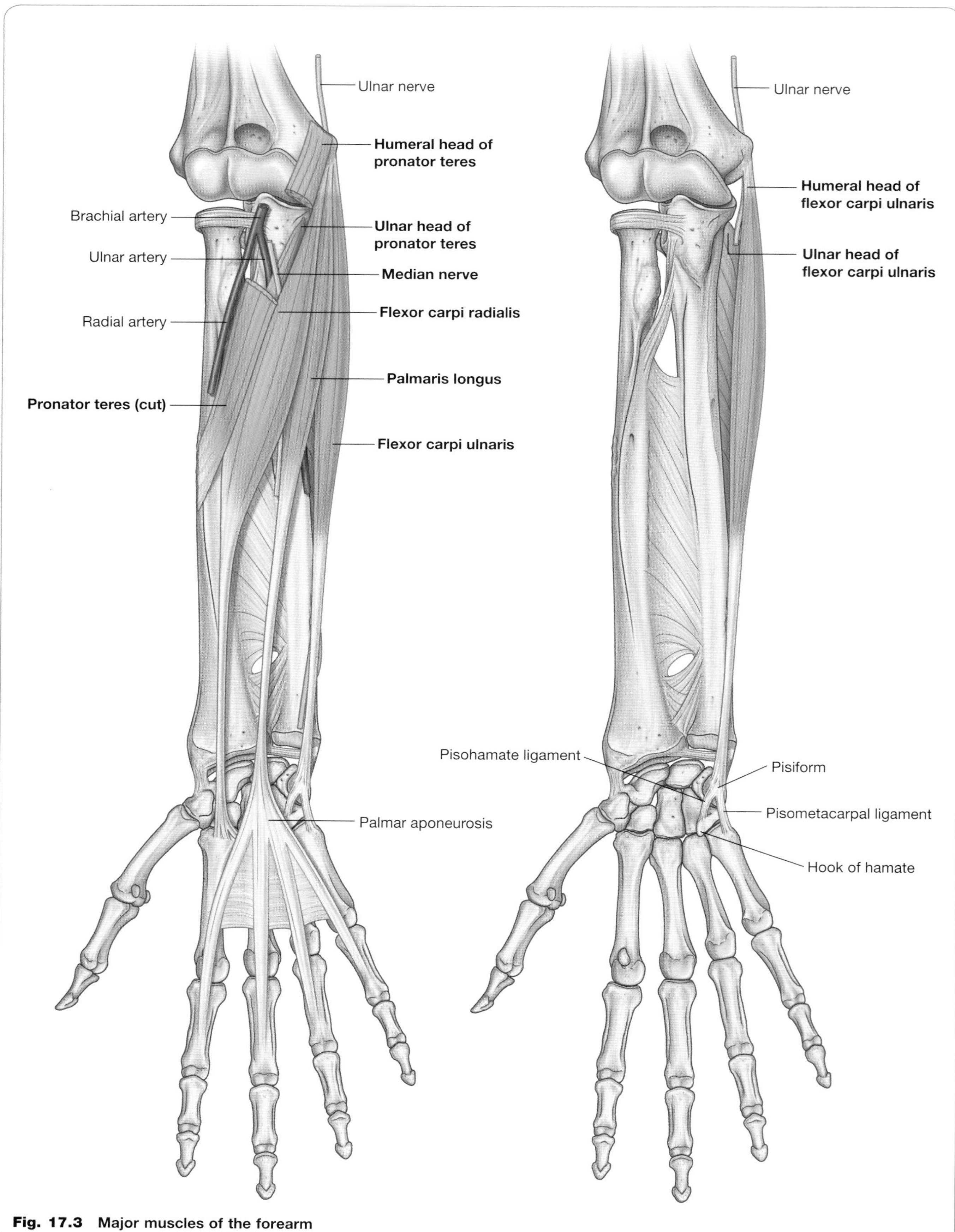

Fig. 17.3 Major muscles of the forearm

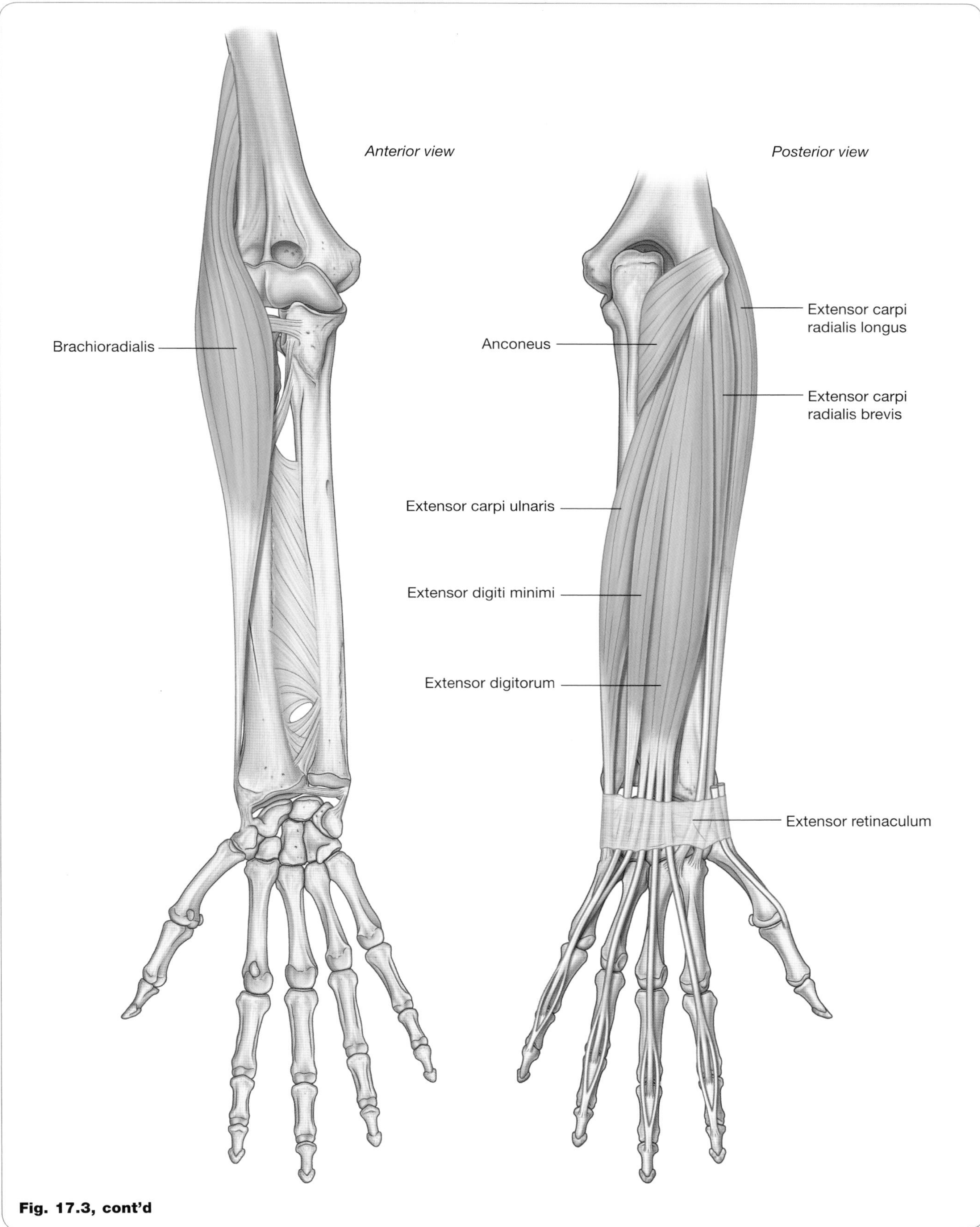

Fig. 17.3, cont'd

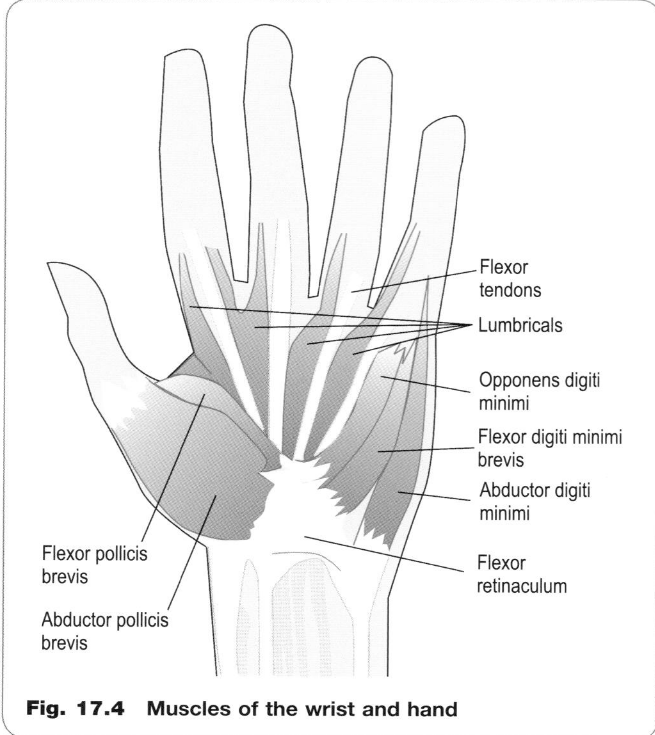

Fig. 17.4 Muscles of the wrist and hand

Assessment of the wrist and hand

1. Case history
2. Outcome measures (e.g. The Patient Specific Scale – see Chapter 2)
3. Postural analysis
4. Functional tests
   Cervical spine
   Active range of motion tests
   Flexion, extension, lateral flexion, rotation
   Glenohumeral joint
   Active range of motion tests
   Flexion, extension, abduction, horizontal adduction, internal rotation, external rotation
   Elbow joint
   Active range of motion tests
   Flexion, extension, supination, pronation
   Wrist and hand
   Active range of motion tests
   Flexion, extension, supination, pronation, adduction, abduction
   Passive range of motion tests
   Flexion, extension, supination, pronation, adduction, abduction
   Resisted range of motion tests
   Flexion, extension, supination, pronation, adduction, abduction
   Resisted and length tests for specific muscles
   Special tests including
   Phalen's test
   Tinel's test
   Finkelstein's test
5. Palpation

History questions should be targeted to include:

- describing the mechanism of the current injury, onset of symptoms, pain, disability and functional impairment and previous injuries to this area. Did the client fall on the outstretched hand? Is there any numbness, tingling, weakness?[8]
- identifying the client's type of work and habitual postures
- identifying red and yellow flags that require referral for further investigation (red flags for serious conditions of the wrist and hand are summarised in Table 17.2)
- identifying the exact location of the symptoms by asking clients to point to the site of pain/symptoms
- determining if the pain is local or referred. Local pain tends to be sharp and well-localised; referred pain tends to be dull and poorly localised. The presence of nerve impingement symptoms like numbness, tingling or weakness suggest referral from lower cervical nerves (C6 nerve root affects the thumb, index finger, radial side of the hand and forearm, C7 affects the middle finger, and C8 affects the ring and little finger, ulnar side of the hand and forearm) (see Figure 17.5 on p 317), or local nerve entrapment (median nerve affects thumb, index and middle fingers, the radial half of the ring finger and the radial half of the palm, ulnar nerve affects the little finger, the ulnar half of the ring finger and the ulnar half of the palm). Other causes of distal paraesthesia include B12 deficiency, hypothyroidism, heavy metal poisoning, diabetes, systemic lupus erythematosus, Sjögren's syndrome[a], malnutrition, HIV and HIV medications.

OUTCOME MEASURES

Outcome measures are questionnaires that are specifically designed to assess clients' level of impairment and to define benefits of treatment. The Patient Specific Scale can be used to measure progress of treatment of clients with any musculoskeletal condition, including conditions of the wrist and hand.

POSTURAL ANALYSIS

Postural analysis enables observation of the whole client and facilitates identification of important features through bilateral comparison. It also facilitates detection of possible predisposing or contributing factors through observing the position of the head, cervical and thoracic spines, glenohumeral joints and scapula. Observe the alignment and symmetry of the upper limbs, carrying angle of the elbow and length of upper limbs in relation to the torso.

Observation of the wrist and hand

Observe the wrist and hand for symmetry, swelling (local or diffuse), colour, bruising, scars and muscle hypertonicity or atrophy.

Common conditions of the hand include:

- Heberden's nodes at distal interphalangeal joints (associated with degenerative joint disease) (see Figure 17.6 on p 317)

[a]Sjögren's syndrome is an autoimmune disease which causes glandular inflammation and is characterised by dry mouth and eyes. It may also be associated with connective tissue diseases like rheumatoid arthritis, systemic lupus erythematosus or scleroderma.

Table 17.1 Muscles of the wrist and hand[7]

Muscle	Origin	Insertion	Action
Forearm Pronators			
• Pronator teres	Medial epicondyle of humerus and coronoid process of ulna	Middle of lateral surface of radius	Pronates forearm at radioulnar joint and weakly flexes forearm at elbow
• Pronator quadratus	Distal portion of shaft of ulna	Distal portion of shaft of radius	Pronates forearm at radioulnar joints
Forearm supinator			
• Supinator	Lateral epicondyle of humerus and supinator crest	Lateral surface of proximal one-third of radius	Supinates forearm at radioulnar joints
Wrist flexors *Superficial flexor compartment of the forearm*			
• Flexor carpi radialis	Medial epicondyle of humerus	Second and third metacarpals	Flexes and abducts hand (radial deviation) at wrist joint
• Palmaris longus	Medial epicondyle of humerus	Flexor retinaculum and palmar aponeurosis	Weakly flexes hand at wrist joint
• Flexor carpi ulnaris	Medial epicondyle of humerus and superior posterior border of ulna	Pisiform, hamate and base of fifth metacarpal	Flexes and adducts hand (ulnar deviation) at wrist joint
• Flexor digitorum superficialis	Medial epicondyle of humerus, coronoid process of ulna and anterior oblique line of radius	Middle phalanx of each finger	Flexes middle phalanx of each finger at proximal interphalangeal joint, proximal phalanx of each finger at metacarpophalangeal joint and flexes hand at wrist joint
Deep flexor compartment of the forearm			
• Flexor pollicis longus	Anterior surface of radius and interosseous membrane (sheet of fibrous tissue that holds shafts of ulna and radius together)	Base of distal phalanx of thumb	Flexes distal phalanx of thumb at interphalangeal joint
• Flexor digitorum profundus	Anterior medial surface of body of ulna	Base of distal phalanx of each finger	Flexes distal and middle phalanges of each finger at interphalangeal joints, proximal phalanx of each finger at metacarpophalangeal joint and hand at wrist joint
Extensors of the wrist and fingers *Superficial extensor compartment of the forearm*			
• Extensor carpi radialis longus	Lateral supracondylar ridge of humerus	Second metacarpal	Extends and abducts hand at wrist joint
• Extensor carpi radialis brevis	Lateral epicondyle of humerus	Third metacarpal	Extends and abducts hand at wrist joint

Continued

Table 17.1 Muscles of the wrist and hand—cont'd

Muscle	Origin	Insertion	Action
• Extensor digitorum	Lateral epicondyle of humerus	Distal and middle phalanges of each finger	Extends distal and middle phalanges of each finger at interphalangeal joints, proximal phalanx of each finger at metacarpophalangeal joint and hand at wrist joint
• Extensor digiti minimi	Lateral epicondyle of humerus	Tendon of extensor digitorum on fifth phalanx	Extends proximal phalanx of little finger at metacarpophalangeal joint and hand at wrist joint
• Extensor carpi ulnaris	Lateral epicondyle of humerus and posterior border of ulna	Ulnar side of fifth metacarpal	Extends and adducts hand at wrist joint
Deep extensor compartment of the forearm			
• Abductor pollicis longus	Posterior surface of middle of radius and ulna and interosseous membrane	First metacarpal	Abducts and extends thumb at carpometacarpal joint and abducts hand at wrist joint
• Extensor pollicis brevis	Posterior surface of middle of radius and interosseous membrane	Base of proximal phalanx of thumb	Extends thumb at carpometacarpal and metacarpophalangeal joints; assists in abduction of the wrist
• Extensor pollicis longus	Middle third of posterior aspect of ulna and interosseous membrane	Base of distal phalanx of thumb	Extends distal phalanx of thumb at interphalangeal joint, assists in extension of metacarpophalangeal and carpometacarpal joints of the thumb and assists in abduction and extenson of the wrist
• Extensor indicis	Posterior surface of ulna	Tendon of extensor digitorum of index finger	Extends distal and middle phalanges of index finger at interphalangeal joints, proximal phalanx of index finger at metacarpophalangeal joint and hand at wrist joint
Intrinsic muscles of the hand			
• Adductor pollicis	Oblique head: capitate and second and third metacarpals Transverse head: third metacarpal	Medial side of proximal phalanx of thumb by a tendon containing a sesamoid bone	Adducts thumb at carpometacarpal and metacarpophalangeal joints
Thenar eminence			
• Abductor pollicis brevis	Flexor retinaculum, scaphoid and trapezium	Lateral side of proximal phalanx of thumb	Abducts thumb at carpometacarpal joint
• Opponens pollicis	Flexor retinaculum and trapezium	Lateral side of first metacarpal (thumb)	Moves thumb across palm to meet little finger (opposition) at the carpometacarpal joint
• Flexor pollicis brevis	Flexor retinaculum, trapezium, capitate and trapezoid	Lateral side of proximal phalanx of thumb	Flexes thumb at carpometacarpal and metacarpophalangeal joints
Hypothenar eminence			
• Abductor digiti minimi	Pisiform and tendon of flexor carpi ulnaris	Medial side of proximal phalanx of little finger	Abducts and flexes the little finger at metacarpophalangeal joint
• Flexor digiti minimi brevis	Flexor retinaculum and hamate	Medial side of proximal phalanx of little finger	Flexes little finger at carpometacarpal and metacarpophalangeal joints

Table 17.1 Muscles of the wrist and hand—cont'd

Muscle	Origin	Insertion	Action
• Opponens digiti minimi	Flexor retinaculum and hamate	Medial side of fifth metacarpal	Moves little finger across palm to meet thumb (opposition) at the carpometacarpal joint
Intermediate midpalmar			
• Lumbricals	Lateral side of tendons and flexor digitorum profundus of each finger	Lateral sides of tendons of extensor digitorum on proximal phalanges of each finger	Flex each finger at metacarpophalangeal joints and extends each finger at interphalangeal joints
• Palmar interossei	Sides of shafts of metacarpals of all digits (except the middle one)	Sides of bases of all proximal phalanges (except the middle one)	Adduct each finger at metacarpophalangeal joints; flex each finger at metacarpophalangeal joints
Dorsal interossei	Adjacent sides of metacarpals	Proximal phalanx of each finger	Abducts fingers at metacarpophalangeal joints; flex fingers at metacarpophalangeal joints; extend each finger at interphalangeal joints

Note: Biceps brachii supinates the forearm. It is described in Chapter 15.

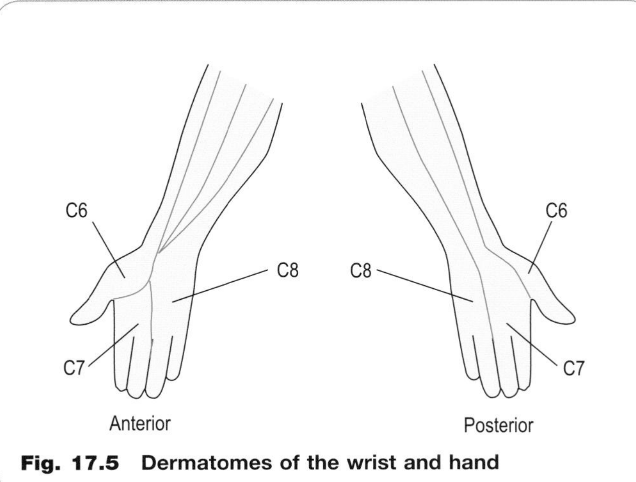

Fig. 17.5 Dermatomes of the wrist and hand

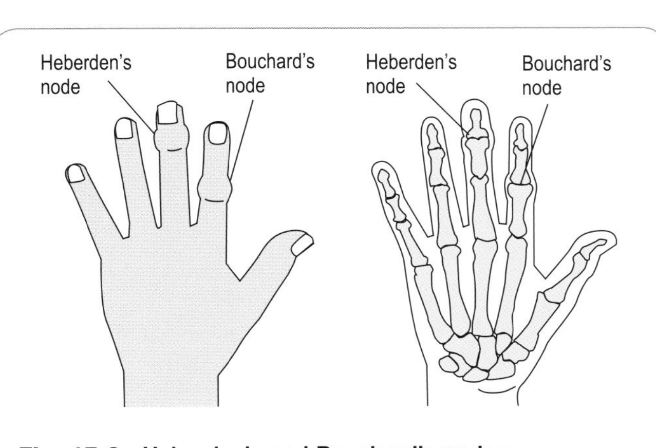

Fig. 17.6 Heberden's and Bouchard's nodes

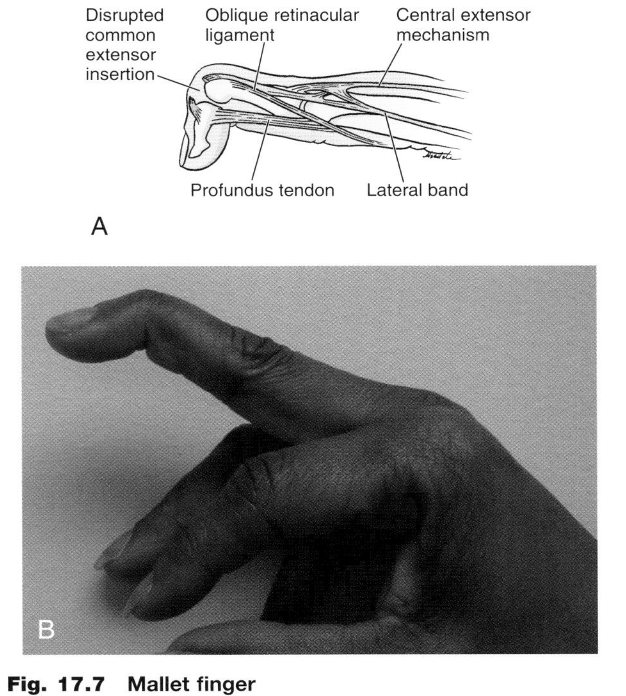

Fig. 17.7 Mallet finger

- Bouchard's nodes at the proximal interphalangeal joint (usually associated with rheumatoid arthritis) (see Figure 17.6)
- Boutonnière deformity at the proximal interphalangeal joint (rupture of the extensor tendon at the middle phalanx, associated with rheumatoid arthritis and severe sprains) (see Figure 17.9 on p 319)
- Mallet finger (rupture of the extensor tendon attachment at the distal phalanx) (see Figure 17.7)

Table 17.2 Red flags for potentially serious wrist and hand conditions[9]

Condition	Red flag – history	Red flag – physical examination
Fracture and/or dislocation	Lunate: History of significant trauma Fall on outstretched hand Generalised wrist pain Scaphoid: History of fall on outstretched hand Prevalent in males 15–30 years and females with osteoporosis Distal radius (Colles' fracture): History of fall on the outstretched arm with forceful wrist extension Young male or older female Radial head: History of fall on the outstretched hand	Deformity consistent with fracture Reduced range(s) of motion Pain with range of motion Significant bruising, if subacute (unusual)
Infection	Recent cut or puncture wound such as a human or animal bite Pain, swelling, redness	Localised heat, swelling, erythema, purulence, erythematous streaks, especially from a portal of entry Systemic signs of infection
Tumour (melanoma)	History of cancer Female <40 years, male >40 years Fair skin, history of sunburns Unintentional weight loss Continuous pain, especially at night and not improved with rest	Asymmetrical or irregular-shaped lesion Borders are notched, scalloped or vaguely defined Colour unevenly distributed or defined Diameter >6 mm
Inflammation	History of gout or pseudogout History of rheumatoid arthritis History of other inflammatory arthritides	Effusion Localised heat, swelling, erythema, tenderness
Rapidly progressive neurological deficit	History of neurological disease Trauma	Abnormal neurological examination Focal or global motor weakness distal to the elbow Weakness may be limited to the distribution of one nerve, such as hand intrinsic muscles
Vascular compromise	History of diabetes mellitus Tobacco use History of fracture or dislocation History of vascular disease of any kind	Decreased or absent peripheral pulses and delayed capillary refill Oedema
Raynaud's phenomenon	Positive family history Women on oestrogen therapy Cold exposure/frostbite injury Underlying collagen vascular disease	Skin pallor, cyanosis, and/or hyperaemic erythema of the fingers Taking medication promoting vasoconstriction such as β-blockers, amphetamines, decongestants and caffeine
Compartment syndrome	History of trauma, surgery or extreme unaccustomed activity Persistent forearm pain and tightness Tingling, burning or numbness	Palpable tenderness and tension of involved compartment Pain intensified with stretch to involved muscles Paraesthesia, paresis and sensory deficits Diminished pulse and prolonged capillary refill
Complex regional pain syndrome (Reflex sympathetic dystrophy)	History of trauma or surgery Severe burning/boring/aching pain out of proportion to the inciting event Pain not responsive to typical analgesics Secondary hyperalgesia/ hypersensitivity	Area swollen (pitting oedema), warm and erythematous Temperature difference between involved and uninvolved extremity, hot or cold

- Dupuytren's contracture (hypertrophic nodular fibroplasia of the palmar aponeurosis producing flexion contracture usually of the ring and little fingers) (see Figure 17.8 on p 319)
- Claw hand (flexion contracture of all digits from ulnar and median nerve palsy)
- Ulnar deviation of fingers and wrist (associated with rheumatoid arthritis) (see Figure 17.9 on p 319)
- Swan neck deformity (proximal interphalangeal joint hyperextension and distal interphalangeal joint flexion associated with severe rheumatoid arthritis) (see Figure 17.9 on p 319)

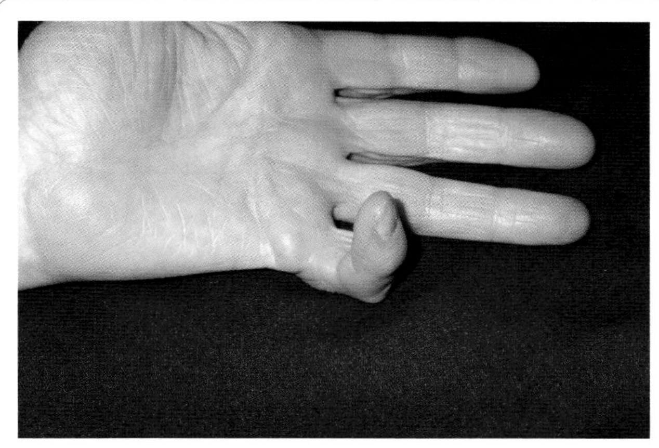

Fig. 17.8 **Dupuytren's contracture**

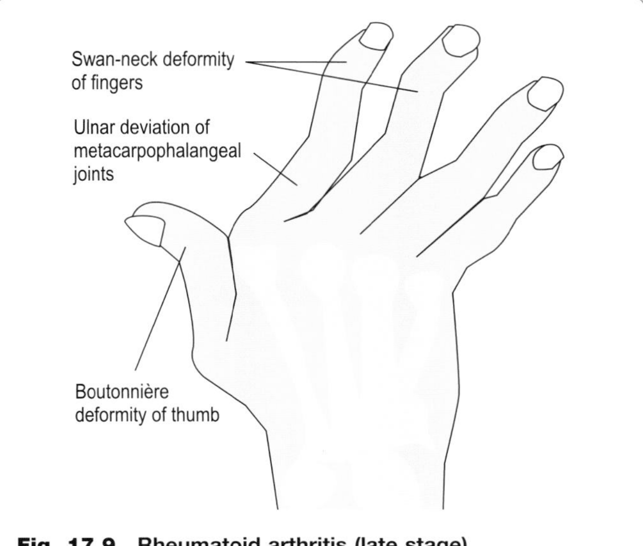

Fig. 17.9 **Rheumatoid arthritis (late stage)**

- Trigger finger (snapping during flexion and extension of the metacarpophalangeal joint which progresses to locking the digit in flexion due to fusiform swelling in flexor digitorum superficialis or flexor pollicis longus just proximal to the metacarpophalangeal joint, associated with degenerative joint disease, rheumatoid arithritis or tendon trauma)
- Ganglia (swellings overlying tendon sheaths or joint capsules occurring commonly in the wrist and hand). Generally no treatment is required.

Observe the fingernails of both hands for signs of certain conditions. Table 17.3 lists some fingernail signs and possible associated conditions.

FUNCTIONAL TESTS

For any tests involving joint movements it is important to compare both sides and take into account any underlying pathology and the age and lifestyle of the client. Measuring wrist range of motion appears to be highly reliable.[7]

Active range of motion of the cervical spine (flexion, extension, lateral flexion and rotation)

Examination of the wrist and hand begins with active range of motion tests of the cervical spine to help rule out brachial plexus injury which may refer pain and other symptoms to the wrist and hand (see Figure 17.5 on p 317). If active range of motion tests of the cervical spine reproduce wrist and hand symptoms, further examination of the cervical spine is indicated (see Chapter 12).

Active range of motion of the glenohumeral joint (flexion, extension, abduction, horizontal adduction, external and internal rotation)

If active range of motion tests of the glenohumeral joint produce symptoms, a full examination of the glenohumeral joint is indicated (see Chapter 15).

Active range of motion of the elbow joint (flexion, extension, pronation and supination)

If the client experiences pain or other symptoms during elbow movement, a full examination of the elbow joint is indicated (see Chapter 16).

Active range of motion of the wrist and fingers[10]

Wrist

Flexion/extension 80°/70°
Supination/pronation 80°/80°
Abduction (radial deviation)/adduction (ulnar deviation) 20°/30°
1st carpometacarpal joint
Flexion/extension 15°/20°
Abduction 70°

Fingers and thumb

Metacarpophalangeal joints
Fingers: Flexion/extension 90°/20°
Thumb: Flexion/extension 50°/0°
Interphalangeal joints
Fingers: PIP flexion/extension 100°/0°
DIP flexion/extension 70°/0°
Thumb: IP flexion/extension 65°/10–20°

Passive range of motion of the wrist and hand

If the client is unable to perform normal AROM in any direction, further investigation is required. PROM testing for the wrist should be performed by stabilising and palpating the wrist with one hand and moving the client's wrist through its ranges of motion with the other. To isolate finger joints, place one contact either side of the joint (e.g. to isolate the PIP, one hand contacts the proximal phalanx, the other contacts the distal phalanx). Palpate for crepitus, capsular pattern and end-feel as the joints are being moved.

CAPSULAR PATTERNS

Wrist joint flexion more limited than extension
1st carpometacarpal joint abduction more limited than extension

Table 17.3 Fingernail signs

Fingernail signs	Associated condition
Clubbing (thickening of end of digits, loss of normal angle between the nailbed and the skin of the distal phalanx)	Chronic decreased oxygen supply to ends of digits; associated with severe respiratory disease, cardiac condition
Spoon nails (thin, concave nails)	Anaemia, local injury, fungal infection, chronic diabetes
Thick, hard, brittle nails	Silica deficiency
Thin, soft, pliable nails	Calcium phosphate deficiency
Lateral ridges (Beau's lines)	Nutritional deficiencies, uncontrolled diabetes, peripheral artery disease, systemic disease, repetitive trauma to nails
White spots	Silica, calcium phosphate, zinc deficiency
White bands under nails	(Muehrcke lines) albumin deficiency (liver and kidney disease) (Mee's lines) arsenic poisoning
Pink-brown bands	Cirrhosis, heart disease, diabetes, cancer
Opaque nails, tip has dark band (Terry's nails)	Congestive heart failure, diabetes, liver disease, malnutrition
Distal half brown	Chronic renal failure
Splinter haemorrhages	Bacterial endocarditis, trauma, glomerulonephritis, vasculitis, cirrhosis, scurvy, psoriasis, trichinosis
No moons	Poor circulation
Blue moons	Naevus (birth mark), argyria (silver poisoning), Wilson's disease
Growths	Fungal infections
Longitudinal ridges	Small or large intestine disease
Pitting (small depressions in nails)	Psoriasis, nail injuries, chronic dermatitis
Yellow nails	Respiratory condition (e.g. chronic bronchitis), lymphoedema

Fingers: metacarpophalangeal joints flexion more limited than extension
Fingers: interphalangeal joints flexion more limited than extension.

Resisted range of motion

RROM tests should also be performed if AROM testing indicates the likelihood of a wrist or hand problem. RROM tests include:

Wrist

Flexion: flexor carpi radialis, flexor carpi ulnaris, palmaris longus, flexor digitorum superficialis and profundus
Extension: extensor carpi radialis longus and brevis, extensor carpi ulnaris, extensor digitorum
Pronation: pronator teres, pronator quadratus
Supination: supinator
Abduction: extensor carpi radialis longus and brevis, flexor carpi radialis
Adduction: flexor carpi ulnaris, extensor carpi ulnaris

Fingers

Flexion: flexor digitorum profundus and superficialis, lumbricals
Extension: extensor digitorum
Abduction: dorsal interossei
Adduction: palmar interossei

Thumb

Flexion: flexor pollicis longus and brevis
Extension: extensor pollicis longus and brevis
Abduction: abductor pollicis longus and brevis
Adduction: adductor pollicis

Resisted tests and length tests for specific muscles[11, 12]

If RROM tests reproduce symptoms, then further tests may be used to help identify specific muscles involved. Refer to Chapter 16 for resisted and length tests of biceps brachii, supinator, pronator teres and pronator quadratus.

1. FLEXOR CARPI RADIALIS

Resisted test

The client holds their wrist flexed towards the radial side, fingers relaxed. Apply pressure to extend their wrist towards the ulnar side. Note that palmaris longus may also be activated during this test (see Figure 17.10).

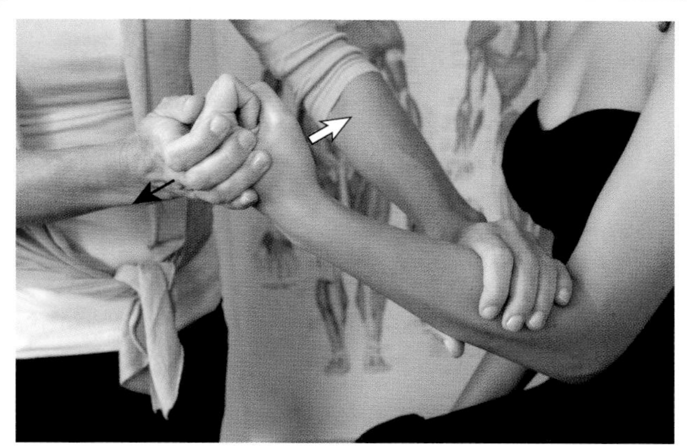

Fig. 17.10 Resisted test for flexor carpi radialis

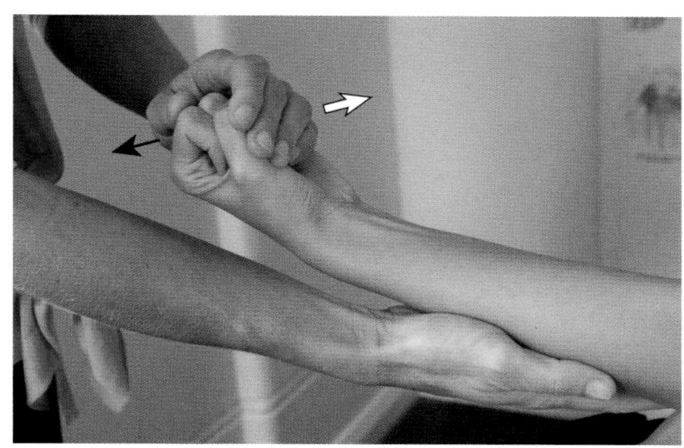

Fig. 17.12 Palmaris longus and brevis resisted test

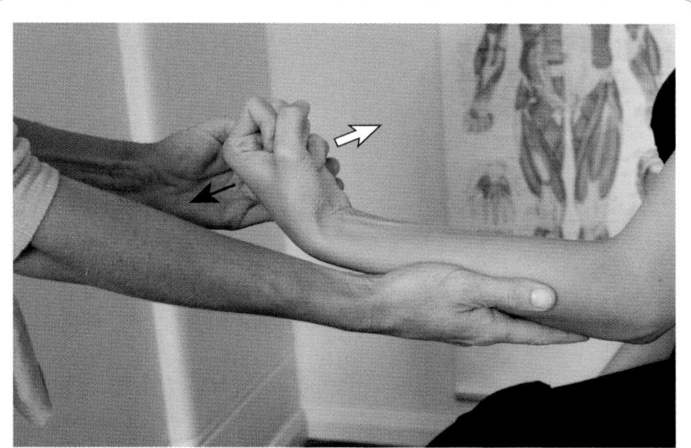

Fig. 17.11 Resisted test for flexor carpi ulnaris

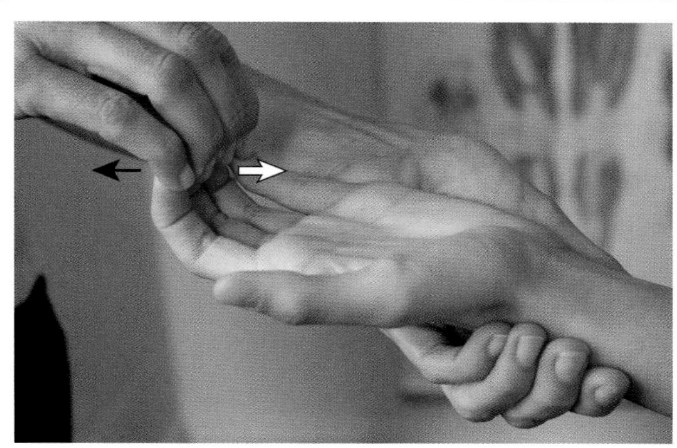

Fig. 17.13 Resisted test for flexor digitorum profundus

Length test

Contracture of flexor carpi radialis prevents the wrist from fully extending and deviating towards the ulnar side.

2. FLEXOR CARPI ULNARIS

Resisted test

The client holds their wrist flexed towards the ulnar side, fingers relaxed. Apply pressure against the hypothenar eminence in the direction of extension towards the radial side (see Figure 17.11).

Length test

Contracture of flexor carpi ulnaris prevents the wrist from fully extending and deviating towards the radial side.

3. PALMARIS LONGUS AND BREVIS

Resisted test

The client strongly cups their palm and flexes their wrist. Apply pressure to both thenar and hypothenar eminences to flatten the hand and extend the wrist as the client tries to hold the position (see Figure 17.12).

Length test

Contracture of palmaris longus and brevis muscles limits the client's ability to open their palm and extend their wrist.

4. FLEXOR DIGITORUM PROFUNDUS

Resisted test

The client flexes the distal interphalangeal joints of the 2nd to 5th digits. Contact the palmar surface of the distal phalanges and try to extend their fingers (see Figure 17.13).

Length test

Contracture of flexor digitorum profundus prevents full extension of the distal phalanges of 2nd to 5th fingers. It can cause a flexion deformity of the distal phalanges of the fingers.

5. FLEXOR DIGITORUM SUPERFICIALIS

Resisted test

This test is similar to the test for flexor digitorum profundus except that pressure is applied at the middle phalanges (see Figure 17.14 on p 322).

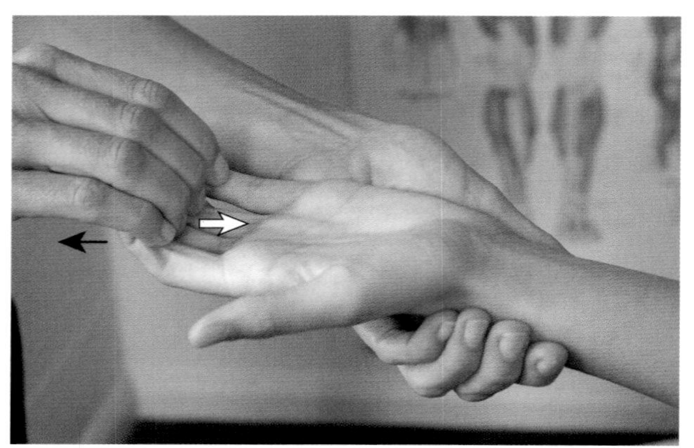

Fig. 17.14 Resisted test for flexor digitorum superficialis

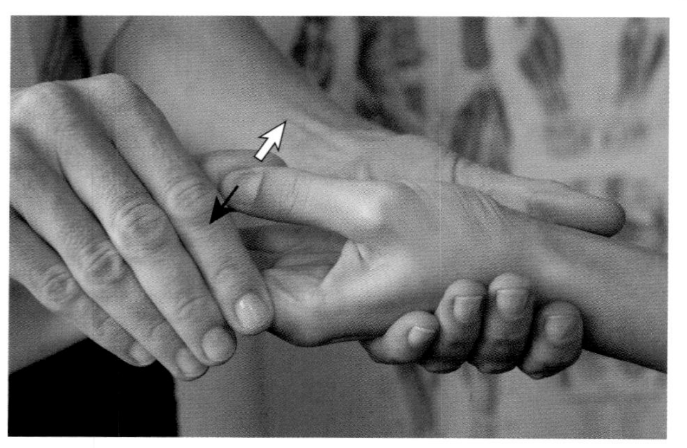

Fig. 17.15 Resisted test for flexor pollicis longus

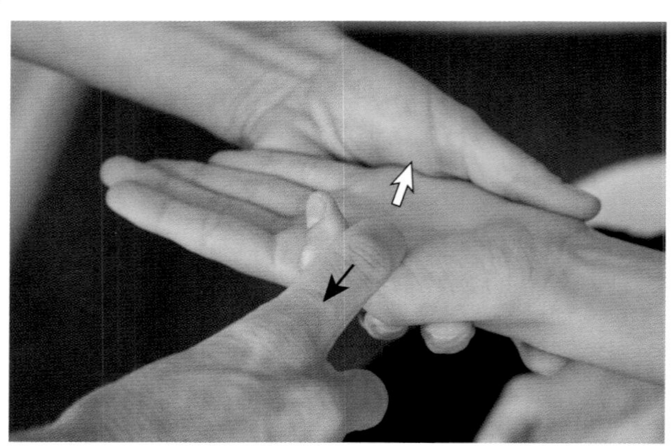

Fig. 17.16 Resisted test for flexor pollicis brevis

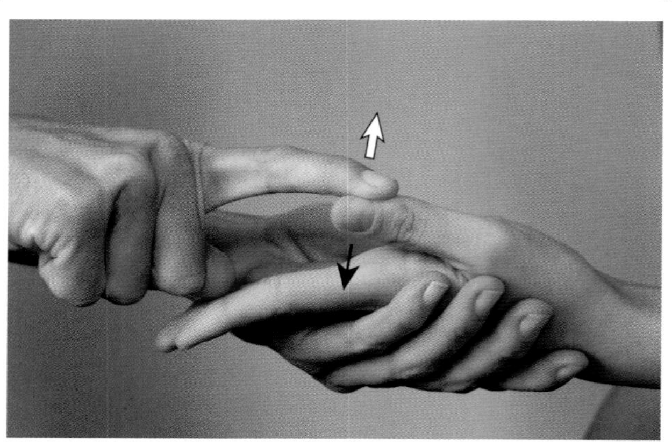

Fig. 17.17 Resisted test for abductor pollicis longus

Length test

Contraction of flexor digitorum superficialis limits extension of the middle phalanges of digits 2 to 5. It can cause flexion of the middle phalanges of the fingers if the wrist is extended or flexion of the wrist if the fingers are extended.

6. FLEXOR POLLICIS LONGUS

Resisted test

The client flexes the distal phalanx of the thumb and holds this position. Contact the palmar surface of the distal phalanx and apply pressure in the direction of extension (see Figure 17.15).

Length test

Contracture of flexor pollicis longus limits extension of the distal phalanx of the thumb. It can cause a flexion deformity of the distal interphalangeal joint of the thumb.

7. FLEXOR POLLICIS BREVIS

This test is similar to the test for flexor pollicis longus except that the client flexes the proximal phalanx of the thumb and the practitioner applies pressure to its palmar surface in the direction of extension (see Figure 17.16).

Length test

Contracture of flexor pollicis brevis limits extension of the proximal phalanx of the thumb. It can cause a flexion deformity of the proximal interphalangeal joint of the thumb.

8. ABDUCTOR POLLICIS LONGUS

The client abducts the thumb. Apply pressure to the lateral surface of the first metacarpal bone in the direction of adduction (see Figure 17.17).

Length test

If abductor pollicis longus is contracted, adduction of the carpometacarpal joint of the thumb is limited. Contracture can cause the first metacarpal to be abducted and slightly extended with slight radial deviation of the hand.

9. ABDUCTOR POLLICIS BREVIS

Resisted test

The test is similar to the test for abductor pollicis longus except that you apply pressure against the proximal phalanx in the direction of adduction towards the palm (see Figure 17.18 on p 323).

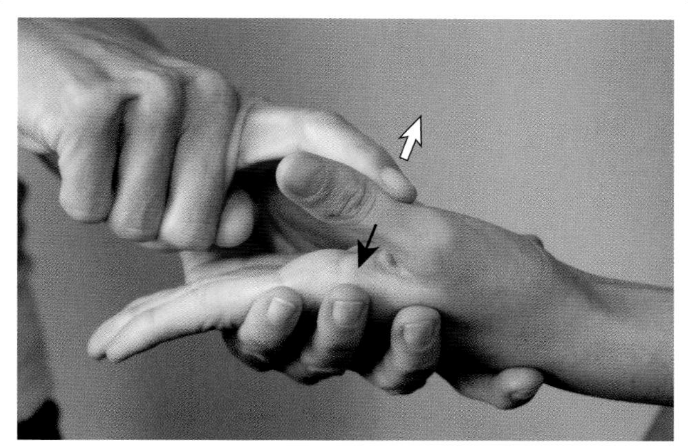

Fig. 17.18 Resisted test for abductor pollicis brevis

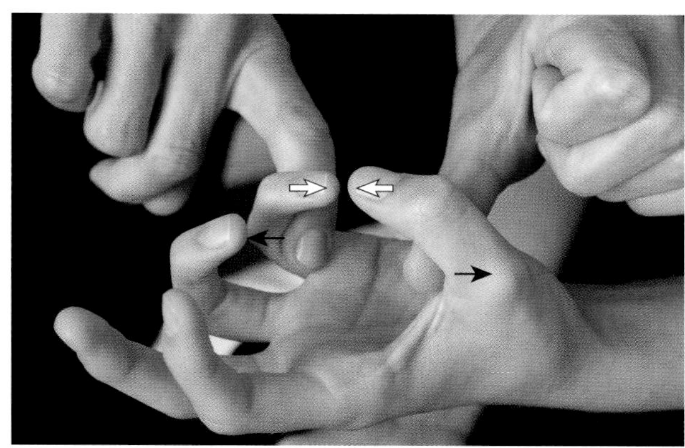

Fig. 17.20 Resisted test for opponens pollicis and opponens digiti minimi

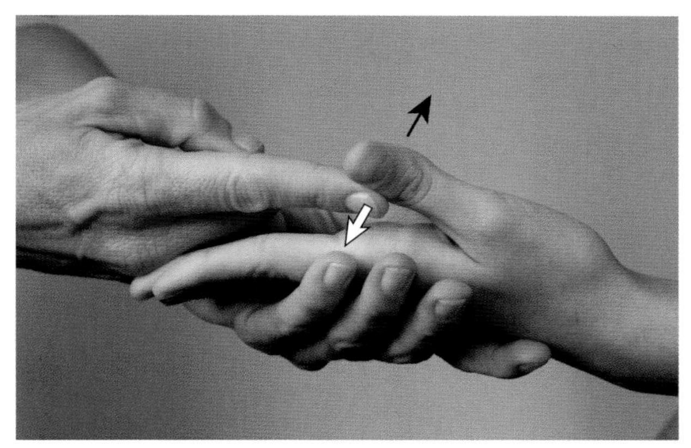

Fig. 17.19 Resisted test for adductor pollicis

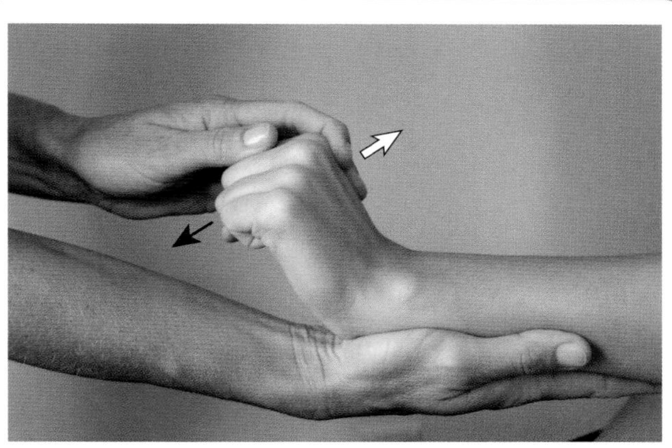

Fig. 17.21 Resisted test for extensor carpi radialis longus and brevis

Length test

If abductor pollicis brevis is contracted, adduction of the carpometacarpal and metacarpophalangeal joints of the thumb is limited.

10. ADDUCTOR POLLICIS

Resisted test

Contact the medial surface of the thumb and resist as the client tries to adduct the thumb towards the palm (see Figure 17.19).

Length test

Contracture of adductor pollicis limits abduction of the thumb and can create an adduction deformity of the thumb.

11. OPPONENS POLLICIS/OPPONENS DIGITI MINIMI

Resisted test

Opponens pollicis and opponens digiti minimi can be tested at the same time. The client touches the tip of their little finger with the tip of their thumb and holds this position as you try to separate finger and thumb (see Figure 17.20).

Length test

Contracture of opponens pollicis limits extension of the carpometacarpal joint of the thumb and contracture of opponens digiti minimi limits extension of the fifth metacarpal.

12. EXTENSOR CARPI RADIALIS LONGUS AND BREVIS

The client extends their wrist towards the radial side and holds the position as you apply pressure against the dorsum of the hand in the direction of flexion towards the ulnar side (see Figure 17.21).

Length test

Contracture of extensor carpi radialis longus and brevis muscles limits flexion and ulnar deviation of the wrist. It can cause the wrist to be held in extension with radial deviation.

13. EXTENSOR CARPI ULNARIS

The client extends their wrist towards the ulnar side and holds the position as you apply pressure against the dorsum of the hand in the direction of flexion towards the radial side (see Figure 17.22 on p 324).

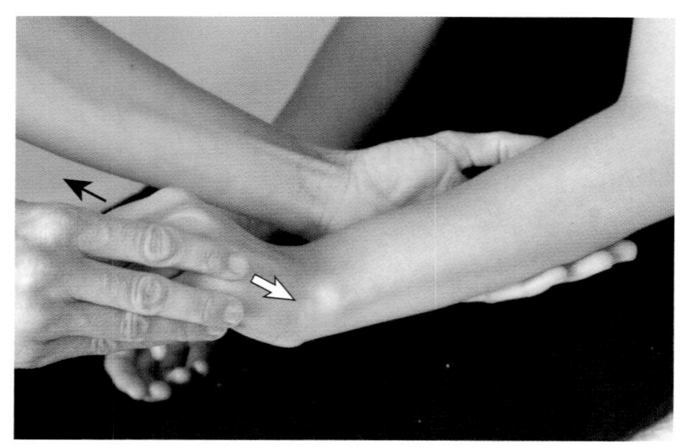

Fig. 17.22 Resisted test for extensor carpi ulnaris

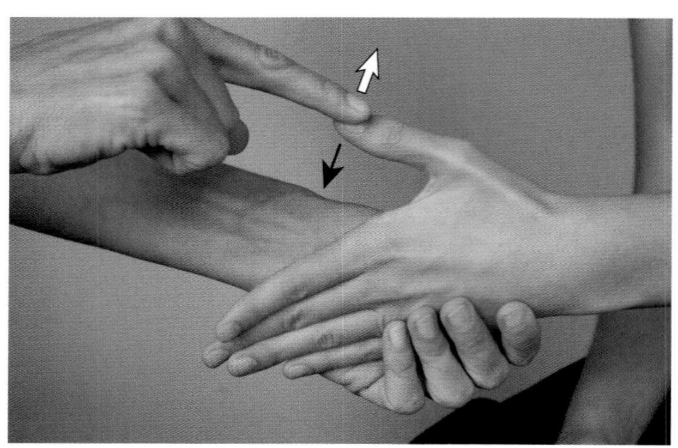

Fig. 17.24 Resisted test for extensor pollicis longus

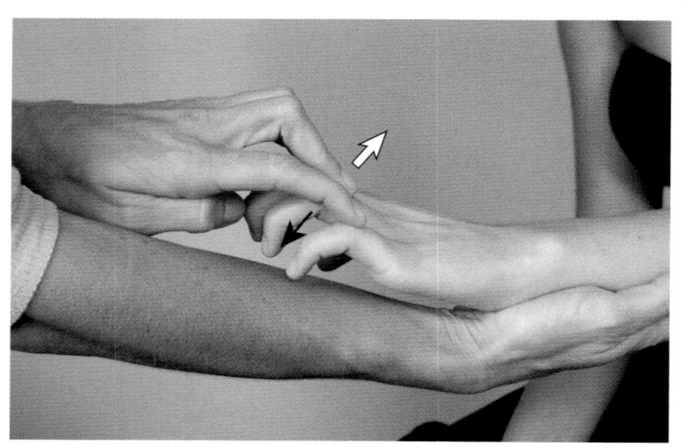

Fig. 17.23 Resisted test for extensor digitorum

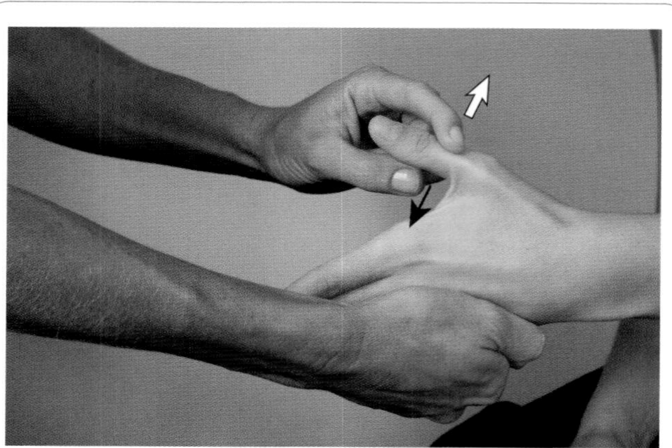

Fig. 17.25 Resisted test for extensor pollicis brevis

Length test

Contracture of extensor carpi ulnaris limits radial deviation and flexion of the wrist. It can cause the wrist to be held in ulnar deviation with slight extension.

14. EXTENSOR DIGITORUM

Resisted test

The client extends the proximal phalanges of the 2nd to 5th digits. The interphalangeal joints are relaxed. Apply pressure against the dorsal surface of the proximal phalanges in the direction of flexion (see Figure 17.23).

Length test

Contracture of extensor digitorum limits flexion of the 2nd to 5th metacarpophalangeal joints. It may create a hyperextension deformity of the metacarpophalangeal joints if the wrist is flexed, or extension of the wrist when the metacarpophalangeal joints are flexed.

15. EXTENSOR POLLICIS LONGUS

Resisted test

The client extends the distal phalanx of the thumb. Apply pressure against the dorsal surface of the distal phalanx of the thumb in the direction of flexion (see Figure 17.24).

Length test

Contracture of extensor pollicis longus limits flexion of the interphalangeal joint of the thumb.

16. EXTENSOR POLLICIS BREVIS

This test is similar to the test for extensor pollicis longus except that you apply pressure against the dorsum of the proximal phalanx of the thumb in the direction of flexion (see Figure 17.25).

Length test

Contracture of extensor pollicis brevis limits flexion and adduction of the carpometacarpal joint and flexion of the metacarpophalangeal joint of the thumb.

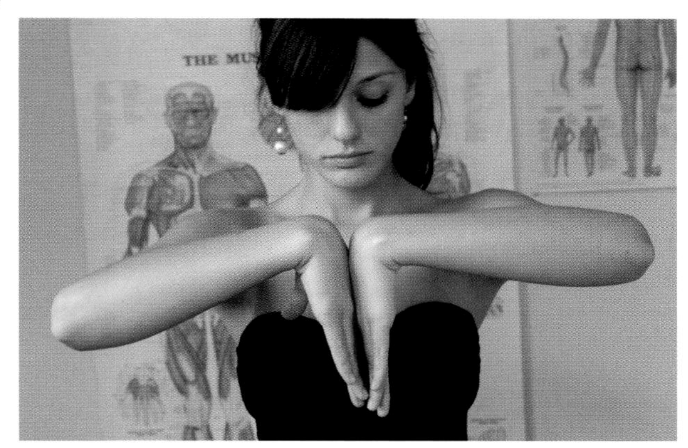

Fig. 17.26 Phalen's test

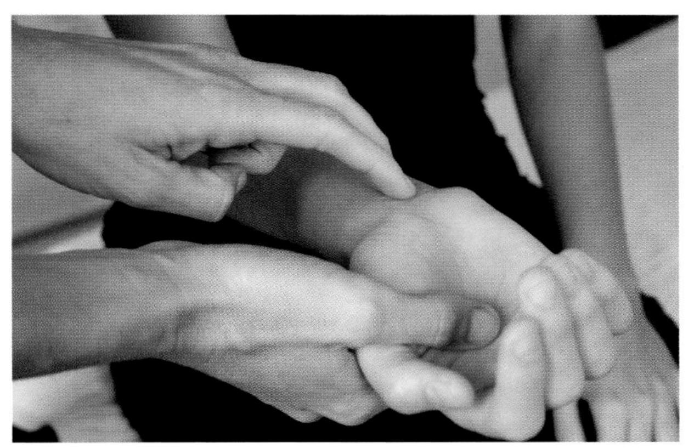

Fig. 17.27 Tinel's sign at the wrist

Special tests

If the client reports symptoms when performing a special test, ask the client to identify the exact location of the symptoms and confirm that they are the same as the symptoms described in the case history. Positive special test results should always be interpreted cautiously and in the context of other clinical findings (see Chapter 2).

PHALEN'S TEST

The client presses the backs of both hands together for up to one minute to maximally flex the wrists. Carpal tunnel is suggested if this position causes numbness and tingling in the thumb, index and middle finger (the median nerve distribution), wrist pain or weakness (see Figure 17.26).

TINEL'S SIGN

Tap over the median nerve in the carpal tunnel with the fingertips. Numbness, tingling or shooting pain into the thumb, index and middle finger (median nerve distribution) suggests median nerve neuropathy (see Figure 17.27).

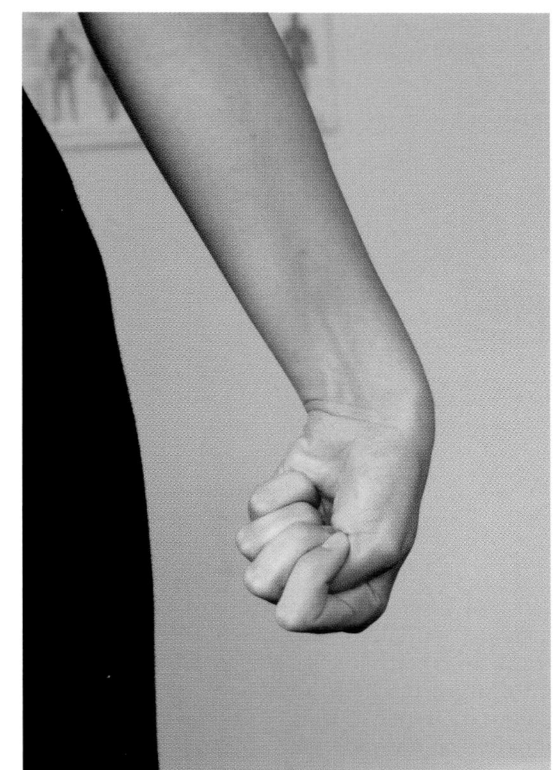

Fig. 17.28 Finkelstein's test

FINKELSTEIN'S TEST

Instruct the client to make a fist with the thumb tucked inside the other fingers and then to move the wrist to the ulnar side. Pain in the area of the abductor pollicus longus and extensor pollicus brevis tendons indicate stenosing tenosynovitis of these tendons of the thumb (de Quervain's tenosynovitis) (see Figure 17.28).

PALPATION

Palpate the radial styloid process on the lateral aspect of the wrist. The depression distal to the radial styloid process is the anatomical snuff box which is bordered posteriorly by the extensor pollicis longus tendon and anteriorly by the extensor pollicis brevis and abductor pollicis longus tendons. Scaphoid and trapezius form the floor. The scaphoid is the most commonly injured carpal bone. Tenderness in the snuffbox could indicate fractured scaphoid or de Quervain's tendinitis.

Medial to the styloid process of the radius on the anterior aspect of the wrist, palpate the radial artery and flexor carpi radialis tendon.

The tubercle on the dorsum of the radius (Lister's tubercle), the lunate, capitate and third metacarpal are in a straight line. This is a useful guide when palpating. The lunate is the most frequently dislocated bone in the wrist and the second most frequently fractured.

Locate the ulnar styloid process, the most prominent structure on the dorsum of the wrist, and the triquetrum in the proximal carpal row. The triquetrum is more easily palpated

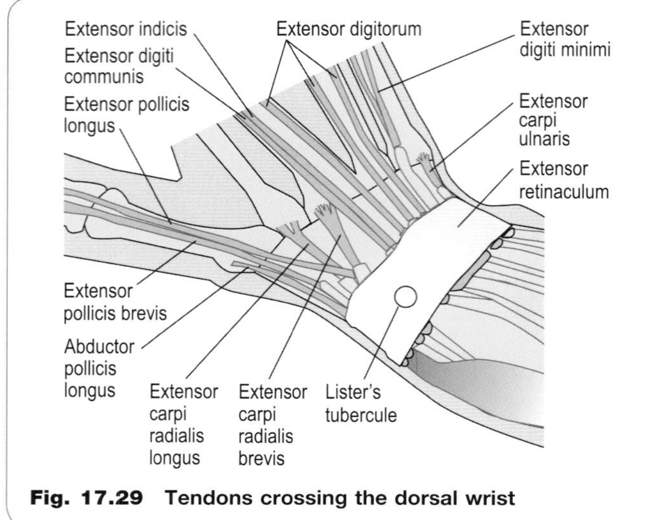

Fig. 17.29 Tendons crossing the dorsal wrist

when the wrist is radially deviated. The pisiform within the flexor carpi ulnaris tendon and the hook of the hamate can be palpated through the hypothenar muscles distal to the ulna. The hook of the hamate forms the lateral border of the tunnel of Guyton which transports the ulnar nerve and artery to the hand. The pulse of the ulnar artery may be felt just proximal to the hook of the hamate.

Palpate the flexor tendons as they cross the palm and any nodules in the palmar fascia. From Lister's tubercle on the dorsum of the distal radius, palpate the tendons of the extensor carpi radialis longus and brevis, abductor pollicis longus and extensor pollicis brevis on the radial side. On the ulnar side of Lister's tubercle, palpate tendons of the extensor pollicis longus, extensor indicis, extensor digitorum communis, extendor digitorum, extensor digiti minimi and extensor carpi ulnaris.

Palpate the thenar and the hypothenar eminences. The thenar muscles are the abductor pollicis brevis, opponens pollicis and flexor pollicis brevis; the hypothenar muscles are the abductor digiti minimi, opponens digiti minimi and flexor digiti minimi brevis.

REMEDIAL MASSAGE TREATMENT

Assessment of the wrist and hand provides essential information for development of treatment plans, including:

- client's suitability for remedial massage therapy
- duration of the condition (i.e. acute or chronic)
- severity of the condition (i.e. grade of injury; mild, moderate or severe pain)
- type(s) of tissues involved
- priorities for treatment if more than one injury or condition are present
- whether the signs and symptoms suggest a common condition of the wrist and hand
- special considerations for individual clients (e.g. client's preference for treatment types and styles, special population considerations).

The wrist and hand have little protection and are easily injured. They are most commonly injured by direct blows, either by falls to the outstretched hand or by catching a ball. Clients presenting for remedial massage therapy within the first 2 to 3 days after an injury should be checked for fracture. However, most clients wait until they are in the subacute and chronic phase before consulting remedial massage therapists for wrist and hand conditions and are often concurrently receiving treatment from other healthcare providers.

Many clients have repetitive strain injuries. Repetitive strain injury does not refer to a single diagnosis but rather encompasses a range of disorders that arise from repetitive movements, often in awkward positions for prolonged periods, including lateral epicondylitis (see Chapter 16), carpal tunnel syndrome, de Quervain's disease and tenosynovitis of the wrist or hand.[13]

OVERVIEW

Develop a short- and a long-term plan for each client. The short-term plan directs treatment to the highest priority (usually determined by symptoms). The long-term plan can be introduced when presenting symptoms have subsided. Long-term treatment focuses on contributing or predisposing factors such as underlying structural features and lifestyle factors. A significant part of both short-term and long-term treatment involves educating clients about likely causal or aggravating factors and guiding the management of these factors. If massage therapy is being used in conjunction with other treatments it is important to communicate with other treating practitioners.

TENDINITIS AND TENOSYNOVITIS

Any of the flexor and extensor tendons around the wrist may become injured with excessive activity, particularly with typing or using a computer mouse. Tendons commonly affected include abductor pollicis longus, extensor pollicis brevis, flexor digitorum superficialis and flexor pollicis longus. It is thought that repeated microtears may occur in the tendon or tendon sheath that initially cause inflammation but with continued overuse eventually lead to degeneration of the collagen fibre structure. However, the pathophysiology remains unclear and some authors have suggested that repetitive strain injuries may be diffuse neuromuscular illnesses involving peripheral tissues and affecting the regulatory structures of the central nervous system.[13, 14]

Assessment

HISTORY

The client presents with pain usually on the dorsum of the hand aggravated by movement. The pain develops gradually and may begin with stiffness after rest. There is usually a history of repetitive overuse (e.g. typing, writing, using a computer mouse).

FUNCTIONAL TESTS

Cervical AROM tests do not reproduce wrist or hand symptoms.

Shoulder AROM tests do not reproduce wrist or hand symptoms.

Key assessment findings for tendinitis/tenosynovitis

- History of repetitive overuse
- Functional tests:
  - AROM painful when the involved muscle contracts
  - PROM painful when involved tendons are passively stretched
  - RROM positive for involved muscles
  - Resisted and length tests positive for involved muscles
  - Special tests: Finkelstein's test positive for de Quervain's tenosynovitis
- Palpation: linear tenderness along the tendon. Fibrotic tissue is usually palpable. Crepitus is often present in tenosynovitis.

Elbow AROM tests do not usually reproduce wrist or hand symptoms.

Wrist tests

AROM is painful when the involved muscles are contracted.
PROM may be painful as the involved muscles are passively stretched.
RROM is painful for involved muscles.
Resisted and length tests are positive for involved muscles.
Special tests: Tinel's sign and Phalen's test are negative.

PALPATION

Tenderness is elicited along the line of the tendon as it crosses the wrist and extends above the wrist. Fibrotic tissue is often palpable in the tendon or tendon sheath. Fine crepitus may be palpated (and heard) when the involved tendon moves.

Overview of treatment and management

Resting the affected tendon by avoiding the responsible activity helps manage symptoms. Acute presentations may require cryotherapy.

A typical remedial massage treatment for subacute or chronic tendinitis or tenosynovitis of the wrist includes:

- Swedish massage therapy to the wrist and hand, upper limb, neck and upper back.
- Remedial massage techniques including (see Table 17.4):
  - deep gliding frictions along the muscle fibres
  - cross-fibre frictions
  - soft tissue releasing techniques
  - deep transverse friction applied directly to the damaged tendon, which may help stimulate collagen production.
  - trigger point therapy
  - muscle stretching.
- Myofascial release including cross-arm techniques and the arm pull (see Chapter 8).
- Thermotherapy may be beneficial for pain relief.
- Other remedial techniques such as wrist joint articulation may also be introduced as required (see Chapter 7):
  - Wrist pronated longitudinal thenar kneading
  - Wrist pronated traction and circumduction
  - Wrist semi-supinated traction and circumduction
  - Wrist overhead traction and supination
  - Metacarpophalangeal and interphalangeal mobilisation

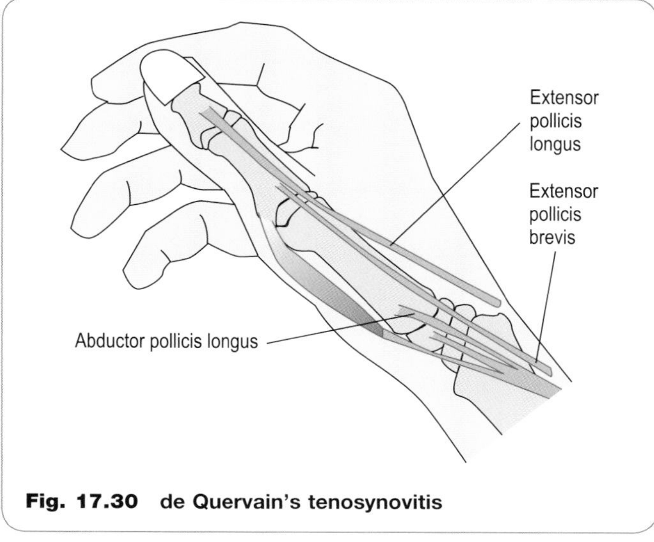

Fig. 17.30 de Quervain's tenosynovitis

  - Metacarpal shearing
  - Rotation and traction of phalanges.

Correct underlying biomechanical and predisposing factors if possible (e.g. upper crossed syndrome, rounded shoulder posture, imbalance of the forearm muscles).

CLIENT EDUCATION

Advise the client to eliminate or avoid all aggravating activities to reduce the stress on the damaged tendons. A wrist splint or brace is sometimes worn to limit wrist movement and rest the affected tendons. Rehabilitative exercises are designed to improve overall strength, endurance and flexibility in the muscles of the entire upper limb kinetic chain. This includes muscles of the neck, shoulder, elbow, wrist and hand. Initially a stretching program is introduced to restore pain-free range of motion. As soon as possible, strengthening exercises are introduced (e.g. using a squeeze ball or stretching an elastic band with the fingers). The emphasis is usually on restoring balance in the muscles that cross the wrist. Ergonomic and posture correction is usually required.

Refer for osseous manipulation and for additional physical therapy modalities such as ultrasound, phonophoresis or electrical stimulation if required.

DE QUERVAIN'S TENOSYNOVITIS

Tenosynovitis of the abductor pollicis longus and/or extensor pollicis brevis is known as de Quervain's tenosynovitis. It is commonly associated with repetitive overuse among people who perform repetitive hand movements, including typists, cashiers, massage therapists and mechanics. It also occurs in sports which involve gripping or throwing. It is sometimes associated with degenerative joint disease or rheumatoid arthritis of the thumb (see Figure 17.30).

Assessment

HISTORY

The onset of pain at the posterolateral aspect of the wrist and thumb is usually insidious. The client reports a history of

Table 17.4 Remedial massage techniques for muscles of the wrist and hand

Muscle	Soft tissue release	Trigger point	Deep transverse friction	Stretch	Corrective action	Home exercise
Abductor pollicis longus and brevis	Practitioner: applies static pressure to the taut band/lesion using fingers or thumbs as the client's thumb is slowly passively or actively abducted and adducted. In the dynamic variant, the practitioner performs a deep glide as the muscle is slowly lengthened (i.e. adducted). 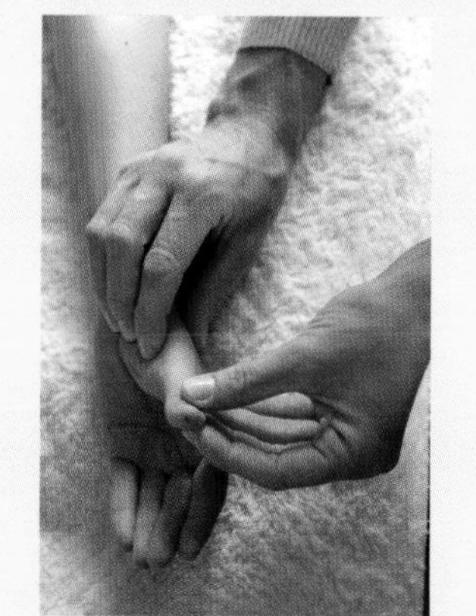 The technique can also be performed with passive or active abduction and adduction of the wrist.	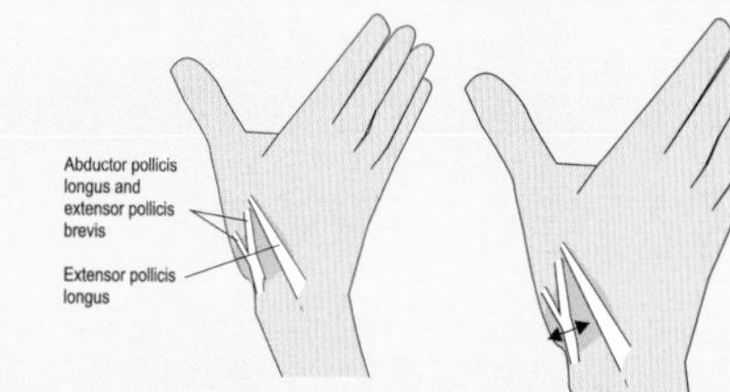 Not yet described		Passive stretch: Flex the client's thumb and adduct the client's wrist to their comfortable limit. Stretch all associated shortened muscles of the wrist and hand, upper limb, upper back and neck. 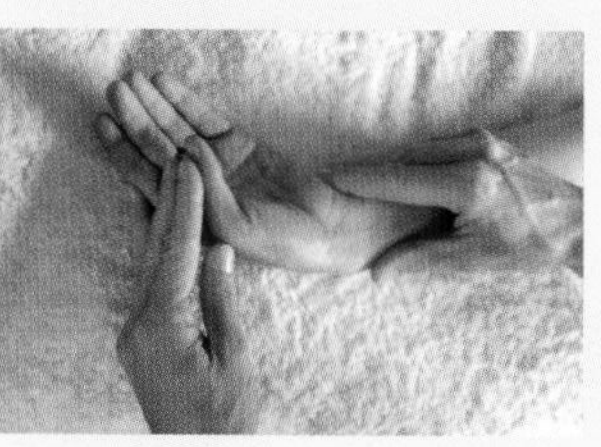	Avoid aggravating activity.	Flex the thumb and adduct the wrist as far as possible within pain tolerance. Hold for up to 30 seconds. Repeat 3 times. General mobilisation and strengthening exercises as indicated: • Gently make a fist and then spread the fingers as far as possible • Gentle mobilisations of the wrist (flexion, extension, rotation, abduction and adduction) • Strengthening exercises including squeeze ball and elastic band exercises 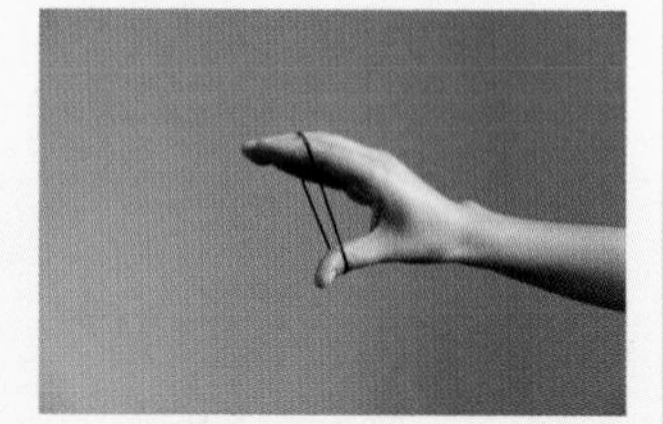

Table 17.4 Remedial massage techniques for muscles of the wrist and hand—cont'd

Muscle	Soft tissue release	Trigger point	Deep transverse friction	Stretch	Corrective action	Home exercise
Extensor pollicis longus and brevis	Practitioner: applies static pressure to the taut band/ lesion using fingers or thumbs as the thumb is slowly passively or actively flexed or and extended. In the dynamic variant, the practitioner performs a deep glide along the muscle as it lengthens (i.e. flexes). The technique can also be performed with passive or active abduction and adduction of the wrist.	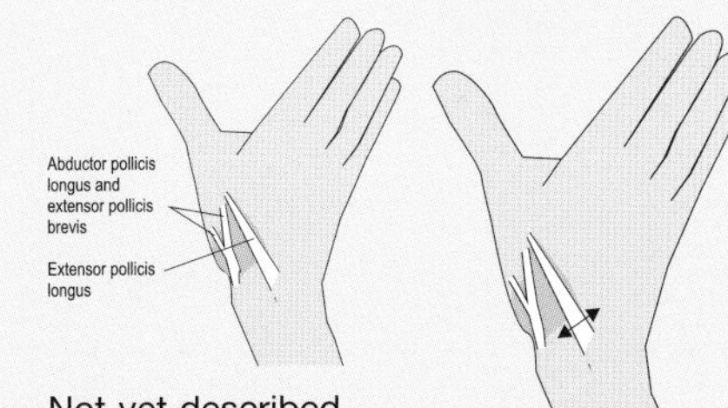 Not yet described		Passive stretch: The thumb is flexed from the carpometacarpal joint and the wrist adducted and flexed. 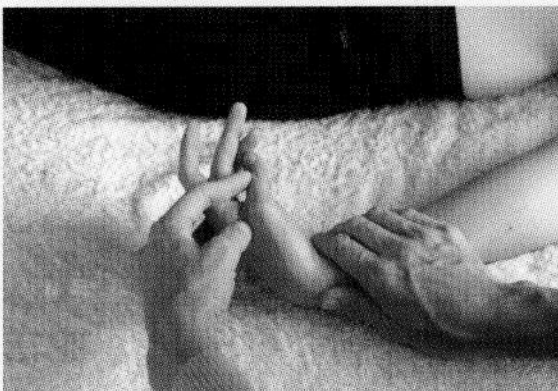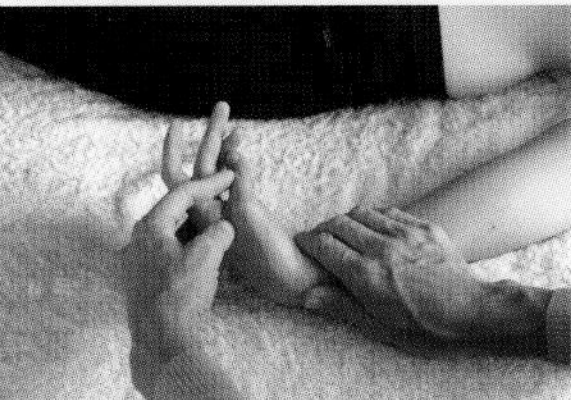 Stretch all associated shortened muscles of the wrist and hand, upper limb, upper back and neck.	Avoid aggravating activities. Correct workplace ergonomics.	Make a fist with the thumb inside and slowly flex and adduct the wrist. Stretch within pain tolerance. Hold for up to 30 seconds. Repeat 3 times. Include general mobilisation and strengthening exercises as indicated.
Flexor pollicis longus	Practitioner: applies static pressure to the taut band/ lesion using fingers or thumbs as the thumb is slowly passively or actively flexed and/or extended. In the dynamic variant, the practitioner performs a deep glide along the muscle as it lengthens (i.e. extends).			Passive stretch: The practitioner extends the thumb from the distal phalanx. Stretch all associated shortened muscles of the wrist and hand, upper limb, upper back and neck. 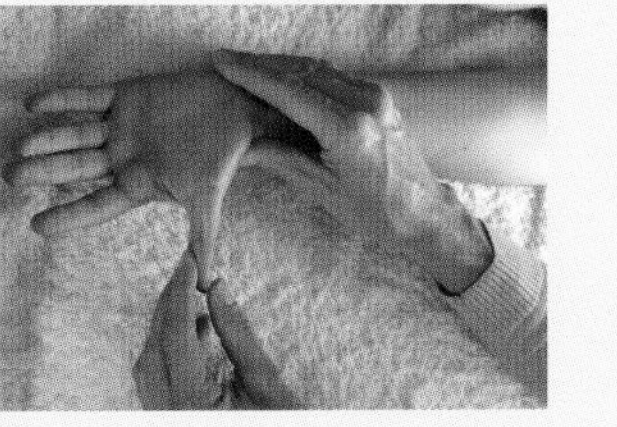	Avoid prolonged tight gripping.	Hold the end of the thumb and stretch it slowly to the side as far as you can comfortably. Hold for up to 30 seconds. Repeat 3 times. Include general mobilisation and strengthening exercises as indicated.

Wrist flexors and wrist extensors are described in Chapter 16.

Key assessment findings for de Quervain's tenosynovitis

- History: insidious onset of pain on the posterolateral aspect of the wrist; pain aggravated by movement of the thumb, relieved by rest; history of repetitive overuse
- Functional tests:
  - AROM painful thumb extension and/or abduction
  - PROM painful thumb flexion and adduction (passive stretch of involved tendon)
  - RROM positive for resisted thumb extension and/or abduction
  - Resisted and length tests positive for involved muscles
  - Special tests: Finkelstein's test positive
- Palpation: local tenderness or pain. Fibrotic tissue (± crepitus) is often palpable.

repetitive overuse such as excessive typing, use of a computer mouse, palm-held computer or mobile phone (Blackberry thumb), playing a keyboard or playing a racquet sport. The pain is described as aggravated by movement of the thumb and relieved by rest and may radiate several centimetres up the forearm.

FUNCTIONAL TESTS

Cervical AROM tests do not reproduce wrist and thumb symptoms.
Shoulder AROM tests do not reproduce wrist and thumb symptoms.
Elbow AROM tests do not reproduce wrist and thumb symptoms.

Wrist and hand tests:

AROM painful for thumb extension and/or abduction. Crepitus may be present.
PROM may be painful for thumb flexion and/or adduction when the tendon is passively stretched.
RROM painful for thumb extension and/or abduction.
Resisted and length tests positive for involved muscles.
Special tests: Finkelstein's test positive.

PALPATION

There is local tenderness on palpation of the involved tendons. Fibrotic tissue is often palpable in extensor pollicis brevis and/or abductor pollicis longus tendons.

Overview of treatment and management

Remedial massage treatment is similar for all cases of tendinitis or tenosynovitis. Advise the client to eliminate or avoid all aggravating activities. Traditionally ice and splints have been prescribed for acute inflammation.

A typical remedial massage treatment for subacute or chronic de Quervain's tenosynovitis includes:

- Swedish massage therapy to the wrist and hand, upper limb, neck and upper back.
- Remedial massage techniques for muscles (see Table 17.4) including:
  - deep gliding frictions along the muscle fibres
  - cross-fibre frictions
  - soft tissue releasing techniques
  - deep transverse friction applied directly to the damaged tendon, which may help stimulate collagen production
  - trigger point therapy
  - muscle stretching.
- Myofascial release including cross-arm techniques and the arm pull (see Chapter 8).
- Thermotherapy may assist with pain relief. Episodes of acute inflammation may require cryotherapy.
- Other remedial techniques such as wrist and thumb joint mobilisation may be introduced as required including (see Chapter 7):
  - wrist pronated longitudinal thenar kneading
  - wrist pronated traction and circumduction
  - wrist semi-supinated traction and circumduction
  - wrist overhead traction and supination
  - metacarpophalangeal and interphalangeal mobilisation
  - metacarpal shearing
  - rotation and traction of phalanges.

Correct any underlying or predisposing factors where possible.

CLIENT EDUCATION

Advise the client to reduce or eliminate aggravating activities. The use of corticosteroid injection may provide short-term relief.[15, 16]

Home exercises

Advise the client to begin stretching and strengthening the wrist muscles as soon as pain permits: stretch the wrist in all directions, stretch the thumb in flexion and opposition and progress to include wrist, thumb and grip-strengthening exercises.[8] Finally exercises to address muscle imbalances of the entire upper limb are introduced.

Refer for osseous manipulation and for additional physical therapy modalities such as ultrasound, phonophoresis or electrical stimulation. Occasionally surgical decompression is required if conservative treatment fails to resolve the symptoms.

CARPAL TUNNEL SYNDROME

The carpal tunnel is the space between the carpal bones and the flexor retinaculum which runs across the anterior aspect of the wrist between the pisiform and the hamate medially and the trapezium and scaphoid laterally. The tunnel transports nine flexor tendons (flexor pollicis longus, four flexor digitorum superficialis tendons and four flexor digitorum profundus tendons) and the median nerve which is the most superficial and consequently most likely to be compressed against the flexor retinaculum[17] (see Figure 17.31 on p 331).

Carpal tunnel syndrome is an entrapment neuropathy of the median nerve as it passes through the carpal tunnel. It may be accompanied by wrist flexor tendinopathy. It occurs most commonly in 40- to 60-year-olds and in females five times more commonly than males.[8] The higher incidence in women than men may be related to women being more highly represented in jobs that are at a high risk for carpal tunnel syndrome like data entry, packing and cleaning. Carpal tunnel syndrome is frequently work-related and may not be solely physiological. Psychosocial, financial and legal issues often play a role in evaluation and management.[18]

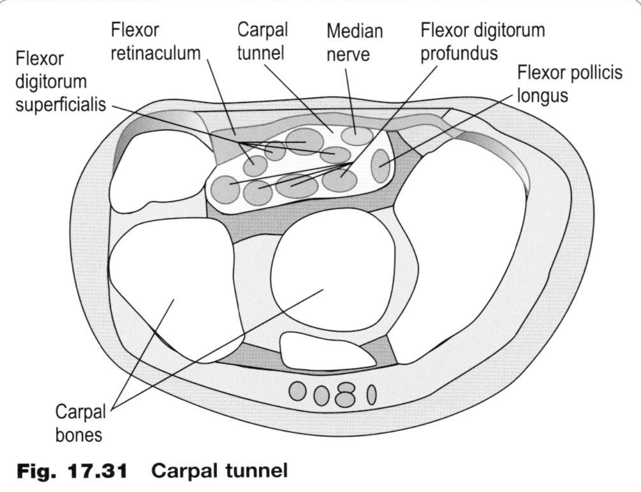

Fig. 17.31 Carpal tunnel

Key assessment findings for carpal tunnel syndrome

- History of intermittent paraesthesia in the thumb, index and middle finger; wrist and hand pain; night pain with morning stiffness, weakness and/or numbness. The client describes shaking their hands to relieve the symptoms.
- Functional tests:
  - AROM positive for wrist flexion and pronation (± crepitus)
  - PROM positive for wrist flexion (± crepitus)
  - RROM negative unless associated wrist flexor tendinopathy
  - Special tests: Phalen's test, Tinel's sign positive
- Palpation: local tenderness or pain. Fibrotic tissue is often palpable.

A number of causes have been identified including:

- Mechanical compression: The flexor tendons are enclosed within a synovial sheath to reduce friction as they bend when the wrist is fully flexed or extended. When overused inflammation or adhesions may develop between the tendons and their synovial sheaths causing tenosynovitis. The increasing size of the tendon sheaths reduces space in the tunnel causing compression of the median nerve. Other causes of mechanical compression include degenerative joint disease, neuroma and ganglia that develop in the tunnel, subluxation of the lunate bone, constant vibration (e.g. using jack hammer) and trauma.
- Fluid retention/metabolic disease (e.g. diabetes, obesity, fluid retention during pregnancy).

Assessment

HISTORY

The most common symptoms of carpal tunnel syndrome include intermittent numbness, paraesthesia and pain in the median nerve distribution of the hand (i.e. the radial half of the palm including the thumb, index and middle fingers). Symptoms are often worse at night because people have a tendency to sleep with their wrists flexed, which increases compression within the tunnel. A wrist splint worn at night often alleviates the symptoms.

As the condition progresses there is likely to be a decrease in tactile sensitivity in the fingertips. Motor symptoms usually develop and are indicated by clumsiness, loss of dexterity and eventually a weakening of hand grip strength. If the condition progresses, it is also common to see a decrease in two-point discrimination ability, further sensory loss, and wasting of the thenar muscles. Sensory symptoms (paraesthesia, numbness and pain) are usually the first to appear because the median nerve at the wrist is composed of over 90% sensory fibres. If motor symptoms are present it is usually an indication of the severity of nerve compression.

FUNCTIONAL TESTS

Cervical AROM tests do not reproduce symptoms.
Shoulder AROM tests do not reproduce symptoms.
Elbow AROM tests do not reproduce symptoms.

Wrist and hand tests

AROM positive for wrist flexion ± pronation. Crepitus may be present.
PROM positive for wrist flexion. Crepitus may be present.
RROM negative unless there is accompanying flexor tendinopathy.
Special tests: Phalen's test, Tinel's sign positive. Note that evidence on the utility of these tests is highly variable.[7]

PALPATION

Swelling may be palpable in the carpal tunnel. In long-standing cases thenar and hypothenar muscles may atrophy.

Overview of treatment and management

Advise the client to eliminate or avoid the aggravating condition. Traditionally, ice and splints are prescribed in the acute presentations. Night splints may be recommended.

A typical remedial massage treatment for subacute or chronic carpal tunnel syndrome includes:

- Swedish massage therapy to the wrist and hand, upper limb, neck and upper back.
- Remedial massage techniques (see Tables 17.4 and 16.5) including:
  - deep gliding frictions along the muscle fibres (e.g. wrist flexors and pronators)
  - cross-fibre friction to the flexor retinaculum and bellies of muscles that pass through the carpal tunnel
  - soft tissue releasing techniques
  - deep transverse friction applied directly to the damaged tendon, which may help stimulate collagen production
  - trigger point therapy
  - muscle stretching, including stretching of the wrist flexor muscles.
- Myofascial release to the flexor retinaculum:
  An example of a stretching technique for the flexor retinaculum is illustrated in Figure 17.32 on p 332: The client's hand is supinated. The practitioner approaches distally and contacts either side of the flexor retinaculum with the pads of the thumbs, fingers resting on the dorsum of the hand. Gentle pressure is maintained for 3–5 minutes. The cross-arm technique and the arm pull (see Chapter 8) may also be beneficial.

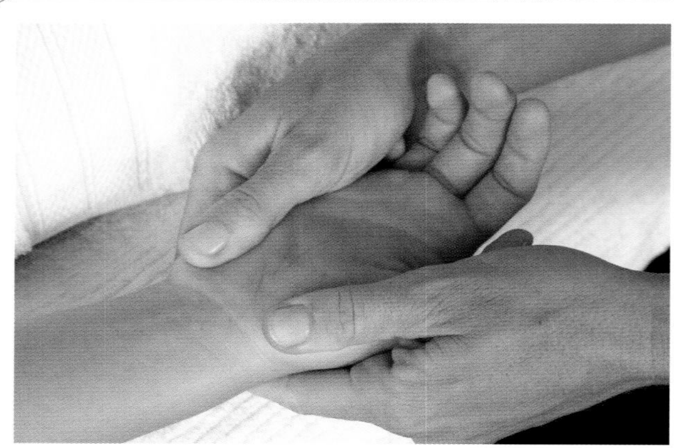

Fig. 17.32 **Myofascial release for the flexor retinaculum**

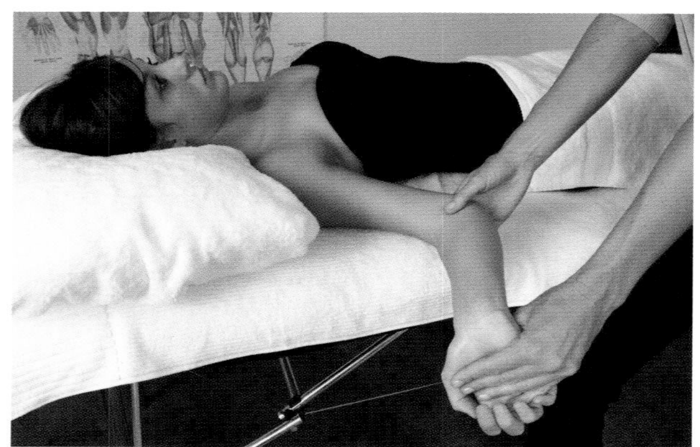

Fig. 17.33 **Median nerve stretch**

- Joint articulation techniques may be useful including (see Chapter 7):
  - wrist pronated longitudinal thenar kneading
  - wrist pronated traction and circumduction
  - wrist semi-supinated traction and circumduction
  - wrist overhead traction and supination
  - metacarpophalangeal and interphalangeal mobilisation
  - metacarpal shearing.
- Neural stretching for median nerve entrapment may be helpful. This procedure is designed to enhance mobility of the median nerve.

  The client is supine with their arms by their side. The wrist is in a neutral position. Take the client's upper limb through the following steps as long as the client remains symptom-free. As soon as symptoms are felt, return to the starting position. Note that this series of procedures can be done actively or passively.

  Begin with upper limb supinated, elbow extended.
  Flex elbow.
  Hyperextend wrist.
  Externally rotate shoulder.
  Repeat the cycle several times.

Caution: The main goal of treatment for carpal tunnel syndrome is to reduce nerve compression. You should be cautious of any techniques that place further pressure on this region. It is also important to evaluate other regions of median nerve entrapment as they may aggravate carpal tunnel syndrome symptoms. These include the lower cervical spine, between the anterior and middle scalene muscles, under the clavicle, under the pectoralis minor muscle, near the anterior aspect of the elbow and between the two heads of the pronator teres muscle (a third of the way along the forearm from the cubital fossa; pronator teres attaches to the medial epicondyle). The absence of night pain usually indicates entrapment in a location proximal to the carpal tunnel.

Correct any underlying or predisposing factors. It is important to address the muscles of the entire upper limb kinetic chain.

CLIENT EDUCATION

If repetitive overuse is a likely causative factor, clients should eliminate or reduce aggravating activities. Many of the carpal tunnel syndrome rehabilitation strategies have focused on work equipment and ergonomics. Interventions proposed include ergonomic re-education, keyboard supports and computer mouse and tool redesign. Diuretics may be used if compression is due to fluid retention. Night wrist splints may be helpful. Surgery is frequently performed, most commonly an incision release of the flexor retinaculum.

Home exercises

Stretching and strengthening the wrist muscles, including stretching the wrist in all directions, stretching the neck, shoulder, elbow, hand and fingers. Progress to include grip-strengthening exercises (e.g. squeeze ball) and strengthening exercises for pronators (except in cases where pronation aggravates symptoms).[8] Exercises to correct muscular imbalances of the entire upper limb, upper back and neck should be introduced as required.

A study by Moraska et al[19] investigated the effects of a general massage protocol for carpal tunnel syndrome compared with a targeted massage treatment. Twenty-seven subjects with carpal tunnel syndrome participated in the 6-week study. The authors found that subjective measures associated with carpal tunnel syndrome improved for both groups, but that improvements in grip strength were only evident in clients in the targeted massage group. Carpal bone mobilisation has also been found to be beneficial.[20, 21]

SPRAINS

Ligament sprains are common in contact sports and falls onto the outstretched hand and most are hyperextension injuries. Because of the pain and swelling it may be difficult to distinguish from a fracture initially.

Assessment

HISTORY

The client describes a traumatic injury to the wrist, often during a contact sport or from a fall onto the outstretched hand. The client may describe popping or tearing at the time of the trauma. Pain is felt immediately and swelling follows approximately one hour later.

Key assessment findings for wrist sprain

- History of trauma, especially hyperextension of the wrist; immediate pain followed by swelling.
- Functional tests:
  - AROM decreased on all wrist movements
  - PROM decreased on all wrist movements
  - RROM negative unless associated muscle strain
  - Special tests: negative
- Palpation: local tenderness or pain. There may be excessive joint movement.

FUNCTIONAL TESTS

Cervical AROM tests do not reproduce wrist symptoms.
Shoulder tests do not reproduce wrist symptoms.
Elbow AROM tests do not reproduce wrist symptoms.

Wrist tests

AROM decreased in all ranges.
PROM decreased in all ranges.
RROM may be positive if there is associated muscle strain.
Resisted and length tests may be positive for affected muscles if there is associated muscle strain.
Special tests negative.

PALPATION

Palpation at the site of injury elicits tenderness or pain. If ligaments have been stretched or completely torn, the affected joints have excessive movement.

Overview of treatment and management

In the acute phase, apply ice, compression and elevation as required to the sprained ligament. The area is usually strapped for 3 to 4 weeks if severe. Commence isometric strengthening exercises as soon as pain permits.

A typical remedial massage treatment for subacute or chronic sprains of the wrist and hand includes:

- Swedish massage therapy to the wrist and hand, upper limb, neck and upper back.
- Remedial massage techniques (caution: make sure that injured ligaments are not stretched during treatment).
- Deep transverse friction to the site of injury.
- Myofascial release techniques (see Chapter 8).
- Joint mobilisation of the wrist and hand as required including (see Chapter 7):
  - wrist pronated traction and circumduction
  - wrist semi-supinated traction and circumduction
  - wrist overhead traction and supination
  - metacarpophalangeal and interphalangeal mobilisation
  - metacarpal shearing
  - rotation and traction of phalanges.
- Thermotherapy may provide pain relief.
- Muscle-specific techniques for associated muscle spasm, including (see Table 16.5 and Table 17.4):
  - deep gliding frictions along the muscle fibres
  - cross-fibre frictions
  - soft tissue releasing techniques
  - trigger point therapy
  - muscle stretching.

Correct any underlying or predisposing factors where possible.

CLIENT EDUCATION

Advise the client to reduce or eliminate aggravating activities. The use of anti-inflammatory medication is controversial. Corticosteroid injection may provide short-term pain relief.[15, 16]

Home exercises

Encourage the client to begin exercises as soon as they can be tolerated. Begin with isometric exercises such as gripping and squeezing a ball. Progress to strengthening exercises of the wrist extensors, flexors, pronators and supinators and exercises for proprioception.

SPRAINED THUMB

The thumb is commonly sprained in sports. For example, the thumb may be forced back during a fend in rugby or a mistimed basketball catch. Firm strapping is required to support the thumb base but it may be modified on return to play to allow some degree of movement and protection without necessarily permitting full abduction. A severe sprain may rupture the ulnar collateral ligament leaving the joint liable to further damage. Surgical repair may be required.

SPRAINED FINGER

A sprained finger may be extremely painful and persist for up to a year. Participation in sporting activities is still permitted, although in contact sports protective strapping may be required as much for confidence as for healing. In cricket, for example, extra padding inside the glove may be required. As a general rule, hand and finger movements are encouraged as soon as possible after injury and there have to be strong medical reasons for immobilising any part of the hand for long periods. In any case, only the affected finger should be immobilised. Stiffness of the fingers may persist after sprains or fractures and can cause considerable disability.

Treatment

Client should make every effort to move the hand. Passive movements and stretches during convalescence are essential and massage is useful.

MALLET FINGER

A blow to the finger, such as can occur in cricket, basketball or goal keeping, may sprain the interphalangeal joints or rupture the extensor tendon insertion into the terminal phalanx. This causes the end of the finger to develop a mallet deformity (see Figure 17.7 on p 317).

Treatment

A straight finger splint worn for about 4 to 6 weeks and followed by persistent exercise ensures recovery with minimal loss of movement. Massage therapy may be beneficial in the rehabilitation phase.

FRACTURES AND DISLOCATIONS

Fractures are usually obvious because of the pain and deformity following injury. Fracture of the distal radius (Colles' fracture) is the commonest of all fractures. It usually occurs as a result of a fall onto the outstretched arm, forcing the hand backwards and upwards. The lower part of the radius is displaced dorsally (dinner fork deformity of the wrist contour). Fracture of the scaphoid, the most common carpal fracture, can also occur from falls onto the outstretched hand. It is a common injury in roller-blading, skating and skiing. Initially fractures may be difficult to distinguish from wrist sprains. Swelling occurs for about 24 hours and then may subside. The most useful diagnostic sign for scaphoid fracture is pain on direct pressure to the floor of the anatomical snuffbox. The blood flow to the scaphoid is easily compromised and fractures tend to heal poorly.

Minor fractures of the fingers are treated simply by taping two adjacent fingers together. Contact sports are excluded but considerable activity and general training can be continued. Some fractures require complex surgical wiring and all suspected fractures should be X-rayed.

The lunate is the most commonly dislocated carpal bone. It usually occurs as a result of a fall onto the thenar eminence which forces the lunate anteriorly as the wrist is forcefully extended. In some cases anterior lunate dislocation is associated with median nerve compression which can cause paraesthesia in the thumb, index and middle fingers. Refer all suspected dislocations for further investigation.

DEGENERATIVE JOINT DISEASE AND RHEUMATOID ARTHRITIS

Both degenerative joint disease and rheumatoid arthritis can affect the wrist and hand. Degenerative joint disease is a common presenting condition in older clients or those with previous significant trauma or history of overuse. The distal interphalangeal joints are most affected and Heberden's nodes may develop in affected joints (see Figure 17.6 on p 317). Treatment involves finding a balance between activity and rest to keep the joints mobile without causing joint inflammation. Remedial massage therapy usually consists of Swedish massage to the entire upper limb and lower cervical and upper thoracic spines, local heat applications (e.g. hot wax treatments), gentle joint articulation, myofascial release techniques and muscle-focused techniques, including muscle stretches. In one study 22 adults with wrist and hand arthritis were randomly assigned to the two groups: one received a 15-minute massage once a week and performed daily self-massage at home for 4 weeks; the other group received standard treatment for arthritis during the period. The massage group had lower anxiety and depressed mood scores, less pain and greater grip strength compared with that of the control group at the end of the study period.[22] Recommendations for arthritis of the wrist and hand include avoiding aggravating conditions, heat applications at home, stretching exercises and referral for dietary modification and supplementation (e.g. glucosamine).

Rheumatoid arthritis affects women more than men and usually begins when the client is between 20 and 40 years of age. The first symptoms are usually in the hands and wrists. Typically the client reports waking with swelling and pain, especially in the proximal and interphalangeal joints. Symptoms occur in both hands and several joints are involved. Swelling and pain are not related to activity. In severe cases, ulnar deviation of the metacarpophalangeal joints and swan-neck deformity may develop (see Figure 17.9 on p 319). Systemic signs such as fatigue and night sweats also accompany joint symptoms. In the subacute and chronic phases, remedial massage therapy is directed to symptomatic relief. Treatments can include Swedish massage, heat applications, gentle joint articulation and myofascial releasing techniques. Clients may be referred to a general medical practitioner, naturopath, herbalist or acupuncturist for further treatment.

A comparison of clinical presentation and treatments of degenerative joint disease and rheumatoid arthritis of the wrist and hand is presented in Table 17.5.

Table 17.5 Comparison of degenerative joint disease and rheumatoid arthritis of the wrist and hand

	Degenerative joint disease	**Rheumatoid arthritis**
Pathology	Breakdown of articular cartilage, subchondral bone sclerosis, osteophyte formation	Autoimmune disease, synovial membrane thickens and produces pannus that corrodes cartilage, joints may fuse
Age of onset	Middle aged and elderly	20 to 40 years
Gender	Males = females	Females > males
Joints affected	Weight-bearing joints asymmetrically In hands, distal interphalangeal joints most affected, Heberden's nodes may be present	Small joints of hands, wrists, elbows symmetrically Metacarpophalangeal and proximal interphalangeal joints most affected. In late stage, Bouchard's nodes, ulnar deviation of fingers and swan neck deformity may be present
Systemic signs	No	Yes
Treatment	Swedish massage, thermotherapy, myofascial release, remedial massage techniques for associated muscle imbalance (weight loss, shock-absorbing footwear is recommended for DJD of the low back and joints of the lower limb), supplementation (e.g. glucosamine, celery seed extract)	In subacute or chronic phase, Swedish massage, thermotherapy, myofascial release, remedial massage techniques for associated muscle imbalance, refer for dietary modification, supplementation, acupuncture

KEY MESSAGES

- Assessment of clients with conditions of the wrist and hand involves case history, outcome measures, postural analysis, functional tests and palpation.
- Assessment findings may indicate the type of tissue involved (contractile or inert: muscle, joint, fascia, ligament), duration of condition (acute or subacute) and severity (grade).
- Assessment findings may indicate a common presenting condition such as tendinitis/tenosynovitis, de Quervain's tendinitis and carpal tunnel syndrome.
- Assessment findings also indicate client perception of injury and preferences for treatment.
- Consider Clinical Guidelines, available evidence and client preferences when planning therapy.
- Although serious conditions of the wrist and hand are rare, be vigilant for red flags (e.g. indications of fractures, dislocations, infections and vascular compromise) during assessment.
- The selection of remedial massage techniques depends on assessment results. Swedish massage to the wrist and hand, upper limb, neck and upper back may be followed by muscle techniques (e.g. deep gliding, cross-fibre frictions, soft tissue releasing techniques, trigger point therapy, deep transverse friction and muscle stretching), joint mobilisation, myofascial release and thermotherapy as indicated.
- Educating clients about likely causal and predisposing factors and exercise rehabilitation are essential parts of remedial massage therapy.
- Over time, increase the client self-help component of treatment wherever possible to reduce likelihood of recurrence and/or to promote health maintenance and illness prevention.

Review questions

1. Name the nine tendons that pass through the carpal tunnel.
2. What is the most commonly fractured bone in the wrist? What is the most useful diagnostic indicator for a fracture of this bone?
3. De Quervain's tendinitis commonly involves strains of:
   a) abductor pollicis longus and brevis
   b) extensor carpi radialis
   c) flexor pollicis longus
   d) extensor pollicis longus and brevis
4. List three conditions that could be classified as repetitive strain injuries.
5. The lunate is the most commonly dislocated bone of the wrist. What is the usual mechanism of injury for its dislocation?
6. A resisted test of the wrist extensor muscles produces pain at the dorsum of the wrist. This result suggests
   a) ligament strain
   b) lateral epicondylitis
   c) wrist extensor tendinitis/tenosynovitis
   d) degenerative joint disease of the wrist
7. Special tests that may reproduce the symptoms of carpal tunnel include:
   a) Apley's test
   b) Tinel's sign
   c) Phalen's test
   d) Finkelstein's test
8. Carpal tunnel syndrome is often caused by mechanical compression of the median nerve. By what other mechanisms can carpal tunnel syndrome occur?
9. The median nerve at the wrist is composed of sensory and motor fibres. Compression of the median nerve in the carpal tunnel can alter:
   i) sensation in ______________________________
   ii) motor activity in ______________________________
10. List three different signs or symptoms that can be useful in distinguishing degenerative joint disease from rheumatoid arthritis of the wrist and hand.
11. List five muscle-specific remedial massage techniques that are commonly used in the treatment of de Quervain's tenosynovitis.
12. What remedial massage techniques are likely to be beneficial for a client with degenerative joint disease of the wrist or finger joints?

REFERENCES

1. Holder N, Clark H, Di Blasio J, et al. Cause, prevalence, and response to occupational musculoskeletal injuries reported by physical therapists and physical therapy assistants. Phys Ther 1999;79(7):642–52.
2. Albert W, Currie-Jackson N, Duncan C. A survey of musculoskeletal injuries amongst Canadian massage therapists. J Bodyw Mov Ther 2008;12(1):86–93.
3. Jang Y, Chi C, Tsauo J, et al. Prevalence and risk factors of work-related musculoskeletal disorders in massage practitioners. J Occup Rehabil 2006;16(3):425–38.
4. McMahon M, Stiller K, Trott P, et al. The prevalence of thumb problems in Australian physiotherapists is high: an observational study. Aust J Physiother 2006;52(4):287–92.
5. Forman T, Forman S, Rose N. A clinical approach to diagnosing wrist pain. Am Fam Physician 2005;72(9):1753–8.
6. Cleland J, Koppenhaver S. Netter's orthopaedic clinical examination: an evidence-based approach. 2nd edn. Philadelphia: Saunders; 2011.
7. Tortora G, Grabowski S. Principles of anatomy and physiology. Stafford, Qld: John Wiley; 2002.
8. Carnes M, Vizniak N. Quick reference evidence-based conditions manual. 3rd edn. Burnaby, BC: Professional Health Systems; 2009.
9. Glass L, editor. Occupational medicine practice guidelines: evaluation and management of common health problems and functional recovery in workers. Beverly Farms, MA: OEM Press; 2004.
10. Reese N, Bandy W. Joint range of motion and muscle length testing. Philadelphia: W.B. Saunders, 2002.
11. Kendall McCreary E, Provance P, McIntyre Rodgers M, et al. Muscles, testing and function, with posture and pain. 5th edn. Philadelphia: Lippincott Williams and Wilkins; 2005.
12. Hislop H, Montgomery J. Daniels and Worthingham's muscle testing: techniques of manual examination. 8th edn. Oxford: Saunders Elsevier; 2007.
13. van Tulder M, Malmivaara A, Koes B. Repetition strain injury: the Lancet 2007;369:1815–22.
14. Barr A. Tissue pathophysiology, neuroplasticity and motor behavioural changes in painful repetitive motion injuries. Man Ther 2006;11: 173–4.
15. McAuliffe JA. Tendon disorders of the hand and wrist. J Hand Surg Am 2010;35(5):846–53; quiz 53.

16. Peters-Veluthamaningal C, Winters JC, Groenier KH, et al. Randomised controlled trial of local corticosteroid injections for carpal tunnel syndrome in general practice. BMC Fam Pract 2010;11:54.
17. Lowe W. Orthopedic massage: theory and technique. Edinburgh: Mosby Elsevier; 2009.
18. Ring D, Kadzielski J, Fabian L, et al. Self-reported upper extremity health status correlates with depression. J Bone Joint Surg Am 2006; 88(9):1983–8.
19. Moraska A, Chandler C, Edmiston-Schaetzel A, et al. Comparison of a targeted and general massage protocol on strength, function, and symptoms associated with carpal tunnel syndrome: a randomized pilot study. J Altern Complement Med 2008;14(3):259–67.
20. O'Connor D, Marshall S, Massy-Westropp N. Non-surgical treatment (other than steroid injection) for carpal tunnel syndrome. Cochrane Database Syst Rev 2003;(1)CD003219.
21. Tal-Akabi A, Rushton A. An investigation to compare the effectiveness of carpal bone mobilisation and neurodynamic mobilisation as methods of treatment for carpal tunnel syndrome. Man Ther 2000;5(4):214–22.
22. Field T, Diego M, Hernandez-Reif M, et al. Hand arthritis pain is reduced by massage therapy. J Bodyw Mov Ther 2007;11(1):21–4.

The hip region 18

The content of this chapter relates to the following Units of Competency:

HLTREM503C Plan remedial massage treatment strategy
HLTREM504C Apply remedial massage assessment framework
HLTREM502C Provide remedial massage treatment
HLTREM505C Perform remedial massage health assessment

Health Training Package HLT07

Learning Outcomes

- Assess clients with conditions of the hip region for remedial massage, including identification of red and yellow flags.
- Assess clients for signs and symptoms associated with common conditions of the hip region (including muscle strains, degenerative joint disease and trochanteric bursitis) and treat and/or manage these conditions with remedial massage therapy.
- Develop treatment plans for clients with conditions of the hip region, taking assessment findings, duration and severity of the condition, likely tissue types, clinical guidelines, the best available evidence and client preferences into account.
- Develop short- and long-term treatment plans to address presenting symptoms, underlying conditions and predisposing factors, and to progressively increase the self-help component of therapy.
- Adapt remedial massage therapy to suit individual client needs based on duration and severity of injury, the client's age and gender, the presence of underlying condition and co-morbidities and other consideration for special population groups.

INTRODUCTION

True hip pathologies are a less common presenting condition to remedial massage clinics than pain referring to the lower limbs from the low back and for this reason assessment protocols should routinely include a scan of the low back. The age of the client is a particularly useful consideration in assessing hip complaints. Generally, older clients with hip pain are likely to have degenerative joint disease of the hip. (The hip is more susceptible to degeneration than to trauma.)[1] Young adults often present with muscle strains. All children presenting with hip or knee pain must be carefully assessed to rule out hip pathologies that require referral (see Table 18.1).

Childhood conditions of the hip are discussed in Chapter 21.

FUNCTIONAL ANATOMY

The hip or acetabulofemoral joint is a synovial ball and socket joint composed of the head of the femur and the acetabulum of the ilium. In normal activities the hip joint carries the greatest load of any joint in the body. In standing, the weight of the upper body is transmitted to the sacrum and then to the iliofemoral ligaments so that the body can remain in equilibrium with minimal muscle activity. The stability of the hip joint is enhanced by the depth of the acetabulum and the presence of the acetabular labrum (cartilaginous ring) and ligamentum teres, which keeps the head of the femur in the socket. Other ligaments of the hip joint include the pubofemoral ligament, ischiofemoral ligament, zona orbicularis and the transverse ligament of the acetabulum.

The pelvis contains five joints: two sacroiliac joints, the symphysis pubis and two acetabulofemoral joints (see Figure 18.1 on p 338). The acetabulofemoral joints are the most mobile joints of the pelvis and problems like degenerative joint disease of the hip or muscle imbalances (e.g. weak gluteus medius, gluteus maximus, quadriceps or hamstrings) disturb the biomechanics of the pelvis and the rate and rhythm of normal gait. The major muscles that move the hip joint include (see Figure 18.2 on p 338):

- Flexion
  - Iliopsoas
  - Rectus femoris
- Extension
  - Gluteus maximus
  - Hamstrings
- Abduction
  - Gluteus medius
  - Gluteus minimus
  - Tensor fasciae latae

Table 18.1 Hip conditions according to age group

Age of onset	Hip pathology
0–5 years	Congenital hip displacement (unilateral or bilateral dislocation, more common in female infants and breech babies)
5–10 years	Perthes' disease (idiopathic aseptic necrosis of the femoral capital epiphysis)
10–15 years	Slipped femoral capital epiphysis (affects tall and thin or obese boys)
20–40 years	Muscle strains
>40 years	Degenerative joint disease
>60 years	Degenerative joint disease, fracture of the neck of femur, Paget's disease (chronic disorder of the adult skeleton which affects normal bone remodelling. Localised areas of bone become soft, enlarged, brittle and prone to fracture)

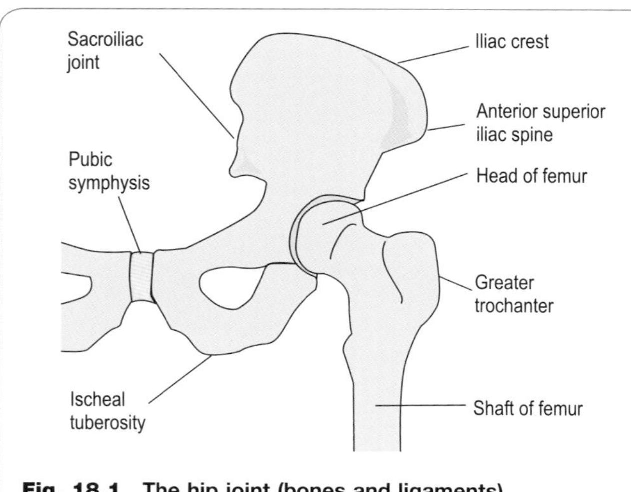

Fig. 18.1 The hip joint (bones and ligaments)

- Adduction
  - Adductor magnus
  - Adductor longus
  - Adductor brevis
  - Gracilis
- Lateral rotation
  - Piriformis
- Medial rotation
  - Gluteus minimus
  - Tensor fasciae latae

Major muscles of the hip are described in detail in Table 18.2.

Blood supply to the femoral head comes from three sources: medial circumflex femoral artery (the most important source), lateral circumflex artery, and artery of the ligamentum teres (a minor blood source in adults). The region is supplied by the femoral nerve (which supplies rectus femoris), the obturator nerve (anterior division of lumbar plexus) and the superior gluteal nerve (which supplies quadratus femoris). Dermatomes covering the region are illustrated in Figure 18.3.

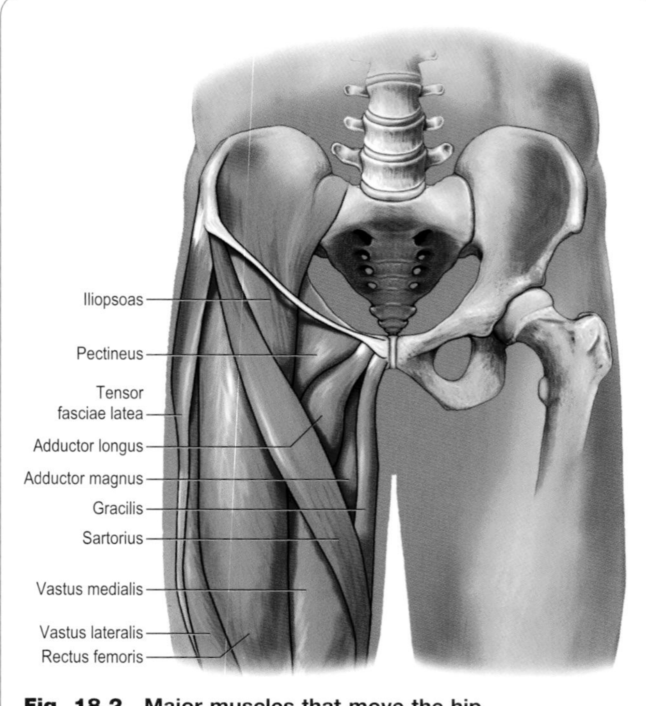

Fig. 18.2 Major muscles that move the hip

ASSESSMENT

The purpose of remedial massage assessment includes:

- determining the suitability of clients for massage (contraindications and red flags)
- determining the duration (acute or subacute), severity and types of tissues involved in the injury/condition
- determining whether symptoms fit patterns of common conditions.

Always refer clients for further assessment and treatment if there is any doubt about their suitability for remedial massage therapy.

Serious conditions of the hip in children and adolescents should not be missed.

- Hip pain in the presence of more than a low-grade fever or in children who appear ill should be assessed for a septic joint.
- Polyarticular pain suggests juvenile rheumatoid arthritis.
- Perthes' disease (avascular necrosis of the femoral head) causes hip pain in children 3 to 12 years old.
- Slipped capital femoral epiphysis occurs most commonly in 10- to 17-year-old boys who are either tall and slim or obese.

Principles of remedial massage assessment are discussed in Chapter 2. This section presents specific considerations for assessment of the hip region.

Table 18.2 Muscles that move the hip[2]

Muscles that move the hip	**Origin**	**Insertion**	**Action**
Hip flexors			
• Psoas major	Transverse processes and bodies of lumbar vertebrae	With iliacus into lesser trochanter of femur	Psoas major and iliacus muscles acting together flex thigh at hip joint, rotate thigh laterally and flex trunk on the hip
• Iliacus	Iliac fossa and sacrum	With psoas major into lesser trochanter of femur	
• Psoas minor	Bodies of T12 and L1 and intervening intervertebral disc	Fascia over psoas major and iliacus	Present in about half the population; when present sits on top of psoas major
• Rectus femoris (this is the only muscle of the quadriceps group that crosses the hip joint)	Anterior inferior iliac spine	Patella via quadriceps tendon and then tibial tuberosity via patellar ligament	Extends leg at knee joint; flexes thigh at hip joint
• Sartorius	Anterior inferior iliac spine	Medial surface of body of tibia	Flexes leg at knee joint; flexes, abducts and laterally rotates thigh at hip joint
Hip extensors			
• Gluteus maximus	Iliac crest, sacrum, coccyx and aponeurosis of sacrospinalis	Iliotibial band of fascia lata and lateral part of linea aspera under greater trochanter (gluteal tuberosity) of femur	Extends thigh at hip joint and laterally rotates thigh
Hamstrings			
• Biceps femoris	Long head arises from ischial tuberosity; short head arises from linea aspera of femur	Head of fibula and lateral condyle of tibia	Flexes leg at knee joint and extends thigh at hip joint
• Semitendinosus	Ischial tuberosity	Proximal part of medial surface of shaft of tibia	Flexes leg at knee joint and extends thigh at hip joint
• Semimembranosus	Ischial tuberosity	Medial condyle of tibia	Flexes leg at knee joint and extends thigh at hip joint
Hip abductors			
• Gluteus medius	Ilium	Greater trochanter of femur	Abducts thigh at hip joint and medially rotates thigh
• Gluteus minimus	Ilium	Greater trochanter of femur	Abducts thigh at hip joint and medially rotates thigh
• Tensor fasciae latae	Iliac crest	Tibia by way of the iliotibial tract	Flexes and abducts thigh at hip joint
Hip lateral rotators			
• Piriformis	Anterior sacrum	Superior border of greater trochanter of femur	Laterally rotates and abducts thigh at hip joint
• Obturator internus	Inner surface of obturator foramen, pubis and ischium	Greater trochanter of femur	Laterally rotates and abducts thigh at hip joint
• Obturator externus	Outer surface of obturator membrane	Deep depression inferior to greater trochanter (trochanteric fossa)	Laterally rotates and abducts thigh at hip joint
• Superior gemellus	Ischial spine	Greater trochanter of femur	Laterally rotates and abducts thigh at hip joint
• Inferior gemellus	Ischial tuberosity	Greater trochanter of femur	Laterally rotates and abducts thigh at hip joint
• Quadratus femoris	Ischial tuberosity	Elevation superior to mid-portion of intertrochanteric crest (quadrate tubercle) on posterior femur	Laterally rotates and stabilises hip joint

Continued

Table 18.2 Muscles that move the hip—cont'd

Muscles that move the hip	Origin	Insertion	Action
Hip adductors • Adductor longus	Pubic crest and pubic symphysis	Linea aspera of femur	Adducts and flexes thigh at hip joint and medially rotates thigh
• Adductor brevis	Inferior ramus of pubis	Superior half of linea aspera of femur	Adducts and flexes thigh at hip joint and medially rotates thigh
• Adductor magnus	Inferior ramus of pubis and ischium to ischial tuberosity	Linea aspera of femur	Adducts thigh at hip joint and medially rotates thigh; anterior part flexes thigh at hip joint, and posterior part extends thigh at hip joint
• Pectineus	Superior ramus of pubis	Pectineal line of femur, between lesser trochanter and linea aspera	Flexes and adducts thigh at hip joint

Assessment of the hip region

1. Case history
2. Outcome measures, e.g. The Patient Specific Scale
3. Postural analysis
4. Gait analysis
5. Functional tests
   Lumbar spine
   Active range of motion tests
   Flexion, extension, lateral flexion, rotation
   Hip joint
   Active range of motion tests
   Flexion, extension, abduction, adduction, internal rotation, external rotation
   Passive range of motion tests
   Flexion, extension, abduction, adduction, internal rotation, external rotation
   Resisted range of motion tests
   Flexion, extension, abduction, adduction, internal rotation, external rotation
   Resisted and length tests for specific muscles, including iliopsoas, rectus femoris, sartorius, gluteus maximus, hamstrings, gluteus medius, gluteus minimus, tensor fasciae latae, adductor muscles, piriformis and lateral hip rotators
   Special tests
   Patrick's/Fabere test
   Thomas test
   Trendelenburg test
   Ober's test
   Modified Ober's test
6. Palpation

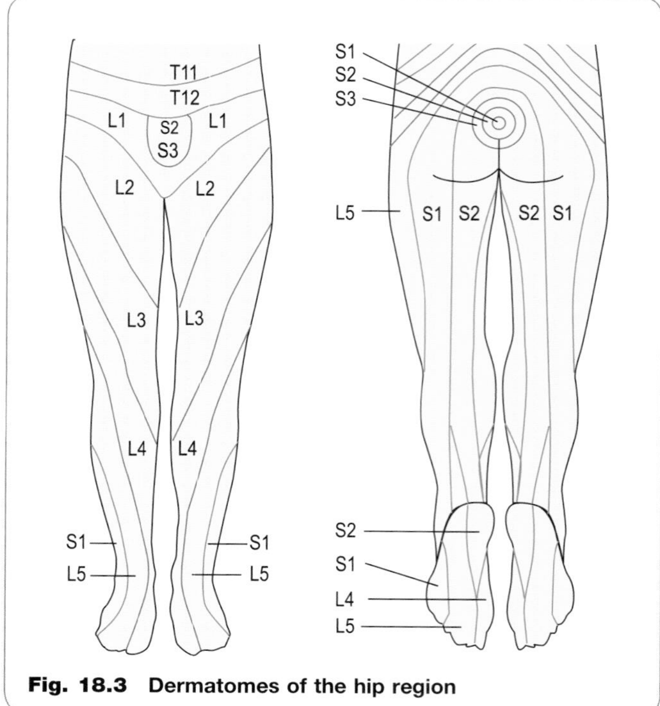

Fig. 18.3 Dermatomes of the hip region

CASE HISTORY

Information from case histories can alert practitioners to the presence of serious conditions requiring referral. Several complaints have also been found to be useful in identifying specific hip pathologies. For example, a complaint of clicking in the hip is strongly associated with acetabular labral tear.[3]

Reports of constant low back/buttock pain and ipsilateral groin pain are moderately helpful in diagnosing osteoarthritis of the hip. Use targeted questioning to collect the most useful and relevant information, including:

- Identifying red and yellow flags that require referral for further investigation (see Table 18.3 for red flags for acute hip pain in adults).
- Identifying the exact location of the symptoms by asking clients to point to the site of pain.
- Determining if the pain is likely to have a mechanical cause. (Is the pain associated with rest or activity, certain

Table 18.3 Red flags for acute hip pain in adults[4]

Feature or risk factor	Condition
Symptoms and signs of infection (e.g. fever, malaise, night sweats) Risk factors for infection (e.g. underlying disease process, immunosuppression, penetrating wound)	Infection (e.g. septic arthritis, osteomyelitis)
History of trauma, fall, motor vehicle accident Sudden onset of pain	Fracture/dislocation
Past history of malignancy Age >50 years Failure to improve with treatment Unexplained weight loss Night pain Pain at multiple sites Pain at rest	Tumour

postures or time of day?) Obtain descriptions of the specific mechanism of the injury and the forces involved. For example, morning pain relieved with daily activity is often associated with arthritis. Enquire about the onset of symptoms, nature of the pain, disability and functional impairment, previous injuries to the area, type of work, typical postures and overuse. Ask clients to demonstrate movements and positions that aggravate or relieve the pain and to be specific with descriptions of aggravating or relieving activities.

- Determining if pain is likely to be associated with visceral function or is neurogenic, or psychosocial (yellow flags). Pain can be referred to the hip from conditions like appendicitis, urinary tract infections, gynaecological conditions and rheumatic conditions like ankylosing spondylitis. Clients with numbness, pins and needles and muscle weakness associated with their hip condition may have referred pain from the lumbar spine or sciatica. Refer all clients with sensory symptoms or muscle weakness for further investigation.

OUTCOME MEASURES

Outcome measures are questionnaires that are specifically designed to assess clients' level of impairment and to define benefits of treatment. The Patient Specific Scale can be used to measure progress of treatment of clients with any musculoskeletal condition, including conditions of the hip.

POSTURAL ANALYSIS

Postural analysis enables observation of the whole client and facilitates identification of important features through bilateral comparison. It also facilitates detection of possible predisposing or contributing factors that may be implicated by observing the position of the thoracic and lumbar spines and pelvis. Observe and compare the lower limbs posteriorly, laterally and anteriorly, noting their symmetry. Observe any bruising, colour changes, swelling, scars and varicose veins. Observe Q-angle,[a] tibial torsion,[b] everted/inverted feet, leg length and muscle hypertonicity or atrophy.

GAIT ANALYSIS

Observe the client walking and note any disturbances in the rate and rhythm of gait. Identify the phase of gait that is altered. Gait disturbances are more evident in stance phase than swing phase, when the hip joint takes the load of the upper body. For example, painful degenerative joint disease can cause clients to reduce the duration of the weight-bearing phase. Weakness of gluteus minimus, gluteus maximus and quadriceps may be manifested as Trendelenburg gait, hip extensor gait and back knee gait respectively.

FUNCTIONAL TESTS

For any tests involving joint movements it is important to compare both sides and to take into account any underlying pathology and the age and lifestyle of the client. Findings from physical examinations should be interpreted in the light of evidence for their diagnostic accuracy. Range of motion tests have been shown to be highly reliable. Limitation in three ranges of motion has been useful in identifying osteoarthritis of the hip (+LR = 4.5 to 4.7). Lateral hip pain during passive abduction is strongly suggestive of lateral tendon pathology (+LR = 8.3); groin pain during hip abduction or adduction suggests osteoarthritis (+LR = 5.7).[3]

Active range of motion (AROM) of the lumbar spine (flexion, extension, lateral flexion and rotation)

Examination of the hip begins with functional tests of the lumbar spine and pelvis to help rule out lumbar radiculopathy which refers pain to the hip region (see Figure 18.3 on p 340). If active range of motion tests of the lumbar spine and pelvis reproduce hip symptoms, further examination of the lumbar spine and pelvis is indicated (see Chapter 10).

Active range of motion (AROM) of the hip joint

The client stands and faces you. The client holds on to the back of a chair, the table or other support if needed. Demonstrate the movements for the client to follow and instruct the client to perform the movements as far as they can comfortably. Note that the knee should be flexed during hip flexion to minimise the influence of hamstring tightness on the range of motion. Examine the following ranges of motion:

- Flexion/extension (120°/20°)[5]
- Internal/external rotation (35–40°/35–40°)
  Instruct the client to turn their whole leg outwards and inwards.
- Abduction/adduction (40–45°/25–30°)

An alternative routine that is commonly used for assessing hip AROM involves asking clients to:

---

[a]The Q-angle is the angle between a line from the ASIS to the middle of the patella and a line from the middle of the patella to the tibial tubercle. In males, the Q-angle is approximately 14° and in females 17°.

[b]Tibial torsion refers to the anatomical twist of the proximal articular axis of the tibia compared to the distal articular axis.

- sit down without using their arms (hip flexion)
- stand up without using their arms (hip extension)
- stand with both feet pointed inwards (hip internal rotation)
- stand with both feet pointed outwards (hip external rotation)
- stand with feet apart as far as they are comfortably able (hip abduction)
- cross one leg over the other to place the lateral border of one foot alongside the medial border of the other (hip adduction).

This quick hip screen enables bilateral comparisons of functional movements.

Passive range of motion (PROM)

If the client is unable to perform normal active range of motion in any direction, further investigation is required. PROM testing should be performed with the client supine and prone, with one hand stabilising and palpating the hip joint while the other hand moves the lower limb. Note that PROM hip tests may be performed with the knee flexed or extended. (Note that hip flexion is usually performed with knee flexion to avoid the complication of hamstring shortness.) Palpate for crepitus, capsular pattern and end-feel (see Table 18.4). The capsular pattern of restriction for the acetabulofemoral joint is internal rotation more limited than extension; extension more limited than abduction.[6]

Resisted range of motion (RROM)

RROM tests should also be performed if AROM testing indicates the likelihood of a hip problem. RROM tests include:

- **flexion**
  iliopsoas, rectus femoris, sartorius
- **extension**
  gluteus maximus, hamstrings
- **abduction**
  gluteus medius and minimus, tensor fasciae latae
- **adduction**
  adductor magnus, gracilis, adductor longus and brevis
- **internal rotation**
  tensor fasciae latae, gluteus medius and minimus
- **external rotation**
  piriformis, quadratus lumborum, superior and inferior gemellus, obturator internus and externus

Table 18.4 Hip joint: end-feel[6]

Normal end-feel	Flexion and adduction	Elastic or tissue approximation
	Extension and abduction	Elastic tissue stretch
	Internal/external rotation	Elastic tissue stretch
Abnormal end-feel	Bony (hard)	Osteoarthrosis
	Late myospasm	Instability
	Empty	Instability or subluxation
	Firm	Contracture or capsular tightness

Resisted tests and length tests for specific muscles[7, 8]

If RROM tests reproduce symptoms, then further tests may be used to help identify specific muscles.

Note that reports of pain during resisted gluteus minimus and medius tests appear to be helpful in identifying lateral tendon pathologies (+LR = 3.27) and that posterior hip pain during a squat is fairly useful in identifying hip osteoarthritis (+LR = 6.1).[3]

1. RECTUS FEMORIS

Resisted test

As a group the quadriceps can be tested with the client seated. Place one hand over the knee and the other over the ankle. Apply resistance at the ankle as the client tries to straighten their leg (see Figure 18.4).

As rectus femoris is the only muscle of the quadriceps group to cross the hip joint, it can be identified from the other muscles in the group by resisting hip flexion. If hip flexion were performed first and found to be painful or weak, resisting knee extension identifies rectus femoris from iliopsoas. Alternatively, if resisted knee extension were found to be painful or weak, resisting hip flexion would differentiate rectus femoris from the other quadriceps muscles.

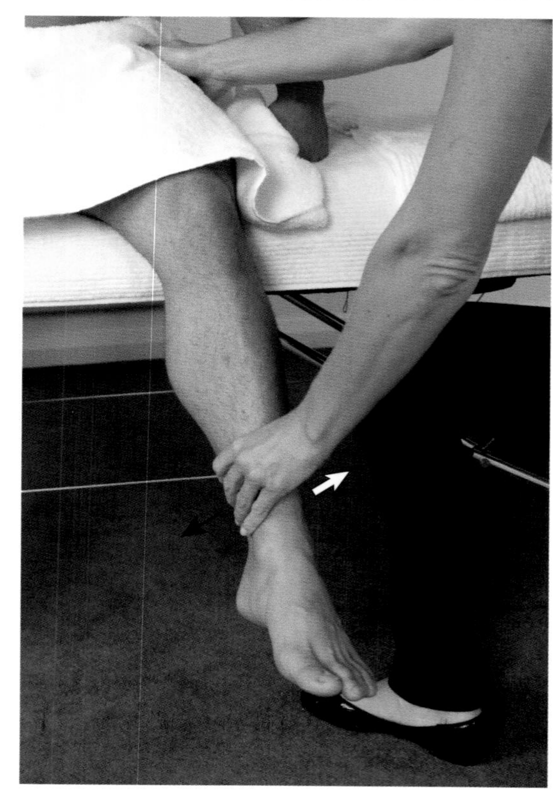

Fig. 18.4 Resisted quadriceps test

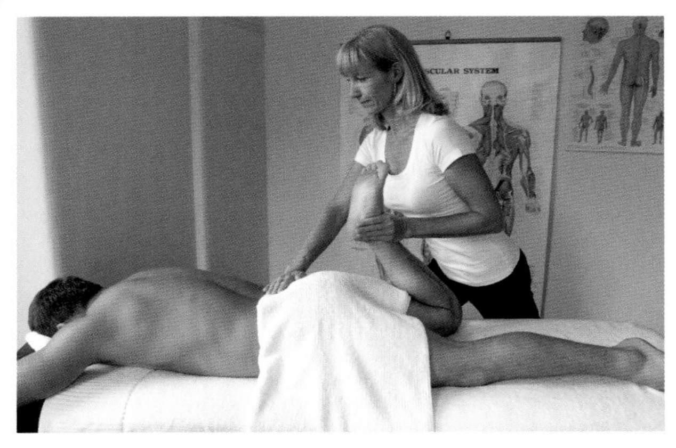

Fig. 18.5 **Length test for quadriceps**

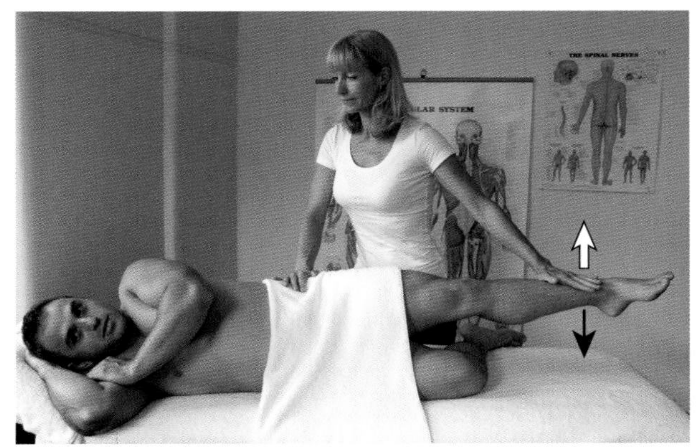

Fig. 18.7 **Resisted test for gluteus medius**

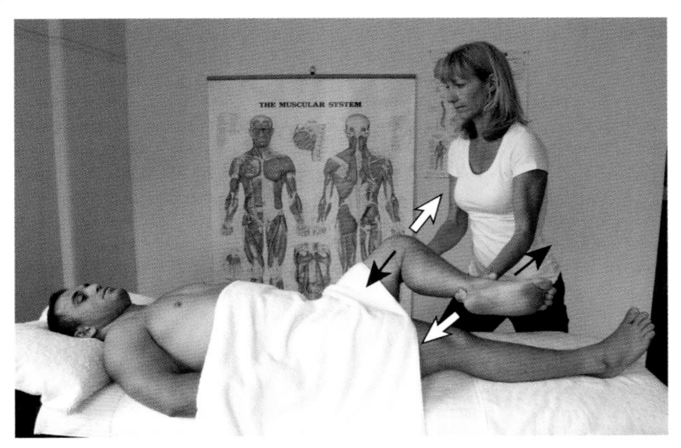

Fig. 18.6 **Resisted test for sartorius**

Length test

Shortening of the quadriceps restricts knee flexion. Shortened rectus femoris can be observed as restricted knee flexion when the hip is extended or restricted hip extension when the knee is flexed (see Figure 18.5).

2. SARTORIUS

Resisted test

The client lies supine with one foot across the knee of the other leg (figure 4 position). Place one hand on the knee and the other on the ankle. Instruct the client to hold this position while you try to straighten the leg (i.e. push knee into extension and adduction and the hip into extension) (see Figure 18.6).

Alternatively, the client may be seated. Kneel at the side of the client and hold the lateral aspect of their knee with one hand and the ankle with the other. Instruct the client to try to place their foot on the opposite knee as you resist the movement.

Length test

The length of sartorius is tested with other hip flexors, abductors and lateral rotators. A short sartorius muscle would limit the client's ability to sit cross-legged. A contracture of sartorius can produce flexion, abduction and lateral rotation deformity of the hip, along with flexion of the knee.

3. GLUTEUS MEDIUS

Resisted test

The client lies on their side with their lower leg flexed at the hip and knee for stability. The client's upper hip is abducted, slightly extended and externally rotated and the knee is extended. Place one hand over the client's upper hip and the other contacts the lateral side of the upper leg proximal to the ankle. The client tries to hold the position as the practitioner applies pressure in the direction of adduction and slight flexion (see Figure 18.7).

Note that the Trendelenburg test (see Figure 18.14 on p 346) also tests gluteus medius strength.

Length test

Shortness of the hip abductors limits hip adduction. Contracture of the hip abductors may be observed as a pelvic drop on the side of tightness and abduction of the lower limb.

4. GLUTEUS MINIMUS

Resisted test

The resisted test for gluteus minimus is similar to the resisted test for gluteus medius except that the client's upper leg is abducted in the neutral position (no flexion, extension or internal or external rotation of the hip). Your pressure is applied in the direction of adduction and very slight extension. (Fig 18.8 on p 344)

Length test

Shortness of gluteus minimus limits hip abduction and lateral rotation. Contracture may be observed as a pelvic drop towards the side of tightness and medial rotation of the hip joint.

5. TENSOR FASCIAE LATAE

Resisted test

The client lies supine and flexes and abducts their straight leg to about 45° and medially rotates the hip. Place one hand on

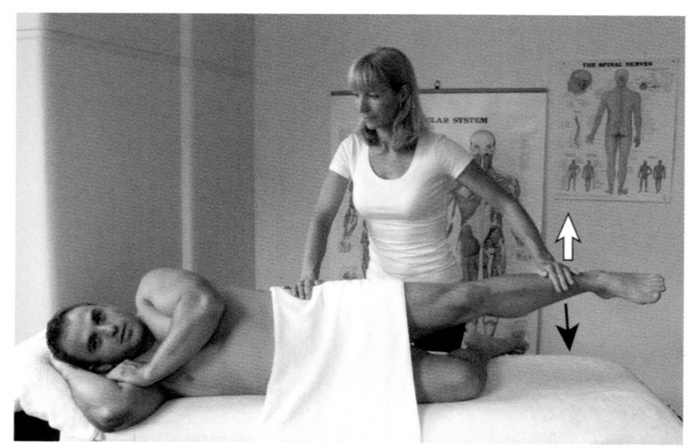

Fig. 18.8 Resisted test for gluteus minimus

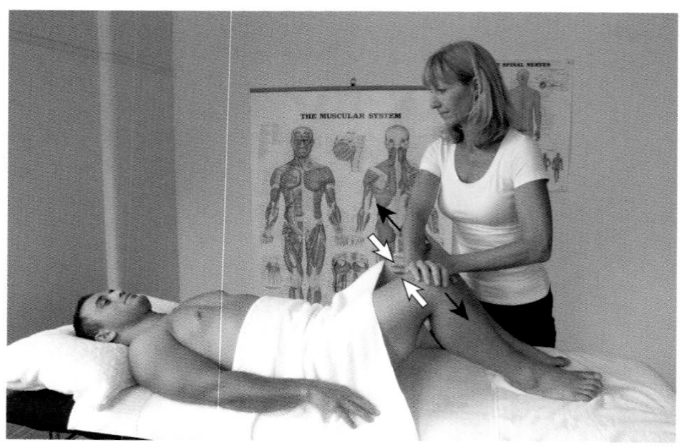

Fig. 18.10 Resisted test for hip adductors

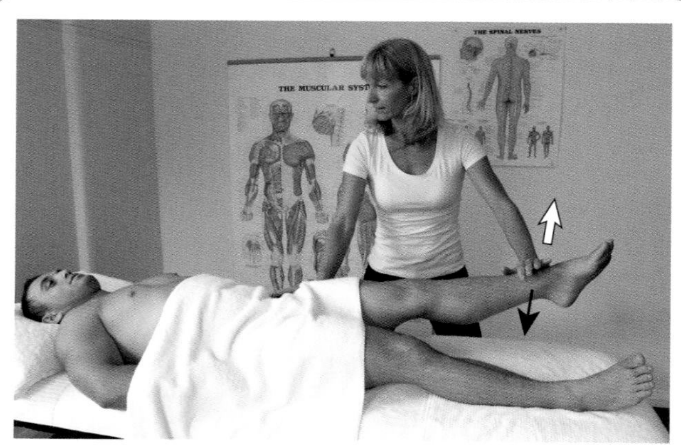

Fig. 18.9 Resisted test for tensor fasciae latae

the lateral pelvis to stabilise the hip, and place the other hand on the lateral aspect of the leg proximal to the ankle. Ask the client to move the leg outwards diagonally in the direction of abduction and flexion as you resist the movement by pushing in the direction of adduction and extension (see Figure 18.9).

Length test

Bilateral contraction of tensor fasciae latae may cause anterior pelvic tilt and occasionally genu valgus. Unilateral tightness of tensor fasciae latae and other hip abductors is associated with pelvic drop to the side of tightness. The knee on the side of tensor fasciae latae tightness tends to genu valgus.

6. HIP ADDUCTORS

Resisted test

The hip adductors (adductor magnus, gracilis, adductor longus, adductor brevis and pectineus) are tested as a group. The client lies supine, knees flexed and feet on the table. Contact the medial aspects of both knees and ask the client to bring their knees together against your resistance (see Figure 18.10).

Length test

Shortened hip adductors limit hip abduction (e.g. sitting cross-legged). Hip adduction contracture is associated with lateral pelvis tilt with the pelvis high on the contracted side. (The knee and hip on the opposite side may be flexed or abducted to compensate.)

7. HIP LATERAL ROTATORS

Resisted test

The lateral rotators of the hip (piriformis, quadratus femoris, obturator internus, obturator externus, gemellus superior and gemellus inferior) are tested as a group. The client sits and flexes their knees over the side of the treatment table. Place one hand on the lateral aspect of the knee; the other on the medial aspect of the leg proximal to the ankle. The client tries to bring their foot towards the midline (i.e. externally rotate their hip) against your resistance (see Figure 18.11 on p 345).

This test can also be performed with the client prone, knee flexed to 90°. The client tries to move their foot medially against your resistance.

Length test

Short lateral rotators of the hip limit internal rotation. Out-toeing gait may be observed.

(Note that the medial rotators of the hip can be tested either as individual muscles (see gluteus medius, gluteus minimus, tensor fasciae latae) or as a group. As a group the medial rotators are tested similarly to the lateral rotators except that the client tries to move their foot laterally against your resistance.)

Special tests

Special tests of the hip have not been demonstrated to be especially helpful in identifying hip pathologies.[3] As with all assessments, findings should be interpreted cautiously and in the context of other clinical findings (see Chapter 2).

PATRICK'S/FABERE TEST

The client is supine and crosses one foot over the other knee in a figure-4 position so that the hip is flexed, abducted and externally rotated. The examiner stabilises the hip on the straight leg side and applies gentle downward pressure to the knee on the opposite side. Inguinal pain is an indication of hip joint pathology or strains in surrounding muscles. (FABERE

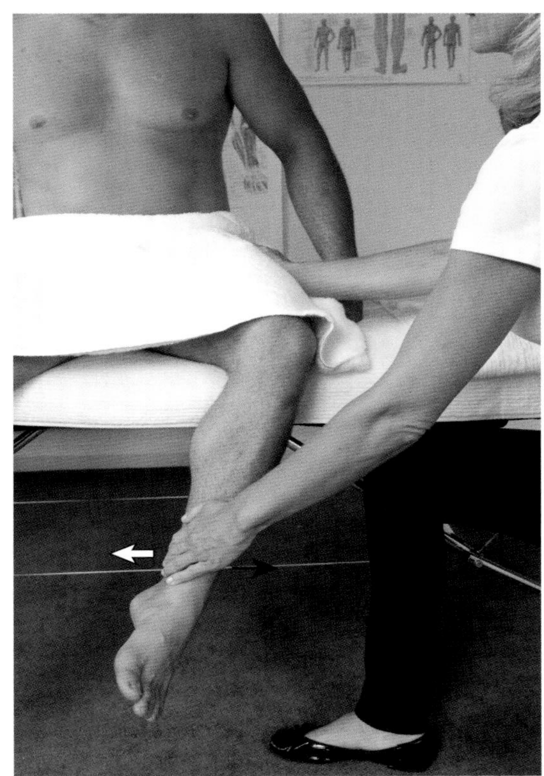

Fig. 18.11 Resisted test for hip lateral rotators

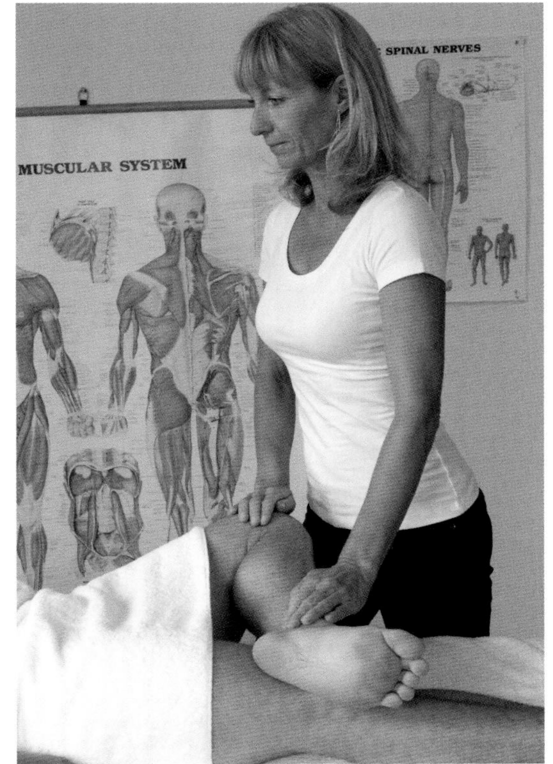

Fig. 18.12 Patrick's test

refers to the testing procedure: flexion, abduction, external rotation and then passive extension.) (See Figure 18.12.)

THOMAS TEST

The client lies supine and brings one knee to their chest keeping the other leg straight. Elevation of the straight leg indicates hip contracture, tight iliopsoas or rectus femoris (see Figure 18.13).

TRENDELENBURG TEST

The patient stands on one leg and the practitioner observes the level of the pelvis. A client with normal hip abductor strength on one side will be able to maintain a level pelvis when they raise the opposite leg off the ground (see Figure 18.14 on p 346).

OBER'S TEST

The client lies on their side with their involved leg uppermost. Hold the client's ankle and flex the knee to 90°, abduct and extend the hip; then internally rotate the hip. Hip pain on this manoeuvre suggests hip joint pathology; trochanteric pain suggests trochanteric bursitis.

(Caution with clients with knee joint pathology.)

MODIFIED OBER'S TEST

The client lies on their side with the involved leg uppermost. Stabilise the client's pelvis with one hand on the upper ilium and adduct the involved leg behind the lower leg. Iliotibial band tightness is suggested if the client is unable to lower the leg to the table (see Figure 18.14 on p 346).

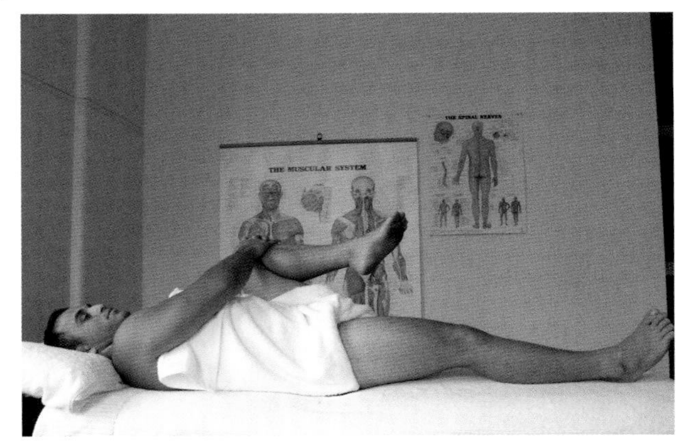

Fig. 18.13 Thomas test

PALPATION

Palpatory findings are interpreted with findings from other assessments and used to guide treatment plans.

In the sidelying position the greater trochanter is palpated at the widest part of the pelvis. Gluteus medius is palpable from its origin just below the iliac crest to its insertion into the upper part of the greater trochanter. Gluteus minimus is

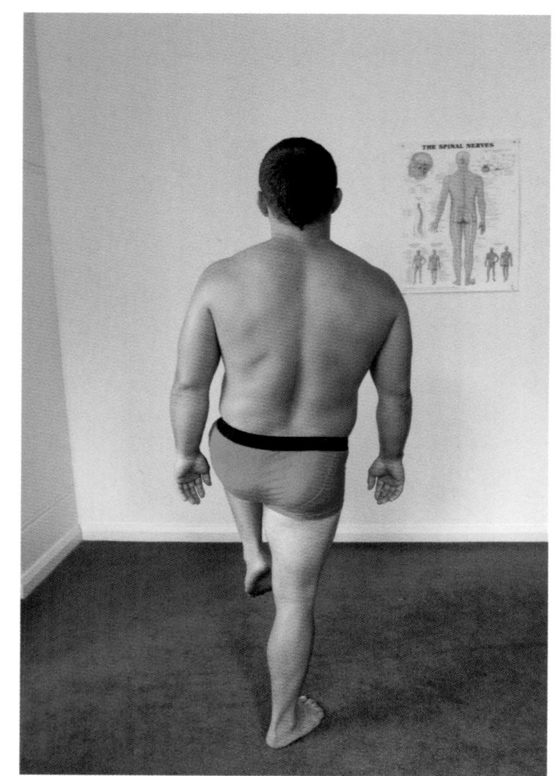

Fig. 18.14 Trendelenburg test

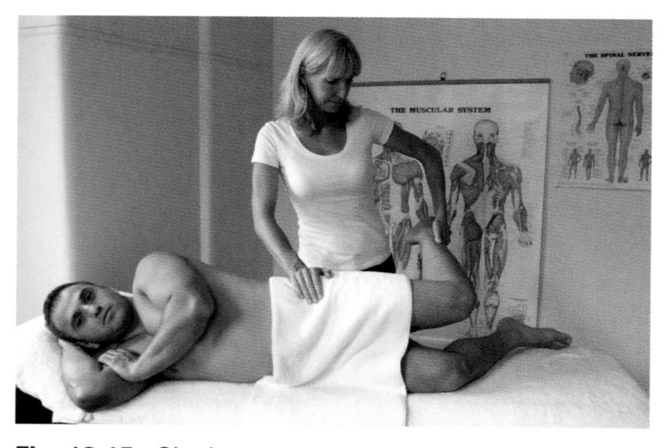

Fig. 18.15 Ober's test

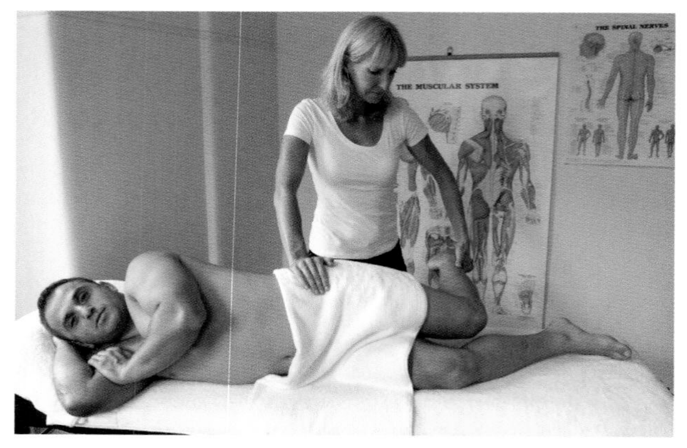

Fig. 18.16 Modified Ober's test

not usually palpable under the gluteus maximus. The trochanteric bursa separates the greater trochanter from the insertions of gluteus medius and minimus. It is palpable only when it becomes inflamed. From the anterior aspect of the iliac crest palpate tensor fasciae latae to its insertion into the iliotibial tract. Palpate the ischial tuberosity posteriorly. The sciatic nerve is palpable in the sidelying position with the knee flexed. It is located halfway between the greater trochanter and the ischial tuberosity.

With the client prone, trace the arc of the iliac crests to the posterior superior iliac spines (PSISs) slightly inferolateral to the dimples of Venus. The PSISs are level with the second sacral segment. The sacroiliac joints are not palpable under the ilia. The gluteus maximus is the largest and most superficial muscle of the pelvis. It runs from the inner upper ilium, sacrum and coccyx to the iliotibial tract and gluteal tuberosity of the femur. Its upper border runs from the PSIS to slightly above the greater trochanter. Its lower border runs from the coccyx to the iliotibial tract. The piriformis is deep to gluteus maximus. It runs from the sacrum to the superior border of the greater trochanter. It can be identified when the client's knee is flexed to 90° and hip lateral rotation is resisted (i.e. the client tries to move their foot towards the midline against your resistance). The sciatic nerve exits below the pirifomis and occasionally through it. The ischial tuberosity is located midway along the gluteal fold. A bursa separates the ischial tuberosity and the overlying gluteal muscle. Palpate the insertion of the hamstrings at the ischial tuberosity. Tenderness over the ischial tuberosity could indicate bursitis or hamstring strain. Palpate the biceps femoris laterally and the semitendinosus and semimembranosus medially.

In the supine position, palpate the iliac crest, greater trochanter and the anterior superior iliac spine (ASIS). The pubic tubercle is located in the midline level with the greater trochanter. The inguinal ligament runs between the ASIS and the pubic tubercle and is not usually palpable. With the client's lower limb in the figure-4 position (i.e. hip abducted and externally rotated, knee flexed and foot placed across the other knee) and appropriately draped, palpate structures in the femoral triangle, which is bounded by the sartorius, adductor longus and inguinal crease (see Figure 18.17 on p 347). The pulse of the femoral artery is palpated halfway along and slightly below the inguinal ligament. The femoral nerve, which runs lateral to the femoral artery, and the femoral vein, which runs medial to the femoral artery, are not palpable. Inguinal lymph nodes are often palpable below and parallel to the inguinal ligament. The iliopsoas may be palpable in the floor of the femoral triangle. Adductor longus is the most superficial muscle of the adductor group. It runs from the symphysis pubis to the middle third of the linea aspera. It forms a prominent cord in the medial upper thigh. The attachment of sartorius is palpable from the ASIS. Rectus femoris arises from the anterior inferior iliac spine and lies lateral to sartorius.

REMEDIAL MASSAGE TREATMENT

Assessment of the hip region provides essential information for development of treatment plans, including:

- client's suitability for remedial massage therapy
- duration of the condition (i.e. acute or chronic)
- severity of the condition (i.e. grade of injury; mild, moderate or severe pain)
- type(s) of tissues involved
- priorities for treatment if more than one injury or condition are present
- whether the signs and symptoms suggest a common condition of the hip region
- special considerations for individual clients (e.g. client's preference for treatment types and styles, special population considerations).

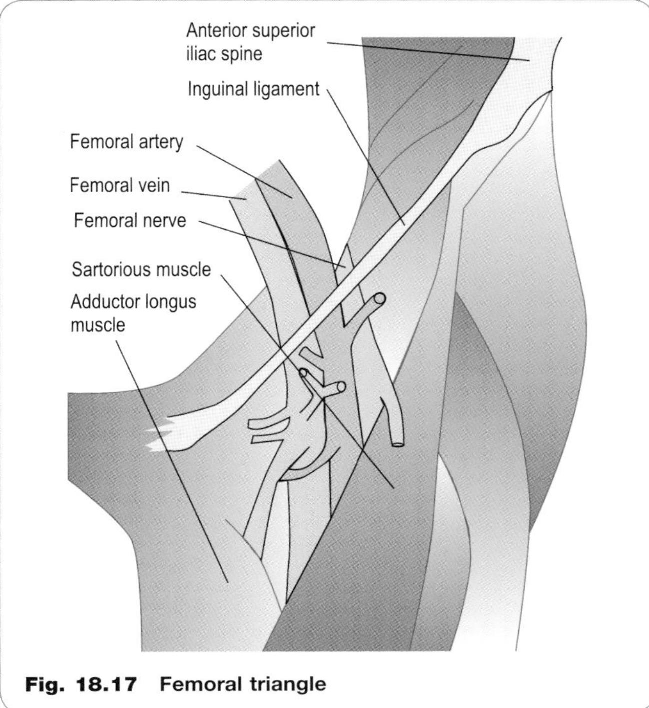

Fig. 18.17 Femoral triangle

Treatment options must always be considered in the context of the best available evidence for treatment effectiveness and clinical practice guidelines where they exist. Little research has been conducted into the effectiveness of massage treatments for conditions of the hip. Some relevant studies are summarised in Table 18.5. Results should be interpreted in light of the variable quality of the trials.

The predominant conditions of the hip treated in remedial massage clinics are mild to moderate thigh muscle strains and degenerative joint disease of the hip and occasionally trochanteric bursitis. Remedial massage treatments for these conditions are described below.

OVERVIEW

Develop a short- and a long-term plan for each client. The short-term plan directs treatment to the highest priority (usually determined by symptoms). The long-term plan can be introduced when presenting symptoms have subsided. Long-term treatment focuses on contributing or predisposing factors such as underlying structural features and lifestyle factors. A significant part of both short-term and long-term treatment involves educating clients about likely causal or aggravating factors and an exercise program to improve or restore normal muscle function. If massage therapy is used in conjunction with other treatments such as corticosteroid injections, it is important to communicate with other treating practitioners and to integrate treatments where possible for the best outcomes.

Table 18.5 Some studies investigating the effectiveness of massage and other treatments for hip osteoarthritis and muscle strains of the thigh

Condition	Summary of studies
Hip osteoarthritis	Electro-acupuncture and hydrotherapy, both in combination with patient education, led to long-term reduced pain and increased functional activity and quality of life in 45 patients with osteoarthritis of the hip.[11] Hoeksma et al[12] compared the effectiveness of a manual therapy program consisting of hip mobilisation and manipulation with an exercise program and concluded that the manual therapy program was more effective than the exercise program in improving hip function in patients with osteoarthritis of the hip. Wegener and Lupke[13] conducted a trial into the effectiveness of devil's claw (harpagophytum procumbens) in the treatment of arthrosis of the hip and knee. According to the authors the results suggest that devil's claw extract has a clinically beneficial effect on pain, stiffness and physical function.
Muscle strains	A study by Hopper et al[14] found that both classic massage and dynamic soft tissue mobilisation had an immediate significant effect on hamstring length in competitive female field hockey players. Chiropractic manual therapy intervention showed a trend towards lower limb injury prevention and a significant reduction in primary lower limb muscle strains and weeks missed from sport due to non-contact knee injuries in 60 semi-elite Australian Rules footballers.[15] A study by Malliaropoulos et al[16] found that an intensive stretching program significantly reduced the time before athletes with second-degree hamstring strains could return to a full training program. A single 8-hour application of a patch containing methyl salicylate and l-menthol provided significant pain relief for 105 men and women diagnosed with mild to moderate muscle strain (including strains of thigh muscles).[17] Mancinelli et al found significant changes in vertical jump displacement and perceived soreness in a group of women collegiate athletes who received a thigh massage.[18]

MUSCLE STRAIN

Muscle strains are usually collagen tears in the connective tissue in and around a muscle.[1] Repair of damaged muscle tissue leads to cross-linkages and adhesions in collagen and the muscle typically shortens and becomes less flexible. Muscle strains occur as a result of direct trauma or from overuse. They are common injuries in sport. For example, in the Australian Football League 2008 Report[19] hamstring strains accounted for 6.6%, groin strains for 3.2% and quadriceps strains for 1.8% of all new injuries per club for the 2008 season. Although research evidence is scarce, anecdotal evidence suggests that massage therapy can be very beneficial for restoring normal structure and function to muscle tissue.

Key assessment findings for muscle strain

- History of trauma or repetitive overuse
- Functional tests of the hip
  - AROM positive in one or more directions
  - PROM may be positive at the end of the range when affected muscle is stretched
  - RROM positive for affected muscle
  - Resisted and length test positive for affected muscle
  - Special tests: positive for specific muscle test (e.g. Thomas test positive, Ober's test)
- Palpation positive for tenderness/pain; ± spasm, myofibril tears/scar tissue

Groin (adductor) strain

Groin strains are relatively common in such activities as soccer, football, water skiing, gymnastics and dancing. They account for 2.5% of all sport-related complaints.[6] Any one of the five adductors (adductor longus, adductor brevis, adductor magnus, pectineus or gracilis) can tear but adductor longus is the most commonly strained. The adductor longus tendon is distinguishable as a prominent cord as it descends from the symphysis pubis. The fibres of the other muscles may be indistinguishable as they blend together near their attachment sites. There are several common causes including a forced abduction of the thigh beyond its flexibility limits (e.g. slipping on a slippery surface, a blocked leg action when kicking a ball with the side of the foot, or a sudden change of direction while running). In soccer, adductor longus appears to be at risk of strain during the transition from hip extension to hip flexion in the kicking leg's swing phase.[20] Groin strains are also associated with overuse activities such as running with increased foot flare, breast stroke and gymnastics. As with any other muscle, adductor strains can be graded as either mild (first degree), moderate (second degree) or severe (third degree). A third-degree strain indicates a complete rupture of the muscle tendon or an avulsion of the tendon from its attachment site on the bone and requires referral.

Hamstring strain

The hamstring muscles are the most commonly injured muscles in the lower limb. A tear can occur in any of the three hamstring muscles (biceps femoris, semitendinosus and semimembranosus) and frequently at or near the musculotendinous junction, the tenoperiosteal junction at the ischial tuberosity or in the muscle belly. However, strains occur most frequently in biceps femoris at the proximal musculotendinous junction. Strain can result from trauma or from overuse (e.g. in sprinters). Injury is common during eccentric contraction and particularly when the muscle is required to stop the leg at the end of its forward swing. Previous hamstring injury also appears to be a significant risk factor for hamstring strain. In one study, previously injured male soccer players had more than twice the risk of sustaining a new hamstring injury than did uninjured players.[21]

There are several possible reasons for the high incidence of hamstring strain:

- strength and flexibility imbalances between the quadriceps and hamstrings
- the hamstrings cross two joints (with the exception of the short head of the biceps femoris) making it more susceptible to injury
- sciatic nerve tension may have a role in hamstring hypertonicity
- muscle fatigue
- insufficient warm-up.

Quadriceps strain

The quadriceps are the most powerful and bulky muscles in the body and injury may result in marked functional disability. Injury often results from sudden contraction of the muscle, especially when it is stretched (e.g. sprinting, jumping or kicking). The injury may be felt as a sudden sharp pain or muscle pull in the anterior thigh during an activity requiring explosive muscle contraction.

Assessment

HISTORY

The client often complains of sudden onset of acute pain at the site of lesion (e.g. near the pubic bone in adductor strain, in the anterior thigh in quadriceps strain) and large areas of bruising may develop. Pain is often aggravated by exercise and relieved by rest. In some cases, the client reports hearing a loud pop or snap when the injury occurs. Symptoms may persist for long periods and re-injury is common.

(In suspected groin strain, it is important to eliminate abdominal causes of groin pain such as appendicitis, urinary tract infection, gynaecological pathology or rheumatoid conditions like ankylosing spondylitis.[22])

FUNCTIONAL TESTS

Lumbar AROM tests do not reproduce symptoms.

Hip tests

AROM: positive in one or more directions.
PROM: may be positive when the affected muscle is passively stretched (e.g. in quadriceps strain the client may have difficulty bringing their heel to their buttock).
RROM: pain and/or weakness in the affected muscles.
Resisted tests and length tests: positive for affected muscles.
Special tests: may be positive (e.g. Thomas test positive for rectus femoris shortening).

PALPATION

Tenderness or pain may be elicited during palpation at the injury site. Spasm and myofibril tears may be evident. In chronic strains, fibrotic tissue may be palpable.

Key indicators of muscle strain:

- Resisted test is painful.
- Muscle stretch is painful.
- Palpation at the site of lesion is painful.

Overview of treatment and management of muscle strains

Treat all acute injuries with RICE and advise the client to avoid or reduce the responsible activity.

In the subacute or chronic phase, remedial massage techniques for muscle strains including Swedish massage to the lumbar spine and hip is followed by:

- muscle pelvis specific techniques (see Tables 10.4 and 18.6).
  - deep gliding frictions along the muscle fibres
  - cross-fibre frictions
  - soft tissue releasing techniques
  - deep transverse friction at the site of the lesion. Deep transverse friction is thought to stimulate collagen production and create mobile scar tissue. Apply the technique for several minutes within the client's pain threshold, alternating with other forms of tissue mobilisation including effleurage, sweeping cross-fibre frictions and stretching.
  - Trigger point therapy
  - Muscle stretching
- Myofascial release including cross-arm techniques and the leg pull (see Figure 18.8).
- Thermotherapy may be beneficial for pain relief.

Note:

i) Treating adductor strains requires appropriate draping. Instruct the client to hold the draping in place to protect modesty.

ii) The femoral artery, vein and nerve travel through the femoral triangle. Care should be taken to avoid compressing these structures when massaging the area.

Other remedial techniques for muscle strains/imbalances include:

- hip passive joint articulation (see Chapter 7)
  - hip rotation
  - hip figure-8

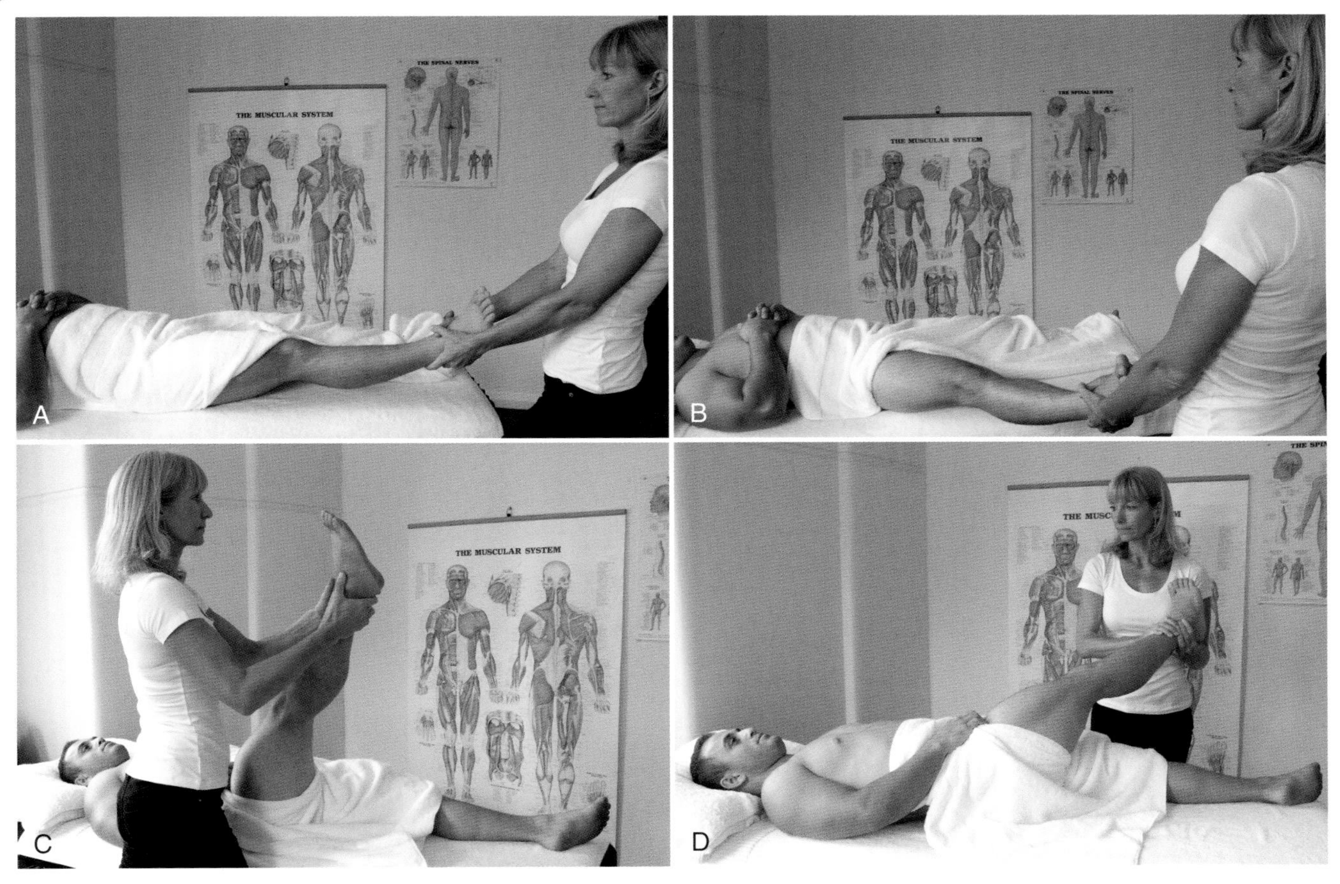

Fig. 18.18 Leg pull

Table 18.6 Remedial massage techniques for muscles of the hip

Muscle	Soft tissue release	Trigger point	DTF	Stretch	Corrective action[9, 10]	Home stretch
Gluteus medius and minimus	Client: Sidelying, towel draped around the upper leg, knee bent or straight as preferred. A pillow may be placed between the client's knees. Practitioner: stands behind the client, contacts the lesion/taut band in the muscle with fingers, thumbs or elbows as the client slowly abducts and adducts the upper leg.	Gluteus medius Gluteus minimus	Gluteus medius	Client supine: flex one knee and place the foot on the table near the outside of the knee of the other leg. Practitioner: stands at side facing towards the client's head. The practitioner stabilises the lateral pelvis with one hand. The other hand contacts the client's flexed knee and slowly moves the knee across the client's body keeping their foot on the table.	Sleep on the uninvolved side with a pillow between the knees. Avoid prolonged immobility.	As for the assisted stretch Alternatively, stand side on to a wall with hand on the wall for support. Place the leg closer to the wall behind the other and slowly lean the pelvis towards the wall. Hold up to 30 seconds. Repeat 3 times.

Table 18.6 Remedial massage techniques for muscles of the hip—cont'd

Muscle	Soft tissue release	Trigger point	DTF	Stretch	Corrective action[9, 10]	Home stretch
Tensor fasciae latae	Client: sidelying, towel draped around the upper leg, knee bent or straight as preferred. A pillow may be placed between the client's knees. Practitioner: stands behind the client, contacts the lesion/taut band in the muscle with fingers, thumbs or pincer grip as the client slowly abducts and adducts the upper leg. 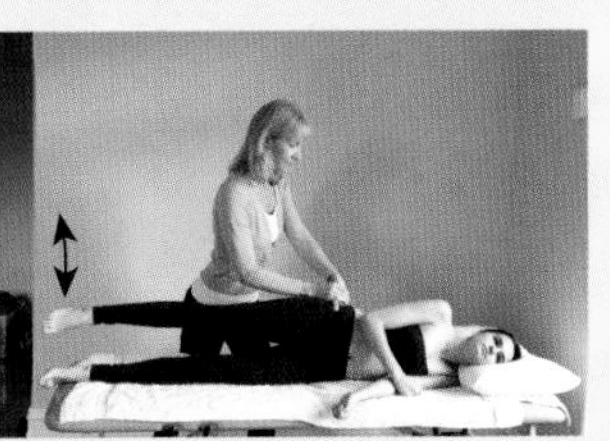 **For iliotibial band** Client: as above. Practitioner: faces cephalad. Using a double thumb contact, interphalangeal joints or knuckles, perform a slow deep glide as the muscle lengthens. In another variation the practitioner performs cross-fibre frictions as the thigh is abducted and adducted.		Tensor fasciae latae	Client: sidelying, back close to the edge of the table, holding the side of the table in front. Practitioner: stands behind the client and gently lowers the top leg over the side of the table. (This stretch can also be performed supine, adducting one leg over the other.) The client tries to abduct their leg against the practitioner's resistance for 6–8 seconds, then relaxes and allows the leg to drop into adduction again. This whole procedure is repeated three times. 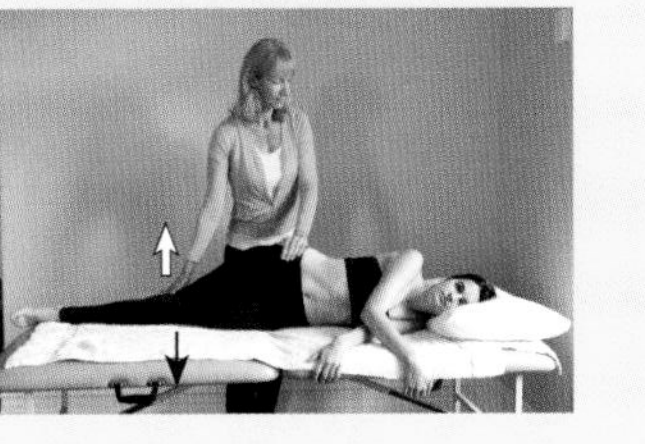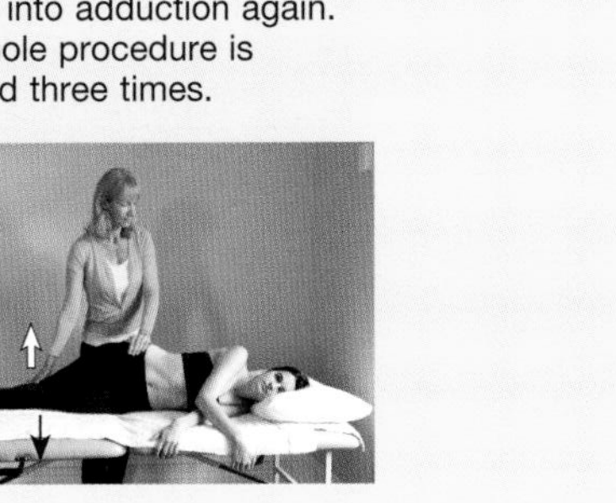	Avoid sitting cross-legged or prolonged hip flexion. Place a pillow between the thighs when sleeping. Adequate warm-up before running. Running technique assessment.	Stand side on to a wall with hand on the wall for support. Place the leg closer to the wall behind the other and slowly lean the pelvis towards the wall. Hold up to 30 seconds. Repeat 3 times.

Continued

Table 18.6 Remedial massage techniques for muscles of the hip—cont'd

Muscle	Soft tissue release	Trigger point	DTF	Stretch	Corrective action[9, 10]	Home stretch
Adductor group	Client: supine, knee flexed, hip slightly abducted (appropriate draping). Practitioner: stands ipsilaterally, facing towards the client's head. The practitioner performs a deep glide over a short range from the proximal knee as the client slowly abducts the thigh to their comfortable limit.			Client: supine. Practitioner: stands to the side of the table, stabilises the pelvis with one hand and abducts the leg as far as possible within the client's comfort. The client tries to adduct the leg against the practitioner's resistance for 6–8 seconds. Next the client relaxes and the practitioner tries to adduct the leg again to its comfortable limit. Repeat the process three times. Alternatively, the same procedure can be performed with the client's hip and knee flexed and the client's foot placed on the table level with the knee of the other leg. 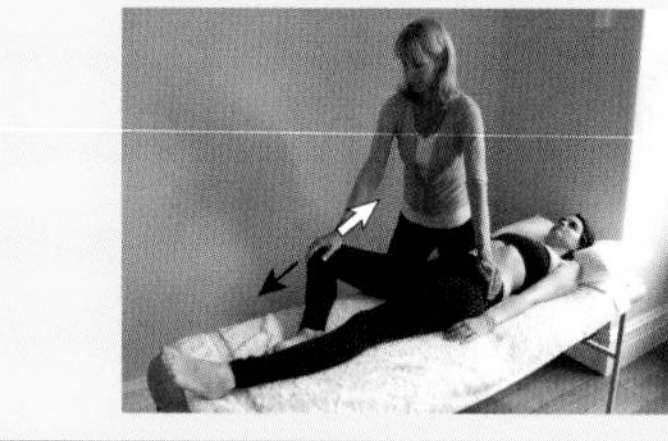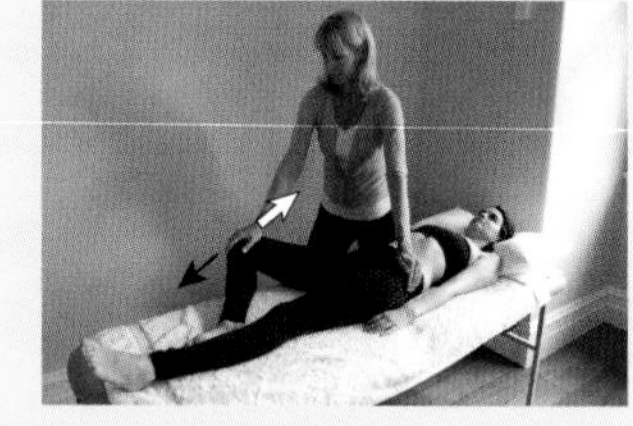	Avoid immobility that places the adductor muscles in a shortened position for long periods. Avoid overuse at the gym. Review skiing, cycling technique.	Sit on the floor with the soles of the feet together. Gently push the knees towards the floor. Hold for 30 seconds and repeat three times.

(Resisted and length tests for iliopsoas, piriformis, gluteus maximus and the hamstring muscles are described in Chapter 10.)

- hip traction
- hip rotation sidelying.

Address any underlying conditions or predisposing factors (e.g scoliosis, ankle pronation, pes planus).

CLIENT EDUCATION

Advise clients of the importance of a rehabilitation program which should be commenced as soon as possible and continued until optimal function has been restored. There are no agreed criteria for return to sport that completely safeguard against recurrence or that maximise performance after muscle strains.[23] Clients may also be referred for manipulation of the low back and pelvis, hip, knee, ankle and foot. Refer any client whose condition worsens or fails to improve within 2 weeks, or shows only slight improvement within 4 weeks.

Home exercise program

A program of progressive rehabilitation should accompany remedial massage treatment. Aim for maximum strength and full length of all major muscles while maintaining general fitness levels. Unresolved strains lead to faulty biomechanics and ultimately to other conditions such as shin splints and plantar fasciitis.

Introduce stretching exercises within 1–2 weeks after injury (depending on severity and pain tolerance). Introduce low-resistance high-repetition exercises as soon as pain permits, including both concentric and eccentric exercises. Progress to functional training and sports-specific skills before returning to sport.

Quadriceps contusion

A quadriceps contusion (charley horse or cork thigh) is a common injury resulting from a direct blow to the anterior thigh. The area becomes swollen and tender. Pain worsens when the muscle is actively contracted or passively stretched.

TREATMENT

The first 24 hours is most important in controlling the haemorrhage. The RICE regimen should be instituted immediately. As with all acute injuries, massage therapy is contraindicated in the first 24 hours but may be useful in restoring range of motion and functional rehabilitation in the subacute phase.

DEGENERATIVE JOINT DISEASE (DEGENERATIVE ARTHRITIS, OSTEOARTHRITIS)

Degenerative joint disease (DJD) of the hip is a common condition affecting the hip joint. It is characterised by progressive degeneration of articular cartilage, subchondral sclerosis and osteophyte formation.[6] The client is usually middle-aged or elderly or has a history of previous significant trauma. Predisposing factors include congenital variants like femoral anteversion, tight fibrotic joint capsule and muscle imbalance. Becoming overweight early in adult life has also been shown to increase the risk of osteoarthritis in the hip and knee.[24] The client complains of chronic pain which is worse after weight-bearing and better with rest. The pain can be felt in the groin, thigh or knee. The pain may be variable with different ranges of motion. Passive internal rotation is usually the most limited movement (capsular pattern of the hip).

Key assessment findings for DJD of the acetabulofemoral joint

- History of chronic hip pain and limitation aggravated by use; deep gnawing pain; stiffness after rest; usually over 50 years old
- Functional tests of the hip:
  - AROM limited ± painful in some directions
  - PROM limited ± painful (capsular pattern); crepitus; hard end-feel
  - RROM usually negative unless associated muscle strain
  - Special tests: Patrick's FABERE test positive
- Palpation may elicit deep pain in the groin, anterior or posterior thigh or referred to the medial thigh and knee

Assessment

HISTORY

The client complains of chronic pain in the groin, thigh and knee and stiffness that is aggravated by use and relieved by rest. The client is usually over 50 years or has a history of significant previous injury or overuse. Stiffness and limited range of motion are common complaints and the client may walk with a limp.

FUNCTIONAL TESTS

Lumbar AROM tests do not reproduce hip symptoms.

Hip tests

AROM positive (limited internal rotation, extension and abduction).

PROM positive (limited internal rotation, extension and abduction), crepitus often present, hard (bony) end-feel.

RROM negative (unless DJD is accompanied by muscle contractures and weaknesses).

Special tests: Patrick's FABERE test positive.

PALPATION

Palpation may elicit deep pain in the groin, posterior or anterior thigh, or pain referred to the thigh and knee.

Treatment of degenerative joint disease of the acetabulofemoral joint

Although degenerative joint disease is a chronic degenerative condition, acute episodes can occur from time to time, usually after over-activity. If acute inflammation is present, treatment could include cryotherapy for analgesia, acupressure, Reiki, reflexology or anti-inflammatory medication. The client should be advised to modify activities to avoid aggravating the condition.

A typical remedial massage treatment for mild or moderate subacute or chronic degenerative joint disease includes:

- Swedish massage therapy to the low back, pelvis and lower limb.
- Remedial massage therapy, which includes heat therapy, myofascial releasing techniques and joint articulation (see Chapter 7) including:
  - hip rotation
  - hip figure-8

  - hip traction
  - hip rotation sidelying.
- Remedial massage techniques (e.g. deep gliding, cross-fibre frictions, soft tissue release and muscle stretching) for associated muscle contractures.

CLIENT EDUCATION

The client should be advised to continue to use heat therapy for pain relief and to modify or avoid all aggravating activities. Range of motion exercises should be commenced as soon as possible within the client's pain tolerance. Stretching and strengthening exercises can be introduced as indicated by assessment findings. Educate clients about the importance of getting the right balance between too little activity (which can lead to capsule and muscle contractures and movement compensations) and too much activity (which can inflame the joint). Non-weight-bearing activities such as water aerobics are often beneficial. Use of shock-absorbing soles and weight loss are recommended.

Nutritional supplements such as glucosamine may be beneficial.[25] Clients may be referred for other supportive therapies including specialist nutritional advice, acupuncture and osseous mobilisation and manipulation of the pelvis and spine.

TROCHANTERIC BURSITIS

The trochanteric bursa lies directly over the greater trochanter and has the role of reducing friction between overlying structures (e.g. iliotibial band, gluteus medius and minimus attachments). The bursa may become inflamed from a direct blow or, more commonly, from chronic compression and friction from the ilitotibial band as it rubs over the greater trochanter during flexion and extension of the hip. Consequently trochanteric bursitis is aggravated by climbing stairs and getting into and out of a car. The condition is often secondary to biomechanical imbalance such as muscle hypertonicity (e.g. tight gluteus maximus or hip abductor muscles) or from overuse injury (e.g. running on a sloped surface). It is more common in the middle to older age groups and more common in women than men.

Assessment

HISTORY

The client complains of aching pain in the region of the greater trochanter, aggravated by direct pressure and by lying on that side in bed or performing activities such as running or climbing stairs. Pain may also refer to the groin or lateral thigh. Note that tendinopathy and myofascial trigger points of the gluteus medius and minimus are often mistaken for trochanteric bursitis. (Caution: rule out other sources of lateral hip pain such as femoral neck stress fracture or hip arthritis.)

FUNCTIONAL TESTS

Lumbar AROM negative.

Hip tests

AROM: positive (flexion and extension).
PROM: positive (flexion and extension).

Key assessment findings for trochanteric bursitis syndrome

- Pain and tenderness posterolateral to the greater trochanter: history of repetitive overuse (e.g. running on sloped surfaces), tight iliotibial band, or trauma: the client is usually a middle-aged female
- Functional tests:
  - AROM positive (flexion and extension)
  - PROM positive (flexion and extension)
  - RROM may be positive for associated muscles (e.g. gluteal and hip abductor muscles)
  - Tests for specific muscles: positive for affected muscles
  - Special tests: negative
- Palpation positive for pain and tenderness posterolateral to greater trochanter. Inflamed bursa may palpate as boggy.

RROM: may be positive for associated muscle strains (e.g. gluteal and abductor muscles).
Resisted tests and length tests may be positive for affected muscles.
Special tests: negative.

PALPATION

Tenderness may be elicited during palpation posterolateral to the greater trochanter. Inflamed bursa may palpate as boggy.

Overview of treatment and management

The aim of treatment is to reduce inflammation in the bursa with rest and ice. Avoid all aggravating activities such as climbing stairs and running on hills, slopes or uneven surfaces. Stretching the gluteal muscles and iliotibial band may be recommended, provided they do not aggravate symptoms.

An indirect approach is required as direct massage will aggravate an inflamed bursa. A typical remedial massage treatment for subacute or chronic trochanteric bursitis includes:

- Swedish massage therapy to the low back, pelvis and lower limb.
- Remedial massage techniques, which are directed to tensor fasciae latae, iliotibial band, gluteus maximus, gluteus minimus and gluteus medius. Sidelying position with the affected side uppermost may provide better access. Muscle-specific techniques include (see Tables 10.4 and 18.6):
  - deep gliding frictions along the muscle fibres
  - cross-fibre frictions
  - soft tissue releasing techniques

    For example: **Soft tissue release for tensor fasciae latae** The client lies on their side close to the edge of the table so that the top leg can be lowered below the level of the table. The client's lower leg is slightly flexed and the client holds on to the side of the table in front of them. Instruct the client to actively abduct the top leg. Apply static pressure to the tensor fasciae latae with thumbs, fingers, knuckles or elbows and instruct the client to actively and slowly lower and raise the leg a number of times while your pressure is maintained (Figure 18.19 on p 355).
  - trigger point therapy
  - muscle stretching.

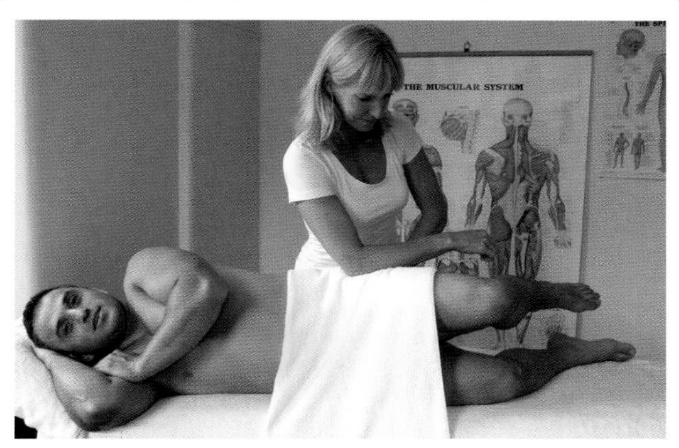

Fig. 18.19 Soft tissue release for tensor fasciae latae

- Myofascial release of the iliotibial band may be beneficial.
- Other remedial techniques including joint articulation may be beneficial (see Chapter 7):
  - hip rotation
  - hip figure-8
  - hip traction
  - hip rotation sidelying.

Correct any underlying or predisposing conditions (e.g. leg length discrepancy) where possible.

CLIENT EDUCATION

Advise the client to avoid all aggravating activities such as climbing stairs or running on uneven surfaces. A rehabilitation exercise program should be started as soon as tolerated by the client. The goal of the program is to restore normal muscle balance to the muscles around the hip joint. This usually involves stretching the tensor fasciae latae/iliotibial band and gluteal muscles. Refer for spinal and hip manipulation.

KEY MESSAGES

- Assessment of clients with conditions of the hip region involves case history, outcome measures, postural analysis, gait analysis, functional tests and palpation.
- Assessment findings may indicate the type of tissue involved (contractile or inert, muscle, joint, fascia, ligament), duration of condition (acute or subacute) and severity (grade).
- Assessment findings may indicate a common presenting condition such as muscle strain, DJD or trochanteric bursitis.
- Assessment findings also indicate client perception of injury and preferences for treatment.
- Consider Clinical Guidelines, available evidence and client preferences when planning therapy.
- Although serious conditions of the hip region are rare, all clients with symptoms of neurological or vascular impairment in the lower limb should be referred for further assessment.
- The selection of remedial massage techniques depends on assessment results. Swedish massage to the hip, lower back, pelvis and lower limb may be followed by muscle techniques (e.g. deep gliding, cross-fibre frictions, soft tissue releasing techniques, trigger point therapy and deep transverse friction), passive joint articulation, myofascial release and thermotherapy as indicated.
- Educating clients about likely causal and predisposing factors and exercise rehabilitation are essential parts of remedial massage therapy.
- Over time, increase the client self-help component of treatment wherever possible (to reduce likelihood of recurrence and/or to promote health maintenance and injury prevention).

Review questions

1. An overweight 14-year-old boy limps in to your clinic complaining of vague knee pain. He must be examined to eliminate the possibility of:
   a) Osteoarthritis of the knee
   b) Perthes' disease
   c) Femoral capital slipped epiphysis
   d) Paget's disease
2. A client's pain is reproduced on resisted hip flexion. A likely assessment is:
   a) Quadriceps muscle strain
   b) Degenerative joint disease of the hip joint
   c) Perthes' disease
   d) Hamstring muscle strain
3. The following diagram represents a stretch for:
   a) Biceps femoris
   b) Vastus lateralis
   c) Rectus femoris
   d) Vastus intermedialis

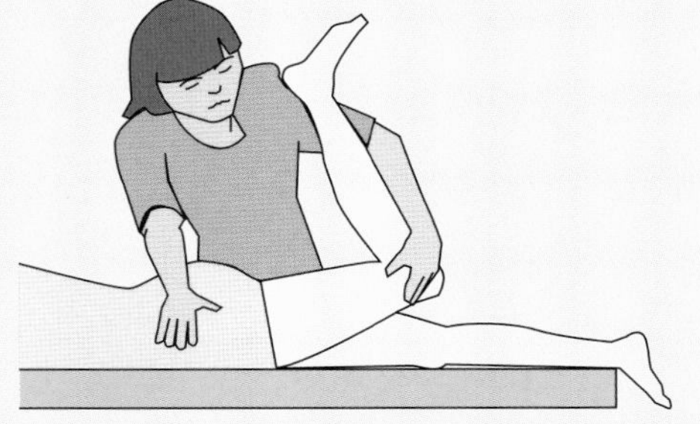

4. The age group usually affected by Perthes' disease of the hip joint is:
   a) 0–5 years
   b) 5–10 years
   c) 10–15 years
   d) 15–20 years

Review questions—cont'd

5. The most limited movement (i.e. the capsular pattern) of an osteoarthritic hip is usually:
   a) extension
   b) abduction
   c) internal rotation
   d) external rotation
6. i) Name all the muscles that attach to the greater trochanter.
   ii) What is trochanteric bursitis?
   iii) Describe the mechanism(s) which contribute to the development of trochanteric bursitis.
7. What anatomical features of the hip joint contribute to its stability?
8. Resisted hip extension produces pain. What resisted test(s) would help determine which specific muscle or muscles are causing the pain?
9. A client presents with pain in the lateral hip region. How will you determine if the client's pain is likely to be related to a lumbar problem or an acetabulofemoral joint problem?
10. Name a muscle that could be implicated if the following special tests are painful:
    i. Trendelenburg test
    ii. Ober's test
    iii. Patrick's test
11. Briefly outline the main features of a remedial massage treatment for degenerative joint disease of the hip.
12. A client has a mild strain of the rectus femoris. List five remedial massage techniques that would be suitable for its treatment.

REFERENCES

1. Hendrickson T. Massage for orthopedic conditions. Baltimore, MD: Lippincott Williams and Wilkins; 2003.
2. Tortora G, Grabowski S. Principles of anatomy and physiology. Stafford, Qld: John Wiley; 2002.
3. Cleland J, Koppenhaver S. Netter's orthopaedic clinical examination: an evidence-based approach. 2nd edn. Philadelphia: Saunders; 2011.
4. Margo K, Drezner J, Motzkin D. Evaluation and management of hip pain: an algorithmic approach. J Fam Pract 2003;52(8):607–17.
5. Reese N, Bandy W. Joint range of motion and muscle length testing. Philadelphia: WB Saunders; 2002.
6. Carnes M, Vizniak N. Quick reference evidence-based conditions manual. 3rd edn. Burnaby, BC: Professional Health Systems; 2009.
7. Kendall McCreary E, Provance P, McIntyre Rodgers M, et al. Muscles, testing and function, with posture and pain. 5th edn. Philadelphia: Lippincott Williams and Wilkins; 2005.
8. Hislop H, Montgomery J. Daniels and Worthingham's muscle testing: techniques of manual examination. 8th edn. Oxford: Saunders Elsevier; 2007.
9. Simons D, Travell J, Simons L. Myofascial pain and dysfunction: The trigger point manual. Volume 1 Upper half of body. 2nd edn. Philadelphia: Williams & Wilkins; 1999.
10. Niel-Asher S. Concise book of trigger points. Berkeley, CA: North Atlantic Books; 2005.
11. Stener-Victorin E, Kruse-Smidje C, Jung K. Comparison between electro-acupuncture and hydrotherapy, both in combination with patient education and patient education alone, on the symptomatic treatment of osteoarthritis of the hip. Clin J Pain 2004;20(3):179–85.
12. Hoeksma H, Dekker J, Ronday H, et al. Comparison of manual therapy and exercise therapy in osteoarthritis of the hip: a randomized clinical trial. Arthritis Care Res 2004;51(5):722–9.
13. Wegener T, Lupke N. Treatment of patients with arthrosis of hip or knee with an aqueous extract of devil's claw (Harpagophytum procumbens DC). Phytother Res 2003;17(10):1165–72.
14. Hopper D, Conneely M, Chromiak F, et al. Evaluation of the effect of two massage techniques on hamstring muscle length in competitive female hockey players. Phys Ther Sport 2005;6(3):137–45.
15. Hoskins W, Pollard H. The effect of a sports chiropractic manual therapy intervention on the prevention of back pain, hamstring and lower limb injuries in semi-elite Australian Rules footballers: a randomised controlled trial. BMC Musculoskelet Disord 2010;11:64.
16. Malliaropoulos N, Papalexandris S, Papalada A, et al. The role of stretching in rehabilitation of hamstring injuries: 80 athletes follow-up. Med Sci Sports Exerc 2004;36(5):756–9.
17. Higashi Y, Kiuchi T, Furuta K. Efficacy and safety profile of a topical methyl salicylate and menthol patch in adult patients with mild to moderate muscle strain: a randomised double-blind parallel-group placebo controlled multicenter study. Clin Ther 2010;32(1):34–43.
18. Mancinelli C, Davis D, Aboulhosn L, et al. The effects of massage on delayed onset muscle soreness and physical performance in female collegiate athletes. Phys Ther Sport 2006;7(1):5–13.
19. Orchard J, Seward H. 17th Annual AFL Injury Report 2008. Online. Available: www.afl.com.au/portals/0/afl_docs/2008_injury_survey.pdf; 2009.
20. Charnock B, Lewis C, Garrett W, et al. Adductor longus mechanics during the maximal effort soccer kick. Sports Biomech 2009;8(3):223–34.
21. Engebretsen A, Myklebust G, Holme I, et al. Intrinsic risk factors for hamstring injuries among male soccer players: a prospective cohort study. Am J of Sports Med 2010;38(6):1147–53.
22. Brukner P, Khan K. Clinical sports medicine. 3rd edn. North Ryde, NSW: McGraw-Hill; 2010.
23. Orchard J, Best T, Verrall G. Return to play following muscle strains. Clin J Sports Med 2005;15(6):436–41.
24. Holiday K, McWilliams D, Maciewicz R, et al. Lifetime body mass index, other anthropometric measures of obesity and risk of knee or hip osteoarthritis in the GOAL case control study. Osteoarthritis Cartilage 2011 Jan;19(1):37–43.
25. McAlindon TE, LaValley MP, Gulin JP, et al. Glucosamine and chondroitin for treatment of osteoarthritis: a systematic quality assessment and meta-analysis. JAMA 2000;283(11):1469–75.

19 The knee

The content of this chapter relates to the following Units of Competency:

HLTREM503C Plan remedial massage treatment strategy
HLTREM504C Apply remedial massage assessment framework
HLTREM502C Provide remedial massage treatment
HLTREM505C Perform remedial massage health assessment

Health Training Package HLT07

Learning Outcomes

- Assess clients with conditions of the knee for remedial massage, including identification of red and yellow flags.
- Assess clients for signs and symptoms associated with common conditions of the knee (including muscle strains, iliotibial band syndrome, patellofemoral pain syndrome, ligament sprains, degenerative joint disease and Osgood-Schlatter's disease), and treat and/or manage these conditions with remedial massage therapy.
- Develop treatment plans for clients with conditions of the knee, taking into account assessment findings, duration and severity of the condition, likely tissue types, clinical guidelines, the best available evidence and client preferences.
- Develop short- and long-term treatment plans to address presenting symptoms, underlying conditions and predisposing factors, and to progressively increase the self-help component of therapy.
- Adapt remedial massage therapy to suit individual client needs based on duration and severity of injury, the client's age and gender, the presence of underlying condition and co-morbidities and other consideration for special population groups.

INTRODUCTION

Knee pain accounts for about one-third of musculoskeletal problems seen in primary care settings in the US, predominantly in physically active patients.[1] In Australia about 12,000 sports-related knee injuries occur each year.[2] Three main mechanisms are responsible for knee injury: (1) overuse injuries, often associated with co-existing predisposing factors like genu valgus, varus or recurvatum; (2) twisting or explosive movements as occur in basketball and soccer; and (3) direct blows to the knee joint. The knee joint is also subject to degenerative changes associated with ageing and with overuse and following injury in sport. In the 2004–2005 National Health Survey, over 3 million Australians (15%) had some form of arthritis. Osteoarthritis was reported most commonly in the knees, neck, lower back, hip and fingers.[3]

FUNCTIONAL ANATOMY

The knee complex consists of:

- knee joint between the lateral and medial condyles of the distal femur and the lateral and medial condyles of the proximal end of the tibia
- patella, a sesamoid bone within the quadriceps tendon, which protects the tendon as it moves across the knee joint and acts as a pully to increase mechanical leverage
- tibial tuberosity, the insertion of the patella ligament
- fibula head which articulates with the lateral tibial condyle.

The knee joint is a modified hinge joint. Its main function is to maintain upright stance with as little energy expenditure as possible. This is achieved by the locking mechanism of the knee and its supporting ligaments. When the femur medially rotates on the tibia during the final stages of extension, the articulating surfaces are in the position of greatest contact and the supporting ligaments are taut. This is also referred to as the close-packed position of the knee. The knee is tight and stable and minimal muscle contraction is required to maintain upright stance (see Figure 19.1 on p 358).

The knee joint capsule (capsular ligament) encloses the patella, ligaments, menisci and bursae. It consists of a synovial and fibrous membrane separated by fat pads. The joint capsule is strengthened by a number of ligaments:

Extra-capsular ligaments

- Patella tendon (ligament), separated from the synovial membrane by an infrapatella fat pad and patella retinaculum (extensions of the aponeuroses of vastus medialis and lateralis).
- Oblique popliteal ligament (under the tendon of semimembranosus), from the medial condyle of tibia to the lateral condyle of femur.

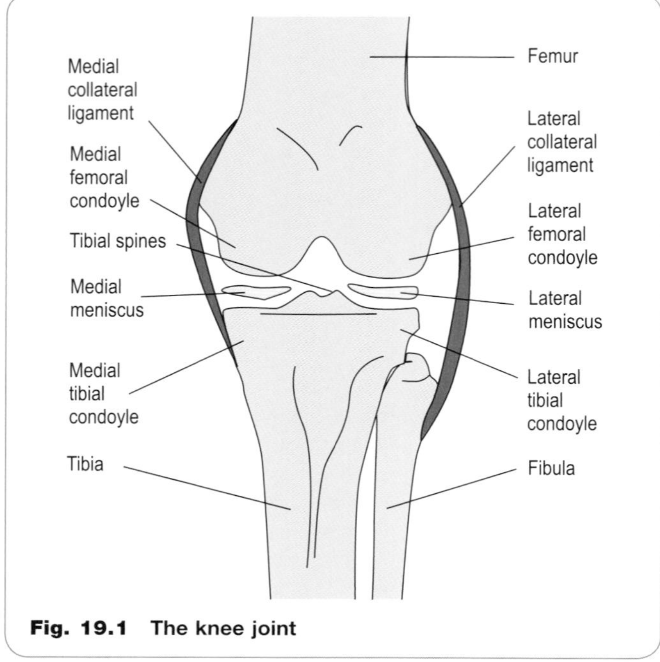

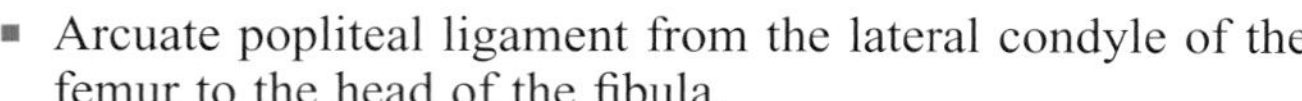

Fig. 19.1 The knee joint

- Arcuate popliteal ligament from the lateral condyle of the femur to the head of the fibula.
- Medial collateral ligament which runs from the medial femoral condyle to the medial tibial condyle. It also attaches to the medial meniscus.
- Lateral collateral ligament which runs from the lateral femoral condyle to the head of the fibula. It is not part of the joint capsule and does not attach to the lateral meniscus (see Figure 19.2).

Intra-capsular ligaments

- Anterior cruciate which runs from the anterior intercondylar area of the tibia to the medial surface of the lateral femoral condyle. It prevents anterior movement of the tibia on the femur or posterior movement of the femur on the tibia.
- Posterior cruciate which runs from the posterior intercondylar area of the tibia to the lateral surface of the medial femoral condyle. It prevents anterior movement of the femur on the tibia and posterior movement of the tibia on the femur. (Note: the anterior and posterior ligaments are named by their tibial attachments.)
- Coronary ligaments are extensions of fibrous capsule that attach the menisci to the tibia.
- Transverse ligament which runs between the anterior horns of the two menisci.

Two fibrocartilaginous discs cover the surface of tibial condyles. They improve the conformity of the articulating surfaces and cushion the joint.

- Lateral meniscus is oval-shaped and thicker and shorter than the medial meniscus. It is more mobile.
- Medial meniscus is C-shaped, thinner and larger. It is less mobile because of its attachment to the medial collateral ligament.

Bursa of the knee include (see Figure 19.3):

- Prepatellar bursa which overlies the patella below the skin.

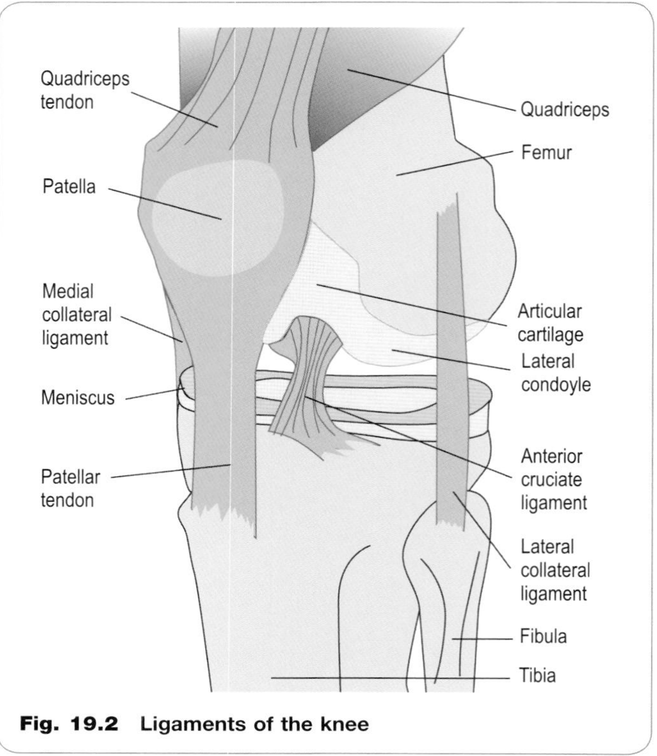

Fig. 19.2 Ligaments of the knee

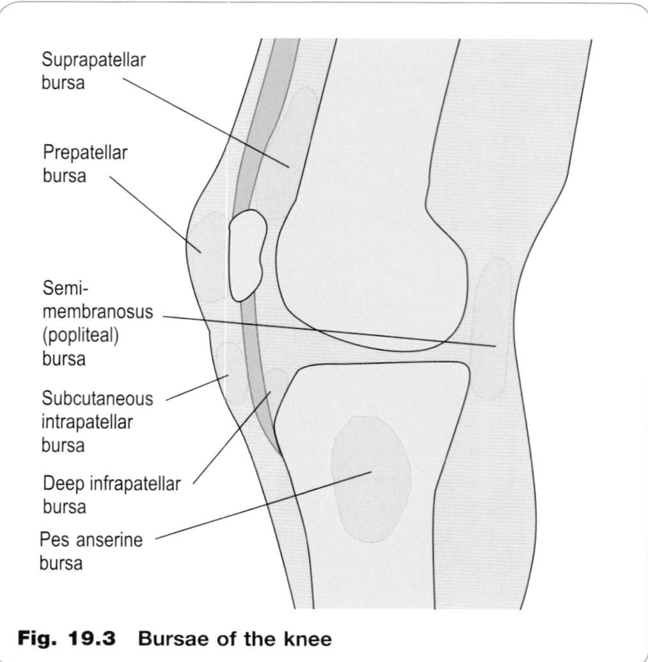

Fig. 19.3 Bursae of the knee

- (Deep) infrapatellar bursa between superior part of tibia and patellar ligament.
- Suprapatellar bursa between inferior part of femur and the quadriceps femoris muscle (communicates directly with the knee joint cavity).
- Popliteal bursa behind the knee joint, a communicating bursa.

Muscles

The prime movers of the knee joint are the quadriceps muscles (knee extension) and the hamstrings (knee flexion). The main function of the popliteus muscle is to unlock the extended (weight-bearing) knee. Popliteus laterally rotates the femur on the tibia and moves the lateral meniscus posteriorly at the beginning of knee flexion. External rotation when the knee is semi-flexed is a function of biceps femoris. Popliteus medially rotates the tibia when the knee is flexed along with sartorius, gracilis and semitendinosus (see Figure 19.4). The major muscles of the knee are described in Table 19.1.

Nerve supply to muscles that move the knee:

- Femoral nerve innervates the quadriceps and sartorius muscle.
- Sciatic nerve innervates the hamstrings and popliteus.
- Obturator nerve innervates gracilis.

Normally the knee joint has a slight valgus. The Q angle measures the angle between a line from the anterior superior iliac spine and the centre of the patella and a line through the centre of the patella and the tibial tuberosity. If the Q angle exceeds 15° to 20° (slightly more in females), the patella is likely to track laterally causing it to rub against

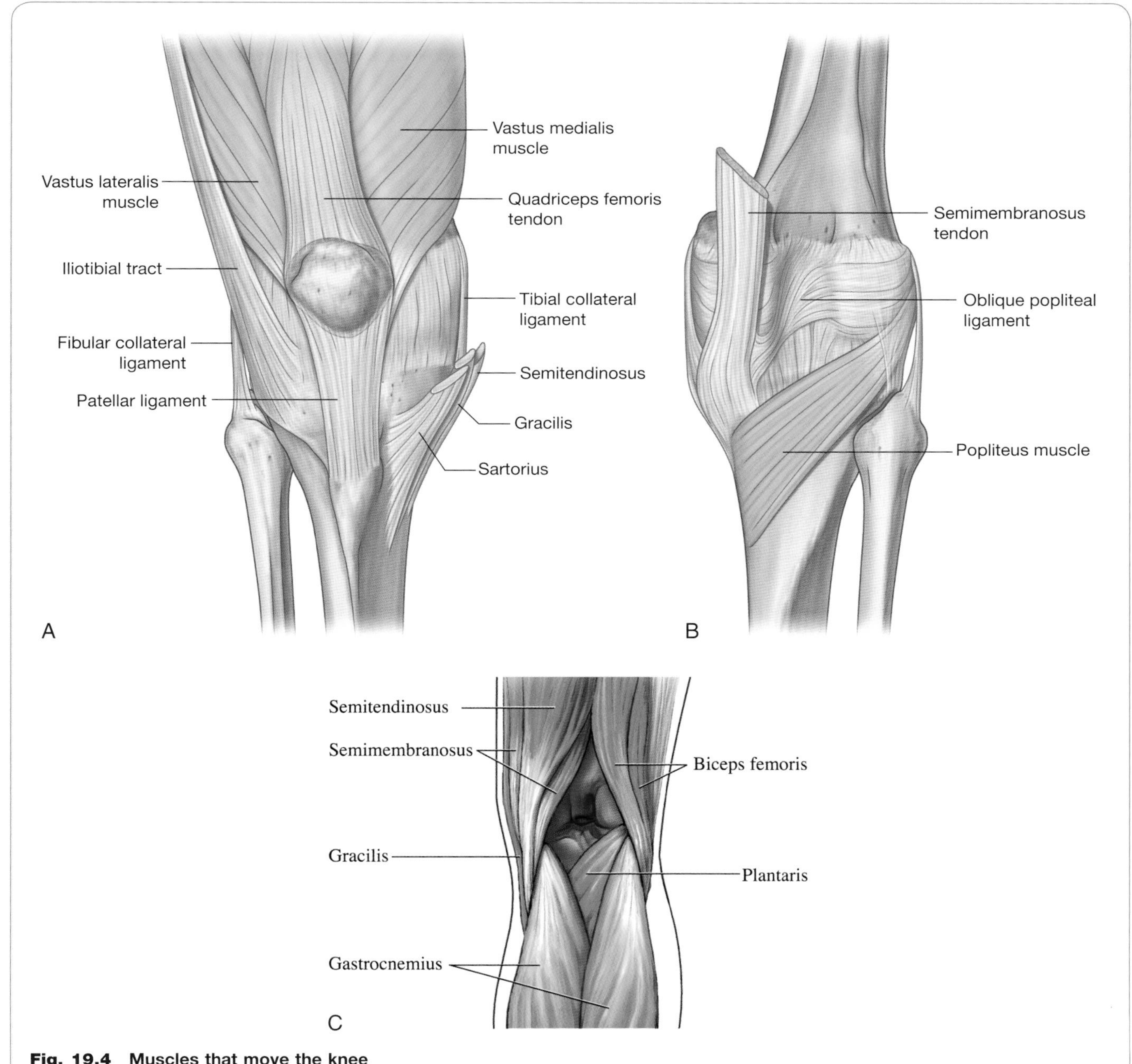

Fig. 19.4 Muscles that move the knee

Table 19.1 Muscles that move the knee[4]

Muscles that move the knee	Origin	Insertion	Action
Anterior compartment of the thigh Quadriceps femoris • Rectus femoris	Anterior inferior iliac spine	Patella via quadriceps tendon and then tibial tuberosity via patellar ligament	Extends leg at knee joint; acting alone also flexes thigh at hip joint
• Vastus lateralis	Greater trochanter and linea aspera of femur	Patella via quadriceps tendon and then tibial tuberosity via patellar ligament	Extends leg at knee joint
• Vastus medialis	Linea aspera of femur	Patella via quadriceps tendon and then tibial tuberosity via patellar ligament	
• Vastus intermedialis	Anterior and lateral surfaces of body of femur	Patella via quadriceps tendon and then tibial tuberosity via patellar ligament	
• Sartorius	Anterior superior iliac spine	Proximal part of medial surface of tibia near anterior border	Flexes leg at knee joint; flexes, abducts and laterally rotates thigh at hip joint; medial rotates tibia when knee is semi-flexed
Posterior compartment of the thigh Hamstrings • Biceps femoris	Long head arises from ischial tuberosity; short head arises from linea aspera and proximal ⅔ of supracondylar line of femur	Lateral side of head of fibula and lateral condyle of tibia	Flexes leg at knee joint and extends thigh at hip joint; externally rotates the knee when it is semi-flexed
• Semitendinosus	Ischial tuberosity	Proximal part of medial surface of shaft of tibia	Flexes leg at knee joint and extends thigh at hip joint; internally rotates tibia on femur when knee is semi-flexed
• Semimembranosus	Ischial tuberosity	Posteromedial aspect of medial condyle of tibia	
• Popliteus	Posterior aspect of lateral femoral condyle and lateral meniscus	Proximal part of posterior surface of tibia	Laterally rotates femur on tibia when the knee is extended: medially rotates tibia on the femur when the knee is flexed

Note: Gastrocnemius assists in flexion of the knee joint. It is described in Chapter 20.

the lateral femoral condyle. Conditions affecting normal alignment, such as genu valgus, genu varum, genu recurvatum and tibial torsion, can predispose the knee to injury (see Figure 19.5 on p 361).

ASSESSMENT

The purpose of remedial massage assessment includes:

- determining the suitability of clients for massage (contraindications and red flags)
- determining the duration (acute or subacute), severity and types of tissues involved in the injury/condition
- determining whether symptoms fit patterns of common conditions.

Principles of remedial massage assessment are discussed in Chapter 2. This section presents specific considerations for assessment of the knee.

CASE HISTORY

Information from case histories can alert practitioners to the presence of serious conditions requiring referral. Little is known about the usefulness of subjective complaints in diagnosing knee conditions.[5] It appears that the absence of weight bearing during trauma may help rule out meniscal tear.

Use targeted questioning to collect the most useful and relevant information, including:

- Identifying red flags requiring immediate referral (e.g. significant trauma, evidence of severe local inflammation, sepsis)[6] (see Table 19.2).
- Identifying yellow flags that require referral for further investigation.
- Identifying the exact location of the symptoms by asking clients to point to the site of pain.
- Determining if the pain is likely to have a mechanical cause. (Is the pain associated with rest or activity, certain postures or time of day?) Obtain descriptions of the

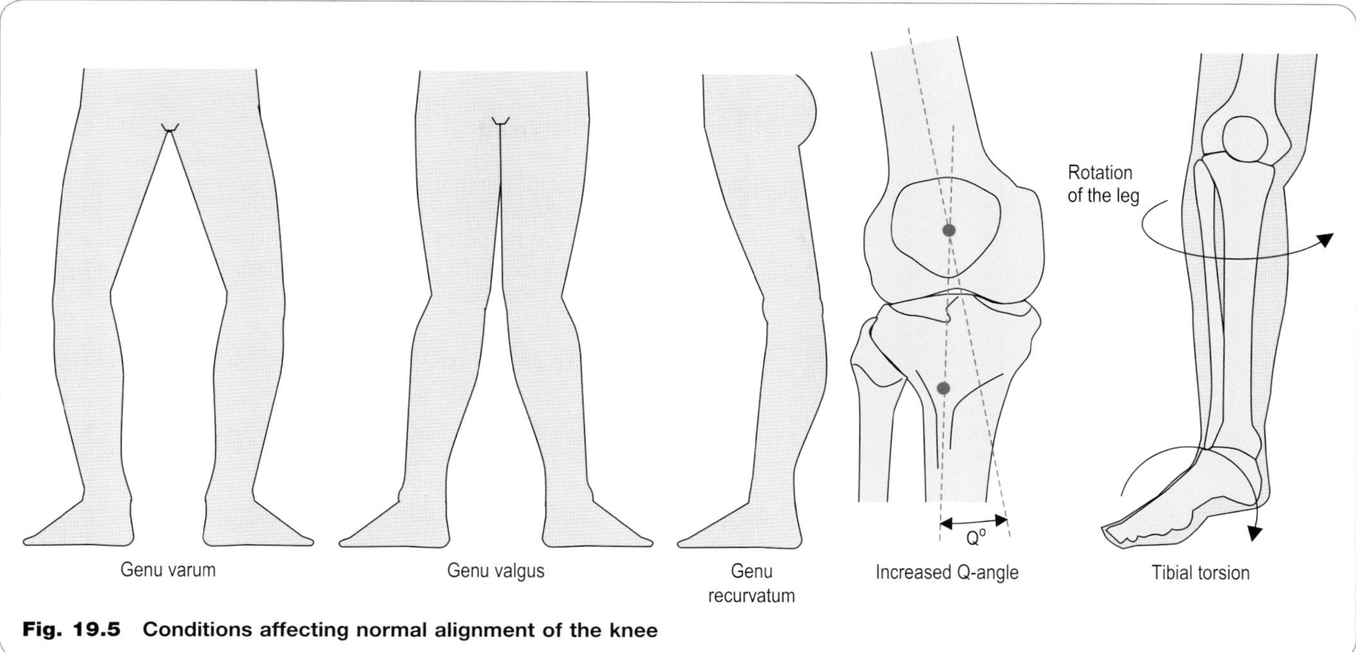

Fig. 19.5 Conditions affecting normal alignment of the knee

Assessment of the knee

1. Case history
2. Outcome measures (e.g. The Patient Specific Scale)
3. Postural analysis
4. Gait analysis
5. Functional tests
   Lumbar spine
   Active range of motion tests
   Flexion, extension, lateral flexion, rotation
   Hip joint
   Active range of motion tests
   Flexion, extension, abduction, adduction, internal rotation, external rotation
   Knee joint
   Active range of motion tests
   Flexion, extension, internal rotation, external rotation
   Passive range of motion tests
   Flexion, extension, internal rotation, external rotation
   Resisted range of motion tests
   Flexion, extension, internal rotation, external rotation
   Resisted and length tests for specific muscles, including:
   Hamstrings, quadriceps, sartorius, popliteus
   Special tests
   Patellofemoral grind test
   Patella apprehension test
   Valgus/varus stress tests
   Anterior/posterior draw tests
   Apley's compression test
6. Palpation

Table 19.2 Red flags for serious conditions associated with anterior knee pain[8]

Feature or risk factor	Condition
Symptoms and signs of infection (e.g. fever, night sweats, large warm effusion) Risk factors for infection (e.g. underlying disease process, immunosuppression, penetrating wound)	Infection
History of trauma Sudden onset of pain Minor trauma if >50 years, history of osteoporosis and taking corticosteroids Note that the Ottawa Knee Rule for Radiography is highly sensitive for knee fracture: if the client is under 55 years, can bear weight and flex the knee to 90°, and has no tenderness on the patella or fibula head, knee fracture can be ruled out (–LR = 0.40).[5, 9]	Fracture/ dislocation
Past history of malignancy Age >50 years Failure to improve with treatment Unexplained weight loss Pain at multiple sites Pain at rest	Tumour

specific mechanism of the injury and the forces involved, including:[7]

- Was the limb weight bearing at the time of injury?
- Was there any valgus or varus stress or rotational force at the time of injury?
- Did the knee contact the ground or an opponent?
- Was there a sound or pop/shift in the knee? (A pop is often associated with a torn anterior cruciate ligament; a shift can occur with anterior cruciate ligament rupture or patella dislocation.)
- What happened after the injury? (Collapse, inability to continue playing, inability to weight bear suggest fracture or serious ligament injury.)
- Did the knee swell and, if so, how quickly did it occur? (Swelling in the first hour suggests haemarthrosis from ruptured cruciate ligament or fracture: swelling

developing more slowly suggests traumatic synovitis associated with meniscal tears and chondral pathology.)
  - Did the knee click, lock or is it unstable? (Painful clicking suggests meniscal tear or chondral pathology.)
- Determining if the client has a history of gout, pseudogout, rheumatoid arthritis or degenerative joint disease.
- Refer any client with evidence of neurological compromise (e.g. change in cutaneous sensation, weakness of foot/toe muscles) or vascular compromise.

OUTCOME MEASURES

Outcome measures are questionnaires that are specifically designed to assess clients' level of impairment and to define benefits of treatment. The Patient Specific Scale can be used to measure progress of treatment of clients with any musculoskeletal condition, including knee conditions.

POSTURAL ANALYSIS

Postural analysis enables observation of the whole client and facilitates identification of important features through bilateral comparison. It also facilitates detection of possible predisposing or contributing factors that may be implicated, observing the position of the cervical, thoracic and lumbar spines, pelvic balance and alignment of the lower limb (e.g. increased Q-angle, genu valgus, genu varum, genu recurvatum and tibial torsion – see Figure 19.5 on page 361). Observe and compare the knees posteriorly, laterally and anteriorly, noting their symmetry. Observe any bruising, colour changes, swelling or bumps. The level of the popliteal creases can indicate leg length. Observe the contour of the thigh and lower leg muscles, noting muscle hypertonicity or atrophy.

GAIT ANALYSIS

During the gait cycles the knee flexes and extends: it flexes to absorb the impact of heel strike (quadriceps eccentrically contracts), extends during mid-stance (quadriceps concentrically contracts) and flexes again for toe-off and swing (gastrocnemius concentrically contracts) (see Chapter 2).

Observe any disturbance to the rate and rhythm of normal gait and the phase of the gait cycle in which it occurs. Impaired knee flexion can result in the trunk being thrust forward at heel strike or manually extending the knee by pressing on their thigh. Impaired knee flexion could prevent the leg from clearing the ground. In this case the pelvis may be hiked up in swing phase. Note any toe-in gait which may be associated with tibial torsion.

FUNCTIONAL TESTS

For any tests involving joint movements it is important to compare both sides and take into account any underlying pathology, previous surgical procedures and the age and lifestyle of the client. Findings from physical examinations should be interpreted in the light of evidence for their diagnostic accuracy. Knee range of motion has consistently been highly reliable but of unknown diagnostic utility.[5] Generally, combining tests seems to be useful for identifying and ruling out various knee conditions. The anterior draw test is useful for identifying anterior cruciate ligament tears (+LR = 9.0–39.3, –LR = 0.08–0.35). Valgus and varus tests are fairly good at ruling out medial collateral ligament tears (–LR = 0.20–0.30). The patella apprehension test appears to be good at identifying and ruling out patella instability. (+LR = 8.3, –LR = 0.00).[5]

Active range of motion (AROM) of the lumbar spine (flexion, extension, lateral flexion and rotation)

Examination of the knee begins with functional tests of the lumbar spine to help rule out conditions which refer pain to the knee. Look for dermatomal distribution of symptoms (see Figure 19.6). If active range of motion tests of the lumbar

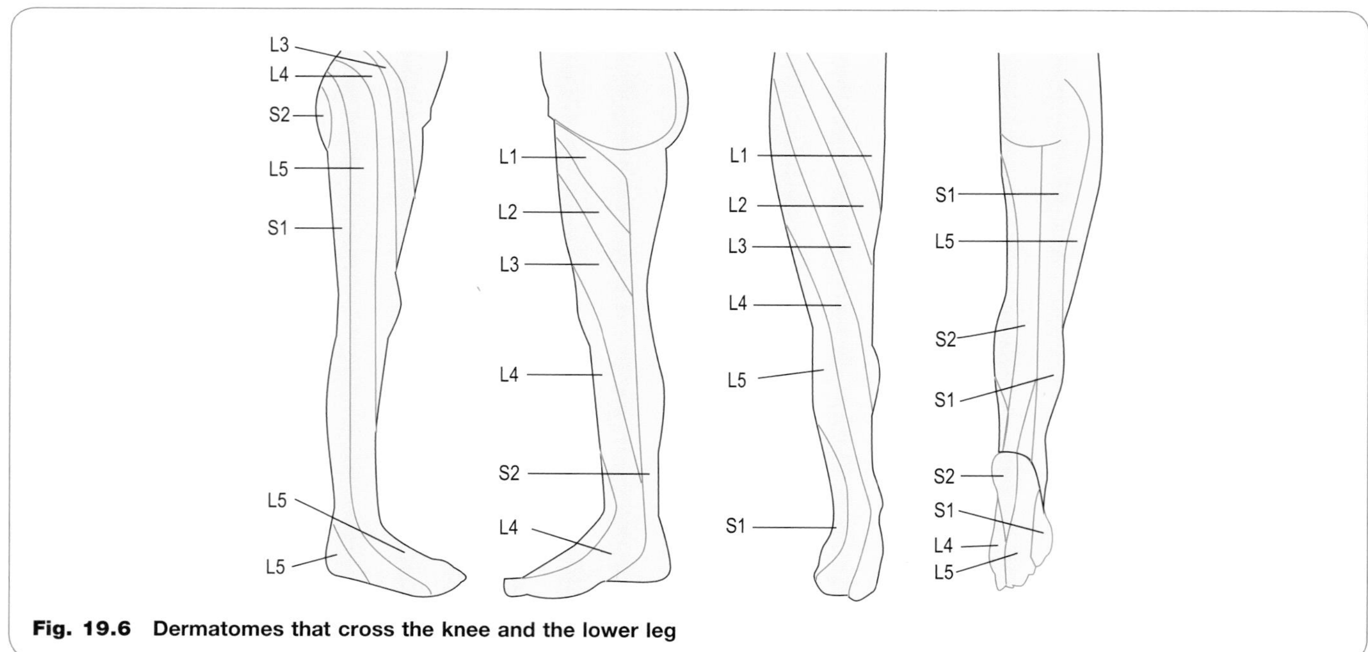

Fig. 19.6 Dermatomes that cross the knee and the lower leg

spine reproduce the lower limb symptoms, further examination of the lumbar spine is indicated (see Chapter 10).

AROM of the hip joint

Examine the hip joint to help rule out hip joint pathology that refers pain to the knee and/or lower leg. If active range of motion tests of the hip joint reproduce the lower limb symptoms, further examination of the hip is indicated (see Chapter 18).

AROM of the knee

The client may be seated on the treatment table. Face the client and demonstrate the movements. Examine the following ranges of motion:

- Flexion/extension (130–150°/0–5[10])
- Internal/external rotation (5°/5°). Stabilise the thigh proximal to the knee and instruct the client to turn their lower leg outwards and inwards.

Passive range of motion (PROM)

If the client is unable to perform normal AROM in any direction, further investigation is required. The client may be seated or supine. Passive flexion and extension should be tested with one hand contacting the front of the knee and the other hand above the ankle. For passive internal and external rotation, stabilise the thigh above the knee and with the other hand holding the leg above the ankle, externally and internally rotate the lower leg. In the supine position, the client's hip and knee are flexed to 90° to perform passive internal and external rotation. Normal end-feel for knee flexion is described as soft tissue compression and for extension elastic/firm capsular.[9] However, assessment of end-feel appears to have low interrater reliability.[5]

Resisted range of motion (RROM)

RROM tests should also be performed if AROM testing indicates the likelihood of a knee or lower leg strain. RROM tests include:

- flexion: hamstrings (semitendinosus, semimembranosus, biceps femoris), sartorius
- extension: quadriceps (vastus medialis, vastus lateralis, vastus intermedius, rectus femoris)
- internal rotation: popliteus with pes anserine muscles (knee flexed)
- external rotation: popliteus (knee extended); biceps femoris (knee flexed).

Resisted tests and length tests for specific muscles[11, 12]

If RROM tests reproduce symptoms, then further tests may be used to help identify specific muscles.

1. HAMSTRINGS

Resisted tests

To test the hamstrings as a group, the client lies prone with their knee flexed to 90°. The client tries to bring their heel towards the buttock against your resistance (see Figure 19.7).

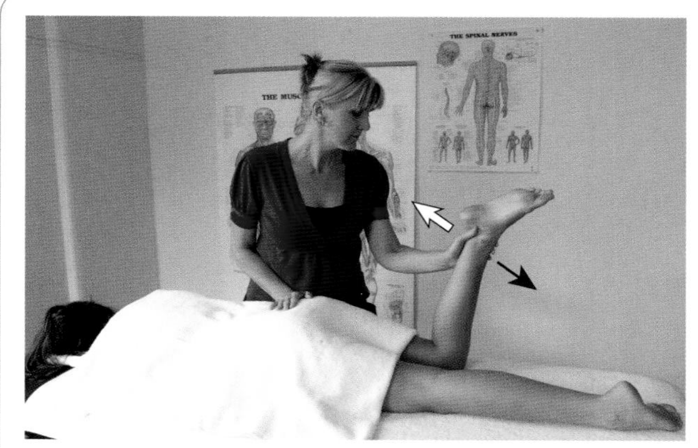

Fig. 19.7 Resisted hamstring test

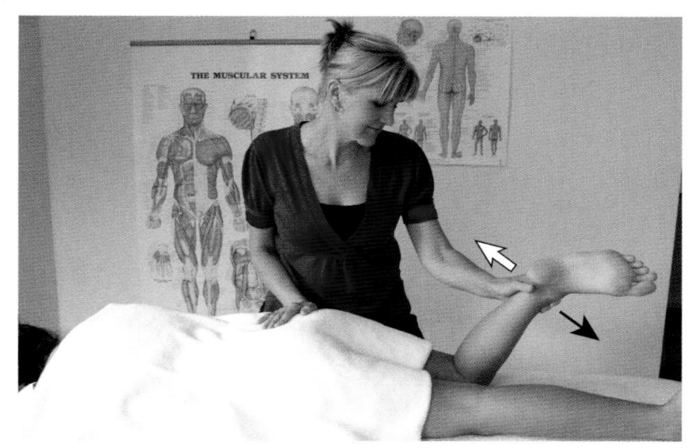

Fig. 19.8 Resisted biceps femoris test

The lateral and medial hamstring muscles may also be tested separately.

Lateral hamstrings (biceps femoris)

The client's knee is flexed to 50° to 70° with the thigh in slight lateral rotation. Apply resistance as the client tries to flex their knee (see Figure 19.8).

Medial hamstrings (semimembranosus, semitendinosus)

This test is similar to the test for biceps femoris except that the client's thigh is placed in slight medial rotation. In this position the client tries to flex their knee against your resistance (see Figure 19.9 on p 364).

Length test

Shortened hamstring muscles restrict knee extension when the hip is flexed or restrict hip flexion when the knee is extended (see Figure 19.10 on p 364).

2. QUADRICEPS

Resisted test

As a group, the quadriceps can be tested with the client seated. Place one hand over the knee and the other over the ankle. Apply resistance as the client tries to straighten their knee.

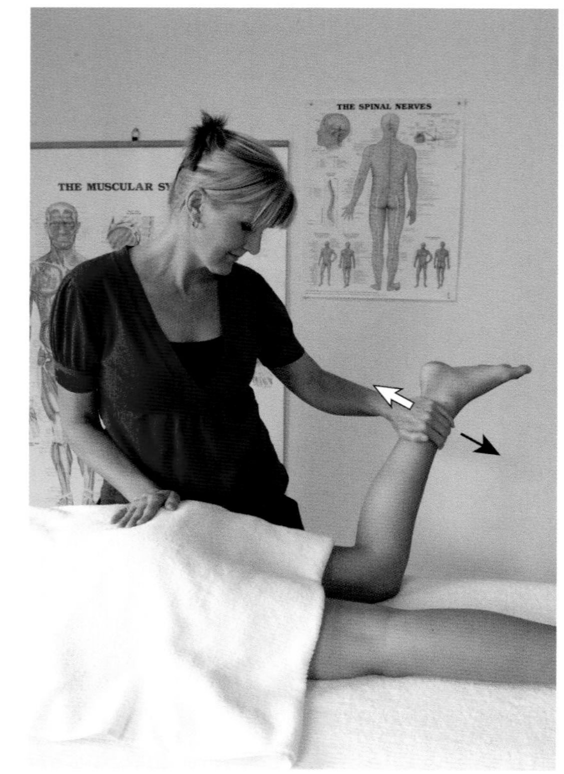

Fig. 19.9 Resisted semimembranosus and semitendinosus test

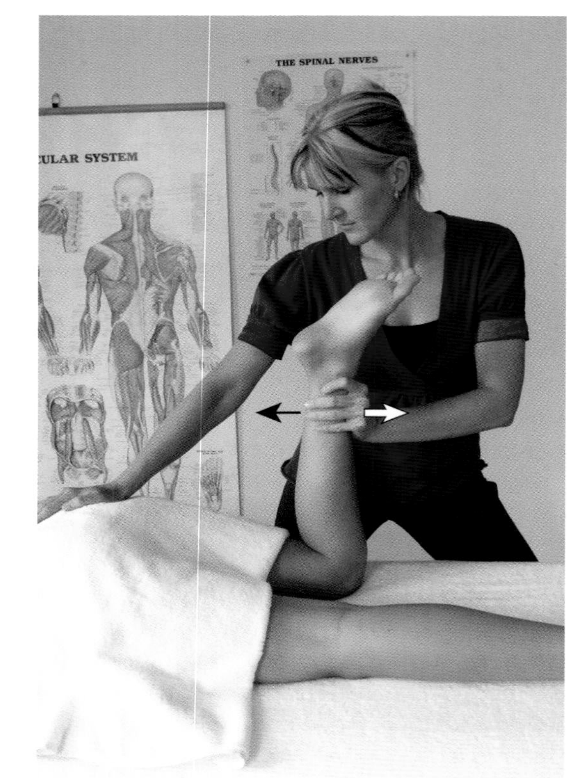

Fig. 19.11 Resisted quadriceps test

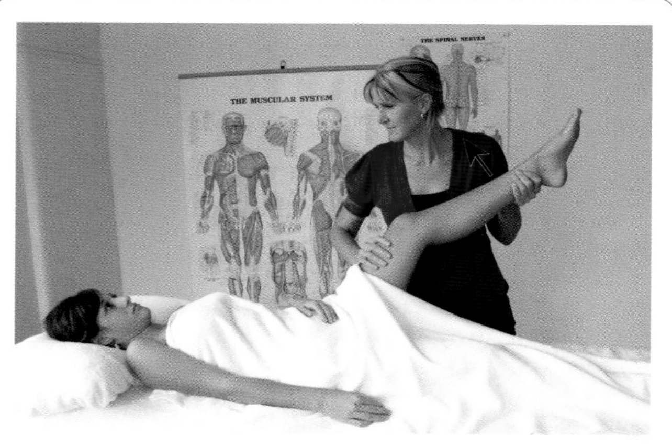

Fig. 19.10 Length test for the hamstring muscles

Quadriceps can also be tested with the client in the prone position. Apply resistance as the client tries to take their heel to their buttock (see Figure 19.11).

Quadriceps activation differs in open chain (non-weight-bearing) and closed chain (weight-bearing) positions. In open chain positions, vastus medialis obliquus is activated last and with smaller amplitude (30% of maximal voluntary contraction) and may be distinguished from other quadriceps muscles by resisting near end range extension. In closed chain positions, there is more activation of vastus medialis obliquus than vastus lateralis at 40° of semisquat with the hip medially rotated 30° degrees.[13] Double leg squat with simultaneous isometric hip adduction may be useful in selectively strengthening vastus medialis obliquus.[14]

Length test

Shortening of the quadriceps restricts knee flexion. Shortened rectus femoris can be observed as restricted knee flexion when the hip is extended or restricted hip extension when the knee is flexed (see Figure 19.12 on p 365).

3. SARTORIUS

Resisted test

The client lies supine with one foot across the knee of the other leg (figure 4 position). Place one hand on the knee and the other on the ankle. The client is instructed to hold this position while you try to straighten the leg (i.e. move the hip into extension, medial rotation and adduction, and the knee into extension) (see Figure 19.13 on p 365).

Alternatively, the client may be seated and instructed to try to place one foot on the opposite knee against your resistance.

Length test

A shortened sartorius muscle limits hip flexion, abduction and external rotation and knee flexion. For example, a client with shortened sartorius muscles has difficulty sitting cross-legged. A contracture of sartorius can produce a flexion, abduction

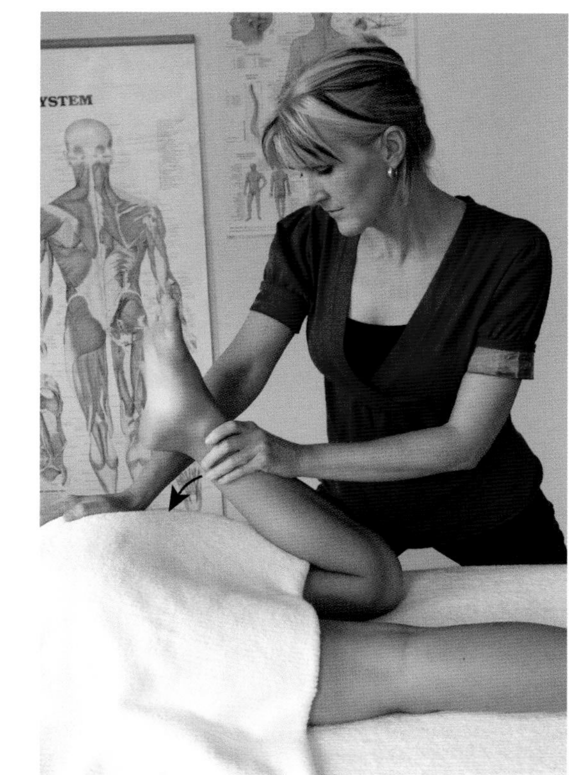

Fig. 19.12 **Length test for rectus femoris**

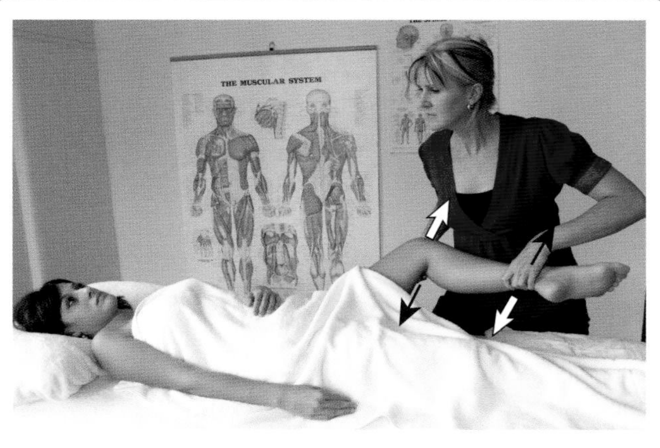

Fig. 19.13 **Resisted test for sartorius**

and lateral rotation deformity of the hip, along with flexion of the knee.

4. POPLITEUS

Resisted test

The client sits with their knee flexed at 90° and is instructed to rotate their leg medially against resistance (see Figure 19.14). Note that weakness in popliteus can lead to hyperextension of the knee and lateral rotation of the tibia against the femur. Popliteus weakness is commonly associated with hamstring imbalance where lateral hamstrings are relatively strong and medial hamstrings weak.[11]

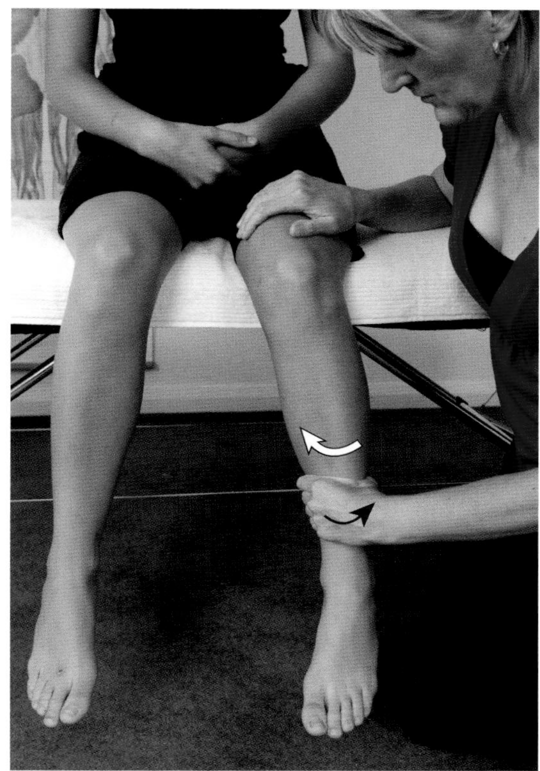

Fig. 19.14 **Resisted test for popliteus**

Test for contracture

Contracture of popliteus results in slight flexion of the knee and medial rotation of the tibia against the femur.

Special tests

Special tests are designed to reproduce the client's symptoms. If symptoms are reported when performing a special test, ask the client to identify their exact location and confirm that they are the same as those described in the case history. Positive special test results should always be interpreted cautiously and in the context of other clinical findings (see Chapter 2).

PATELLA

Patellofemoral grind test

The client is supine, legs extended. Gently compress the patella onto the femur using one palm on top of the other. Maintaining the pressure, gently move the patella inferiorly. Pain and/or crepitus suggests patellofemoral syndrome, degenerative joint disease or osteochondritis of the patella (see Figure 19.15 on p 366).

Patella apprehension test

This test is designed to determine if the patella is prone to lateral dislocation. The client lies supine. Gently move the patella laterally while observing the client for signs of apprehension. A positive test suggests patella instability (see Figure 19.16 on p 366).

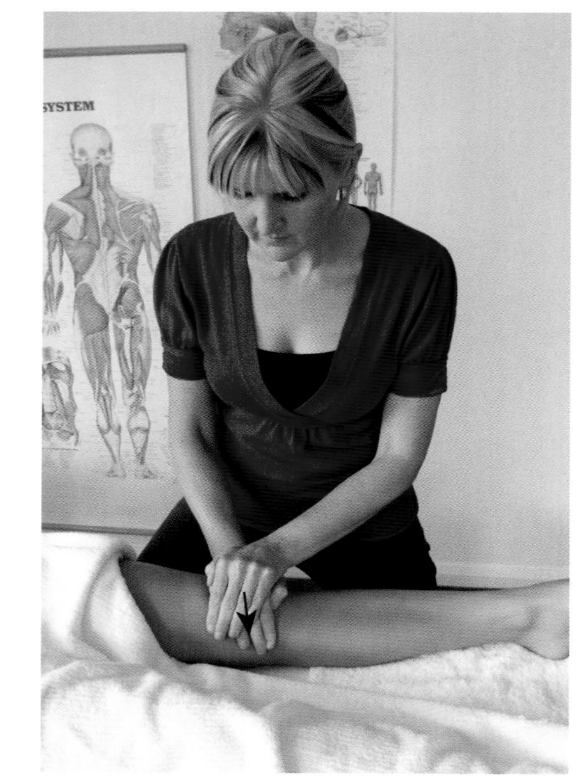

Fig. 19.15 Patellofemoral grind test

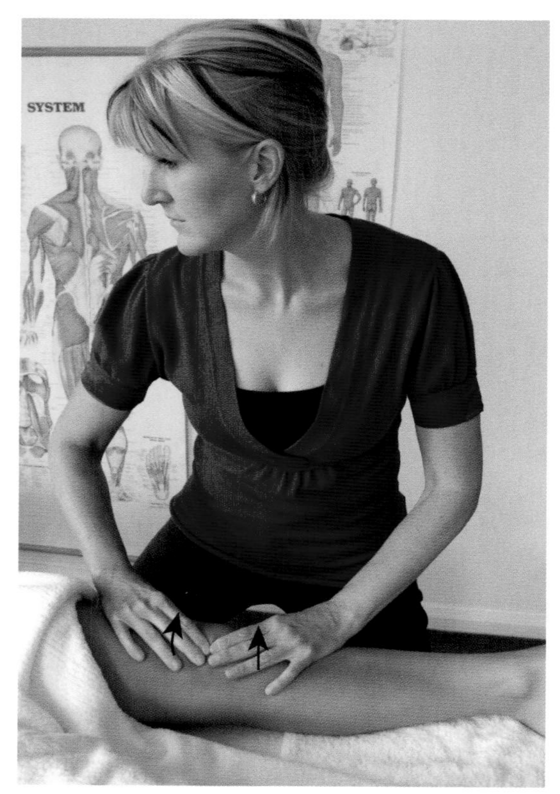

Fig. 19.16 Patella apprehension test

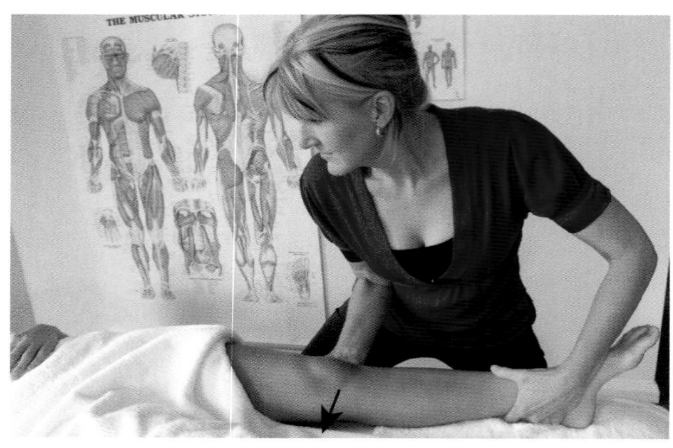

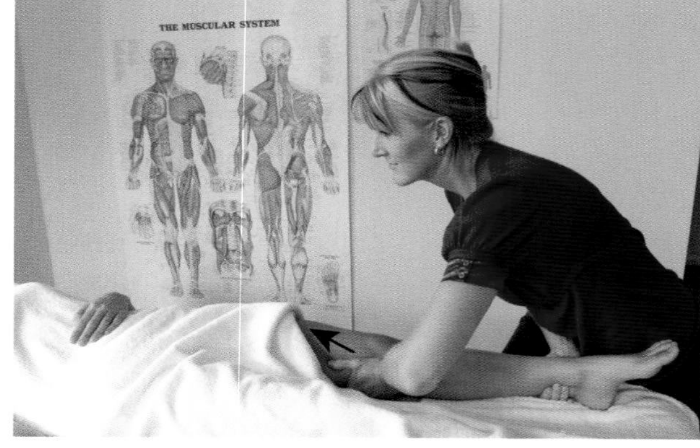

Fig. 19.17 Valgus/varus stress tests

LIGAMENTS

Valgus/varus stress tests

The client lies supine, legs extended. Stand at the side of the table just below the knee and stabilise the medial ankle with one hand. With the other hand apply lateral to medial (valgus) pressure at the knee. This tests the integrity of the medial collateral ligament. To test the lateral collateral ligament, the lateral ankle is stabilised and medial to lateral (varus) stress is applied to the knee (see Figure 19.17).

Anterior/posterior draw test

The client lies supine with the knee flexed to 90° and the foot flat on the table. Place a folded towel across the client's foot and sit on the end of the table to stabilise the client's foot. Place both your hands around their leg just distal to the knee joint and gently draw the proximal tibia forward. Pain during the test suggests anterior cruciate ligament sprain; excessive movement suggests rupture.[15]

The client maintains the same position for the anterior and posterior draw tests. In the posterior draw test the proximal tibia is pushed posteriorly to test the integrity of the posterior cruciate ligament. Pain during the procedure suggests ligament sprain; excessive movement suggests rupture (see Figure 19.18 on p 367).

MENISCUS

Apley's compression test

The client lies prone with knee flexed to 90°. Place both hands on the plantar surface of the foot and apply sufficient

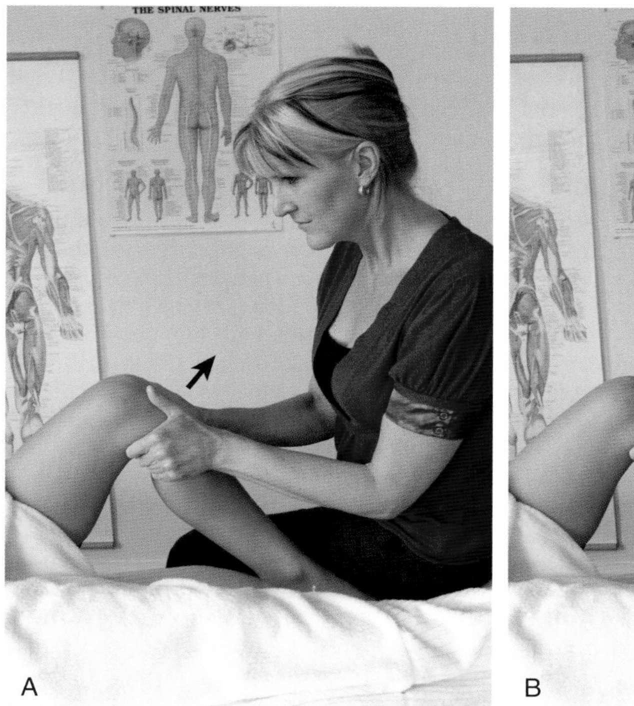

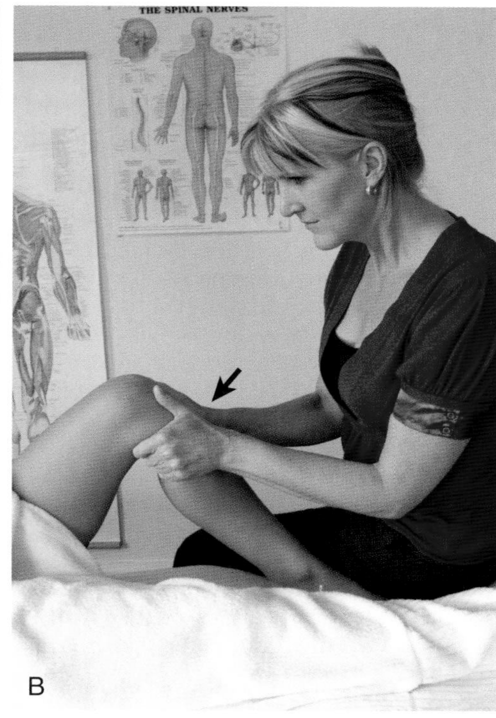

Fig. 19.18 Anterior/posterior draw tests

pressure to compress the medial and lateral menisci between the tibia and femur. The pressure is maintained while the tibia is internally and externally rotated on the femur. Pain on this manoeuvre suggests meniscal damage (see Figure 19.19).

Note: Apley's distraction test can help distinguish between meniscal and ligamentous or capsular lesions. The client's position is the same as for Apley's compression test. Stabilise the knee by placing one knee on the client's mid thigh. Using both hands, hold the ankle and apply traction to the leg while rotating the tibia internally and externally. This manoeuvre reduces pressure on the meniscus and puts strain on the coronary ligaments and joint capsule.

PALPATION

Palpatory findings along with findings from other assessments are used to guide treatment plans.

With the client supine, palpate the patella which lies entirely above the level of the knee joint. To palpate its underside move the patella gently from side to side. Palpate the quadriceps muscle just proximal to the patella and compare the lateral and medial muscles. (In patellofemoral syndrome, vastus lateralis is hypertonic and vastus medialis palpates as hypotonic or atrophied.)

Palpate the patella tendon inferior to the patella and its attachment to the tibial tuberosity. Tenderness at the tibial tuberosity suggests quadriceps tendinitis or, in an athletic child, Osgood-Schlatter's disease. The superficial infrapatellar bursa and prepatellar bursa are normally not palpable although they may palpate as boggy when inflamed.

Bend the client's knee and place their foot on the table. From the depression at the side of the infrapatellar tendon,

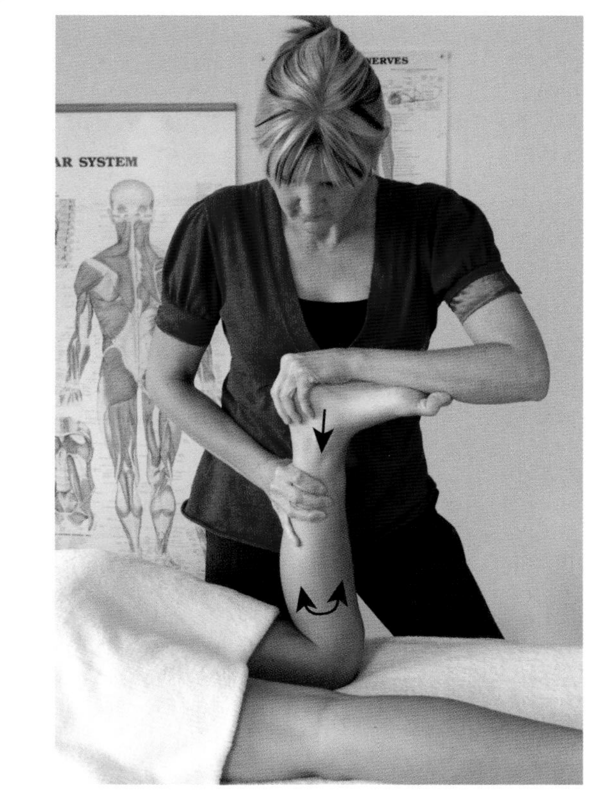

Fig. 19.19 Apley's compression

palpate medially to the upper edge of the medial tibial plateau and the attachment point of the medial meniscus. Move superiorly to palpate the medial femoral condyle immediately medial to the patella. Palpate the medial femoral epicondyle and the attachment of the medial collateral ligament. Trace the medial collateral ligament to the medial surface of the tibia.

The adductor tubercle is a useful landmark. Grasp the medial side of the proximal lower leg and press laterally and inferiorly with the thumb. Resisting hip adduction makes the tendon of adductor magnus become prominent. Sartorius, gracilis and semitendinosus muscles attach to the tibia at the pes anserine insertion. Palpate the posterior medial knee and resist knee flexion to detect the prominent semitendinosus.

From the depression at the side of the infrapatellar tendon, palpate the lateral tibial plateau and the lateral tubercle just below it. Palpate the lateral femoral condyle and epicondyle. The lateral collateral ligament runs between the lateral femoral condyle and the fibular head. It may be more easily palpated by placing the client's foot on the knee of the other leg. In this position it is palpated as a cord in front of the biceps tendon under the client's flexed knee.

The head of the fibula is inferior and posterior and approximately level with the tibial tuberosity. The common peroneal nerve crosses the neck of the fibula. Avoid heavy pressure on the nerve which can cause pain and/or paraesthesia. With the knee extended the anterior border of the iliotibial tract becomes prominent. When the client flexes their knee against resistance the iliotibial tract is palpable lateral to the patella.

With the client's knee bent, resist knee flexion. Feel the biceps tendon laterally and trace it to the head of the fibula. Palpate the prominent semitendinosus tendon medially. Biceps femoris forms the superior lateral border of the popliteal fossa and semimembranosus and semitendinosus form its superior medial border. The two heads of gastrocnemius form its inferior borders. The posterior tibial nerve bisects the fossa vertically. The popliteal vein and artery are medial to the tibial nerve.

REMEDIAL MASSAGE TREATMENT

Assessment of the knee provides essential information for development of treatment plans, including:

- client's suitability for remedial massage therapy
- duration of the condition (i.e. acute or chronic)
- severity of the condition (i.e. grade of injury; mild, moderate or severe pain)
- type(s) of tissues involved
- priorities for treatment if more than one injury or condition are present
- whether the signs and symptoms suggest a common condition of the knee region
- special considerations for individual clients (e.g. client's preference for treatment types and styles, special population considerations).

Treatment options must always be considered in the context of the best available evidence for treatment effectiveness and clinical practice guidelines where they exist. Treatments for osteoarthritis of the knee have been the subjects of a number of systematic reviews. For example, one systematic review examined the evidence for the use of thermotherapy in the treatment of osteoarthritis of the knee.[16] Firm conclusions could not be drawn because of the small size and low quality of the studies. However, the authors concluded that there is silver level evidence that ice massage could be used to improve range of motion and strength of the knee in people with osteoarthritis of the knee and that cold packs may be used to decrease swelling. Silver level evidence was also found in another systematic review for the use of a brace and a lateral wedge insole for osteoarthritis of the knee. There was no evidence whether a brace or insole was more effective. Aquatic exercises were found to have some beneficial short-term effects for patients with hip and/or knee osteoarthritis.[17] An updated systematic review could still not confirm the effectiveness of transcutaneous electrostimulation for pain relief in patients with osteoarthritis of the knee.[18] However, an updated systematic review on the effectiveness of therapeutic ultrasound found more promising results.[19]

A number of randomised controlled trials have examined the effectiveness of massage on muscles. A study by Hunter et al[20] examined the effect of lower limb massage on electromyography and force production of the knee extensors. The study of ten healthy males measured isokinetic concentric contractions of the knee extensors at speeds of 60°, 120°, 180° and 240°/second before and after a 30-minute massage and found a significant decrease at contractions of 60°/sec and a trend for a decrease at contractions of 120°/sec as a result of massage compared with passive rest. The authors suggest that this was because massage influenced muscle architecture. In another small study, sports massage was not found to reduce girth or pain in the lower leg after eccentric exercise within 72 hours.[21] In contrast, massage and dynamic soft tissue manipulation (massage targeted to the areas of muscle tightness including deep gliding and soft tissue release) were shown to have an immediate and significant effect on hamstring length in competitive female field hockey players.[22]

A study by Loghmani and Warden[23] examined the effects of instrument-assisted cross-fibre friction massage on tissue-level healing of knee medial collateral ligament injuries. The authors concluded that instrument-assisted cross-fibre massage accelerated ligament healing, possibly through enhanced collagen formation and organisation, although there appeared to be minimum effects on the final outcome of healing. Aromatherapy massage was also examined in a study by Yip and Tam.[24] The authors found promising results for the short-term relief of moderate to severe knee pain among 59 elderly clients in Hong Kong with the use of massage with aromatic ginger and orange essential oil.

Current research on interventions for anterior knee pain are summarised in Table 19.3.

OVERVIEW

Develop a short- and a long-term plan for each client. The short-term plan directs treatment to the highest priority (usually determined by symptoms). The long-term plan can be introduced when presenting symptoms have subsided. Treatment of all knee problems should include attention to contributing or predisposing factors such as underlying structural features, especially of the lower back, pelvis, hip, ankle and foot, and lifestyle factors. A significant part of both short-term and long-term treatment is educating clients

Table 19.3 Evidence for interventions for anterior knee pain[8]

Evidence of benefit	• Advice to stay active: maintenance of normal activity has a beneficial effect on patellofemoral pain compared to no treatment and to the use of patellofemoral orthoses. • Injection therapy: Injection therapy (treatment and placebo saline) appears to be effective for the management of patellofemoral pain in the short term compared to no injection therapy. • Foot orthoses: Foot orthoses in combination with quadriceps and hamstring exercises are effective compared to placebo insoles in women with patellofemoral pain. • Exercises: A six-week regimen of quadriceps muscle retraining, patellofemoral joint mobilisation, patella taping and daily home exercises significantly reduces patellofemoral pain compared to placebo in the short term. • Eccentric quadriceps exercises produce better functional outcomes compared to standard quadriceps strengthening exercises.
Conflicting evidence	• Patellofemoral orthoses: There is conflicting opinion about the effectiveness of patellofemoral orthoses compared to other interventions and no treatment for patellofemoral pain.
Insufficient evidence	• Acupuncture • Analgesics • Electrical stimulation to the quadriceps muscle • Non-steroidal anti-inflammatory drugs (NSAIDs) • Patella taping • Progressive resistance braces • Therapeutic ultrasound
Evidence of no benefit	• There is evidence that low-level laser therapy provides similar effect to sham laser in the management of patellofemoral pain.

about likely causal or aggravating factors and guiding their management of these factors. If massage therapy is used in conjunction with other treatments it is important to communicate with other treating practitioners. Health conditions can be complex and do not always conform to assessment protocols. Working with other practitioners provides an opportunity to develop integrative treatment practices for the best outcomes for clients.

MUSCLE STRAIN

Muscle imbalances arise when muscles develop shortness and tightness or become inhibited and weak. These imbalances cause dysfunctional movement patterns.[25] Muscles of the low back, pelvis and lower limb can affect knee function:
Muscles that tend to be tight and short:

- Iliopsoas, tensor fasciae latae, rectus femoris, quadratus lumborum, pectineus, gracilis, hip adductors, hamstrings (lateral hamstrings more than medial), soleus, gastrocnemius, piriformis and other external rotators of the hip.

Key assessment findings for muscle strain

- History of repetitive overuse
- Functional tests of the knee:
  - AROM: positive in one or more directions
  - PROM: may be positive at end of range (passive muscle stretch)
  - RROM: positive for affected muscle(s)
  - Resisted and length tests: positive for affected muscle(s)
- Palpation positive for tenderness/pain. Muscle spasm and myofibril tears/scar tissue may also be evident.

Muscles that tend to be weak:

- Gluteus maximus, hip abductors, hip internal rotators (gluteus minimus and medius), vastus lateralis, intermedius and especially vastus medius obliquus, dorsiflexors of the ankle, especially tibialis anterior.

Quadriceps tendinitis at the knee

Quadriceps muscle strains tend to occur at three common sites: (1) tenoperiosteal junction at the superior aspect of the patella, (2) infrapatella tendon (jumper's knee) and (3) the quadriceps expansion.[25] The client presents with pain at the front of the knee after excessive or sudden contraction of the quadriceps (e.g. running, hiking, dancing, squats or repetitive deep knee bends in weight lifting).

Hamstring tendinitis at the knee

Hamstring strain is a common muscle strain in activities and sports that involve excessive eccentric contractions of the hamstrings such as running, kicking and dancing. The muscle is vulnerable to strain when it is eccentrically contracting to fully extend the knee at heel strike, particularly when a fuller or more intense stretch than usual is required (e.g. running on slippery or hilly surfaces). Ankle pronation and hip anteversion may predispose to hamstring tendinitis. Pain is felt at the medial or lateral tenoperiosteal insertions of the hamstring muscles either side of the knee.

Assessment

HISTORY

The client complains of localised knee pain that is aggravated by activity and relieved by rest. There is a history of repetitive overuse (e.g. excessive running, kicking, dancing) or an episode that required more than usual intensity of muscle contraction (e.g. running on slippery or hilly surfaces).

FUNCTIONAL TESTS

Lumbar AROM tests do not reproduce knee symptoms.
Hip AROM tests do not reproduce knee symptoms (except for resisted hip flexion for rectus femoris strains and resisted hip extension for hamstring strains).

Knee tests

AROM: positive in one or more directions.
PROM: positive at the end of the range of motion when the affected muscle is passively stretched.
RROM: positive for affected muscles.

Resisted tests and length tests positive for affected muscles.
Special tests: Negative.

PALPATION

Tenderness or pain may be elicited during palpation at the site of lesion. Muscle spasm, myofibril tears or scar tissue may be evident.

Overview of treatment for muscle strains

For acute muscle strains the RICE regimen is recommended. Advise the client to avoid the responsible activity. An elastic knee brace with cutout and horseshoe pad may be useful, especially if patellar tracking correction is required. Pain-free stretches and isometric exercises of the affected muscle should be introduced as soon as possible.

A typical treatment for grades 1 or 2 muscle strains includes:

- Swedish massage to the lower limb including ankle and foot, low back and pelvis.
- Remedial massage techniques for muscle strains include (see Table 19.4):
  - deep gliding frictions along the muscle fibres
  - cross-fibre frictions
  - soft tissue releasing techniques
  - deep transverse friction
  - trigger point therapy
  - muscle stretching.
- Myofascial release including cross-arm techniques and the leg pull (see Chapter 8).

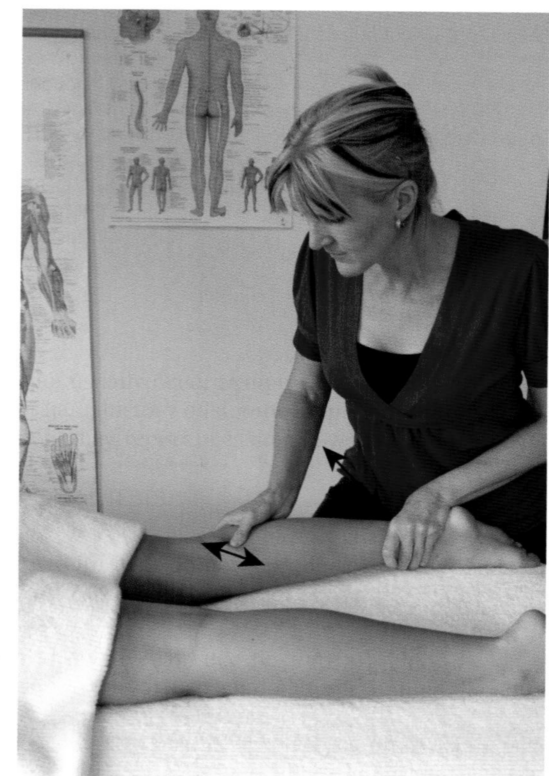

Fig. 19.20 Popliteus release

Other remedial techniques for muscle strains/imbalances include:

- The popliteus release.
  The client lies prone and flexes the affected knee to 80–90°. Palpate the popliteus in the popliteal fossa just inferior to the knee joint under the heads of the gastrocnemius. Slowly glide the fingers across the muscle, keeping the depth within the client's pain tolerance. The knee can also be passively or actively flexed and extended during the technique (see Figure 19.20).
- Knee passive joint articulation may be introduced after the acute phase including (see Chapter 7):
  - Knee articulation inferior approach
  - Knee articulation lateral approach.

Address any underlying conditions or predisposing factors (e.g. ankle pronation, hip anteversion, scoliosis).

CLIENT EDUCATION

Advise clients about stretching, warm-up and graduated return to activity. Runners may need to replace inappropriate or worn-out footwear. Rehabilitation exercises usually involve pain-free isometric and later isotonic contractions of the affected muscles and stretching of quadriceps, hamstrings, iliotibial band, gastrocnemius, soleus and iliopsoas as required.

Clients may be referred for manipulation of the low back, pelvis, knee, ankle and foot.

ILIOTIBIAL BAND SYNDROME

Iliotibial band syndrome is an overuse syndrome that leads to inflammation of the distal iliotibial band near the lateral femoral condyle and in some cases to the bursa between the ilitotibial band and the condyle.[9] At full knee extension the iliotibial band is anterior to the lateral condyle but when the knee is flexed to 30° or more, the iliotibial band moves posterior to the condyle. Excessive running or cycling can cause inflammation of the iliotibial band as it rubs over the lateral condyle.

Assessment

HISTORY

The client complains of diffuse knee pain during activity and there is often a history of repetitive overuse (e.g.

Key assessment findings for iliotibial band syndrome

- History of repetitive overuse (e.g. excessive downhill running, cycling)
- Functional tests of the knee:
  - AROM: positive (hip adduction)
  - PROM: positive (hip adduction)
  - RROM: positive for associated muscles
  - Resisted and length tests positive for associated muscles (e.g. hamstring, quadriceps, gluteal muscle)
  - Special test: Modified Ober's test positive
- Palpation positive for pain in iliotibial band approximately 3 cm above the knee joint line; possible crepitus or snapping with knee flexion and extension; myospasm may be present in gluteal muscles or tensor fasciae latae.

Table 19.4 Remedial massage techniques for muscles that move the knee

Muscle	Soft tissue release	Trigger point	Deep transverse friction	Stretch	Corrective action	Home exercise
Hamstring	Client: prone, knee flexed to 90° Practitioner: Using knuckles of one hand glide along the muscle fibres or apply pressure at the site of the muscle lesion while the other hand holds the ankle and slowly flexes and extends the client's leg. Active: as above but the client flexes and extends their leg unassisted 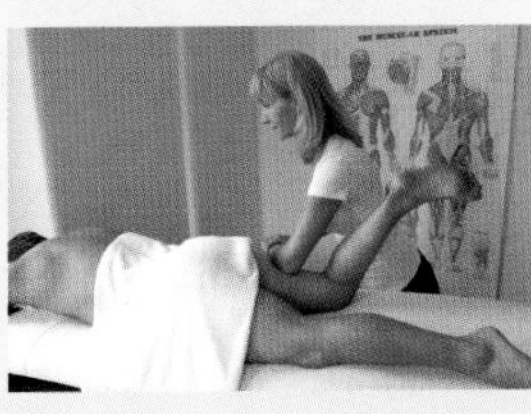	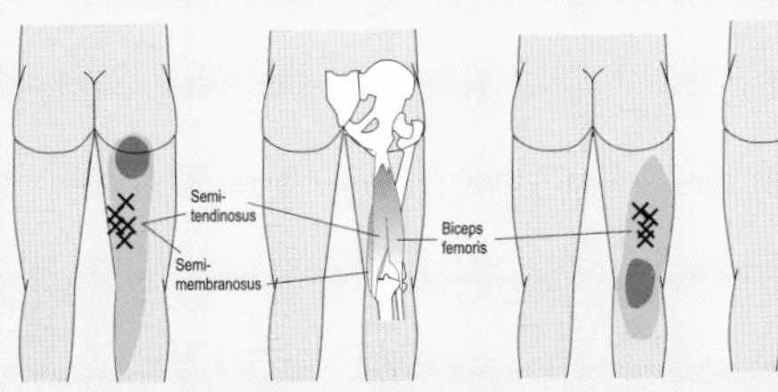 	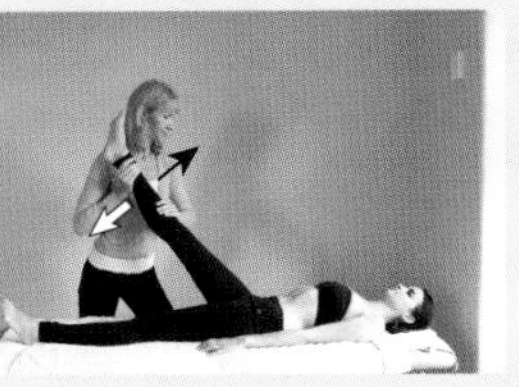	Client: supine and raises their leg until they feel the muscle stretch. Practitioner: Using hands or shoulder, the practitioner resists the client as they attempt to return their leg to the table. Hold the resistance for 6–8 seconds. The client tries to raise their leg further within the pain-free range. Repeat the whole procedure three times. 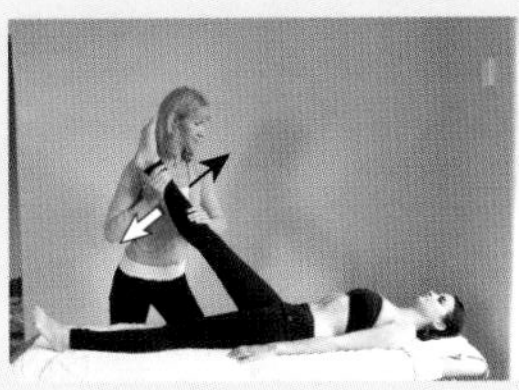	Use chairs that match the client's leg length and a seat with a well-rounded and padded edge. Use a foot stool when seated. Take frequent breaks during long-distance driving.	There are a number of ways to stretch the hamstrings including: i) The client sits with their legs straight out in front of them or with one leg bent. The foot of the bent leg is placed on the floor alongside the thigh of the other leg and the knee rests on the floor. The client reaches forward towards their toes. ii) The client stands or kneels with one leg straight out in front. The client leans forward from their hips towards their toes. 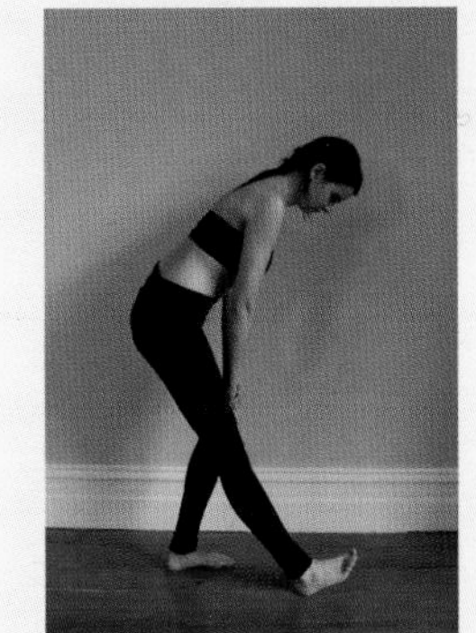 Hold stretches for up to 30 seconds and repeat three times.

Continued

Table 19.4 Remedial massage techniques for muscles that move the knee—cont'd

Muscle	Soft tissue release	Trigger point	Deep transverse friction	Stretch	Corrective action	Home exercise
Quadriceps	Client: supine, towards the side of the table, with knee flexed and leg over the side of the table. Practitioner: applies pressure to the muscle lesion with fingers, thumbs, knuckles or elbows and glides along the muscle fibres. Ask the client to slowly straighten and bend their leg as the technique is applied. 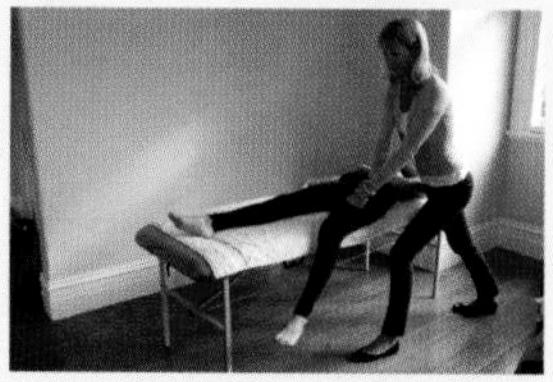	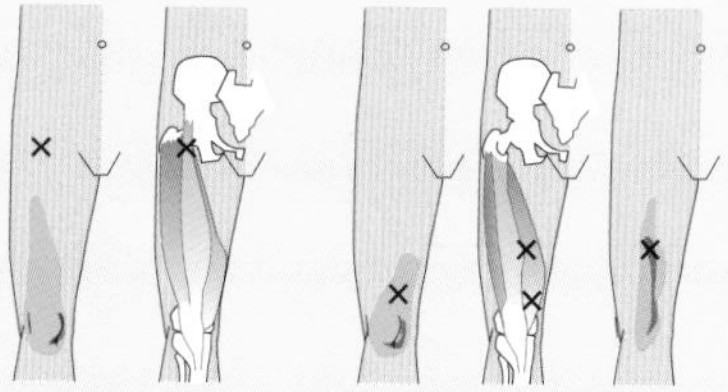	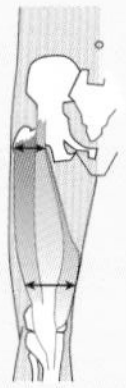	Client prone. Knee flexed to their comfortable limit Practitioner: Faces cephalad, holding the client's ankle. The practitioner applies resistance as the client tries to straighten their leg for 6–8 seconds. After the contraction the client tries to take their heel to their buttocks again. Repeat the procedures three times. Alternatively the practitioner can sit on the side of the table and apply resistance with their medial shoulder.	Avoid shortening and/or prolonged immobilisation of the quadriceps muscles. Avoid deep knee bends and complete squats. Avoid prolonged sitting with hips at 90°. Avoid full flexion of the hip when sleeping on the side.	Lying prone or standing, take the heel towards the buttocks. Hold the stretch for up to 30 seconds and repeat three times. 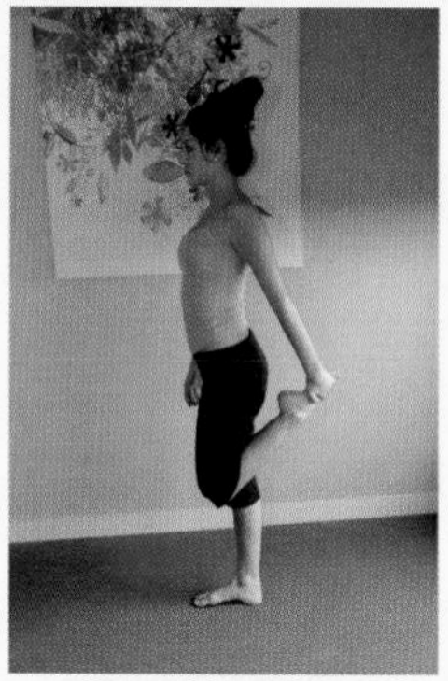

excessive running, cycling). Pain may be aggravated by downhill running. Occasionally the client reports crepitus or snapping during walking and running.

FUNCTIONAL TESTS

Lumbar AROM tests do not reproduce symptoms.
Hip AROM tests do not reproduce symptoms (may be positive for passive stretch).

Knee tests

AROM: may be positive as iliotibial band rubs across the condyle during flexion/extension.
PROM: may be positive as iliotibial band rubs across the condyle during flexion/extension.
RROM: may be positive in abduction due to associated myospasm.
Resisted tests and length tests for specific muscles may be positive for affected muscles (e.g. gluteal muscles, tensor fasciae latae, hamstrings, quadriceps).
Special tests: Modified Ober's test positive (see Chapter 18).

PALPATION

Tenderness may be elicited during palpation of the iliotibial band approximately 3 cm above the knee joint line.

Overview of treatment for iliotibial band syndrome

In the acute phase, the RICE regimen is recommended. Advise the client to decrease the intensity of exercise and avoid aggravating activities like downhill running.

A typical treatment for subacute or chronic iliotibial band syndrome includes:

- Swedish massage to the lower limb including ankle and foot, low back and pelvis.
- A range of remedial massage techniques including the following:
  - Deep transverse friction and cross-fibre frictions to the iliotibial band. Sidelying position provides easy access to the iliotibial band and tensor fasciae latae.
  - Myofascial release including cross-arm techniques and the leg pull (see Chapter 8).
  - For associated myospasm, deep gliding frictions along the muscle fibres, cross-fibre frictions, soft tissue releasing techniques, trigger point therapy (see Table 19.4).
  - Knee and hip passive joint articulation (see Chapter 7).

Address any underlying conditions or predisposing factors (e.g. ankle over-pronation and under-pronation).

CLIENT EDUCATION

Advise clients about stretching, warm-up and graduated return to activity. Poor shock-absorbing shoes should be replaced. Hard surfaces, hills and uneven surfaces should be avoided. Cyclist may need to lower the bicycle seat and adjust the pedals. Rehabilitation exercises include stretching and strengthening of tensor fasciae latae, gluteal muscles, hamstrings and quadriceps as required.

Clients may be referred for manipulation of the low back, pelvis, knee, ankle and foot.

PATELLOFEMORAL PAIN SYNDROME

Patellofemoral pain reportedly affects around 7% of young active adults[26] and accounts for between 2 and 30% of presentations to sports medicine clinics.[27] The term is used to describe anterior knee pain that may originate from a variety of causes. (Chondromalacia patellae is sometimes used as a synonym for patellofemoral pain syndrome, although patellofemoral pain syndrome is really a precursor for it.) Patellofemoral pain syndrome is characterised by anterior knee pain that is worse with knee extension in activities like ascending or descending stairs. The primary cause of the problem appears to be related to the tracking of the patella during knee extension movements.

The patella is embedded in the quadriceps tendon. Its primary function is to improve the angle of pull of the quadriceps on the proximal tibia. The patella is pulled superiorly during quadriceps contraction along the line of the pull of the quadriceps. The degree to which this pull deviates from a vertical line is indicated by the Q angle, that is the angle between a line that connects the tibial tuberosity and the midpoint of the patella, and a line that connects the midpoint of the patella and the anterior superior iliac spine (see Figure 19.5 in p 361). An excessive Q angle is considered to be >15° for women and >10° for men.

A number of factors play a role in the development of patellofemoral pain syndrome:

- A large Q angle is one of the most common factors that lead to patella tracking disorders.
- Vastus medialis obliquus, the distal portion of the vastus medialis muscle, is important in counteracting the tendency of the other quadriceps to pull the patella in a lateral direction. Imbalances between the strength of the vastus medialis obliquus, vastus lateralis and iliotibial band, with its lateral patella expansion, can contribute to tracking disorders.
- Intrinsic factors such as patella alta (a hypermobile and unstable patella that is displaced proximally) and patella baja (a patella that is displaced distally so that the articular surfaces are incongruent) may also be involved.

Assessment

HISTORY

The client complains of anterior knee pain that is aggravated by activities like ascending or descending stairs or squatting. Clients also complain of knee pain on standing after a prolonged period of sitting. Prolonged sitting with knee flexion maintains the quadriceps in a stretched position and a sudden change in position may elicit knee pain (the movie sign).

Key assessment findings for patellofemoral pain syndrome

- History of repetitive activity (e.g. running)
- Functional tests of the knee:
  - AROM positive knee extension
  - PROM may be positive in knee flexion
  - RROM positive knee extension
  - Resisted and length tests positive for affected muscles.
- Palpation of the patella positive for pain; atrophy of vastus medialis obliquus may be present.

Clients sometimes report the knee giving way which may be due to reflex muscular inhibition in response to strong pain sensation in the knee extensors.[28]

FUNCTIONAL TESTS

Lumbar AROM tests do not reproduce symptoms.
Hip AROM tests do not reproduce symptoms.

Knee tests

AROM: positive extension.
PROM: may be positive in flexion.
RROM: pain on resisted knee extension.
Resisted tests and length tests for specific muscles positive for affected muscles.
Special tests: Patellofemoral compression test positive.

PALPATION

Tenderness may be elicited during palpation on the undersurface of the patella (palpate by pushing the patella medially and laterally). Muscle imbalance may also be palpated in the vastus lateralis and vastus medialis obliquus: vastus lateralis may be hypertonic and vastus medialis obliquus may be hypotonic or atrophied.

Overview of treatment and management

Conservative treatment includes eliminating or avoiding responsible activities, bracing and quadriceps strengthening exercises. Since a significant part of the problem with patellofemoral pain syndrome appears to originate from the soft tissues around the knee, massage is helpful in treating this problem. Changes may not be immediate as altered biomechanical patterns have usually been established for some time. However, the client should feel some improvement in 3 to 4 treatments. A typical remedial massage treatment for mild or moderate patellofemoral pain syndrome includes:

- Swedish massage therapy to the knee, anterior and posterior thigh, hip, lower back and pelvis.
- Remedial massage techniques, which are aimed at addressing the muscle imbalance in the quadriceps and iliotibial band tightness. Techniques (especially to vastus lateralis) include the following:
  - Deep gliding frictions along the muscle fibres. Short stripping strokes can be performed in several directions on the quadriceps retinaculum
  - Cross-fibre frictions.
  - Active and passive soft-tissue releasing techniques. In later stages of treatment, resistance to the eccentric contraction of the quadriceps during their elongation can enhance the active techniques further. Additional eccentric load can be added with resistance bands, weights or with your hand.
  - Deep transverse friction. The patella may be displaced to the medial and lateral sides for better access to the tissues just adjacent to it. Although the retinacular fibres are mostly oriented in a superior/inferior direction, stripping in several directions will help improve the overall mobility in the retinaculum.
  - Trigger point therapy (include all quadriceps muscles).
  - Muscle stretches.

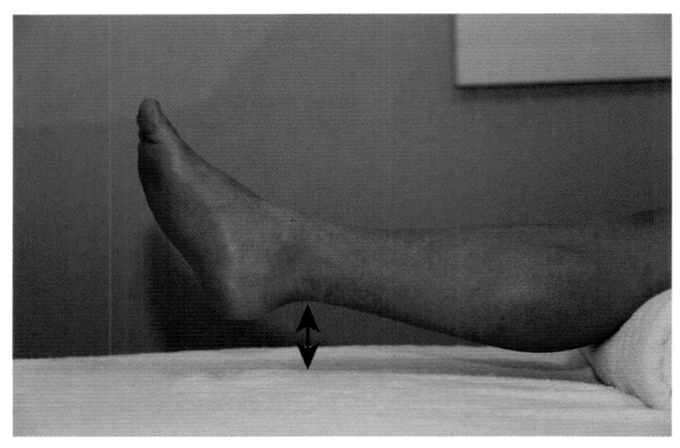

Fig. 19.21 Strengthening vastus medialis obliquus

Passive joint articulation (see Chapter 7) and thermotherapy may be helpful. Address causative and predisposing factors where possible, including muscle imbalances in the lower back, pelvis and hip.

CLIENT EDUCATION

Advise clients to avoid all aggravating activities and on progressive and gradual return to activities. Strengthening vastus medialis obliquus may offset the tendency of the other quadriceps to pull the patella laterally. Vastus medialis obliquus may be most active in the last 20–30° of knee extension. Recommend repeated short arc quadriceps extension exercises over the last 20–30° of knee extension against some resistance (see Figure 19.21). Begin by repeating the exercise to fatigue twice a day and progressively increase the number of repetitions and the resistance. Stretching lateral quadriceps muscles may also help restore quadriceps muscle balance.

Patella taping has also been used to facilitate improved patella tracking. Two factors seem to predict favourable response to off-the-shelf foot orthoses and activity modification:[5]

- Foot valgus $\geq 2°$
- Hallux extension $\leq 78°$

Refer for osseous manipulation where indicated. Surgical intervention may be called for if conservative methods are unsuccessful. Surgical options include articular cartilage procedures and lateral retinacula release which involves cutting the retinacula to reduce the lateral pull on the patella. There is little research to support the use of many current treatments for patellofemoral pain syndrome and further high-quality studies are needed.

CHONDROMALACIA PATELLA

Patellofemoral pain syndrome is a likely precursor for chondromalacia patella. In chondromalacia clients describe pain under the patella whereas in patellofemoral pain syndrome pain the pain is described more superficially in the front of the knee. In chondromalacia patella the hyaline cartilage on the underside of the patella becomes eroded as a result of friction that occurs when the patella fails to track properly in the groove between the two femoral condyles. The client is likely to report crepitus (grating or grinding sensations) during flexion and extension of the knee. Pain may be experienced anteriorly and deep to the patella. The actual pain source is not the cartilage but subchondral bone just below the surface of the cartilage.

TREATMENT

Assessment and treatment approaches for patellofemoral pain syndrome and chondromalacia are similar. Treatment focuses on avoiding all aggravating activities, bracing and an exercise program to address muscle imbalances, especially strengthening vastus medialis obliquus by resisting the last 20–30° of knee extension. Compressive knee braces may encourage activation of specific muscles. Surgical remodelling of the cartilage on the undersurface of the patella may be considered in persistent cases.

Remedial massage techniques approach are similar to those for patellofemoral syndrome. Caution should be taken to avoid undue pressure directly on the patella.

PATELLA DISLOCATION

Patella dislocation occurs when the patella moves laterally onto the lateral femoral condyle. It is usually the result of a twisting injury, such as sudden turning in football sports. It often reduces spontaneously. Predisposing factors include femoral anteversion, shallow femoral groove, genu valgus, loose medial retinaculum, tight lateral retinaculum, congenital absence of vastus medialis, increased Q angle and excessive subtalar pronation. The client often reports a sensation of something 'popping out' in the knee, severe pain and an episode of instability.[7]

Treatment

Arthroscopy may be required to inspect the articular surfaces and remove any osteochondral fragments. The most important aim of rehabilitation is to minimise recurrence. Strengthening vastus medialis and stretching the lateral structures is required. Prolonged taping may also be required.

LIGAMENT SPRAIN

The most common ligament sprain in the body is that of the medial collateral ligament[25] but the anterior cruciate ligament is the most common severe sprain or rupture.[9] The terrible triad (or unhappy triad) which consists of the anterior cruciate ligament, the medial collateral ligament and the medial meniscus was so named because of the frequency with which these structures were injured together from a single injury, usually involving a strong valgus or rotary force to the knee. The new unhappy triad (anterior cruciate and medial collateral ligaments and the lateral meniscus) has been found to occur more frequently in athletes than the originally described triad.[29] When assessing and treating ligament injuries it is important to be aware that the medial collateral ligament is often injured along with other structures in the knee and that anterior cruciate ligament ruptures almost always require surgery and 9 to 12 months rehabilitation.[7]

Medial collateral ligament sprain

The medial collateral ligament is the larger of the two collateral ligaments. Its function is to enhance medial stability of the knee. It runs from the medial epicondyle to the medial side of the tibia about 2.5 cm below the condyle, just posterior to the pes anserine insertion (the common insertion of sartorius, gracilis and semitendinosus). Its deep part is firmly attached to the medial meniscus. Consequently injury to the medial collateral ligament may cause damage to the joint capsule and damage to the medial meniscus. (The lateral collateral ligament is not connected to the joint capsule or the lateral meniscus and injuries to this ligament are rarely as severe as injuries to the medial collateral ligament.) The pes anserine muscles cross over the lower part of the medial collateral ligament and are separated from it by the pes anserine bursa.

Anterior cruciate ligament sprain

The anterior cruciate ligament runs from the anterior part of the intercondylar area of the tibial plateau to the medial side of the lateral femoral condyle. It is a primary knee stabiliser preventing forward displacement of the tibia on the femur (or preventing the femur slipping backwards on the tibia). Anterior cruciate ligament sprains are relatively common, especially in strenuous physical activities. Excessive loads on the anterior cruciate ligament may be incurred during sharp deceleration, deceleration before a change in direction or from landing from a jump or other activity. Anterior cruciate ligament sprains occur more often to women than men, possibly due to the role of oestrogen in ligamentous relaxation and their greater Q angle.[28] Other predisposing factors include narrowness of the intercondylar notch, weak hamstrings relative to quadriceps and pes planus.

Posterior cruciate ligament sprain

The posterior cruciate ligament runs from the back of the intercondylar area of the tibia to the lateral surface of the medial femoral condyle. Sprains of the posterior cruciate are much less common than anterior cruciate ligament or medial collateral ligament. It is usually injured by a direct blow to the tibia, often when the knee is bent (e.g. dashboard injury) or by falls that hyperflex the knee. Clients report a sense of popping or giving way. The posterior cruciate ligament is mostly extracapsular, has a good blood supply and good healing capacity.

Assessment

HISTORY

- Collateral ligament sprains: History of valgus or varus stress through the flexed knee. Pain ± instability in the medial or lateral knee, especially with change of direction.
- Anterior cruciate ligament sprains: History of heavy landing on an extended or slightly flexed knee with internal tibial rotation. Sensation of popping or shifting. Immediate severe pain. Swelling develops rapidly.
- Posterior cruciate ligament sprains: History of fall onto knee with impact to the anterior tibia. May have instability descending stairs and walking downhill.

FUNCTIONAL TESTS

Lumbar AROM tests do not reproduce knee symptoms.
Hip AROM tests do not reproduce knee symptoms.

Assessment findings for ligament sprains

- History of direct trauma. Collateral ligament sprains usually produce well-localised pain at the medial/lateral knee. Anterior cruciate ligament damage usually leads to immediate pain and swelling in the anterior knee ± a 'pop' or 'shift' in the knee; posterior cruciate ligament may lead to pain and swelling around the knee.
- Functional tests of the knee:
  - AROM limited and painful
  - PROM limited and painful
  - RROM may be positive if associated muscle injury
  - Resisted and length tests may be positive for affected muscles
  - Special tests: valgus/varus stress tests, anterior/posterior drawer tests positive for specific ligament sprain
- Palpation positive for collateral ligament sprains and other palpable injured structures; joint effusion

Knee tests

AROM: positive for limitation and pain.
PROM: limited and painful.
RROM: Protective muscle spasm may accompany sprains. Resisted and length tests may be positive for associated muscle strain or protective muscle spasm (e.g. hip adductors in medial collateral ligament sprain, quadriceps and hamstrings in cruciate ligament sprains).
Special tests: Ligament stress tests positive (e.g. valgus stress positive for medial collateral ligament sprain; anterior draw test positive for anterior cruciate ligament sprain and posterior drawer test for posterior cruciate).

Overview of treatment and management

Medial collateral ligament sprains are often treated non-operatively with good success. Treatment immediately after injury includes cryotherapy, anti-inflammatory medication, splints or hinged knee braces and elastic wrap. Range of motion and resistance exercises for muscles that stabilise the joint (e.g. quadriceps and pes anserine muscles) should be commenced as soon as possible.

The anterior cruciate ligament is inaccessible to manual treatment. In the acute phase protective weight-bearing (e.g. using crutches, knee brace or splints), reducing weight-bearing, ice, elastic wrap and electrotherapy are used. More severe injuries may require surgical intervention including total reconstruction of the ligament using part of the patella tendon. The length of rehabilitation to full levels of activity is usually 6 months. The hamstring muscles act as synergists to the anterior cruciate ligament and strengthening exercises for the hamstring muscles provide important support for the damaged ligament.

Appropriate rehabilitation can return good results for posterior cruciate ligament sprains. Acute sprains are treated with ice, elastic wrap and, if severe, a knee splint may be required. Range of motion exercises should be introduced as soon as possible.

A typical remedial massage treatment for mild or moderate ligament sprain includes:

- Swedish massage therapy to the knee, lower limb, back and pelvis.
- Remedial massage therapy including the following:
  - Deep transverse friction. The most tender part of the ligament is usually the primary site of tissue damage. Deep transverse friction is applied to promote collagen production and to prevent the formation of adhesions to surrounding tissue. Deep transverse friction could be applied for 2–3 minutes working at a pain level of 4 or 5 out of 10. (Note that the cruciate ligaments are not accessible for direct massage techniques.)
  - Muscle-focused techniques address imbalances of muscles that cross the joint (e.g. hypertonic hip adductors associated with medial collateral ligament sprain, hypertonic hamstring muscles associated with anterior cruciate ligament sprain). Techniques include:
    - deep gliding along the muscle fibres
    - cross-fibre frictions
    - muscle stretches provided they do not stress the ligament
    - soft tissue releasing techniques
    - trigger point therapy.

  Note that in some cases increased muscle tone may stabilise the joint while the ligament heals.
- Other remedial techniques include heat therapy, myofascial release and passive joint articulation (e.g. knee articulation inferior approach and knee articulation lateral approach). Clients may also require treatment of the lower back, pelvis, lower leg, ankle and foot. Some clients may benefit from referral for osseous manipulation and/or acupuncture.

CLIENT EDUCATION

The client should be advised to use ice/heat therapy for pain relief. A typical rehabilitation program for grade 1 or 2 medial collateral ligament sprain would be:

First weeks post injury

The aim is to decrease pain and swelling. Initially depending on severity weight bearing should be avoided or minimsed. The joint is protected with a hinged knee brace. Commence active range of motion as soon as possible within the client's pain tolerance. Progress to isometric exercises for quadriceps, hamstrings and hip abductors. Swimming to maintain fitness. After the first few days introduce stationary bicycle.

Second week post injury

Improve mobility and flexibility. Full weight bearing with brace is encouraged. Increase stationary bicycle work. Introduce light leg press, squats and jogging. Commence isotonic quadriceps and hamstring exercises.

Third week post injury

Re-establish co-ordination and proprioception. Increase strengthening exercises. Commence agility skill (skipping, hopping, running longer distances and at a higher speed). Use brace only for jogging and agility work.

Four weeks post injury

Functional training. Increase proprioceptive tasks (e.g. wobble board). Begin sport-specific skills. Use brace only for agility work and return to sport drills.

Key assessment findings for meniscal injuries

- History of trauma, often characterised by a sudden twinge over medial or lateral joint line with clicking, catching or locking.
- Functional tests of the knee:
  - AROM limited and painful, especially extension
  - PROM limited and painful, especially extension
  - RROM may be positive if associated muscle strain
  - Resisted and length tests may be positive for affected muscles
  - Special tests: positive Apley's compression.
- Palpation positive for joint line tenderness.

Table 19.5 Management of meniscal injury

Minor injury	Major injury
Conservative treatment	Surgery required
Symptoms develop 24–48 hours post injury	Unable to continue playing
Able to bear weight (no locking)	Joint locking
Minimal swelling	Swelling
Pain at end of range of motion	Little improvement with conservative treatment after 3 weeks or worsening over time

MENISCAL INJURY

The two fibrocartilaginous menisci help shock absorption and provide a larger contact surface between the femur and the tibia. They also help counteract the tendency of the femur to roll off the top of the tibial plateau. When a meniscus is removed or severely damaged, degenerative joint disease often follows.

The meniscus may be damaged by trauma or degeneration. Compressive forces can break, chip or tear the meniscus; tensile forces such as acute valgus injury can tear the meniscus. The medial meniscus is attached to the deep fibres of the medial collateral ligament which restricts its movement and makes it more readily injured than the more mobile lateral collateral ligament. In fact, the medial meniscus is involved in 75% of meniscal injuries, particularly to the posterior horn.[9] In some instances, pieces of meniscus become separated and cause the knee to lock from time to time as they move around the joint.

Assessment

HISTORY

Traumatic meniscal damage is characterised by a twinge or sudden pain over the medial or lateral joint line with clicking, catching or locking. Swelling occurs in about 50% of cases. Meniscal damage can also be the result of degenerative changes which may be without symptoms and progress to recurring pain, crepitus, catching ± swelling.

FUNCTIONAL TESTS

Lumbar AROM tests do not reproduce the knee symptoms.
Hip AROM tests do not reproduce the knee symptoms.

Knee tests

AROM: limited and painful, especially extension.
PROM: limited and painful, especially extension.
RROM: positive if associated muscle strains.
Resisted and length tests: positive for affected muscles.
Special tests: Apley's compression test positive.
Palpation: positive for joint line tenderness.

Overview of treatment and management

If the meniscal damage is not severe, physical therapy will often be successful. Tears that occur on the outer third of the meniscus, which has a good vascular supply, have a better chance of healing; tears on the inner two-thirds and deep regions of the posterior horn are poorly vascularised and may require surgery (see Table 19.5).

In the subacute phase, remedial massage treatment focuses on restoring muscle balance around the joint. Muscle techniques include cross-fibre friction on the joint line followed by ice application if required.[9] Heat packs may be beneficial after the first post-injury week.

CLIENT EDUCATION

Avoid sudden changes of speed and direction, rotation of the knee and prolonged standing on hard surfaces. Refer to an osteopath, chiropractor or physiotherapist for manipulation. Refer for correction of ankle pronation if necessary. Advise clients that extensive rehabilitation is required.

Home exercises

Pain-free activities including stretching and strengthening hamstrings, quadriceps, gastrocnemius, tibialis anterior, hip abductors and rotators. Discontinue exercise if pain or swelling occurs during or after exercises. Gradually resume ballistic movements, high impact, direction changes and twisting. Progressively increase strengthening and stretching program.

DEGENERATIVE JOINT DISEASE (DEGENERATIVE ARTHRITIS, OSTEOARTHRITIS)

Degenerative joint disease (DJD) of the knee is very common in older clients, those with a history of a significant previous trauma to the knee or those whose work or sport involves repetitive loads to the knee. It is characterised by progressive degeneration of articular cartilage, subchondral sclerosis and osteophyte formation (see Figure 19.22 on p 378).[9]

Assessment

HISTORY

The client complains of chronic knee pain and stiffness that is aggravated by use and relieved by rest. Symptoms are usually better in the morning and worsen as the day progresses

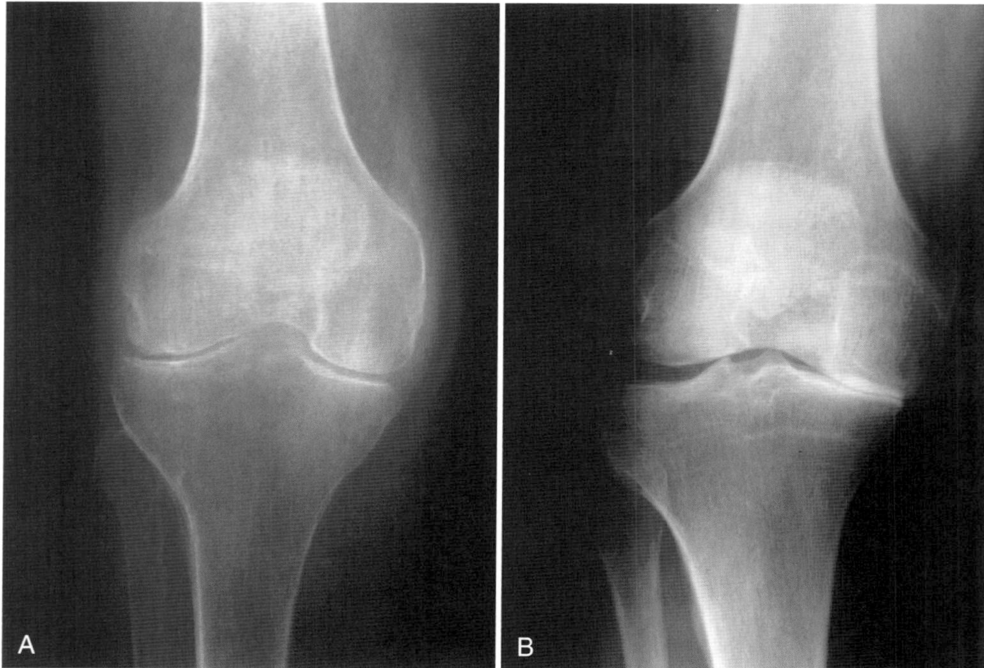

Fig. 19.22 Radiographs of degenerative joint disease of the knee *(Source: Goldman: Cecil Medicine, 23rd edn.* Copyright © 2007 Saunders).

Key assessment findings for DJD of the knee joint

- History of chronic pain and limitation worse after weight bearing and relieved by rest. Occasional swelling. Usually over 50 years old.
- Functional tests of the knee:
  - AROM limited ± painful, especially in flexion
  - PROM limited ± painful in flexion (capsular pattern), hard end-feel
  - RROM usually negative.
- Palpation positive for crepitus and hard or capsular end-feel.

but do not usually occur at night. The client is usually over 50 years or has a history of significant previous injury or overuse. The client may report occasional swelling.

FUNCTIONAL TESTS

Lumbar AROM tests do not reproduce knee symptoms.
Hip AROM tests do not reproduce knee symptoms.

Knee tests

AROM positive (limited flexion).
PROM positive (capsular pattern: limited flexion), hard end-feel, crepitus often present.
RROM negative (Note that DJD is often accompanied by capsule tightening and muscle contractures. In such cases, passive muscle stretching is often painful and limited.)
Special tests usually negative.

PALPATION

Crepitus and abnormal hard or capsular end-feel are usually palpated. Client reports tenderness at several sites around the joint.

Treatment of DJD of the knee joint

Although DJD is a chronic degenerative condition acute episodes occur from time to time, usually after over-activity. If acute inflammation is present, treatment could include cryotherapy for analgesia, acupressure, Reiki, reflexology or anti-inflammatory medication. The client should be advised to modify activities to avoid aggravating the condition.

A typical remedial massage treatment for mild or moderate subacute or chronic DJD includes:

- Swedish massage therapy to the knee, lower limb, ankle and foot, lower back and pelvis.
- Remedial massage therapy includes:
  - heat therapy
  - passive joint articulation (see Chapter 7):
    - knee articulation inferior approach
    - knee articulation lateral approach
  - myofascial releasing techniques (see Chapter 8)
  - remedial massage techniques (e.g. deep gliding, cross-fibre frictions, soft tissue releasing techniques, trigger point therapy and muscle stretching) to address any associated muscle contractures.

CLIENT EDUCATION

The client should be advised to continue to use heat therapy for pain relief and to modify or avoid all aggravating activities. Weight loss and the use of shock-absorbing soles in shoes may reduce the load on the joint and provide symptom relief. Home exercises should be commenced as soon as pain permits. Stretching and strengthening exercises can be introduced as indicated by assessment findings. Educate clients about the importance of getting the right balance between too little activity (which can lead to capsule and muscle contractures and movement compensations) and too much activity (which can inflame the joint). Non-weight-bearing activities such as swimming are often beneficial.

Nutritional supplements such as glucosamine may be beneficial.[30] Clients may be referred for other supportive therapies including specialist nutritional advice and acupuncture.

BURSITIS

Bursae are fluid-filled sacs located at sites where tissues move across one another. Their function is to minimise friction between the tissues as they move. Bursitis (inflammation of a bursa) can arise from friction with repetitive motion or direct trauma. Five common sites where bursitis occurs in the knee are the prepatellar bursa, pes anserine bursa, gastrocnemius bursa, popliteal bursa and iliotibial band bursa (see Figure 19.3 on p 358).

Prepatellar bursitis

Prepatellar bursitis (housemaid's knee) is common. A painless or slightly painful swelling is localised over the anterior aspect of the patella and the patellar tendon. (If there is redness, significant tenderness or a nearby break in the skin, the swelling must be tapped to rule out infection.) It is usually the result of prolonged kneeling, kneeling on a hard surface or from direct trauma from a fall.

TREATMENT

In the acute phase, bursitis is managed with RICE. The client should avoid kneeling or use a knee pad. The bursitis usually resolves when the aggravating activity is removed. In the subacute phase, heat, massage to the surrounding area and electrophysical therapy may be useful. Note that friction massage applied directly to the bursa is contraindicated.

OSGOOD-SCHLATTER'S DISEASE

Osgood-Schlatter's disease is a traction apophysitis of the tibial tuberosity in active children and young adolescents which causes pain at the tibial tuberosity. It is three times more common in males than females. It is caused by excessive traction on the soft apophysis of the tibial tuberosity by the powerful patellar tendon. It is associated with high levels of activity during a period of rapid growth.

Assessment

HISTORY

The client is an active young male (10–15 years old) or female (8–13 years old) who complains of pain at the tibial tuberosity. Pain may be felt during walking up or down hills and stairs or kneeling.

FUNCTIONAL TESTS

Lumbar AROM tests do not reproduce knee symptoms.
Hip AROM tests do not reproduce knee symptoms.

Key assessment findings for Osgood-Schlatter's disease

- Pain at the tibial tuberosity in an active child or young adolescent.
- Functional tests of the knee:
  - AROM painful in extension
  - PROM painful in flexion (passive quadriceps stretching)
  - RROM painful extension
  - Resisted and length tests positive for quadriceps femoris.
- Palpation: pain and tenderness on palpation at the tibial tuberosity.

(Note: knee pain can be the main presenting complaint of a child with a serious disease of the hip.)

Knee tests

AROM positive, especially on extension.
PROM positive with passive knee flexion (stretching quadriceps).
RROM positive on extension.
Resisted and length tests positive for quadriceps.
Special tests negative.

PALPATION

Clients report pain and tenderness at the tibial tuberosity. There may be local swelling.

Treatment

In the acute phase, recommend RICE and rest, or at least reduced participation in the responsible activity for at least two weeks. Ice and taping to reduce the pull of the quadriceps on the tibial tuberosity are often beneficial. In the chronic phase, heat and massage therapy may help reduce pain but the most important factor is reduction of activity until the end of the rapid growth phase. Avoid vigorous quadriceps stretching until the tibial tuberosity fuses to the tibia at about 16 years of age. After fusion, stretching and strengthening quadriceps and hamstrings as required to restore normal knee biomechanics.

KEY MESSAGES

- Assessment of clients with conditions of the knee involves history, outcome measures, postural analysis, gait analysis, functional tests and palpation.
- Assessment findings may indicate the type of tissue involved (contractile or inert, muscle, joint, fascia, ligament), duration of condition (acute or subacute) and severity (grade).
- Assessment findings may indicate a common presenting condition such as muscle strain, patellofemoral syndrome, ligament sprains, meniscal injury, degenerative joint disease, bursitis and Osgood-Schlatter's disease.
- Assessment findings also indicate client perception of injury and preferences for treatment.
- Consider Clinical Guidelines, available evidence and client preferences when planning therapy.

- Conditions requiring referral are common (e.g. acute knee injuries such as ligament sprains and meniscal tears). Refer all clients with symptoms of neurological or vascular impairment in the lower limb for further assessment (e.g. decreased sensation, muscle atrophy, unexplained swelling, discolouration of the lower limb, diminished dorsalis pedis pulse, delayed capillary refilling after compression).
- The selection of remedial massage techniques depends on assessment results. Swedish massage to the lower limb, lower back and pelvis may be followed by muscle techniques (e.g. deep gliding, cross-fibre frictions, soft tissue releasing techniques, trigger point therapy and deep transverse friction), passive joint articulation, myofascial release and thermotherapy as indicated.
- Educating clients about likely causal and predisposing factors and exercise rehabilitation are essential parts of remedial massage therapy.
- Over time, increase the client self-help component of treatment wherever possible to reduce likelihood of recurrence and/or to promote health maintenance and illness prevention.

Review questions

1. Match the ligaments in Column A with the characteristics in Column B.

Column A	Column B
Medial collateral ligament	Prevents anterior movement of the femur on the tibia
Lateral collateral ligament	Resists valgus stress
Anterior cruciate ligament	Attaches to the tibial tuberosity
Posterior cruciate ligament	Attaches to the head of the fibula
Patellar ligament	Runs between the posterior intercondylar area of the tibia to the lateral surface of the medial femoral condyle

2. The popliteus can act as both a medial rotator and a lateral rotator of the knee. Explain how this can occur.
3. Describe resisted tests for the following muscles:
   i) Quadriceps as a group
   ii) Rectus femoris
   iii) Vastus medialis obliquus
4. Name a special test which could suggest the following conditions:
   i) Damage to the medial collateral ligament of the knee
   ii) Rupture to the anterior cruciate ligament of the knee
   iii) Torn cartilage (meniscus)
5. What is the movie sign? What condition does it suggest?
6. The prognosis of a meniscal tear depends on the location of its damage. What is the prognosis of a meniscal tear affecting its outer third?
7. Name the three structures of the knee that are referred to in the 'unhappy triad'.
8. Which statement does NOT accurately describe the lateral meniscus:
   a) Oval shaped
   b) Larger than the medial meniscus
   c) More mobile than the medial meniscus
   d) Not attached to the lateral collateral ligament
9. The effect of weak knee flexor muscles on gait can include:
   a) trunk thrown forwards over the centre of gravity
   b) lifting the hip during swing phase
   c) in-toeing gait
   d) manually pushing the knee into extension
10. The pes anserine muscles include all of the following except:
    a) sartorius
    b) semimembranosus
    c) semitendinosus
    d) gracilis
11. A runner is diagnosed with patellofemoral pain syndrome.
    i) Briefly describe the pathogenesis of the condition.
    ii) List three factors which can predispose to patellofemoral pain syndrome.
    ii) What is the usual focus of remedial massage treatment for patellofemoral pain syndrome?
12. Briefly describe the home advice that would be beneficial for a client with degenerative joint disease of the knee.

REFERENCES

1. Calmbach W, Hutchens M. Evaluation of patients presenting with knee pain: Part 1: History, physical examination, radiographs and laboratory tests. Am Fam Physician 2003;68(5):907–12.
2. Britt H, Miller G, Charles J, et al. General practice activity in Australia 2007-08. Canberra: Australian Institute of Health and Welfare; 2008.
3. Australian Bureau of Statistics. National Health Survey: Summary of Results 2004-5. Canberra: Australian Bureau of Statistics; 2005 [cited 2007 29 January]. Online. Available: www.abs.gov.au/austats/abs@.nsf/Latestproducts.
4. Tortora G, Grabowski S. Principles of anatomy and physiology. Stafford, Qld: John Wiley; 2002.
5. Cleland J, Koppenhaver S. Netter's orthopaedic clinical examination: an evidence-based approach. 2nd edn. Philadelphia: Saunders; 2011.
6. Mallen C, Peat G, Porcheret M. Chronic knee pain. Br Med J 2007;335(7614):303.
7. Scotney B. Sports knee injuries: Assessment and management. Aust Fam Physician 2010;39(1/2):30–4.
8. Australian Acute Musculoskeletal Pain Guidelines Group. Evidence-based management of acute musculoskeletal pain: a guide for clinicians. Bowen Hills, Qld: Australian Academic Press; 2004.
9. Carnes M, Vizniak N. Quick reference evidence-based conditions manual. 3rd edn. Burnaby, BC: Professional Health Systems; 2009.
10. Reese N, Bandy W. Joint range of motion and muscle length testing. Philadelphia: W.B. Saunders; 2002.
11. Kendall McCreary E, Provance P, McIntyre Rodgers M, et al. Muscles, testing and function, with posture and pain. 5th edn. Philadelphia: Lippincott Williams and Wilkins, 2005.
12. Hislop H, Montgomery J. Daniels and Worthingham's muscle testing: techniques of manual examination. 8th edn. Oxford: Saunders Elsevier; 2007.
13. Mattheson J, Kernozek T, Fater D, Davies G. Electromyographic activity and applied load during seated quadriceps exercises. Med Sci Sports Exerc 2001;33(10):1713–25.
14. Irish S, Millward A, Wride J, Haas B, Shum G. The effect of closed-kinetic chain exercises and open-kinetic chain exercise on the muscle activity of vastus medialis oblique and vastus lateralis. J Strength Condit Res 2010;25(5):1256–62.
15. Vizniak N. Physical assessment. Burnaby, B.C.: Professional Health Systems; 2008.

16. Brosseau L, Yonge KA, Welch V, et al. Thermotherapy for treatment of osteoarthritis. Cochrane Database Syst Rev [Systematic Review]. 2003;(4):CD004522.
17. Bartels E, Lund H, Hagen K, et al. Aquatic exercise for the treatment of knee and hip osteoarthritis. Cochrane Database Syst Rev [serial on the Internet]. 2007;(4):CD005023.
18. Rutjes A, Nüesch E, Sterchi R, et al. Transcutaneous electrostimulation for osteoarthritis of the knee. Cochrane Database Syst Rev [serial on the Internet]. 2009;(4):CD002823.
19. Rutjes A, Nüesch E, Sterchi R, et al. Therapeutic ultrasound for osteoarthritis of the knee and hip. Cochrane Database Syst Rev [serial on the Internet]. 2010;(1):CD003132.
20. Hunter A, Watt J, Watt V, et al. Effect of lower limb massage on electromyography and force production of the knee extensors. Br J Sports Med 2006;40:114–18.
21. Hart J, Swanik C, Tierney R. Effects of sports massage on limb girth and discomfort associated with eccentric exercise. J Athl Train 2005;40(3):181–5.
22. Hopper D, Conneely M, Chromiak F, et al. Evaluation of the effect of two massage techniques on hamstring muscle length in competitive female hockey players. Phys Ther Sport 2005;6(3):137–45.
23. Loghmani M, Warden S. Instrument-assisted cross-fiber massage accelerates knee ligament healing. J Orthop Sports Phys Ther 2009;39(7):506–14.
24. Yip B, Tam A. An experimental study on the effectiveness of massage with aromatic ginger and orange essential oil for moderate-to-severe knee pain among the elderly in Hong Kong. Complement Ther Med 2008;16:131–8.
25. Hendrickson T. Massage for orthopedic conditions. Baltimore, MD: Lippincott Williams and Wilkins; 2003.
26. Witvrouw E, Lysens R, Bellemans J, et al. Intrinsic risk factors for the development of anterior knee pain in an athletic population: a two-year prospective study. Am J Sports Med 2000;28: 480–9.
27. Baquie P, Brukner P. Injuries presenting to an Australian sports medicine centre: a 12-month study. Clin J Sports Med 1997;7:28–31.
28. Lowe W. Orthopedic massage: Theory and technique. Edinburgh: Mosby Elsevier; 2009.
29. Shelbourne K, Nitz P. The O'Donoghue triad revisited. Combined knee injuries involving anterior cruciate and medial collateral ligament tears. Am J of Sports Med 1991;19(5):474–7.
30. McAlindon TE, LaValley MP, Gulin JP, et al. Glucosamine and chondroitin for treatment of osteoarthritis: a systematic quality assessment and meta-analysis. JAMA 2000;283(11): 1469–75.

20 The leg, ankle and foot

The content of this chapter relates to the following Units of Competency
- HLTREM503C Plan remedial massage treatment strategy
- HLTREM504C Apply remedial massage assessment framework
- HLTREM502C Provide remedial massage treatment
- HLTREM505C Prove remedial massage health assessment

Health Training Package HLT07

Learning Outcomes

- Assess clients with conditions of the leg, ankle and foot for remedial massage, including identification of red and yellow flags.
- Assess clients for signs and symptoms associated with common conditions of the leg, ankle and foot (including muscle strains, shin splints, inversion sprains and plantar fasciitis) and treat and/or manage these conditions with remedial massage therapy.
- Develop treatment plans for clients with conditions of the leg, ankle and foot, taking assessment findings, duration and severity of the condition, likely tissue types, clinical guidelines, the best available evidence and client preferences into account.
- Develop short- and long-term treatment plans to address presenting symptoms, underlying conditions and predisposing factors, and to progressively increase the self-help component of therapy.
- Adapt remedial massage therapy to suit individual client needs based on duration and severity of injury, the client's age and gender, the presence of underlying conditions, and other consideration for special population groups.

INTRODUCTION

Ankle ligaments are perhaps the most commonly injured ligaments in the body and gastrocnemius strains and Achilles tendinopathy are the most common athletic injuries of the region.[1] The foot is prone to degenerative problems and is also subject to systemic diseases like diabetes mellitus. Of particular importance to remedial massage therapists is deep venous thrombosis of the leg. Clients with suspected deep venous thrombosis should be referred for medical investigation.

DEEP VENOUS THROMBOSIS

In many cases the most significant indicator is history of recent surgery or a long plane or bus trip. Suspect deep venous thrombosis when the client has constant pain, tenderness, increased temperature and swelling in the calf. Homan's sign (passive dorsiflexion of the ankle) may reproduce pain (but would also be painful for calf muscle strains). The presence of deep venous thrombosis may be confirmed by Doppler scan and venography. Serious complications include pulmonary embolism and postphlebitic syndrome. Treatment consists of anticoagulant therapy, elevation of the limb, fibrinolytic therapy and sometimes thrombectomy.

FUNCTIONAL ANATOMY

The ankle (talocrural) joint is made up of the lateral malleolus of the fibula, the medial malleolus of the tibia and the talus. The distal ends of the tibia and fibula form a mortise into which the dome of the talus fits to form a hinge for plantarflexion and dorsiflexion of the foot. There are seven tarsal bones: talus, calcaneus, cuboid, navicular and the three cuneiform bones. The medial aspect of the ankle joint is supported by the deltoid ligament: three lateral ligaments (anterior talofibular, posterior talofibular and calcaneofibular ligament) support the lateral side (see Figure 20.1 on p 383).

The foot can be divided into three regions: the hindfoot, midfoot and forefoot. The hindfoot contains the calcaneus, the largest of the tarsal bones, and the talus which rests on top. About half the body weight is transmitted to the calcaneus, the other half to the other tarsal bones. The subtalar joint between the calcaneus and the talus is bound by several talocalcaneal ligaments and supported by part of the medial and lateral ligaments of the ankle. There are no muscle attachments to the talus. The sinus tarsi is a channel between the two bones just anterior to the lateral malleous. On the posteromedial aspect of the calcaneus is the sustentaculum tali, a shelf-like projection for the attachment of flexor hallucis longus. The Achilles tendon attaches to the calcaneal tuberosity. A fibroelastic fat pad cushions the heel when weight bearing. Anteriorly the calcaneus articulates with the cuboid bone.

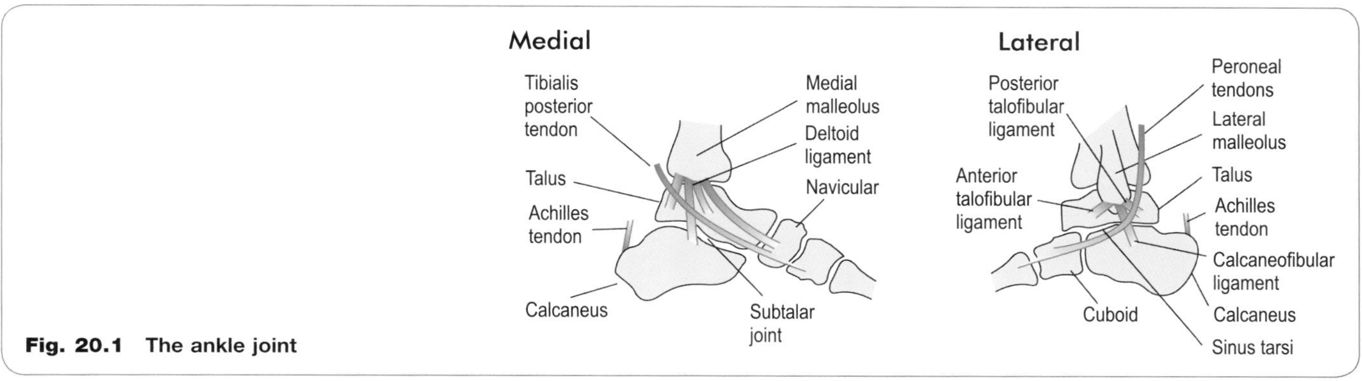

Fig. 20.1 The ankle joint

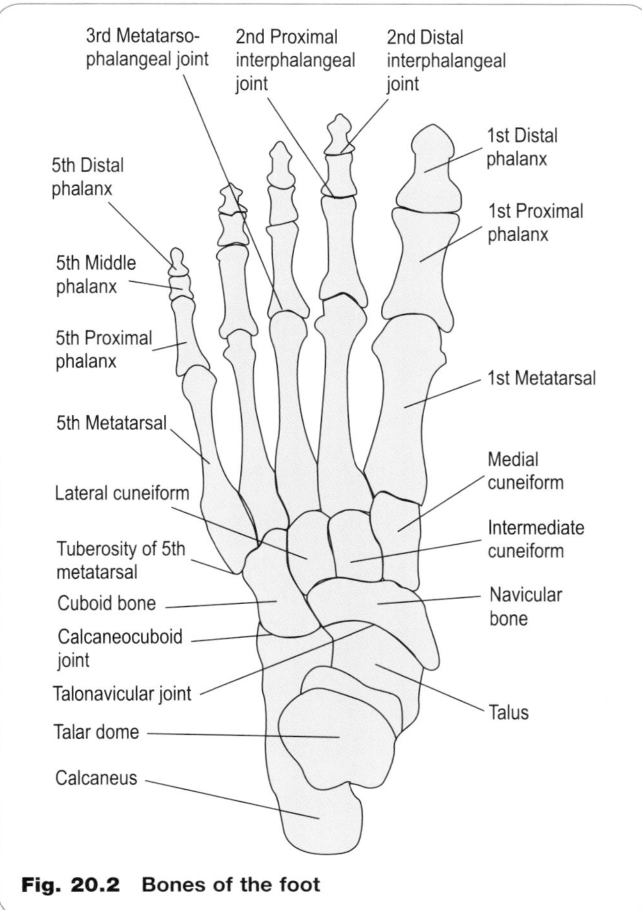

Fig. 20.2 Bones of the foot

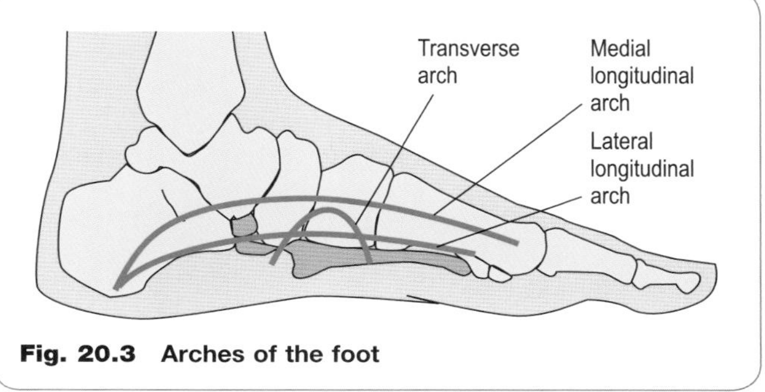

Fig. 20.3 Arches of the foot

The midfoot is made up of five of the seven tarsal bones which are arranged in two rows, the cuboid occupying both rows. The proximal row contains the navicular medially and the cuboid laterally. The distal row contains the three cuneiforms medially and the cuboid laterally. The tarsometatarsophalangeal joints form the boundary between the midfoot and the forefoot. The cuneiform bones articulate with the first, second and third metatarsals; the cuboid articulates with the fourth and fifth metatarsals (see Figure 20.2). Tibialis posterior attaches to the tuberosity on the medial surface of the navicular bone. No muscles attach to the cuboid although the peroneus tendon crosses the cuboid tuberosity. The cuboid also provides attachment for the long plantar ligament and the calcaneocuboid ligament.

The five metatarsals and phalanges make up the forefoot. The first metatarsal bone is thicker than the other metatarsals because it bears more weight and is important in the push-off phase of gait. The first metatarsal also provides attachments for tibialis anterior and peroneus longus. Two sesamoid bones are located in the flexor hallucis brevis tendon on its plantar surface. Peroneus brevis tendon attaches to the lateral side of the fifth metatarsal. Several ligaments connect the metatarsophalangeal joints and the interphalangeal joints. The interphalangeal and metatarsophalangeal joints can plantarflex and dorsiflex. Abduction and adduction of the toes are functions of metatarsophalangeal joints.

All the joints in the hindfoot and midfoot from the subtalar joint to the tarsometatarsal joints contribute to inversion and eversion of the foot. These are complex movements: inversion involves both medial rotation and supination; eversion involves lateral rotation and pronation.

The arches of the foot are important for weight bearing and propulsion. They are usually developed by 12 or 13 years of age. Pliability to adapt to uneven surfaces is provided by the multiple bones and joints of the foot. The arches are maintained by the irregular and interlocking shape of the bones, supporting ligaments and muscles and tendons of the foot. The three arches are (see Figure 20.3):

- medial longitudinal arch: calcaneus, talus, navicular, cuneiform bones and first three metatarsals
- lateral longitudinal arch: calcaneus, cuboid, fourth and fifth metatarsals
- transverse arch: wedge-shaped cuneiforms, cuboid and bases of the five metatarsal bones.

The deep fascia of the foot forms the plantar fascia that extends from the tuberosity of the calcaneus to the heads of the metatarsal bones. The plantar aponeurosis which encloses the flexor tendons of the foot forms the central part of the plantar fascia. It supports the longitudinal arch of the foot.

The muscles of the foot are classified as intrinsic or extrinsic. Intrinsic muscles are located within the foot itself. They are responsible for movements of the toes and provide support for the arches of the foot. The extrinsic muscles arise in the lower leg. Their long tendons cross the ankle and insert into bones of the foot. They are responsible for movements of the ankle and toes and provide some support for the foot arches. Muscles of the leg and foot are described in Table 20.1 (see Figure 20.4).

NERVE SUPPLY TO MUSCLES OF THE LEG, ANKLE AND FOOT

- Deep peroneal nerve: tibialis anterior (L4, L5), extensor hallucis longus (L5) and extensor digitorum longus (L5)
- Superficial peroneal nerve: peroneus longus and brevis (L5, S1)
- Tibial nerve: gastrocnemius (S1, S2), soleus (S1, S2), flexor hallucis longus (L5), flexor digitorum longus (L5) and tibialis posterior (L5)

ASSESSMENT

The purpose of remedial massage assessment includes:

- determining the suitability of clients for massage (contraindications and red flags)
- determining the duration (acute or subacute), severity of injury and types of tissues involved in the injury/condition
- determining whether symptoms fit patterns of common conditions.

Principles of remedial massage assessment are discussed in Chapter 2. This section presents specific considerations for assessment of the leg, ankle and foot.

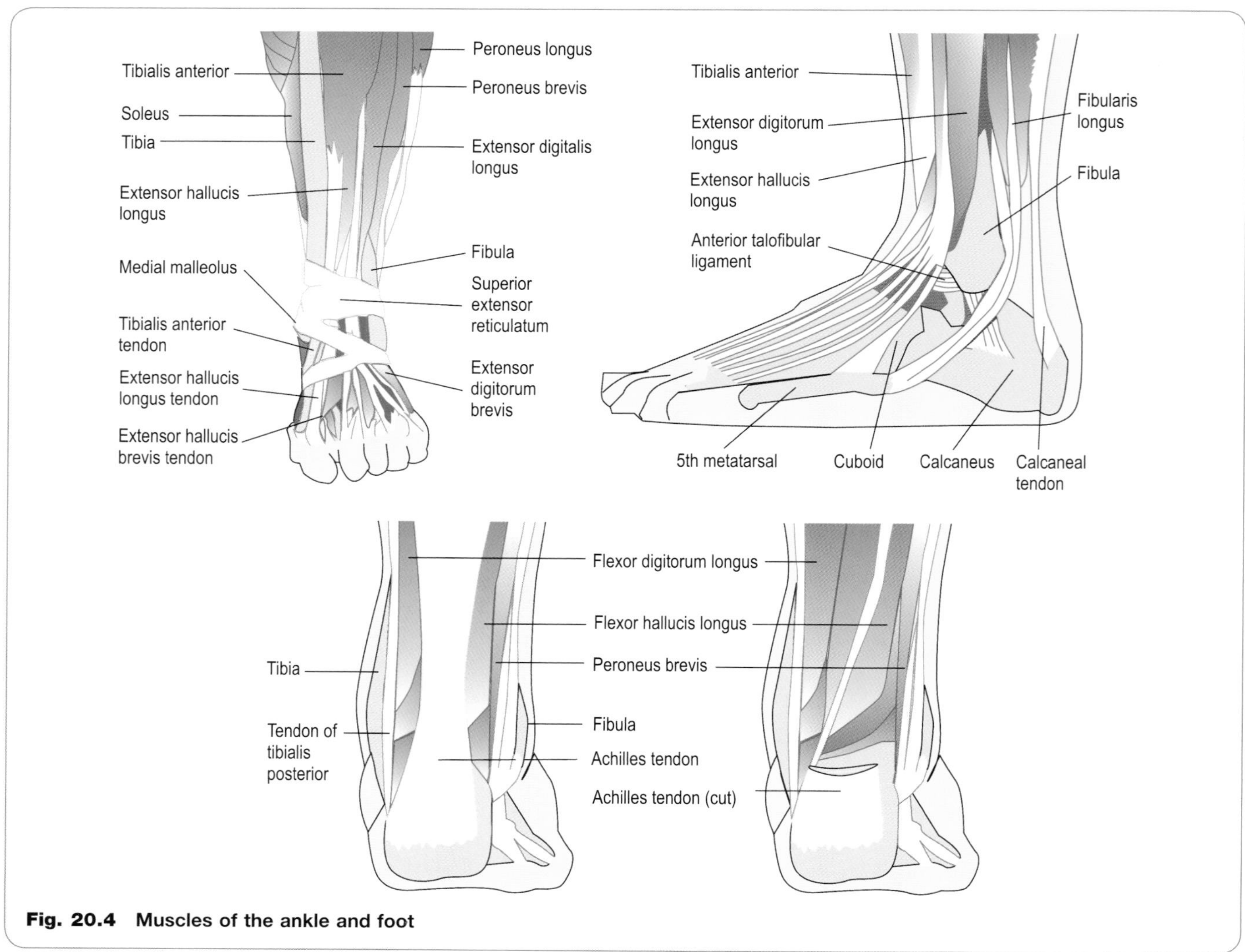

Fig. 20.4 Muscles of the ankle and foot

Table 20.1 Muscles of the leg and foot

Muscles that move the foot and toes	Origin	Insertion	Action
Anterior Compartment of the Leg			
• Tibialis anterior	Lateral condyle and body of tibia and interosseous membrane	First metatarsal and first (medial) cuneiform	Dorsiflexes foot at ankle joint and inverts foot at intertarsal joints
• Extensor hallucis longus	Anterior surface of fibula and interosseous membrane	Base of distal phalanx of great toe	Dorsiflexes foot at ankle joint and extends proximal phalanx of great toe at metatarsophalangeal joint
• Extensor digitorum longus	Lateral condyle of tibia, proximal ⅔ of anterior surface of fibula and interosseous membrane	Middle and distal phalanges of toes 2–5	Dorsiflexes foot at ankle joint and extends distal and middle phalanges of each toe at interphalangeal joints and proximal phalanx of each toe at metatarsophalangeal joint
• Fibularis (Peroneus) tertius	Distal third of fibula and interosseous membrane	Base of fifth metatarsal	Dorsiflexes foot at ankle joint and everts foot at intertarsal joints
Lateral (Fibular) Compartment of the Leg			
• Fibularis (Peroneus) longus	Head and body of fibula and lateral condyle of tibia	Base of first metatarsal and first cuneiform	Plantar flexes foot at ankle joint and everts foot at intertarsal joints
• Fibularis (Peroneus) brevis	Lateral distal ⅔ of body of fibula	Lateral aide of base of fifth metatarsal	Plantar flexes foot at ankle joint and everts foot at intertarsal joints
Superficial Posterior Compartment of the Leg			
• Gastrocnemius	Lateral and medial condyles of femur and capsule of knee	Calcaneus via calcaneal (Achilles) tendon	Plantar flexes foot at ankle joint and flexes leg at knee joint
• Soleus	Posterior surface of head of fibula and medial ⅓ of its body, and middle ⅓ of medial border of tibia	Calcaneus via calcaneal (Achilles) tendon	Plantar flexes foot at ankle joint
• Plantaris	Distal part of lateral supracondylar ridge, adjacent popliteal surface and oblique popliteal ligament	Calcaneus via calcaneal (Achilles) tendon	Plantar flexes foot at ankle joint and flexes leg at knee joint
Deep Posterior Compartment of the Leg			
• Popliteus	Lateral condyle of femur	Proximal to soleal line on posterior tibia	Flexes leg at knee joint and medially rotates tibia to unlock the extended knee
• Tibialis posterior	Lateral part of posterior tibia, proximal ⅔ medial fibula and interosseous membrane	Metatarsals 2–4, navicular, all three cuneiforms and cuboid	Plantar flexes foot at ankle joint and inverts foot at intertarsal joints
• Flexor digitorum longus	Posterior surface of tibia	Bases of distal phalanges of toes 2–4	Plantar flexes foot at ankle joint; flexes middle and distal phalanges of each toe at interphalangeal joints and proximal phalanx of each toe at metatarsophalangeal joint
• Flexor hallucis longus	Posterior surface of distal ⅔ of fibula, interosseous membrane and intermuscular septum	Base of distal phalanx of great toe	Plantar flexes foot at ankle joint; flexes distal phalanx of great toe at interphalangeal joint and proximal phalanx of great toe at metatarsophalangeal joint

Continued

Table 20.1 Muscles of the leg and foot—cont'd

Muscles that move the foot and toes	Origin	Insertion	Action
Intrinsic muscles of the foot **Dorsal** • Extensor digitorum brevis	Anterior and lateral surfaces of calcaneus and inferior extensor retinaculum	Tendons of extensor digitorum longus on toes 2–4 and proximal phalanx of great toe Note: The tendon that inserts into the proximal phalanx of the great toe is also described as extensor hallucis brevis.	Extends toes 2–4 at interphalangeal joints Extensor hallucis brevis extends great toe at metatarsophalangeal joint
Plantar First Layer (most superficial)			
• Abductor hallucis	Medial process of tuberosity of calcaneus, plantar fascia and flexor retinaculum	Medial side of proximal phalanx of great toe with the tendon of the flexor hallucis brevis	Abducts and flexes great toe at metatarsophalangeal joint
• Flexor digitorum brevis	Medial process of tuberosity of calcaneus and plantar fascia	Sides of middle phalanges of toes 2–5	Flexes toes 2–5 at proximal interphalangeal and metatarsophalangeal joint
• Abductor digiti minimi	Medial process of tuberosity of calcaneus and plantar fascia	Lateral side of proximal phalanx of little toe with the tendon of the flexor digiti minimi brevis	Abducts and flexes little toe at metatarsophalangeal joint
Second Layer • Quadratus plantae	Medial head: medial surface of calcaneus Lateral head: lateral border of plantar surface of calcaneus	Tendon of flexor digitorum longus	Assists flexor digitorum longus to flex toes 2–5 at metatarsophalangeal joints
• Lumbricals	Tendons of flexor digitorum longus	Tendons of extensor digitorum longus on proximal phalanges of toes 2–5	Extends toes 2–5 at interphalangeal joints and flexes toes 2–5 at metatarsophalangeal joints
Third Layer • Flexor hallucis brevis	Medial plantar surface of cuboid and 3rd (lateral) cuneiform	Medial and lateral sides of base of proximal phalanx of great toe	Flexes great toe at metatarsophalangeal joint
• Adductor hallucis	Metatarsals 2–4, ligaments of 3–5 metatarsophalangeal joints, and tendon of peroneus longus	Lateral side of proximal phalanx of great toe	Adducts and flexes great toe at metatarsophalangeal joint
• Flexor digiti minimi brevis	Base of 5th metatarsal and tendon of peroneus longus	Lateral side base of proximal phalanx of little toe	Flexes little toe at metatarsophalangeal joint
Fourth layer (deepest) • Dorsal interossei	Adjacent side of metatarsals	Proximal phalanges: both sides of 2nd toe and lateral side of toes 3 and 4	Abduct and flex toes 2–4 at metatarsophalangeal joints and extend toes at interphalangeal joints
• Plantar interossei	Bases and medial sides of metatarsals 3–5	Medial side of bases of proximal phalanges of toes 3–5	Adduct and flex proximal metatarsophalangeal joints and extend toes at interphalangeal joints

CASE HISTORY

Information from case histories can alert practitioners to the presence of serious conditions requiring referral. Reliability or diagnostic utility of subjective complaints of ankle and foot pain remain to be determined.[2] Information from case histories needs to be integrated with findings from other assessments and interpreted with caution. Questioning should be targeted to include:

- description and mechanism of current injury, onset of symptoms, pain, disability and functional impairment, previous injuries to this area. Was there a popping sound? Is

Assessment of the leg, ankle and foot

1. Case history
2. Outcome measures (e.g. The Patient Specific Scale)
3. Postural analysis
4. Gait analysis
5. Functional tests
   Lumbar spine and pelvis
   Active range of motion tests
   Flexion, extension, lateral flexion, rotation
   Hip joint
   Active range of motion tests
   Flexion, extension, abduction, adduction, internal rotation, external rotation
   Knee joint
   Active range of motion tests
   Flexion, extension, internal rotation, external rotation
   Ankle joint and foot
   Active range of motion tests
   Flexion, extension, inversion, eversion
   Passive range of motion tests
   Flexion, extension, inversion, eversion
   Resisted range of motion tests
   Flexion, extension, inversion, eversion
   Resisted and length tests for specific muscles, including:
   gastrocnemius, soleus, tibialis anterior, tibialis posterior, peroneus longus and brevis, extensor digitorum longus and brevis, flexor digitorum longus and brevis
   Special tests
   Anterior/posterior draw
   Lateral ligament stability
   Morton's foot test
6. Palpation

there bruising and swelling, or numbness, tingling or weakness?[3]

- type of work, footwear, wear patterns on shoes
- identifying red and yellow flags that require referral for further investigation (red flags for serious causes of ankle and foot pain are summarised in Table 20.2)
- eliminating other conditions that can cause symptoms in the ankle and foot (e.g. diabetes, Raynaud's phenomenon[a])
- identifying the exact location of the symptoms by asking clients to point to the site of symptoms
- determining if pain is local or referred. Local pain tends to be sharp and well localised; referred pain tends to be dull and poorly localised. Is there any numbness, tingling or weakness? The presence of nerve impingement symptoms suggests local nerve entrapment or referral from the lumbosacral radiculopathy. Dermatomes of the foot indicate the level of impingement (see Figure 20.5 on p 388). Other causes of distal paraesthesia include B12 deficiency, hypothyroidism, heavy metal poisoning, diabetes, systemic lupus erythematosus, malnutrition, HIV, HIV medications.

OUTCOME MEASURES

Outcome measures are questionnaires that are specifically designed to assess clients' level of impairment and to define benefits of treatment. The Patient Specific Scale is a generic assessment tool that can be used to measure progress of treatment of clients with any musculoskeletal condition, including leg, ankle and foot conditions.

[a]Raynaud's phenomenon is characterised by impaired blood flow to the fingers, toes, ears and nose. Cold temperatures or strong emotions cause sudden constriction of blood vessels.

Table 20.2 Red flags for potentially serious conditions of the leg, ankle and foot[4]

Condition	Red flag – history	Red flag – physical examination
Fracture and/or dislocation	History of recent trauma, crush injury, motor vehicle accident, falls from heights, sports injuries, osteoporosis in the elderly	Joint effusion, haemarthrosis, bruising, swelling, throbbing pain, point tenderness, unwilling to bear weight on involved leg
Infection (septic arthritis)	History of recent infection, surgery, injection, immunosuppressive disorder	Constant ache and/or throbbing pain, joint swelling, tenderness, warmth May have fever
Peripheral arterial occlusive disease	Age >55 years, history of type II diabetes, ischaemic heart disease, smoking, sedentary lifestyle, intermittent claudication	Unilateral cool extremity, prolonged capillary refill time (>2 sec), decreased pulses in arteries below level of occlusion
Deep venous thrombosis	Recent surgery, malignancy, pregnancy, trauma or leg immobilisation (e.g. long plane or bus trip)	Calf pain, oedema, tenderness, warmth. Pain increases with standing or walking, relieved by rest and elevation. Possible pallor and loss of dorsalis pedis pulse
Cellulitis	History of recent skin ulceration or abrasion, venous insufficiency, congestive heart failure or cirrhosis	Pain, skin swelling, warmth, advancing irregular margin of erythema/reddish streaks Fever, chills, malaise, weakness
Compartment syndrome	History of blunt trauma, crush injury, or recent participation in rigorous unaccustomed exercise	Severe persistent leg pain that is aggravated by stretching the involved muscles Swelling, exquisite tenderness and palpable tension/hardness of involved compartment Paraesthesia, paresis, absence of pulse

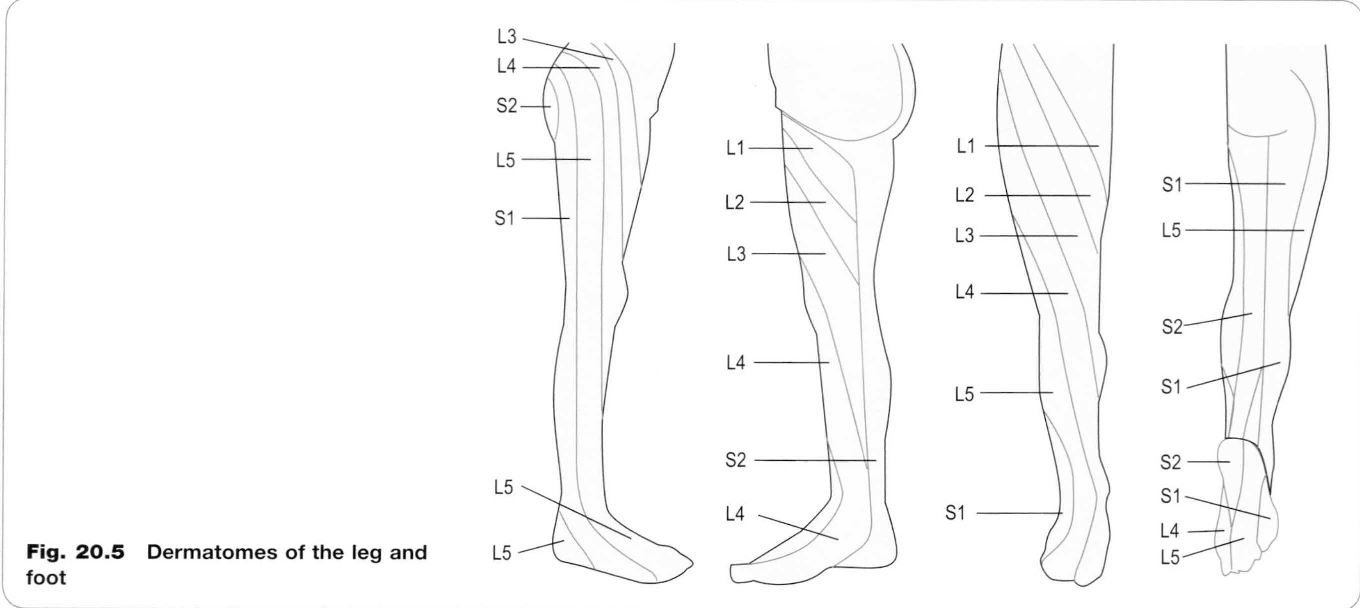

Fig. 20.5 Dermatomes of the leg and foot

POSTURAL ANALYSIS

Postural analysis enables observation of the whole client and facilitates identification of important features through bilateral comparison. It also facilitates detection of possible predisposing or contributing factors that may be implicated by observing the position of the thoracic and lumbar spines, pelvis and lower limbs. Note in particular the presence of scoliosis, femoral anteversion or retroversion, excessive Q angle, tibial torsion, genu valgus, varum or recurvatum (see Chapter 19), ankle pronation, pes cavus or planus and any abnormalities of the toes.

Observing the ankles and feet

Observe the ankles and feet for symmetry, swelling (local or diffuse), colour, bruising, scars and muscle hypertonicity or atrophy.

Common conditions of the ankles and feet include:

- Ankle pronation: Observe the Achilles tendons. Medial deviation suggests ankle pronation (see Figure 20.6). Pronation syndrome accounts for approximately 90% of all soft tissue injuries treated by podiatrists. Management is directed to correction of the underlying causes which include forefoot varus, rearfoot varus, tibia varum, genu varum and valgus, gastrocnemius and soleus contracture, hallux valgus, leg length asymmetry and spinal or pelvic asymmetry.[3]
- Pes planus: absent or reduced medial longitudinal arch of the foot (flat foot). The talus displaces medially and towards the plantar surface of the foot. Pes planus affects approximately 33% of adults.[3] Management includes wearing shoes with shock-absorbing soles, strengthening intrinsic muscles of the foot (e.g. picking up objects with toes), strengthening quadriceps and hamstrings, stretching gastrocnemius and soleus and referral for orthotics (see Figure 20.7 on p 389).
- Pes cavus: Abnormally high arches, often associated with claw toes. Pes cavus occurs in approximately 20% of adults.[3] The foot is rigid and absorbs shock poorly. Management includes mobilisation and manipulation of the foot, shock-absorbing shoes and stretches to gastrocnemius, plantar fascia and toe flexors (see Figure 20.8 on p 389).

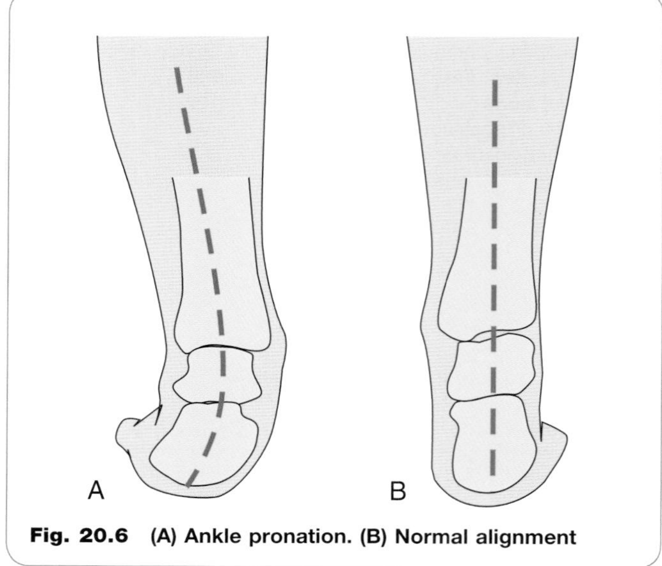

Fig. 20.6 (A) Ankle pronation. (B) Normal alignment

- Hallux valgus: an anatomical variant involving abduction of the 1st metatarsal and adduction of the proximal phalanx of the hallux, often associated with bunion formation. Management includes padding, wide shoes with a low heel, mobilisation and manipulation, stretches to abduct the big toe.
- Hallux rigidus: decreased dorsiflexion of the matatarsophalangeal joint of the hallux, usually from degenerative arthritis. Management includes mobilisation, massage and referral for orthotics (see Figure 20.9 on p 389).
- Claw toes: hyperextension of the metatarsophalangeal joint and hyperflexion of the proximal and distal interphalangeal joints, often accompanies pes cavus. Management includes padding, appropriate shoes, manipulation and mobilisation of the foot and ankle (see Figure 20.10 on p 389).

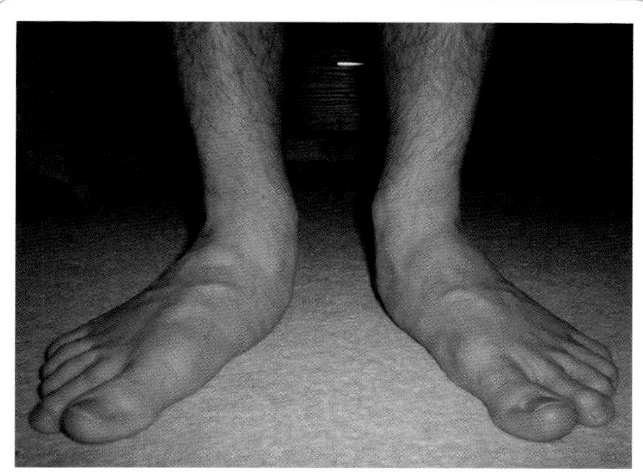

Fig. 20.7 Pes planus

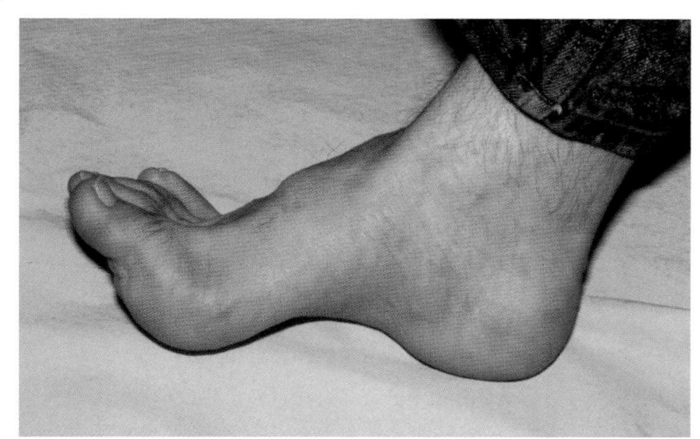

Fig. 20.8 Pes cavus

- Hammer toes: hyperflexion of the proximal interphalangeal joint, some extension of the metatarsophalangeal joint, often at the 2nd toe. The best prognosis occurs when hammer toe is treated in childhood. Later treatment includes padding, appropriate shoes, splinting and surgery (see Figure 20.11 on p 390).
- Morton's foot: the 2nd metatarsal is longer than the first (approximately 20% of the population). Clients should be advised to wear proper-fitting shoes. Morton's foot is associated with pronation-related injuries.

GAIT ANALYSIS

During the gait cycle the ankle dorsiflexes and plantarflexes. The ankle dorsiflexors, particularly tibialis anterior, concentrically contract during the swing phase so that the foot clears the ground. Tibialis anterior eccentrically contracts to control the lowering of the foot to the ground. The ankle plantarflexors are responsible for push-off along with eccentrically contracting toe extensors (see Chapter 2).

Observe any ankle over-pronation and over-supination as the foot takes the weight of the body. Compare the duration of stance phase for both lower limbs. A shortened time in stance phase (antalgic gait) can occur in any condition causing pain on weight bearing. Avoiding heel strike suggests retrocalcaneal bursitis or heel spurs. Weak tibialis anterior may cause drop foot gait. Walking on the balls of the toes suggests gastrocnemius or soleus shortening or strain, or heel or foot pain. A flat foot gait which avoids forceful push-off suggests weak gastrocnemius, soleus or hallux rigidis. Steppage gait in swing phase suggests weak dorsiflexors. Limited ankle movement is observed in clients with degenerative joint disease of the ankle.

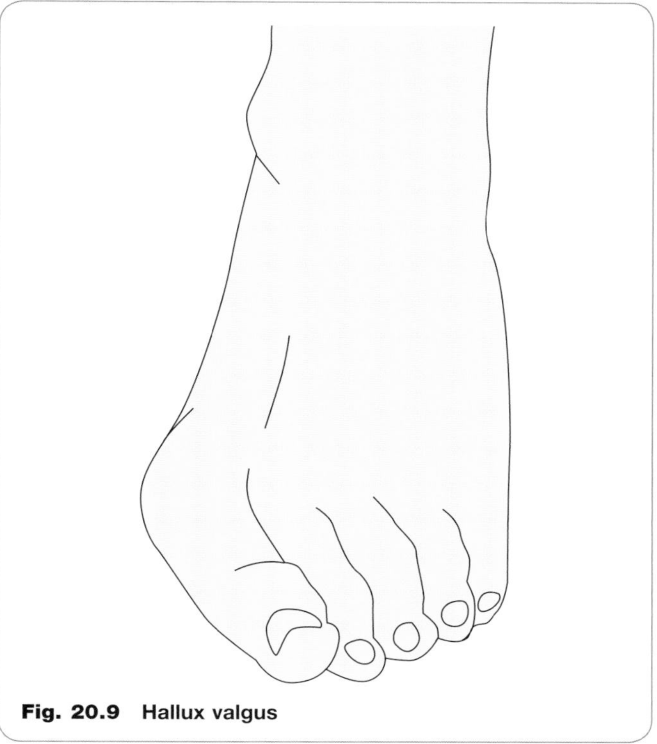

Fig. 20.9 Hallux valgus

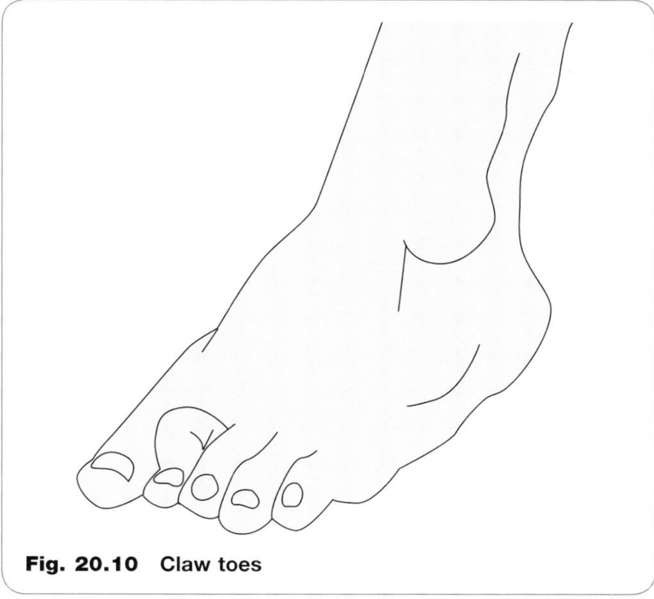

Fig. 20.10 Claw toes

FUNCTIONAL TESTS

For any tests involving joint movements it is important to compare both sides and take into account any underlying

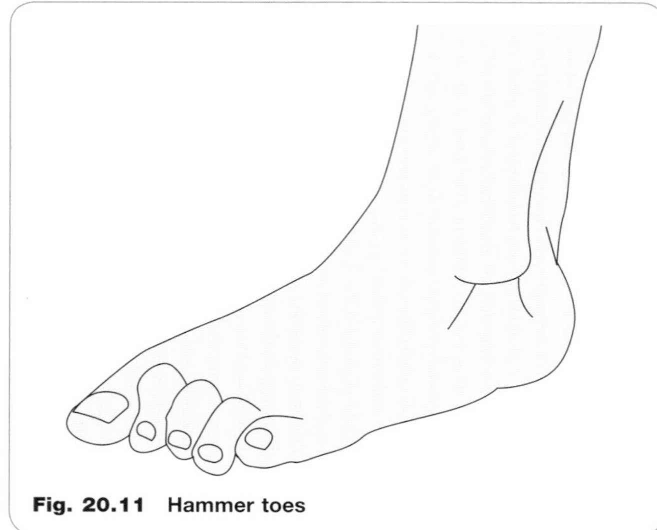

Fig. 20.11 Hammer toes

pathology and the age and lifestyle of the client. Measuring ankle range of motion has been shown to be highly reliable when measured by the same person.[2]

Active range of motion of the lumbar spine and pelvis (flexion, extension, lateral flexion and rotation)

Examination of the leg, ankle and foot begins with active range of motion tests of the lumbar spine and pelvis to help rule out lumbosacral radiculopathy which may refer pain and other symptoms to the lower limb. If active range of motion tests of the lumbar spine and pelvis reproduce leg, ankle or foot symptoms, further examination of the lumbar spine and pelvis is indicated (see Chapter 10).

Active range of motion of the hip joint (flexion, extension, abduction, adduction, external and internal rotation)

If active range of motion tests of the hip joint reproduce leg, ankle or foot symptoms, a full examination of the hip joint is indicated (see Chapter 18). Note that hip disease often manifests as knee pain.

Active range of motion of the knee joint (flexion, extension, internal and external rotation)

If the client experiences pain or other symptoms during knee movement, a full examination of the knee joint is indicated (see Chapter 19).

Active range of motion of the ankle and foot[5]

Talotibial joint
Dorsiflexion/plantarflexion 15–20°/40–50°
Subtalar and midtarsal joints
Inversion/eversion 30–35°/20°
1st metatarsophalangeal joint
Flexion/extension 20°/80°
2nd–5th toes metatarsophalangeal joints
Flexion/extension 75°/35°
2nd–5th toes interphalangeal joints
Flexion/extension ~60°/20°

Ankle and foot active range of motion is often tested using functional movements. Ask the client to:

- Walk on toes.
- Walk on heels.
- Walk on the outsides of their feet.
- Walk on the insides of their feet (see Figure 20.12 on p 391).

Passive range of motion of the ankle and foot

If the client is unable to perform normal AROM in any direction, further investigation is required. PROM testing for the ankle and foot may be performed with the client supine. For the toes, isolate the joint by placing one contact proximal and the other distal to the joint (e.g. to isolate the proximal interphalangeal joint, one hand contacts the proximal phalanx, the other contacts the distal phalanx). Palpate for crepitus, capsular pattern and end-feel. Capsular patterns of restriction of the ankle and foot are:[3]

- talotibial joint: plantar flexion more limited than dorsiflexion
- subtalar joint: varus and valgus equally limited
- midtarsal joints: dorsiflexion more limited than plantarflexion
- 1st metatarsophalangeal joint: flexion more limited than extension
- 2nd–5th metatarsophalangeal joints: variable
- interphalangeal joints: flexion more limited than extension.

Resisted range of motion

RROM tests should also be performed if AROM testing indicates the likelihood of a leg, ankle or foot problem. RROM tests include:

ANKLE

Dorsiflexion: tibialis anterior, extensor digitorum longus, extensor hallucis longus
Plantarflexion: Soleus, gastrocnemius, tibialis posterior, flexor digitorum longus, flexor hallucis longus
Inversion: tibialis anterior, tibialis posterior
Eversion: fibularis longus, brevis and tertius

HALLUX

Flexion: flexor hallucis longus and brevis
Extension: extensor hallucis longus and brevis
Abduction: abductor hallucis
Adduction: adductor hallucis

2ND TO 5TH TOES

Flexion: flexor digitorum longus and brevis, lumbricals
Extension: extensor digitorum longus and brevis
Abduction: dorsal interossei, abductor digiti minimi
Adduction: plantar interossei

Resisted tests and length tests for specific muscles

If RROM tests reproduce symptoms, further tests may be used to help identify specific muscles.

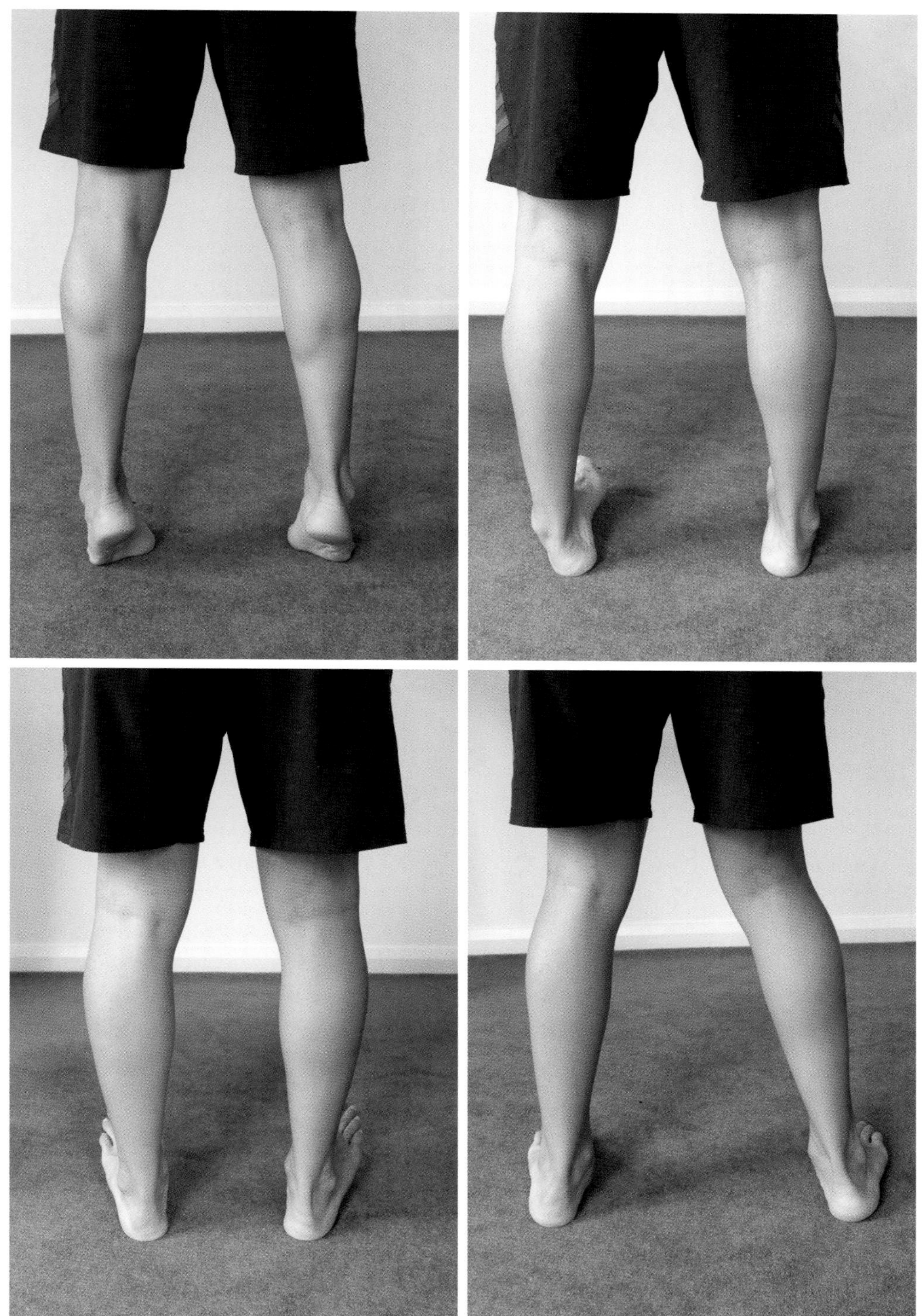

Fig. 20.12 Functional active range of motion test of the ankle joint

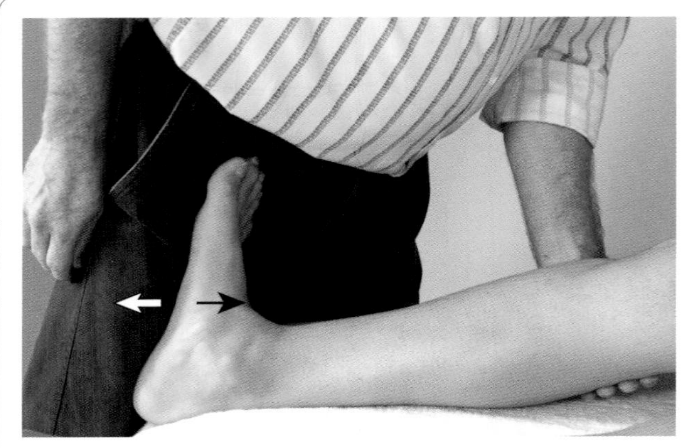

Fig. 20.13 Resisted test for gastrocnemius

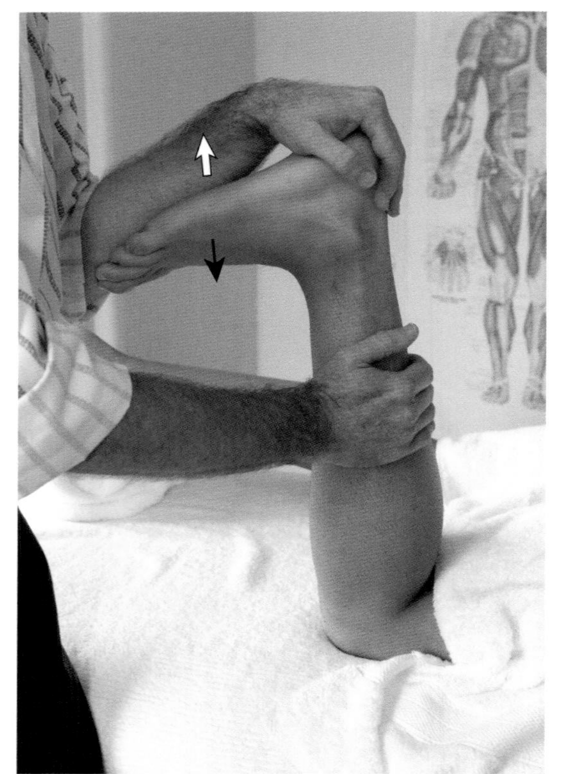

Fig. 20.14 Resisted test for soleus

1. GASTROCNEMIUS

Resisted test

The client lies supine, knees straight, and tries to point their toes against your resistance (see Figure 20.13). Alternatively, ask the client to stand on their toes while resistance is applied by pushing down on their shoulders.

2. SOLEUS

Resisted test

The client lies prone with their knee flexed to 90°. Apply resistance as the client tries to plantarflex their ankle (see Figure 20.14).

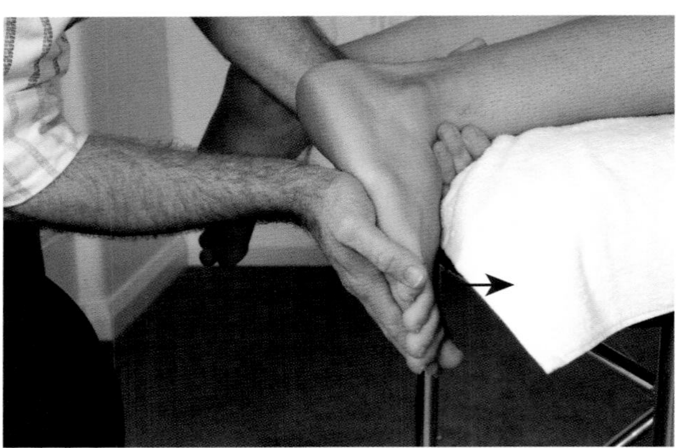

Fig. 20.15 Length test for ankle plantarflexors

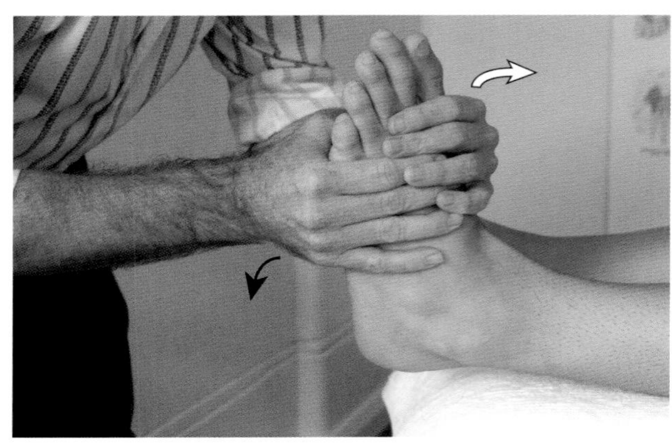

Fig. 20.16 Resisted test for tibialis anterior

Length test for ankle plantarflexors

Shortened gastrocnemius and soleus limit ankle dorsiflexion. When walking, it can interfere with heel strike and the client may tend to walk on their toes (see Figure 20.15).

3. TIBIALIS ANTERIOR

Resisted test

The client's foot is placed in inversion and dorsiflexion. Instruct the client to hold this position while resistance is applied in the direction of flexion and eversion (see Figure 20.16).

Length test

Contracted tibialis anterior limits plantarflexion and eversion (see Figure 20.17 on p 393). In some cases contracture may cause inversion of the foot (calcaneovarus).

4. TIBIALIS POSTERIOR

Resisted test

Plantarflex and invert the client's foot and instruct the client to hold this position. Apply resistance against the medial and plantar surface of the foot in the direction of dorsiflexion and eversion (see Figure 20.18 on p 393).

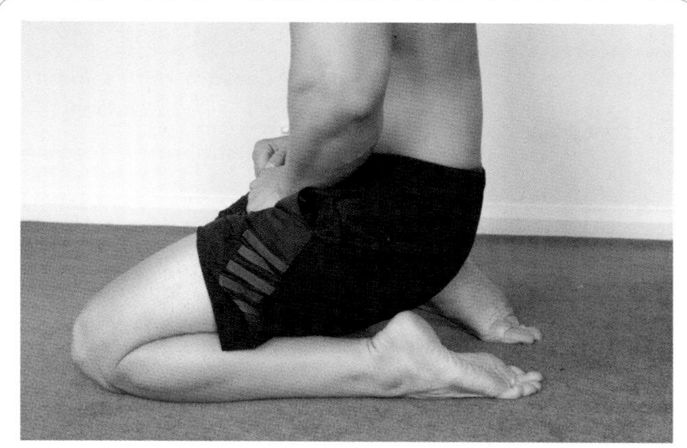

Fig. 20.17 Length test for tibialis anterior

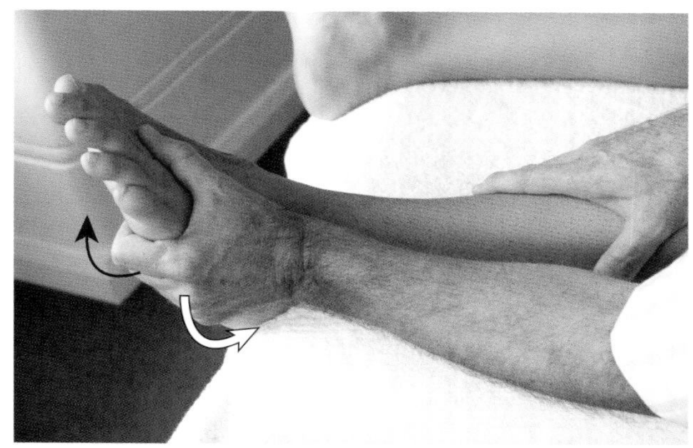

Fig. 20.19 Resisted test for fibularis longus and brevis

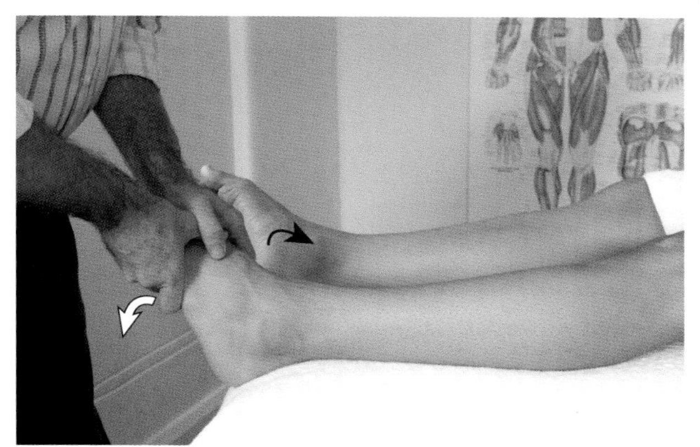

Fig. 20.18 Resisted test for tibialis posterior

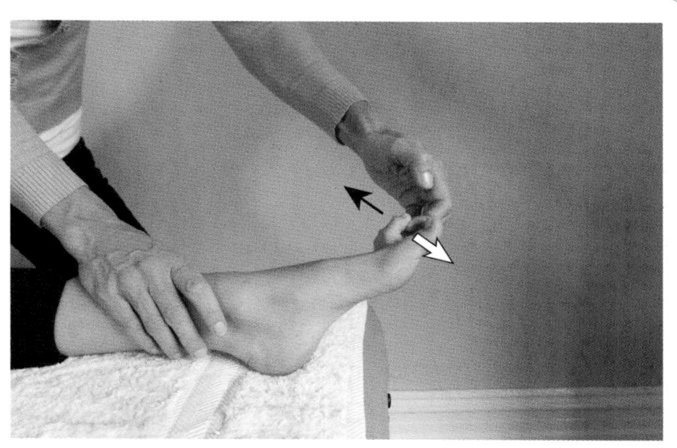

Fig. 20.20 Resisted test for flexor digitorum longus

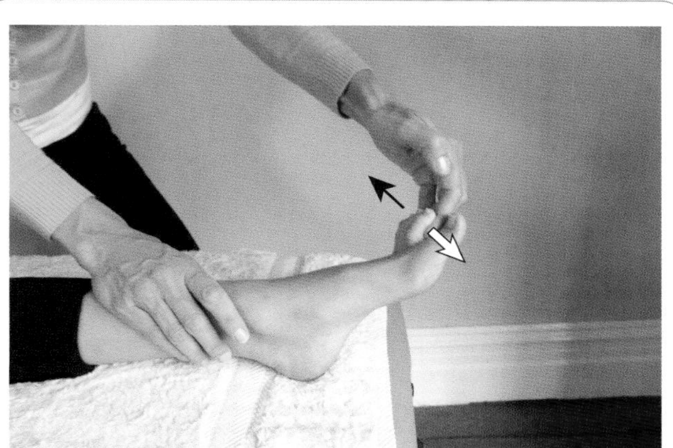

Fig. 20.21 Resisted test for flexor digitorum brevis

Length test

Contraction of tibialis posterior limits dorsiflexion and eversion.

5. FIBULARIS (PERONEUS) LONGUS AND BREVIS

Resisted test

Plantarflex and evert the client's foot and instruct them to hold the position while pressure is applied to the lateral border and sole of the foot in the direction of inversion and dorsiflexion (see Figure 20.19).

Length test

Contraction of fibularis longus and brevis limits inversion. In some cases contraction causes an everted or valgus position of the foot.

6. FLEXOR DIGITORUM LONGUS

Resisted test

The client flexes the distal phalanges of toes 2 to 5. Pressure is applied against the plantar surface of the distal phalanges of toes 2 to 5 in the direction of extension (see Figure 20.20).

Length test

Contracture of flexor digitorum longus can cause flexion deformity of the distal phalanges of toes 2 to 5.

7. FLEXOR DIGITORUM BREVIS

Resisted test

This test is similar to the test for flexor digitorum longus except that the client flexes the proximal phalanx of toes 2 to 5 and you apply pressure to their plantar surface in the direction of extension (see Figure 20.21).

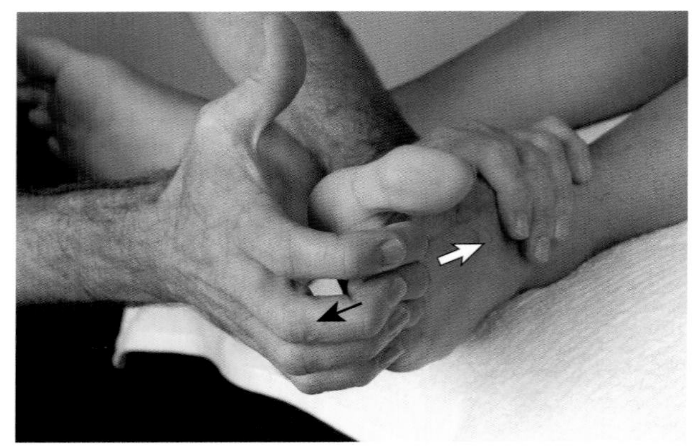

Fig. 20.22 **Resisted test for extensor digitorum longus and brevis**

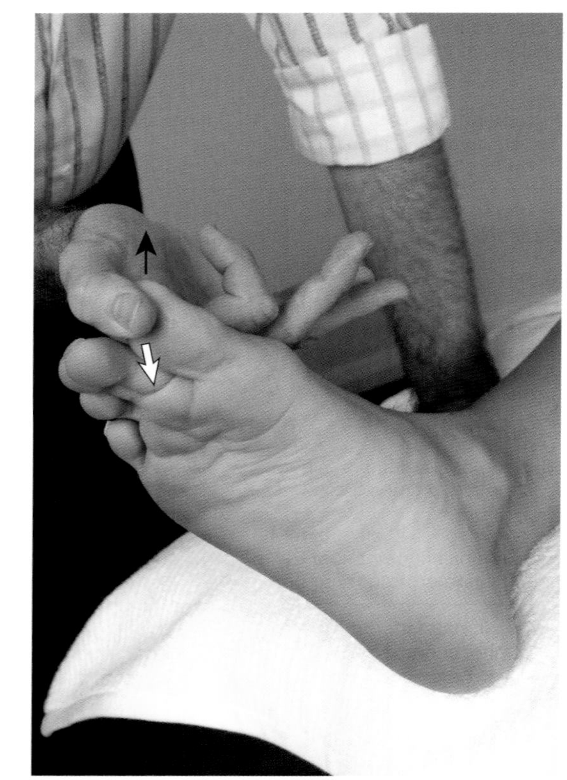

Fig. 20.23 **Resisted test for flexor hallucis longus**

Length test

Shortened flexor digitorum brevis limits extension of the proximal interphalangeal and metatarsophalangeal joints of toes 2 to 5.

8. EXTENSOR DIGITORUM LONGUS AND BREVIS

Resisted test

Extensor digitorum longus and brevis are tested together, as their tendons fuse, extending all joints of toes 2 to 5. To perform a resisted test on the muscles, pressure is applied against the dorsal surface of toes 2 to 5 in the direction of flexion (see Figure 20.22).

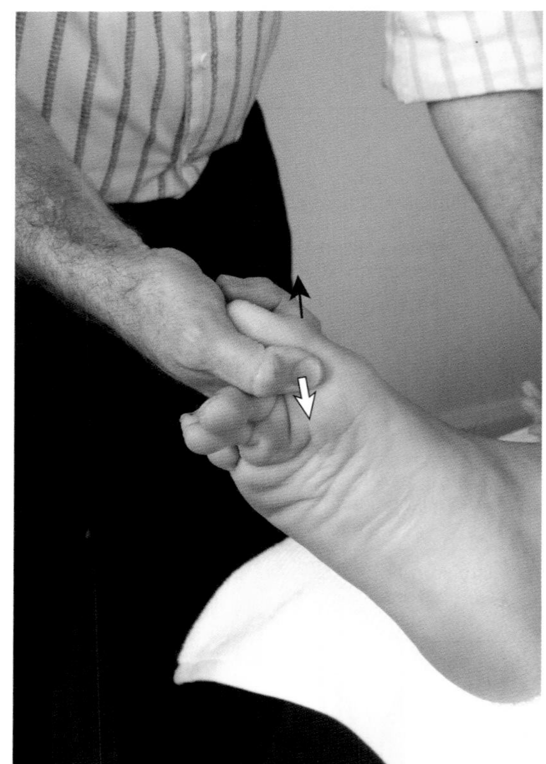

Fig. 20.24 **Resisted test for flexor hallucis brevis**

Length test

Shortened extensor digitorum longus and brevis muscles limit flexion of all joints of toes 2 to 5. Contracture of extensor digitorum longus and brevis leads to hyperextension of the metatarsophalangeal joints.

9. FLEXOR HALLUCIS LONGUS

Resisted test

Pressure is applied against the plantar surface of the distal phalanx of the big toe in the direction of extension (see Figure 20.23).

Length test

Contracture of flexor hallucis longus can cause a hammer toe deformity of the big toe.

10. FLEXOR HALLUCIS BREVIS

Resisted test

This test is similar to the test for flexor hallucis longus except that you contact the plantar surface of the proximal phalanx of the big toe and apply pressure in the direction of flexion (see Figure 20.24).

Length test

Contracture holds the proximal phalanx of the big toe in flexion.

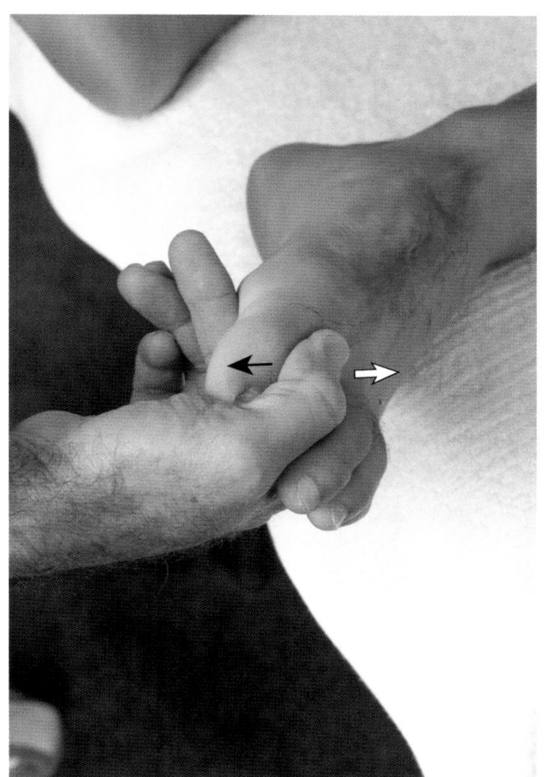

Fig. 20.25 Resisted test for extensor hallucis longus and brevis

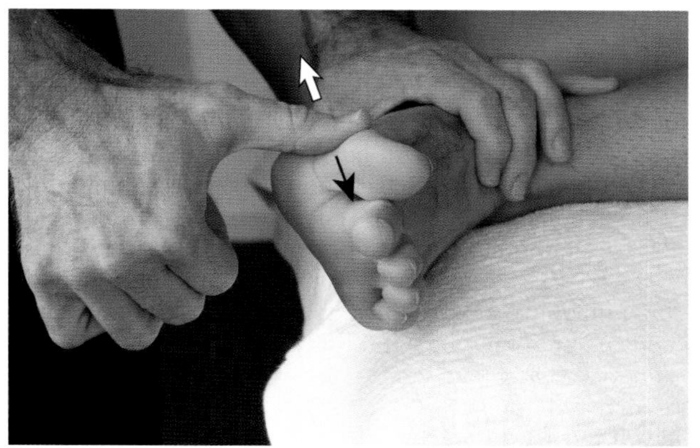

Fig. 20.26 Resisted test for abductor hallucis

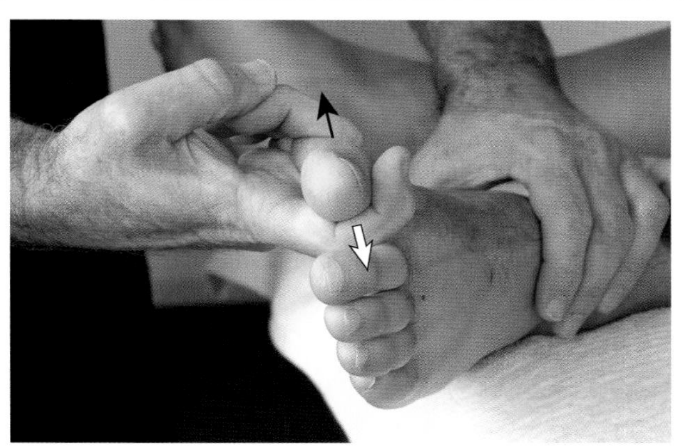

Fig. 20.27 Resisted test for adductor hallucis

11. EXTENSOR HALLUCIS LONGUS AND BREVIS

Resisted test

Extensor hallucis brevis extends the proximal phalanx of the big toe; extensor hallucis longus extends both distal and proximal phalanges. Both muscles are tested simultaneously. The client tries to extend the metatarsophalangeal joints and interphalangeal joints of the big toe against your resistance (see Figure 20.25).

Length test

Contraction of extensor hallucis longus and brevis causes extension of the big toe.

12. ABDUCTOR HALLUCIS

Resisted test

The client is asked to resist pressure applied against the medial side of the proximal phalanx of the big toe (see Figure 20.26).

Length test

If abductor hallucis is contracted, the big toe is abducted and the forefoot is pulled into varus.

13. ADDUCTOR HALLUCIS

Resisted test

The client is asked to resist pressure applied against the lateral side of the proximal phalanx of the big toe (see Figure 20.27).

Test for contracture

Contracture of adductor hallucis can cause hallux valgus.

Special tests

If symptoms are reported when performing a special test, ask the client to identify their exact location and confirm that they are the same symptoms described in the case history. Functional tests have varying level of reliability and diagnostic utility and test results should always be interpreted cautiously and in the context of other clinical findings (see Chapter 2).

ANKLE DRAW TESTS

- Anterior draw: The client is supine with the knee on the involved side flexed and foot flat on the table. Stabilise the foot with one hand and hold the leg just proximal to the ankle with the other. Push the leg posteriorly (i.e. the foot becomes relatively anterior). Pain or excessive movement suggests anterior talofibular sprain or laxity (LR+ = 3.1, LR− = 0.29) (see Figure 20.28 on p 396).
- Posterior draw: This test is similar to the anterior draw except that the leg is pulled anteriorly (i.e. the foot becomes relatively posterior). Pain or excessive movement suggests posterior talofibular ligament sprain or laxity (see Figure 20.28 on p 396).

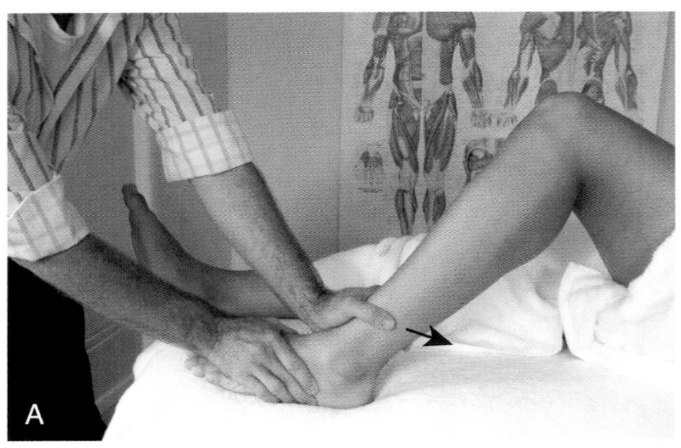

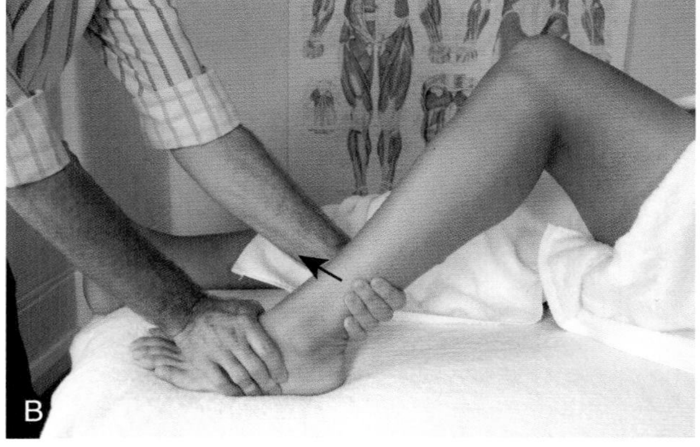

Fig. 20.28 (a) Ankle anterior and (b) posterior draw

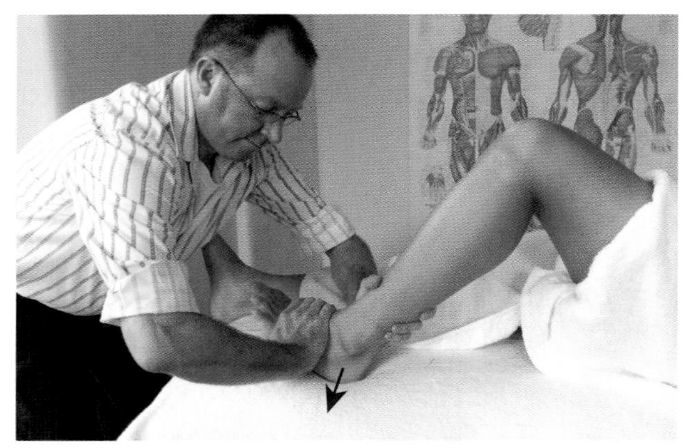

Fig. 20.29 Lateral ligament stability test

LATERAL LIGAMENT STABILITY TEST (TALAR TILT TEST)

The client is supine with knee and hip flexed. Invert the calcaneus by applying lateral pressure on the medial malleolus. Pain or excessive movement could suggest sprain or laxity of the calcaneofibular ligament and anterior talofibular ligament (see Figure 20.29).

MORTON'S TEST

With the client supine, squeeze the client's foot medially and laterally across the metatarsal heads. Pain on this manoeuvre suggests Morton's neuroma, metatarsal joint arthritis or fracture of the metatarsal heads (see Figure 20.30).

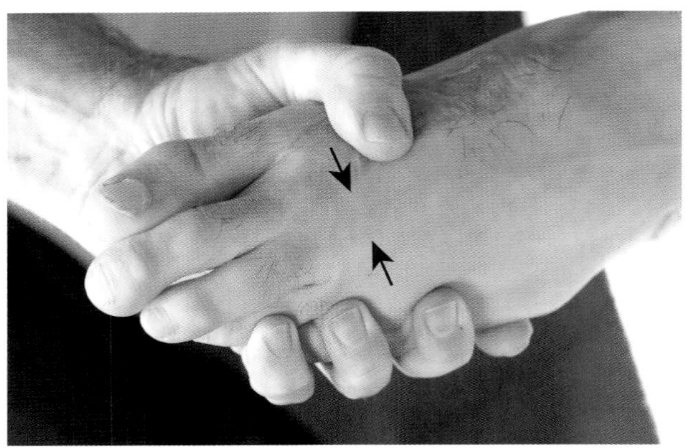

Fig. 20.30 Morton's test

PALPATION

The client lies supine. Palpate the anterior border of the tibia from above the tibial tuberosity to below the medial malleolus. Palpate the muscles of the anterior compartment (tibialis anterior, extensor digitorum longus, extensor hallucis longus and peroneus tertius) lateral to the tibial border. Further lateral, palpate the lateral compartment (peroneus longus and brevis). Palpate the head of the fibula posterolateral to the knee. The common peroneal nerve runs along the lateral aspect of the head of the fibula. Palpate the circumference of the lateral malleolus at the distal end of the fibula. Compare the blunt end of the medial malleolus at the distal end of the tibia to the sharp end of the lateral malleolus. The level of the lateral malleolus is just below and slightly posterior to the level of the medial malleolus.

Medial aspect of the ankle and foot

- The first metatarsophalangeal joint is easily located. This is a common site of bunion formation, often as a result of lateral deviation of the proximal phalanx of the big toe, and of gouty arthritis, which is usually associated with redness, heat and pain. Palpate the sesamoids under the head of the first metatarsal as they slide when the big toe is passively articulated.
- Palpate the navicular tubercle, the large bony prominence on the medial side of the midfoot.
- The talar head is found approximately halfway between the medial malleolus and the navicular tubercle. Everting the foot makes the talar head more prominent.
- The sustentaculum tali of the calcaneus is palpated more than a finger's breadth below the medial malleolus posteriorly. Approach from below and press upwards. Tibialis posterior tendon and the spring ligament run from the sustentaculum tali to the navicular bone.
- The medial collateral ligament (deltoid ligament) lies under tibialis posterior and flexor digitorum longus. It can be mapped as a triangle with its apex at the medial malleolus and its base extending from the navicular to the sustentaculum tali.

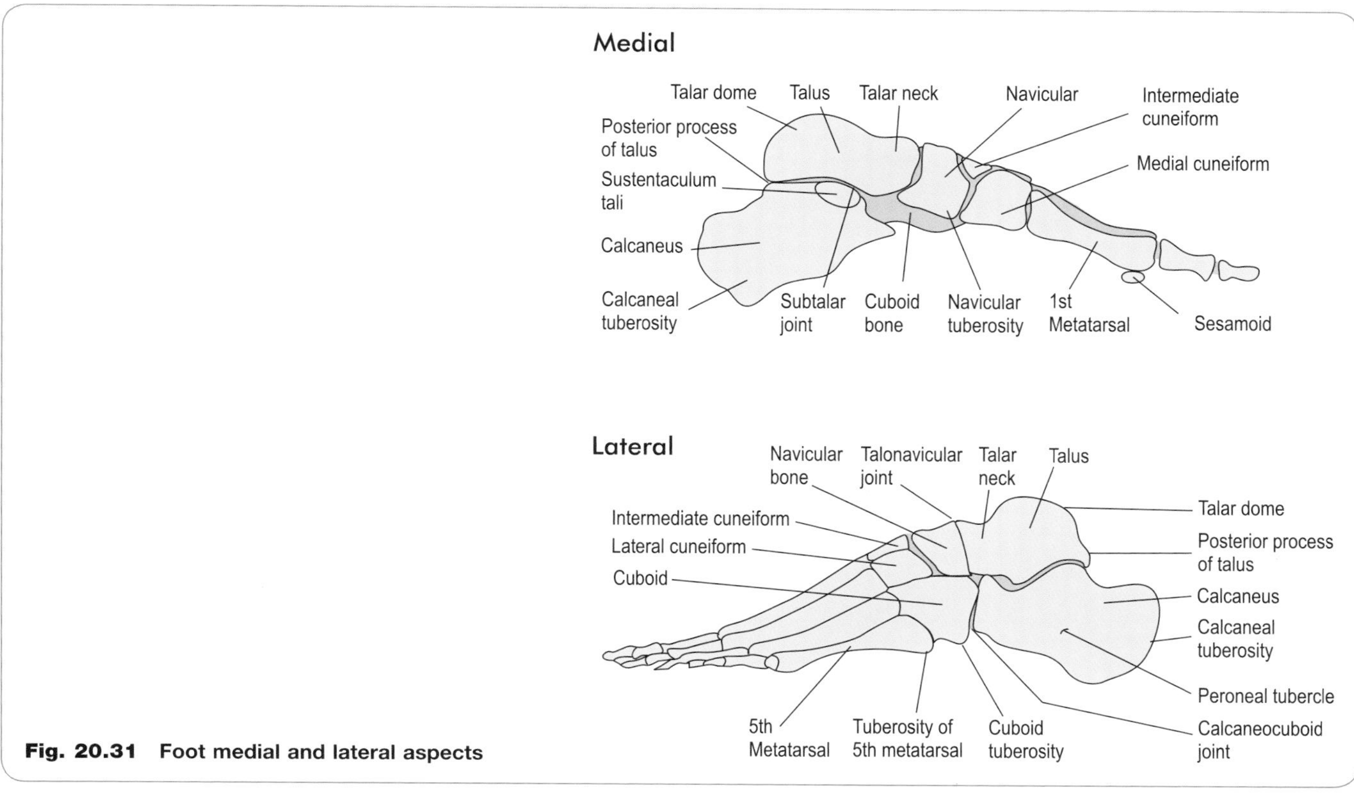

Fig. 20.31 Foot medial and lateral aspects

- From the medial malleolus to the Achilles tendon palpate, in order, tendons of tibialis posterior and flexor digitorum longus, the posterior tibial artery and nerve and flexor hallucis longus.
- Abductor hallucis occupies the concavity of the instep (see Figure 20.31).

Lateral aspect of the ankle and foot

- Palpate the styloid process of the fifth metatarsal bone. This is the attachment site for peroneus brevis.
- Move posteriorly to the cuboid. Peroneus longus tendon winds around the lateral malleolus and runs in a groove under the cuboid towards its insertion at the medial cuneiform and first metatarsal.
- Palpate the tendons of peroneus longus and brevis (brevis is more anterior).
- Palpate the calcaneus and the peroneal tubercle (where peroneus longus and brevis tendons separate) distal to the lateral malleolus.
- Palpate the sinus tarsi area, a depression just anterior to the lateral malleolus. The talar dome is palpable here when the client's foot is plantarflexed.
- Abductor digiti minimi forms the lateral border of the foot (see Figure 20.31).
- The lateral collateral ligament is made up of three ligaments:
  - Anterior talofibular ligament runs from the anterior aspect of the lateral malleolus to the lateral talus. Tenderness and swelling in the sinus tarsi usually indicate a sprain of the anterior talofibular ligament.
  - Calcaneofibular ligament runs from the inferior lateral malleolus to the lateral calcaneus.
  - Posterior talofibular ligament runs from the posterior lateral malleolus to the posterior talus (see Figure 20.1 on p 383).

Posterior aspect of the ankle

- Palpate the Achilles tendon from the lower third of the calf to the calcaneus. Trace the belly of the gastrocnemius up the calf and palpate the two heads to their insertions into the medial and lateral condyles of the femur. When the client stands on their toes the gastrocnemius muscle becomes prominent with the soleus bulging on either side of it.
- The subcutaneous calcaneal bursa (between the Achilles insertion and the skin) and retrocalcaneal bursa (between the Achilles tendon and the superior angle of the calcaneus) are normally not palpable. When inflamed they often feel warm and palpate as boggy.

Dorsal aspect of the ankle and foot

- Ask the client to invert the foot and dorsiflex the ankle to bring tibialis anterior into prominence. Trace its insertion to the first metatarsal base and first cuneiform.
- Extensor hallucis longus is made prominent when the client extends their big toe.
- The anterior tibial artery runs from the neck of the fibula to midway between the malleoli. It lies lateral to the tibialis anterior and extensor hallucis longus and medial to extensor digitorum longus and peroneus tertius. Identify these tendons when the client dorsiflexes the ankle. The dorsalis pedis artery (the continuation of the anterior tibial artery) continues to the proximal end of the first intermetatarsal space.

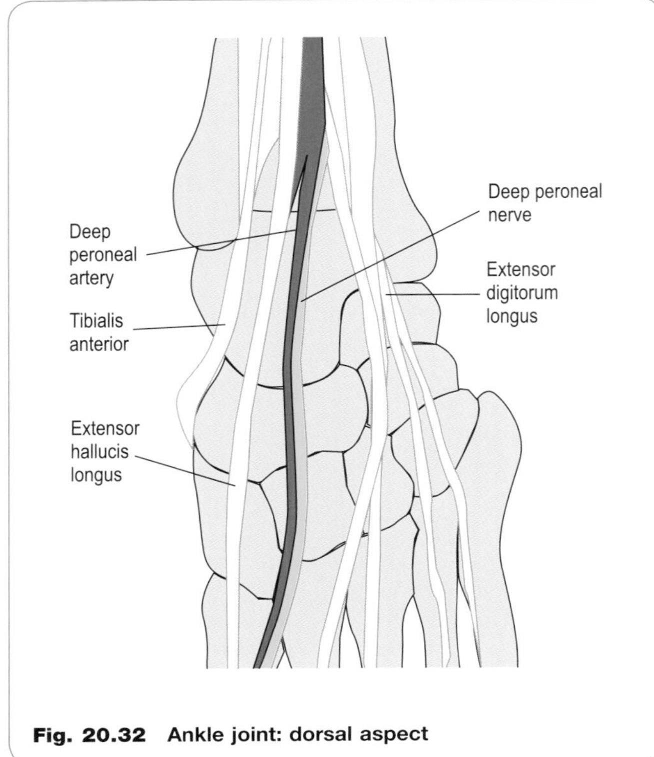

Fig. 20.32 Ankle joint: dorsal aspect

- The superior extensor retinaculum is a broad band connecting the anterior border of the tibia to the anterior border of the fibula just above the malleoli. It forms the upper part of the anterior annular ligament.
- Palpate extensor digitorum brevis in front of the lateral malleolus when the foot is at 90° to the ankle (see Figure 20.32).

Plantar surface of the foot

- Palpate the metatarsal heads and note the integrity of the transverse arch.
- The plantar fascia consists of bands of fascia that run from the medial tuberosity of the calcaneus to the metatarsal heads. In plantar fasciitis tenderness is often elicited when the anteromedial aspect of the calcaneus is palpated.
- Most of the muscles of the plantar surface of the foot originate from the calcaneus.

Phalanges

- Palpate each tarsometatarsal and interphalangeal joint. Note any swelling, tenderness and abnormal alignment.

REMEDIAL MASSAGE TREATMENT

Assessment of the leg, ankle and foot provides essential information for development of treatment plans, including:

- client's suitability for remedial massage therapy
- duration of the condition (i.e. acute or chronic)
- severity of the condition (i.e. grade of injury; mild, moderate or severe pain)
- type(s) of tissues involved
- priorities for treatment if more than one injury or condition are present
- whether the signs and symptoms suggest a common condition of the leg, ankle or foot
- special considerations for individual clients (e.g. client's preference for treatment types and styles, special population considerations).

OVERVIEW

Develop a short- and a long-term plan for each client. The short-term plan directs treatment to the highest priority (usually determined by symptoms). The long-term plan can be introduced when presenting symptoms have subsided. Long-term treatment focuses on contributing or predisposing factors such as underlying structural features and lifestyle factors. Treatment should also include associated functional impairments in other parts of the kinetic chain (foot/ankle/knee/hip/low back). A significant part of both short-term and long-term treatment involves educating clients about likely causal or aggravating factors and guiding their management of these factors. If massage therapy is used in conjunction with other treatments such as corticosteroid injections, it is important to communicate with other treating practitioners and to integrate treatment for the best outcome for the client.

LEG

MUSCLE STRAINS OF THE LEG

Muscle strains in the leg include gastrocnemius strain (tennis leg), tibialis anterior and posterior strain and strains of the peroneal muscles. Assessment and treatment of all muscle strains follow similar procedures. Tennis leg is presented here and can be used as a guide for treatment of other muscle strains of the leg.

GASTROCNEMIUS STRAIN (TENNIS LEG)

This injury tends to occur in older athletes (30 to 50 years) following a sudden explosive push off from a stationary position, climbing a slope or suddenly changing direction. It is often associated with a cold environment.

Assessment

HISTORY

The client is usually an older athlete (30–50 years old). Sudden onset of pain in the medial head of gastrocnemius is

Key assessment findings for gastrocnemius strain (tennis leg)

- History of sudden acceleration from stationary position or uphill running in a cold environment; client 30–50 years old
- Functional tests:
  - AROM: painful ankle plantarflexion
  - PROM: painful dorsiflexion (passive stretch of gastrocnemius)
  - RROM: positive plantarflexion
  - Resisted and length tests: positive for gastrocnemius
- Palpation: tender in belly ~5 cm superior and medial to musculotendinous junction; muscle defect may be palpable

characteristic. The client sometimes reports a sudden stinging or popping sensation in the calf.

FUNCTIONAL TESTS

Lumbar AROM tests do not reproduce symptoms.
Hip AROM tests do not reproduce symptoms.
Knee AROM tests do not reproduce symptoms.

Ankle tests

AROM: painful plantarflexion
PROM: painful dorsiflexion (passive stretch of gastrocnemius)
RROM: positive plantarflexion
Resisted and length tests: positive for gastrocnemius
Special tests: negative

PALPATION

The client usually reports tenderness in the muscle belly approximately 5 cm superior and medial to musculotendinous junction. In severe cases muscle defects may be palpable.

Overview of treatment and management

In the acute phase the RICE regimen is recommended. Crutches may be necessary. A heel raise may be used on both legs to limit full muscle lengthening. Gentle stretching to pain tolerance may be commenced soon after injury.

A typical remedial massage treatment for a subacute/ chronic mild or moderate gastrocnemius tear includes:

- Swedish massage therapy to the lower limb, lumbar spine and pelvis.
- Remedial massage techniques including (see Table 20.3):
  - deep gliding frictions along the muscle fibres
  - cross-fibre frictions
  - soft tissue releasing techniques
  - deep transverse friction applied directly to the injury site to help stimulate collagen production
  - trigger point therapy
  - muscle stretching.
- Myofascial release including cross-arm techniques and the leg pull (see Chapter 8).
- Other remedial techniques such as knee and ankle joint articulation may also be introduced as required (see Chapter 7).
- Correct underlying biomechanical and predisposing factors if possible (e.g. ankle pronation, pes planus, muscle imbalance of the lower limb).

CLIENT EDUCATION

Advise the client to rest from aggravating activities to reduce the stress on the injured muscle. A progressive strengthening and stretching program for the gastrocnemius should be commenced as soon as pain permits. Strengthening exercises can begin with isometric contractions, progressing to concentric bilateral calf raises and to unilateral calf raises, gradually adding weights. Finally add eccentric calf lowering over a step. Stretches should include both gastrocnemius and soleus. The client should also stretch and strengthen hamstrings, quadriceps and tibialis anterior.

Refer for osseous manipulation and for additional physical therapy modalities such as ultrasound and electrophysical therapies.

Key assessment findings for shin splints

- History of anterolateral or posteromedial shin pain related to excessive exercise, repetitive impacts, downhill walking or running (anterior shin splints) or overpronation of the ankle (posterior shin splints)
- Functional tests:
  - AROM: painful
  - PROM: painful due to passive stretch
  - RROM: positive for involved muscles
  - Resisted and length tests: positive for involved muscles (e.g. tibialis anterior, tibialis posterior, flexor digitorum longus, soleus)
  - Special tests: negative
- Palpation: pain on palpation at the site of inflammation; small lumps or nodules may be palpable along muscle attachments to the tibia

SHIN SPLINTS

Shin splints is a term used to describe shin pain due to repetitive overuse such as running or dancing. Long periods of standing on a concrete floor or other hard surface in hard-soled shoes has also been implicated. There are two main types of shin splints:

- Anterior/lateral shin splints: tibialis anterior strain, tendinopathy or periostitis. Anterior shin splints is associated with excessive eccentric dorsiflexion (e.g. downhill walking or running)
- Posterior shin splints: tibialis posterior strain, tendinopathy or periostitis. Flexor digitorum longus and soleus may also be involved. It is associated with overpronation or incorrect running stride.

Assessment

HISTORY

The client describes anterolateral or posteromedial leg pain after exercise (e.g. downhill running or running on uneven surfaces, long-distance running, repeated impacts on a hard surface or with poor footwear). Pain is initially relieved by rest but can progress to constant pain.

FUNCTIONAL TESTS

Lumbar AROM tests do not reproduce symptoms.
Hip AROM tests do not reproduce symptoms.
Knee AROM tests do not reproduce symptoms.

Ankle tests

AROM: painful (e.g. dorsiflexion and inversion for tibialis anterior, plantarflexion and inversion for tibialis posterior).
PROM: painful as the involved muscle is passively stretched.
RROM: positive for involved muscles.
Resisted and length tests: positive for involved muscles (e.g. tibialis anterior and posterior may be weak).

PALPATION

Pain is elicited on palpation of the affected soft tissue and along the medial tibial border. Small nodules are often palpable in the muscle attachments to the medial tibia.

Table 20.3 Remedial massage techniques for muscles of the leg and foot[6, 7]

Muscle	Soft tissue release	Trigger point	Deep transverse friction	Stretch	Corrective action[6]	Home exercises
Gastrocnemius	Client: prone, leg extended and abducted so that the foot is off the side of the table. Practitioner: stands at the foot of the table, facing cephalad. The practitioner applies pressure to the injury site or performs a deep longitudinal glide with fingers, thumbs or knuckles as the client slowly plantarflexes and dorsiflexes their ankle.	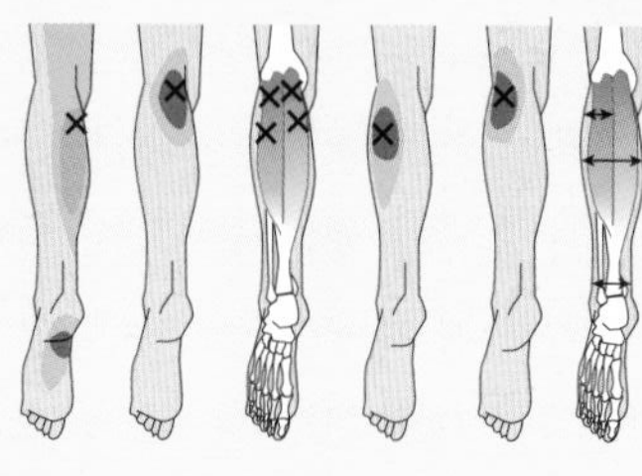		Client: supine, knee extended and heel overhanging the end of the table. Practitioner: standing or kneeling at the foot of the table. The practitioner holds the ankle with both hands and dorsiflexes the client's foot as far as possible. The client tries to plantarflex their ankle for 6–8 seconds against the practitioner's resistance. Next the practitioner dorsiflexes the client's ankle as far as possible. This whole procedure is repeated three times. Alternatively, the client's foot can be placed on the practitioner's anterior thigh and the ankle passively dorsiflexed as the practitioner transfers their weight to their front foot. 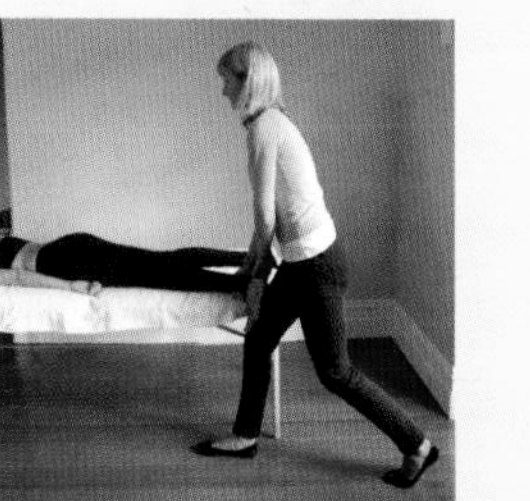	Avoid high-heeled shoes. Change running shoes regularly. Use a footrest if heels do not reach the floor when seated.	Stretch: 1. Stand with one foot in front of the other and bend the front knee. Keep the heel of the back foot on the ground to stretch gastrocnemius. 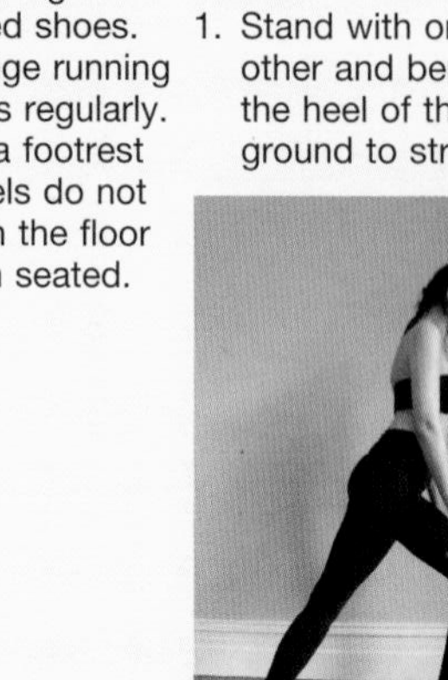 2. Stand on the end of a step with both feet and lower the heel of one foot off the step while keeping the other foot on the step. 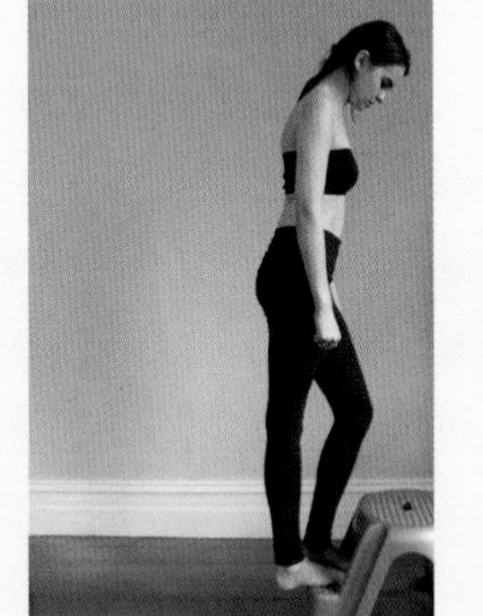 Strengthen: Calf raise (standing heel raise) Leg curls.

Table 20.3 Remedial massage techniques for muscles of the leg and foot—cont'd

Muscle	Soft tissue release	Trigger point	Deep transverse friction	Stretch	Corrective action[6]	Home exercises
Soleus	Client: prone, knee flexed and bolster placed under leg proximal to the ankle. Practitioner: stands at side of the table, facing cephalad. The practitioner applies pressure to the injury site or performs a deep longitudinal glide with thumbs, knuckles or elbow as the client slowly plantarflexes and dorsiflexes their ankle.			Client: prone, knee flexed to 90°. Practitioner: stands at the side of the table facing across the client. The practitioner holds the calcaneus with the caudal hand and places their forearm on the sole of the client's foot. The other hand holds the leg just proximal to the ankle. The practitioner dorsiflexes the ankle as far as comfortable with the caudal hand. The client tries to plantarflex their ankle for 6–8 seconds against the practitioner's resistance. Next the practitioner dorsiflexes the client's ankle as far as possible again. This whole procedure is repeated three times.	Modify activities that overload or maintain a fixed shortened position (e.g. use a footrest, avoid high-heeled shoes). Change running technique and surface. Correct leg length inequality	Stretch: Stand with one foot in front of the other. Bend both knees. Strengthen: Calf raise (standing heel raise) Leg curls.

Continued

Table 20.3 Remedial massage techniques for muscles of the leg and foot—cont'd

Muscle	Soft tissue release	Trigger point	Deep transverse friction	Stretch	Corrective action[6]	Home exercises
Tibialis anterior	Client: supine. Practitioner: stands at the side of the table facing caudad. The practitioner applies pressure to the injury site or performs a deep longitudinal glide with fingers, thumbs or knuckles as the client slowly plantarflexes and dorsiflexes their ankle.			Client: supine. Practitioner: at foot of table. The practitioner plantarflexes (± everts) the client's foot and holds the stretch for up to 30 seconds. Repeat three times.	Eliminate prolonged shortening of the muscle (e.g. avoid long car trips (use of pedal)). Avoid prolonged walking on sloping surfaces.	Stretch: 1. Kneel and sit on your heels. Lift one knee. Hold 6–8 seconds and repeat three times. 2. Sit in a chair and flex the knee so that the dorsum of the toes touch the ground. Strengthen: Foot flat, raise the toes and forefoot leaving heel on the ground.

Table 20.3 Remedial massage techniques for muscles of the leg and foot—cont'd

Muscle	Soft tissue release	Trigger point	Deep transverse friction	Stretch	Corrective action[6]	Home exercises
Tibialis posterior	As for gastrocnemius or soleus Or Client: sidelying. Practitioner: standing or sitting, facing towards the client's head. The practitioner applies pressure to the medial border of the tibia as the client plantarflexes and dorsiflexes their ankle.			As for gastrocnmenius or soleus.	When running or jogging use a full arch support, run only on smooth flat surfaces. May require referral for orthotics.	As for gastrocnemius or soleus.

Continued

Table 20.3 Remedial massage techniques for muscles of the leg and foot—cont'd

Muscle	Soft tissue release	Trigger point	Deep transverse friction	Stretch	Corrective action[6]	Home exercises
Fibularis longus and brevis	Client: sidelying. Practitioner: Standing behind the client. The practitioner applies pressure to the injury site as the client plantarflexes and dorsiflexes their ankle. 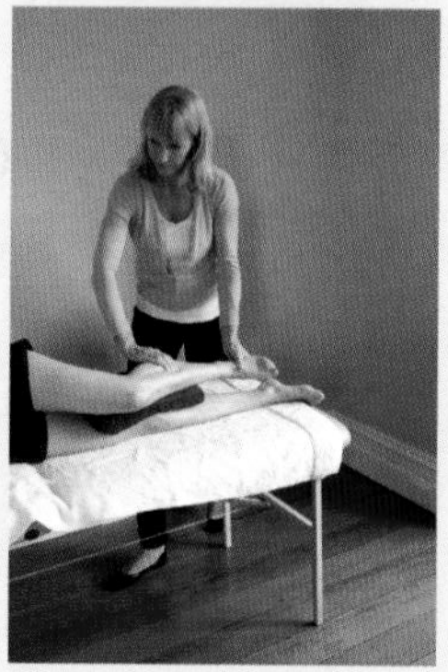 Or Client: supine. Practitioner at the side of the table facing cephalad. The practitioner contacts the taut band/lesion in the muscle as the client plantarflexes/everts and dorsiflexes/inverts. The practitioner can perform a deep glide from behind the lateral malleolus to the fibular head as the muscle lengthens (i.e. dorsiflexes/inverts the ankle).	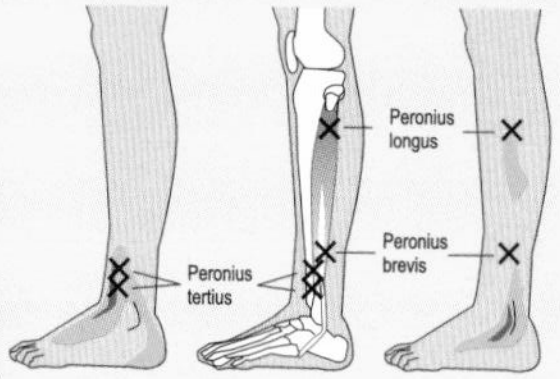 Peronius tertius Peronius longus Peronius brevis	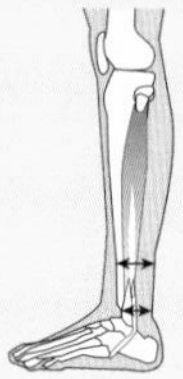	Client: supine. Practitioner: stands at foot of table. The practitioner passively dorsiflexes and inverts the client's ankle as far as comfortable for the client. The client then tries to plantarflex and evert their foot against the practitioner's resistance for 6–8 seconds. When the resistance is released, the practitioner passively dorsiflexes and inverts the foot as far as comfortable for the client. Repeat the procedure three times. 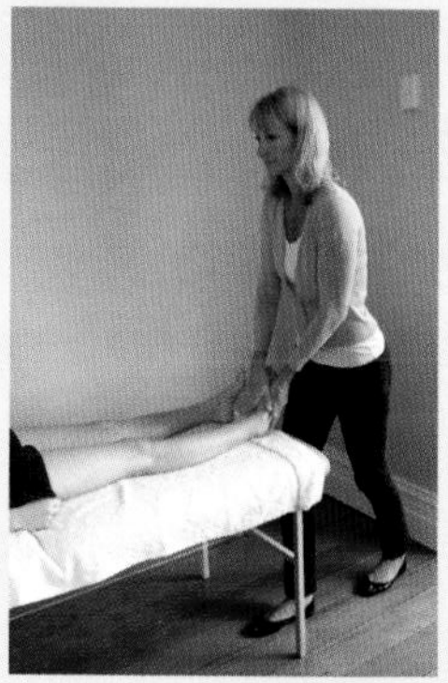	Avoid high-heeled shoes. Ensure that footwear is appropriate for the foot shape (e.g. Morton's foot). May require referral for orthotics.	Stretch: As for gastrocnemius and soleus. Strengthening: calf raises.

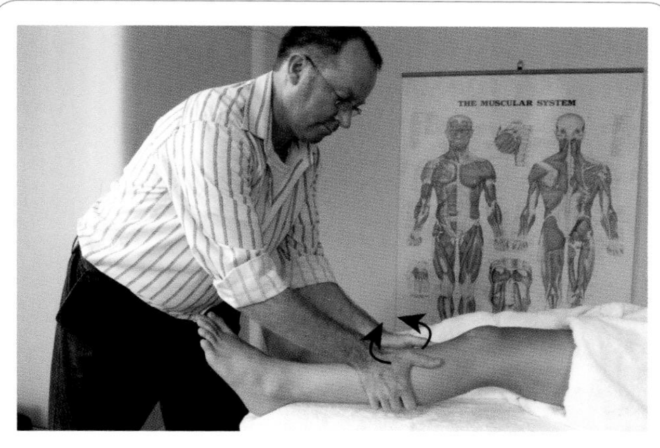

Fig. 20.33 Shin splints technique

Overview of treatment and management

In the acute phase, the RICE regimen is recommended. Advise the client to rest from aggravating activities such as exercise on hard, uneven surfaces. Gentle stretching should be commenced as soon as possible within pain tolerance. The client may be referred for mobilisation and manipulation of the low back, hip, knee, ankle and foot. Referral for orthotics may also be required.

In chronic presentations, massage therapy is directed towards reducing hypertonicity in affected muscles. A typical remedial massage treatment for subacute or chronic shin splints includes:

- Swedish massage therapy to the lower limb, lumbar spine and pelvis. Avoid all techniques that pull on the tibial attachments of muscles. A useful technique involves compressing muscles back onto the bone (see Figure 20.33).

SHIN SPLINTS TECHNIQUE

The client lies supine with the knee extended. Stand to the side of the foot of the table facing the client and hold the leg, with one hand on either side, just proximal to the ankle. Using both hands draw the leg muscles anteriorly, compressing them onto the tibia with the thenar eminences. This drawing and compressing movement is repeated, progressing from the ankle to just below the knee. Alternatively, the same movement can be performed with the client lying supine with their knee flexed and their foot flat on the table.

- Remedial massage techniques including (see Table 20.4):
  - deep gliding frictions along the muscle fibres (including soleus, popliteus)
  - cross-fibre frictions
  - soft tissue releasing techniques – for example, for tibialis posterior and soleus muscles, with the client sidelying, apply pressure to the medial border of the tibia as the client plantarflexes and dorsiflexes their ankle
  - deep transverse friction applied directly to the injury site may help stimulate collagen production
  - trigger point therapy
  - muscle stretching.
- Myofascial release including cross-arm techniques and the leg pull (see Chapter 8 and Figure 20.34 on p 406).
- Heat therapy is usually beneficial.
- Other remedial techniques such as ankle joint articulation may also be introduced as required (see Chapter 7):
  - ankle prone circumduction
  - calcaneus prone circumduction
  - tarsals prone plantarflexion
  - ankle traction
  - metatarsal shearing
  - phalanges mobilisation.
- Correct underlying biomechanical and predisposing factors where possible (e.g. overpronation of ankles, foot flare, externally rotated hips, apparent leg length inequality, tight quadriceps, hamstrings, hip flexors or abductors as indicated).

CLIENT EDUCATION

Advise the client to rest from aggravating activities such as downhill running or excessive impacts on hard surfaces. Gentle stretching should be introduced as soon as pain permits and continued throughout the rehabilitation. Weakness and/or tightness of tibialis anterior and posterior, gastrocnemius, soleus, quadriceps, hamstrings, hip flexors and hip abductors should be addressed in a progressive strengthening and stretching program. The client may need to change shoes and may need to be referred for orthotics.

Clients may also develop chronic recurrent shin splints which limits their full participation in sports.[8] Refer for osseous manipulation and for additional physical therapy modalities such as electro-acupuncture if required. If the condition does not improve within two weeks, refer for further assessment for possible stress fracture.

CHRONIC COMPARTMENT SYNDROME

The leg has four compartments separated by fascial sheets: anterior, lateral, superficial posterior and deep posterior (see Figure 20.35 on p 406).

Compartment syndrome occurs most commonly in the anterior compartment which contains tibialis anterior, extensor digitorum longus, extensor hallucis longus, the tibial artery and vein and the deep peroneal nerve.

Note: In acute anterior compartment syndrome, elevated pressure from tissue fluid/blood within the compartment causes ischaemia.[3] This is a medical emergency and requires immediate referral. Refer any client with persistent pain in the anterior leg with visible swelling or 'stocking' numbness or tingling for immediate surgical decompression.

Lateral compartment syndrome involves the peroneal muscles and may be associated with paraesthesia or a trickling pain on the outer lower border of the leg. This is due to compression of the superficial peroneal nerve usually from increased pressure in both the lateral and the posterior compartments. Refer any client with persistent pain and numbness or tingling in the leg and foot.

Remedial massage therapy may be beneficial for clients with chronic compartment syndrome when symptoms are mild to moderate and transient.

Assessment

HISTORY

Signs and symptoms of chronic compartment syndrome may be difficult to differentiate from shin splints. Clients describe crampy pain after exercise, relieved by rest and transient

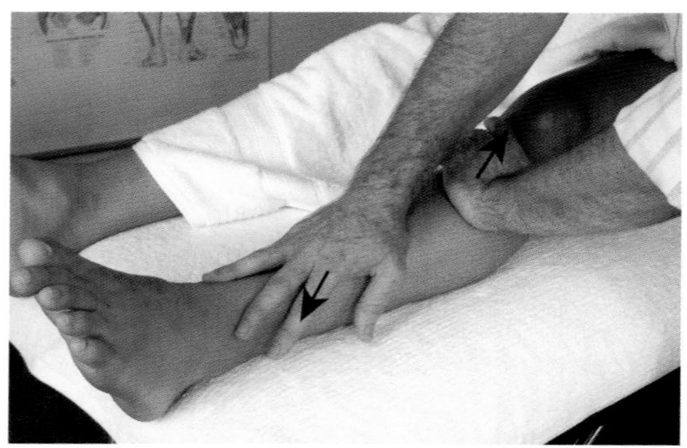

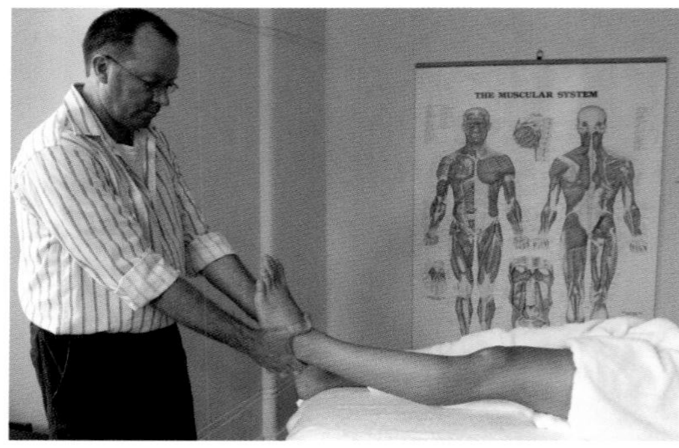

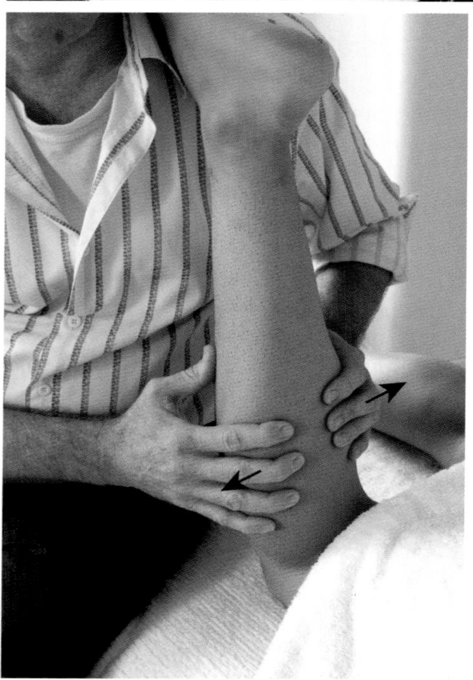

Fig. 20.34 Myofascial release techniques for the leg

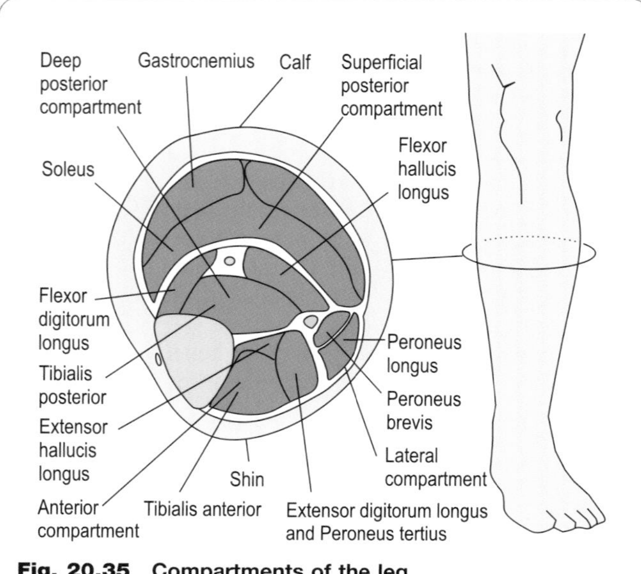

Fig. 20.35 Compartments of the leg

Key assessment findings for chronic compartment syndrome

- Client complains of crampy pain brought on by exercise, relieved by rest and transient neurological and vascular signs
- Functional tests:
  Ankle
  - AROM: limited and painful
  - PROM: limited and painful
  - RROM: positive for involved muscles (pain, weakness)
  - Resisted and length tests positive for involved muscles.
  - Special tests: negative
- Palpation: pain on palpation of the muscles in the involved compartment; muscle tightness is evident.

colour changes in the limb, sensations of coldness in the extremity or feet. Nerve compression produces numbness, tingling or motor loss to the dorsiflexors of the foot. One of the most significant distinguishing features of compartment syndrome is that the level of pain is out of proportion for that normally associated with shin splints.

Table 20.4 Characteristics of shin splints, compartment syndrome and tibial stress fracture[9]

Shin splints	Compartment syndrome	Stress fracture
Excessive activity (e.g. running on hard or uneven ground), overtraining, poor shoes, repeated impacts on a hard surface.	Activity induced, repeated episodes, fails to respond to conservative treatment.	Following prolonged activity (e.g. marching, skiing, running), especially in a hard-soled shoe/boot.
Pain anterolateral or posteromedial border tibia.	Crampy ache, tightness, swelling in the legs. Anterior compartment – pain on dorsiflexion; lateral. Compartment – pain on eversion.	Severe anterior shin pain. Acute, sharp.
Pain decreases as the muscle warms up.	Increases with exercise (can continue to increase for a short time after exercise).	Constant, increasing with exercise. Worse with impact.
Pain worse in morning and after exercise.	Occasionally muscle weakness or sensory symptoms.	Night ache. May be worse in morning.
Palpatory tenderness over a wide region of the tibia and involved muscle.	Tightness evident on palpation.	Palpation elicits localised pain.

FUNCTIONAL TESTS

Lumbar AROM do not reproduce symptoms.
Hip AROM do not reproduce symptoms.
Knee AROM do not reproduce symptoms.

Ankle tests

AROM: painful and limited.
PROM: painful and limited.
RROM: positive for involved muscles (pain or weakness).
Resisted and length tests: positive for involved muscles.
Special tests: negative.

PALPATION

Palpating muscles in the affected compartment elicits pain and muscle tightness is evident.

Overview of treatment and management

Treatment of chronic compartment syndrome requires vigilance for any change in signs or symptoms of neurological and vascular compression that indicate progression from transient symptoms to persistent ones which require immediate referral.

The most important massage therapy techniques for chronic compartment syndrome are myofascial release (Chapter 8) and lymphatic drainage (Chapter 9). Note: Massage techniques that increase blood flow to the compartments are contraindicated, as is the application of ice on compromised circulation. Stretching of the whole lower limb kinetic chain may be useful. Discontinue treatment if symptoms are aggravated.

When pain level is reduced, articulation of the ankle, especially the talotibial articulation, can assist in the restoration of proper function of the lower limb (see Chapter 7).

- Ankle prone circumduction
- Calcaneus prone circumduction
- Tarsals prone plantarflexion
- Ankle traction
- Metatarsal shearing
- Phalanges mobilisation.

STRESS FRACTURE OF THE TIBIA

Stress fracture of the tibia is a hairline break that occurs without history of trauma. Chronic shin splints may be a precursor. It usually occurs after prolonged activity such as running, skiing or marching on a hard surface or in a hard-soled boot. Stress fracture can also occur from osteoporosis in female long-distance runners. Stress fractures require referral for medical assessment. They are diagnosed by X-ray or bone scan. Table 20.4 highlights some characteristics of shin splints, compartment syndrome and stress fracture that may be useful for determining appropriate treatment.

VARICOSE VEINS AND SPIDER VEINS

Varicose veins occur when valves in veins are damaged causing blood to pool. They commonly occur in the saphenous veins of the legs. Spider veins (telangiectasia) are small dilated blood vessels that lie close to the surface of the skin or mucous membranes. Their formation is associated with venous hypertension within varicose veins. Common locations include the face (nose, cheeks, chin), upper thigh and ankle.

Pregnancy and prolonged sitting or standing predispose to the formation of varicose veins and spider veins. Note that massage directly on varicose veins or spider veins is contraindicated.

ANKLE

It is important to rule out fracture for any traumatic ankle or foot injury. The Ottawa ankle rules have been developed to indicate when radiographs are required. They have been shown to be highly sensitive for ankle and midfoot fracture in adults and children.[10] Refer any client for radiographic examination of the foot or ankle if there has been a traumatic ankle injury and any of the following are met:

- the client is unable to bear weight for four successive steps (two with each foot)
- localised tenderness along the posterior aspect of lateral or medial malleolus

Key assessment findings for Achilles tendinopathy

- Achilles tendon pain, history of repetitive overuse (e.g. running, jumping)
- Functional tests:
  - AROM: painful plantarflexion
  - PROM: painful dorsiflexion as the muscle is passively stretched
  - RROM: positive for plantarflexion
  - Resisted and length tests tests positive for gastrocnemius ± soleus
  - Special tests: negative
- Palpation: tenderness and pain along the tendon, usually 2–6 cm above calcaneus.

- localised tenderness over the navicular, cuboid or base of 5th metatarsal

ACHILLES TENDINOPATHY

The Achilles tendon is commonly injured in running and sports that involve jumping. The client complains of pain and tenderness along the Achilles tendon most commonly where the tendon becomes hypovascular at about 2–6 cm above its calcaneal insertion.[3] Overloading is crucial in the development of tendinopathy.[11] It is associated with shoes with heels that are too low, excessive dorsiflexion on uphill areas, tight calf muscles, shoes with insufficient flexibility in the soles, overpronation of the ankle or excessive activity on hard surfaces. Most of the histological findings in tendinopathy suggest chronic degeneration, regeneration and microtears in the tendon and the absence of evidence of acute inflammation. However, much uncertainty remains as other studies indicate that an inflammatory process may be related to the development of tendinopathy and chronic tendinopathy.[11–13]

Assessment

HISTORY

The client presents with pain in the Achilles tendon above the heel. Pain increases with activity and stretching and decreases with rest. Morning pain is common in chronic cases. There is usually a history of repetitive overuse (e.g. running, jumping).

FUNCTIONAL TESTS

Lumbar AROM tests do not reproduce symptoms.
Hip AROM tests do not reproduce symptoms.
Knee AROM tests do not reproduce symptoms.

Ankle tests

AROM: painful plantarflexion.
PROM: painful dorsiflexion as the muscles are passively stretched.
RROM: positive for plantarflexion.
Resisted and length tests for specific muscles: positive for gastrocnemius and soleus.
Special tests: negative. (Note: squeezing the Achilles from the sides increases pain.)

PALPATION

Tenderness is elicited in the tendon above the heel.

Overview of treatment and management

If acute, use RICE to decrease inflammation. Advise the client to avoid any aggravating activities. Using a small heel lift or using higher-heeled shoes is often useful for decreasing pain. Commence range of motion exercises as soon as pain permits.

A typical remedial massage treatment for subacute or chronic Achilles tendinopathy includes:

- Swedish massage therapy to the lower limb, low back and pelvis.
- Remedial massage techniques including (see Table 20.3):
  - deep gliding frictions along the muscle fibres
  - cross-fibre frictions
  - soft tissue releasing techniques (see Figure 20.36)
  - deep transverse friction applied directly to the site of lesion, which may help stimulate collagen production
  - trigger point therapy
  - muscle stretching.
- Focus treatment on agonists, antagonists and any muscle imbalances to restore optimal range of motion (e.g. gastrocnemius, soleus, hip external rotators).
- Myofascial release including cross-arm techniques and the leg pull (see Chapter 8).
- Other remedial techniques such as ankle joint articulation may also be introduced as required (see Chapter 7):
  - ankle prone circumduction
  - calcaneus prone circumduction
  - tarsals prone plantarflexion
  - ankle traction
  - metatarsal shearing
  - phalanges mobilisation.

Correct underlying biomechanical and predisposing factors if possible (e.g. excessive ankle pronation, muscle imbalances).

CLIENT EDUCATION

Advise the client to rest from aggravating activities to reduce the stress on the damaged tendons. Replace low-heeled or

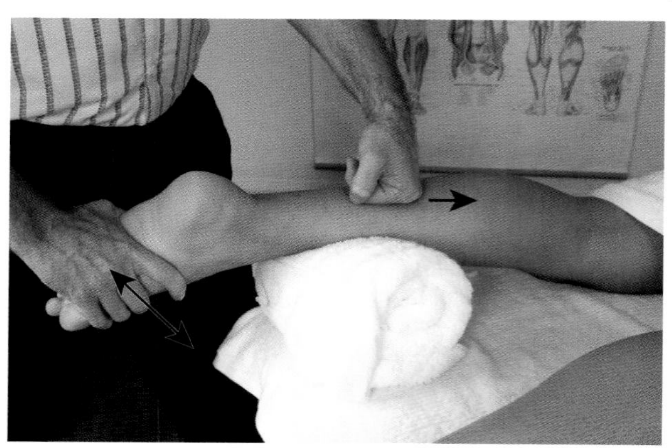

Fig. 20.36 Soft tissue release for Achilles tendinitis

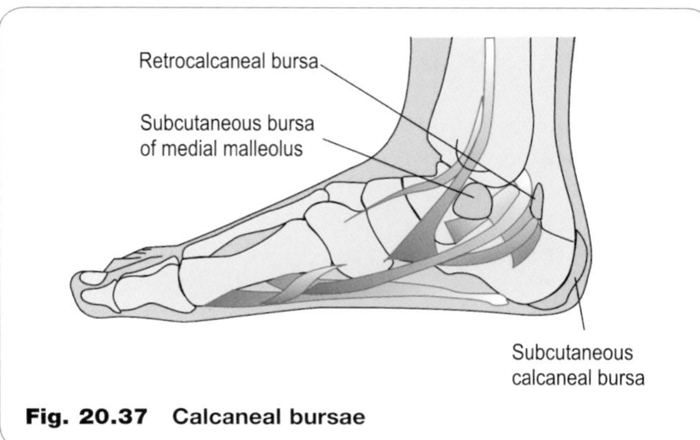

Fig. 20.37 Calcaneal bursae

worn-out shoes. Adequate warm-up/stretching of the calf muscles is required before exercise. Gradually introduce toe and forefoot raises and eccentric exercises (e.g. standing on edge of a step and dropping the heel below the level of the step). Refer for osseous manipulation and for additional electrophysical therapies such as electro-acupuncture or therapeutic ultrasound if required.

CALCANEAL BURSITIS

The bursa which cushions the insertion of the Achilles tendon at the heel can become inflamed, usually from direct rubbing from shoes in which the upper border heel counter is too tight, too loose or convex (see Figure 20.37). Bursitis can also follow a direct impact on the heel. The client complains of pain at the Achilles insertion which may be swollen.

Treatment

The RICE regimen is recommended until the inflammation subsides. A heel pad may be worn to protect the area from further rubbing. Avoid wearing the offending shoes. In the subacute phase, the remedial massage approach prescribed for Achilles tendinopathy may be applied.

SEVER'S DISEASE

Sever's disease is a common foot problem in active children aged 8 to 15 years. It is a traction apophysitis at the Achilles insertion into the calcaneus that often occurs during rapid growth spurts when bone growth can cause muscles and tendons to become tight.

Assessment

HISTORY

The client is a physically active adolescent (8 to 15 years) who complains of heel pain, which is aggravated by activity and relieved by rest.

FUNCTIONAL TESTS

Lumbar AROM tests do not reproduce symptoms.
Hip AROM tests do not reproduce symptoms.
Knee AROM tests do not reproduce symptoms.

Key assessment findings for Sever's disease

- The client is a physically active adolescent (8 to 15 years); history of pain at the Achilles insertion that is aggravated by activity and relieved by rest
- Functional tests:
  - AROM: painful plantarflexion
  - PROM: painful dorsiflexion as the calf muscles are passively stretched
  - RROM: positive for ankle plantarflexion
  - Resisted and length tests: postitive for ankle plantarflexors
  - Special tests: negative
- Palpation: tenderness and swelling at the Achilles insertion

Ankle tests

AROM: painful plantarflexion.
PROM: painful dorsiflexion as the muscles are passively stretched.
RROM: positive for plantarflexion.
Resisted and length tests for specific muscles: positive for gastrocnemius and soleus.
Special tests: negative.

PALPATION

Palpation at the Achilles insertion elicits tenderness or pain. Swelling may be present. Palpation may reveal tightness in the gastrocnemius and soleus muscles.

Overview of treatment and management

Advise the client to reduce the level of physical activity for one to two weeks. Ice application after exercise may help control inflammation. Shoes should be replaced when they become too small or if the heel counter is too tight. The condition can become chronic and persist until about 16 years of age. Massage therapy in chronic cases focuses on restoring muscle balance, especially of gastrocnemius, soleus and tibialis anterior.

ANKLE SPRAIN

The ankle is a hinge joint supported by ligament on either side. The medial deltoid ligament is the strongest of the ankle ligaments. Consequently eversion sprains are rare and when they do occur often involve fractures or ligament avulsions. Any client with an eversion sprain should be referred for further investigation. Inversion sprains account for 85% of ankle sprains.[14] The lateral collateral ligaments, from weakest to strongest, are the anterior talofibular ligament, the calcaneofibular ligament and the posterior talofibular ligament (see Figure 20.38 on p 410).

Sprains can occur as a result of improper landing on the foot, muscle imbalance or proprioception deficit. Inversion sprains are likely to be worse if the foot is both inverted and plantar flexed. Bruising will often occur after the injury and is likely to remain for some weeks.

Assessment

HISTORY

The client reports rolling onto the lateral side of the ankle. This may be accompanied by a popping or tearing. Swelling

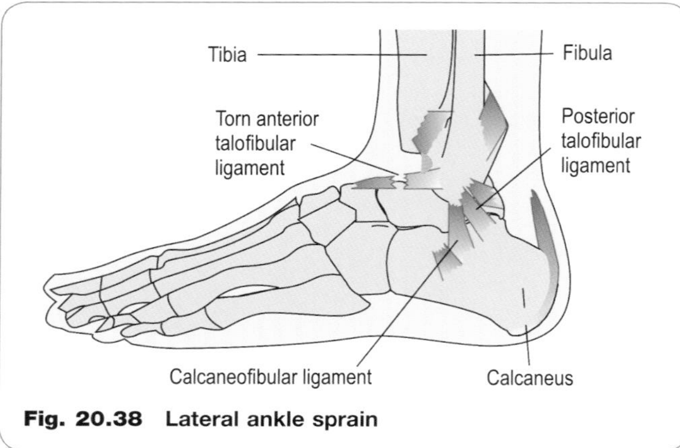

Fig. 20.38 Lateral ankle sprain

Key assessment findings for inversion ankle sprain

- History of rolling onto the outside of the ankle; may be accompanied by a popping or tearing sensation; swelling.
- Functional tests:
  - AROM: painful inversion
  - PROM: painful inversion
  - RROM: negative (unless associated muscle strain)
  - Special test: positive (ankle anterior drawer, posterior drawer and/or lateral ligament stability)
- Palpation: tenderness and swelling at the site of ligament damage

occurs over the anterior talofibular ligament. Bruising may follow in the next day or two.

FUNCTIONAL TESTS

Lumbar AROM tests do not reproduce symptoms.
Hip AROM tests do not reproduce symptoms.
Knee AROM tests do not reproduce symptoms.

Ankle tests

AROM: painful inversion.
PROM: painful inversion.
RROM: negative unless the injury is accompanied by muscle strain.
Resisted and length tests for specific muscles: negative (unless associated muscle strain).
Special tests: positive ankle anterior draw (anterior talofibular ligament sprain), posterior draw (posterior talofibular ligament sprain), lateral ligament stability (calcaneofibular ligament).

PALPATION

Tenderness is elicited anterior to the lateral malleolus in anterior talofibular sprain and inferior to the malleolus in calcaneofibular sprain. Swelling is usually evident. Suspect fracture if tenderness is present posterior or superior to the lateral malleolus.

Overview of treatment and management

The treatment goal immediately after the injury is to decrease pain, increase pain-free range of motion and to protect the ankle from further damage. Immediate mobilisation and functional treatment is widely regarded as the best treatment strategy.[15] Acute sprains require RICE. Ankle splints and taping provide protection for the joint. Reduce weight bearing (crutches may be required). Commence pain-free range of motion exercises as soon as pain permits. Refer for electrophysical therapy. (Note that the extent and quality of available evidence for the use of ultrasound for acute ankle sprains is limited. One Cochrane review concluded that the use of ultrasound is not supported by current evidence.)[16]

A typical remedial massage treatment for subacute or chronic ankle inversion sprain includes:

- Swedish massage therapy to the lower limb, low back and pelvis.
- Remedial massage techniques including:
  - light lymphatic drainage to promote reduction of swelling
  - deep transverse friction at the site of lesion to help prevent adhesion formation. This should be performed within the client's pain tolerance. Recommendations vary as to how long to perform deep transverse friction. Good results have been obtained with short applications (20–30 seconds) interspersed with active movement and other massage strokes.
- Massage techniques for associated muscle strains (e.g. peroneal muscles) or imbalances include (see Table 20.3):
  - deep gliding frictions along the muscle fibres
  - cross-fibre frictions
  - soft tissue releasing techniques
  - trigger point therapy
  - muscle stretching.

Use the client's pain threshold as a guide for when to progress to more vigorous massage techniques.

- Myofascial release including cross-arm techniques (see Chapter 8).
- Other remedial techniques such as ankle joint articulation may also be introduced as required (see Chapter 7). Note that initially active movement is preferred to passive movements for safety.

Longer-term management involves correcting underlying biomechanical and predisposing factors where possible (e.g. genu varum, weak ankle everters and/or tight ankle inverters).

Client education

Early mobilisation is important to stimulate collagen production. Most ankles regain functional mobility within several weeks. However, full structural recovery takes longer (1–2 months for Grade 1 sprains, 6–12 months for Grade 2 sprains and up to 1 year for Grade 3 sprains).[3, 17] Grade 1 injuries require RICE for 2 or 3 days and then complete weight bearing can commence. Rehabilitation of Grade 2 and 3 sprains is generally divided into three phases:[15]

1. RICE, non-weight-bearing according to pain.
2. Rehabilitation of movement, strength and proprioception of the ankle: Rehabilitation begins with isometric exercises of the ankle everters, active pain-free ankle range

of motion. Progressively increase walking distance and speed. Resisted theraband/elastic tubing exercises for ankle everters, dorsiflexors and eventually inverters are gradually introduced. Calf muscle strengthening exercises and balance drills can be introduced. Restoring neuromuscular control appears to be vital for functional stability of the joint.[18] To improve proprioception, for example, the client can trace the letters of the alphabet in the air with their big toe.

3. Exercises and retraining of specific skills. In the late rehabilitation phase clients can use wobble boards, hopping and sports-specific drills including running forward and backward, sudden stopping and zig-zagging.

For some clients laxity of ligaments permits recurrent inversion sprain. This is thought to occur because of neuromuscular deficits such as impaired balance, reduced joint position sense, slower firing of peroneal muscles, slower nerve conduction velocity, impaired cutaneous sensation, strength deficits and decreased dorsiflexion range of motion.[18, 19] Rehabilitation should therefore address restoration of neuromuscular function as well as mechanical stability. Encourage clients to continue active proprioceptive training and massage therapy for optimal muscle balance and neuromuscular control. A study of track and field athletes undergoing the same rehabilitation program found that athletes with grades 1 and 2 lateral ankle sprain were at a higher risk of re-injury than those with high-grade acute lateral ankle sprains.[20]

DEGENERATIVE JOINT DISEASE OF THE ANKLE

Degenerative joint disease is common in older patients or those with significant previous trauma. Clients complain of limited range of motion and chronic pain which is aggravated by weight-bearing activity.

Assessment

HISTORY

The client is older or has a history of previous significant trauma and complains of limited range of motion and/or chronic pain. Pain is aggravated by weight-bearing activity and slight swelling may be present. The client may complain of morning stiffness.

FUNCTIONAL TESTS

Lumbar AROM do not reproduce symptoms.
Hip AROM do not reproduce symptoms.
Knee AROM do not reproduce symptoms.

Key assessment findings for ankle degenerative joint disease

- History of limited range of motion and chronic pain aggravated by weight-bearing activity; older client or client with history of previous significant trauma, morning stiffness.
- Functional tests:
  - AROM: limited ± painful (plantarflexion/dorsiflexion)
  - PROM: limited ± painful (plantarflexion/dorsiflexion)
  - RROM: negative (unless associated muscle strain)
  - Special tests: negative
- Palpation: variable diffuse tenderness

Ankle tests

AROM: limited ± painful (plantarflexion/dorsiflexion).
PROM: limited ± painful (plantarflexion/dorsiflexion); hard end-feel and crepitus.
RROM negative unless the injury is accompanied by muscle strain or contracture.
Resisted and length tests for specific muscles: negative (unless associated muscle strain or contracture).
Special tests: negative.

PALPATION

Diffuse tenderness may be elicited on palpation around the joint.

Overview of treatment and management

Degenerative joint disease is a chronic condition of the ankle. Episodes of acute inflammation can occur after excessive weight-bearing activity and require RICE treatment.

A typical remedial massage treatment for chronic degenerative joint disease of the ankle includes:

- Swedish massage therapy to the lower limb, low back and pelvis.
- Remedial massage techniques including:
  - joint articulation (see Chapter 7)
  - ankle prone circumduction
  - calcaneus prone circumduction
  - tarsals prone plantarflexion
  - ankle traction
  - metatarsal shearing
  - phalanges mobilisation.
- Heat therapy.
- Myofascial release (see Chapter 8).
- Massage techniques for associated muscle strains (e.g. peroneal muscles) or imbalances include (see Table 20.3):
  - deep gliding frictions along the muscle fibres
  - cross-fibre frictions
  - soft tissue releasing techniques
  - trigger point therapy
  - muscle stretching.

Correct underlying biomechanical and predisposing factors where possible (e.g. pes planus, leg length inequality).

Client education

Advise the client of the importance of range of motion exercises and muscle stretching. Heat packs may be useful for pain relief. Recommend weight loss if clients are overweight and shock-absorbing soles should always be worn.

FOOT

Many remedial massage clients suffer with foot pain, often the result of poor biomechanics from congenital problems (e.g. pes planus or cavus, hallux valgus or ankle pronation) or from many years of poor-fitting shoes. Remedial massage usually consists of Swedish massage, passive joint articulation to the ankles and toes and advice about weight loss and supportive shoes. A common condition encountered in remedial massage practice is plantar fasciitis.

Key assessment findings for plantar fasciitis

- History of overuse (e.g. distance running) in athletes: non-athletic middle-aged women. Client complains of pain at the front of the heel on the sole of the foot on the first few steps after rising
- Functional tests:
  - AROM: painful plantarflexion
  - PROM: painful dorsiflexion, extension of toes
  - RROM: may be positive for toe flexors (flexor digitorum brevis)
  - Resisted and length tests may be positive for affected muscles
  - Special tests: negative
- Palpation: tenderness or pain at the medial tubercle of the calcaneus

PLANTAR FASCIITIS (HEEL SPUR)

Plantar fasciitis is the most common cause of painful feet and it occurs more often in women than men. The plantar fascia contributes to arch support and shock absorption of the foot. It attaches proximally to the anterior calcaneus and distally to the fascia that crosses the metatarsal heads and extends into the toes. Biomechanical dysfunction in the foot, particularly associated with excessive pronation and lowered longitudinal arch or with pes cavus, places excessive tension on the plantar fascia at the medial tubercle of the anterior calcaneus. Prolonged tensile stress on the periosteum may lead to the development of a bony spur. A spur may also develop in the insertion of the Achilles tendon to the superior part of the calcaneus (dancer's heel).

Assessment

HISTORY

Two types of clients are typical: (1) non-athletic middle-aged women, and (2) distance runners and basketball players. Pain on the sole of the foot at the front of the heel is the main complaint. The pain commonly radiates forward to the middle of the foot. The pain is worse on the first few steps on standing and improves as walking continues but worsens again at the end of the day or the next morning. Plantar fasciitis may be associated with standing for prolonged periods on a hard floor.

FUNCTIONAL TESTS

Lumbar AROM tests do not reproduce symptoms.
Hip AROM tests do not reproduce symptoms.
Knee AROM tests do not reproduce symptoms.

Ankle tests

AROM: painful plantarflexion.
PROM: painful dorsiflexion of ankle, extension of toes.
RROM: may be positive for toe flexion.
Resisted and length tests: may be positive for flexor digitorum brevis.
Special tests: negative.

PALPATION

Pain is elicited on palpation at the medial tubercle of the calcaneus.

Overview of treatment and management

In the acute phase, apply the RICE regimen. A small heel lift or wearing a shoe with a slightly elevated heel helps decrease the pain. Refer for electrophysical therapies, osseous manipulation and acupuncture.

A typical remedial massage treatment for subacute or chronic plantar fasciitis includes:

- Swedish massage therapy to the lower limb, low back and pelvis.
- Remedial massage techniques including:
  - myofascial release (see Chapter 8)
    - gentle myofascial release (see Figure 20.39)
    - deep myofascial release

    For example, longitudinal gliding of the plantar fascia (glide towards the calcaneus to avoid additional stress on the fascia), and cross-fibre frictions on the fascia, avoiding pressure on the medial tubercle (see Figure 20.40 on p 413).
  - passive joint articulation (see Chapter 7)
    - ankle prone circumduction
    - calcaneus prone circumduction
    - tarsals prone plantarflexion
    - ankle traction
    - metatarsal shearing
    - phalanges mobilisation.
- Techniques for associated muscle tightness (especially flexor digitorum brevis, gastrocnemius, soleus and tibial muscles) include (see Table 20.4):
  - deep gliding frictions along the muscle fibres
  - cross-fibre frictions
  - soft tissue releasing techniques
  - trigger point therapy
  - muscle stretching.

Correct underlying biomechanical and predisposing factors (e.g. pes planus, leg length inequality) where possible.

Client education

Advise the client of the importance of restoring normal biomechanics of the foot. Stretching the fascia by standing on a step and dropping the heels below the level of the step or rolling the foot over a tennis or golf ball may be useful.

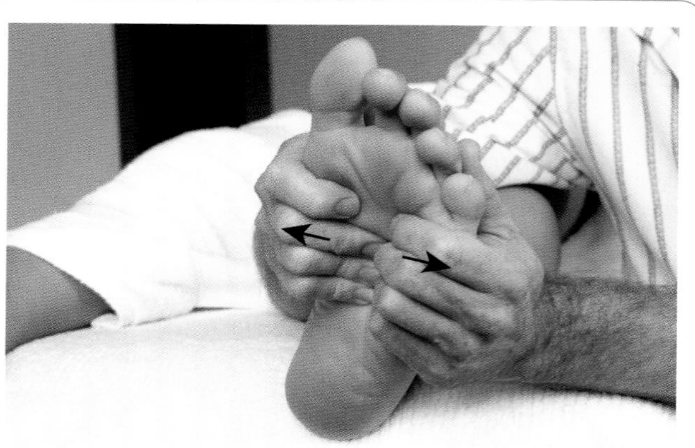

Fig. 20.39 Myofascial release for the foot

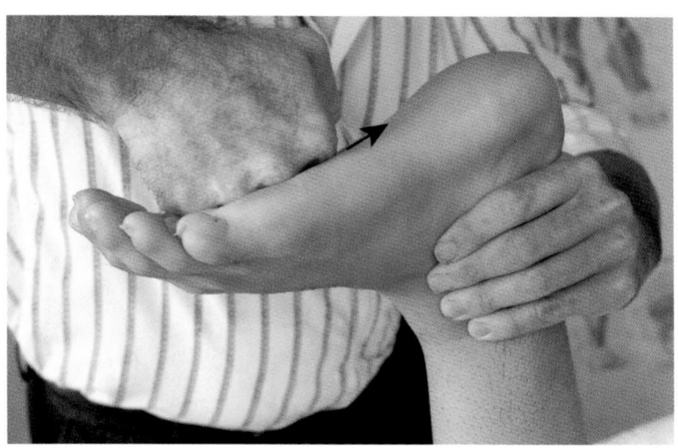

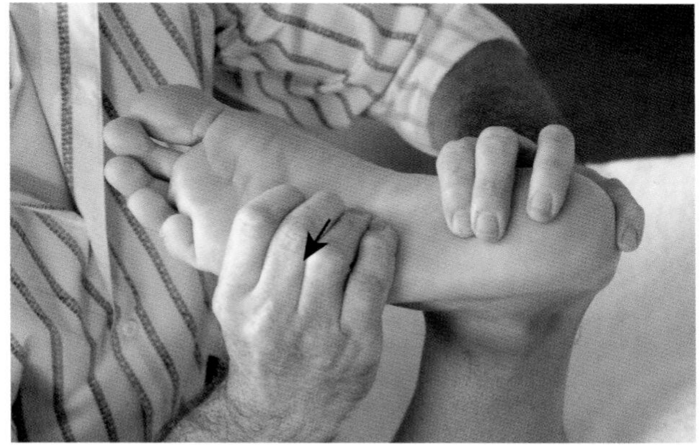

Fig. 20.40 Deep myofascial release for plantar fasciitis

Progressively introduce a program of stretching and strengthening exercises to address muscle imbalances of the lower limb. Recommend weight loss if clients are overweight. Shock-absorbing soles should always be worn. Refer clients for orthotics if required. Kinesiotaping could also be considered. In a randomised controlled trial of 52 subjects, kinesiotaping of the gastrocnemius and plantar fascia was worn continuously for one week in addition to their usual daily physiotherapy treatment of ultrasound and low-frequency electrotherapy. The authors concluded that continuous kinesiotaping for one week might alleviate the pain of plantar fasciitis better than a traditional physical therapy program only.[21]

FOREFOOT

METATARSALGIA

Metatarsalgia refers to tenderness under the 2nd and 3rd (occasionally 3rd and 4th) metatarsal heads following collapse of the transverse metatarsal arch. Often a callus develops under the foot. Chronic foot biomechanical dysfunction causes changes in weight bearing from the heel and 1st metatarsal to the 2nd to 4th metatarsals. Metatarsalgia is associated with prolonged standing on a hard surface, pes planus, pregnancy, hallux valgus, high heels, pes cavus, short gastrocnemius and poor footwear. Often a change of shoes, especially to a higher heel, triggers the condition.

Treatment

The purpose of remedial massage is to improve the biomechanics of the foot. Massage therapy includes Swedish massage and a range of remedial massage techniques designed to address muscle imbalance and to mobilise the ankle and foot, such as passive joint articulation (see Chapter 7), myofascial release, deep gliding, cross-fibre frictions, soft-tissue release techniques, trigger point therapy and muscle stretching. Correct underlying biomechanical and predisposing factors where possible.

CLIENT EDUCATION

Advise the client to wear supportive shoes and to avoid high-heeled shoes. A metatarsal bar (transverse arch support) may be worn under the metatarsal heads. Exercises to strengthen intrinsic foot muscles and stretches for gastrocnemius and hamstrings are recommended. Referral to a podiatrist, chiropractor, osteopath or physiotherapist may be required.

MORTON'S NEUROMA (INTERDIGITAL NEUROMA)

A fusiform swelling develops on the interdigital nerve following chronic compression by the metatarsal heads, most commonly between the 3rd and 4th metatarsal heads. The client complains of tenderness at the site and may report numbness in the interdigital space distal to the neuroma. Symptoms are relieved by removing the shoe.

Treatment

Advise the client to wear shoes that are wide enough to avoid compressing the metatarsal heads. Remedial massage treatment focuses on improving the biomechanics of the foot using such techniques as myofascial release, passive joint articulation (see Chapter 7) and muscle techniques for reducing muscle tightness (see Table 20.3).

KEY MESSAGES

- Assessment of clients with conditions of the leg, ankle and foot involves history, outcome measures, postural analysis, gait analysis, functional tests and palpation.
- Assessment findings may indicate the type of tissue involved (contractile or inert, muscle, joint, fascia, ligament), duration of condition (acute or subacute), and severity (grade).
- Assessment findings may indicate a common presenting condition such as ankle sprains, shin splints and plantar fasciitis.
- Assessment findings also indicate client perception of injury and preferences for treatment.
- Consider Clinical Guidelines, available evidence and client preferences when planning therapy.
- Although serious conditions of the lower limb, ankle and foot are rare, be vigilant for red flags during assessment.

- The selection of remedial massage techniques depends on assessment results. Swedish massage to the lower limb, low back and pelvis may be followed by muscle techniques (e.g. deep gliding, cross-fibre frictions, soft tissue releasing techniques, trigger point therapy, deep transverse friction and muscle stretching), passive joint articulation, myofascial release and thermotherapy as indicated.
- Educating clients about likely causal and predisposing factors and exercise rehabilitation are essential parts of remedial massage therapy.
- Over time, increase the client self-help component of treatment wherever possible (to reduce likelihood of recurrence and/or to promote health maintenance and illness prevention).

Review questions

1. The symptoms of anterior compartment syndrome include:
   a) a dull ache along the anteromedial border of the tibia which is aggravated by activity
   b) weakness of the dorsiflexors of the foot
   c) night ache
   d) pain and paraesthesia in the sole of the foot
2. Which test is likely to reproduce symptoms in a client with tennis leg?
   a) resisted ankle plantarflexion
   b) posterior drawer test
   c) passive ankle plantarflexion
   d) resisted ankle dorsiflexion
3. Which statement does not apply to plantar fasciitis?
   a) Pain is increased with dorsiflexion of the foot.
   b) Tenderness is felt at the posteromedial aspect of the calcaneus.
   c) Pain is worse with the first few steps on rising.
   d) Tenderness is felt on the sole of the foot between the 3rd and 4th metatarsal heads.
4. The most commonly sprained ankle ligament is:
   a) anterior talofibular ligament
   b) calcaneofibular ligament
   c) talofibular ligament
   d) deltoid ligament
5. Heel pain in a very active 10-year-old boy is most likely to be:
   a) Osgood-Schlatter's disease
   b) Sever's disease
   c) Achilles tendinitis
   d) Retrocalcaneal bursitis
6. i) What are shin splints?
   ii) How would you differentiate shin splints from a stress fracture of the tibia?
   iii) What treatment (including advice) would you give a client with shin splints?
7. Where would you palpate the anterior talotibial ligament?
8. Describe your treatment for lateral ankle sprain:
   i) in the acute phase
   ii) in the chronic phase
9. Name some common predisposing or causative factors of plantar fasciitis.
10. A client presents with calf pain. List three signs or symptoms that would make you suspect deep venous thrombosis.

REFERENCES

1. Hendrickson T. Massage for orthopedic conditions. Baltimore, MD: Lippincott Williams and Wilkins; 2003.
2. Cleland J, Koppenhaver S. Netter's orthopaedic clinical examination: an evidence-based approach. 2nd edn. Philadelphia: Saunders; 2011.
3. Carnes M, Vizniak N. Quick reference evidence-based conditions manual. 3rd edn. Burnaby, BC: Professional Health Systems; 2009.
4. Klingman R, Godges J. Red flags for potentially serious conditions in patients with knee, leg, ankle and foot problems. Online. Available: xnet.kp.org/socal_rehabspecialists/ptr_library/09FootRegion/01MedicalScreening-KneeLegAnkleandFootRegions.pdf; 2009.
5. Reese N, Bandy W. Joint range of motion and muscle length testing. Philadelphia: WB Saunders; 2002.
6. Simons D, Travell J, Simons L. Myofascial pain and dysfunction: The trigger point manual. Volume 1 Upper half of body. 2nd edn. Philadelphia: Williams & Wilkins; 1999.
7. Niel-Asher S. Concise book of trigger points. Berkeley, CA: North Atlantic Books; 2005.
8. Ugalde V, Batt M. Chir MBB. Shin splints: current theories and treatment. Critical Reviews in Physical and Rehabilitation Medicine 2001;13(2–3):217–53.
9. Brukner P, Khan K. Clinical sports medicine. 3rd edn. North Ryde, NSW: McGraw-Hill; 2010.
10. Bachmann L, Kolb E, Koller M, et al. Accuracy of Ottawa ankle rules to exclude fractures of the ankle and mid-foot: systematic review. BMJ 2003;326: 326–32.
11. Fredberg U, Stengaard-Pedersen K: Chronic tendinopathy tissue pathology, pain mechanisms, an etiology with a special focus on inflammation. Scand J Med Sci Sports 2008;18(1):3–15.
12. Cilli F, Khan M, Fu F, et al. Prostaglandin E2 affects proliferation and collagen synthesis by human patellar tendon fibroblasts. Clin J Sport Med 2004; 14:232–6.
13. Khan K, Li Z, Wang J. Repeated exposure of tendon to prostaglandin-E2 leads to localized tendon degeneration. Clin J Sport Med 2005;15: 27–33.
14. Valderrabano V, Hintermann B, Horrisberg M, et al. Ligamentous posttraumatic ankle osteoarthritis. Am J Sports Med 2006;34(4):612–20.
15. Guirao C, Pleguezuelos C, Perez M. Functional treatment and sprained ankle. Rehabil 2004;38(4): 182–7.
16. van der Windt D, van der Heijden GJ, Van den Berg S, et al. Therapeutic ultrasound for acute ankle sprains. Cochrane Database Syst Rev 2002;(1): CD001250.
17. Hubbard TJ, Hicks-Little CA, Hubbard TJ, et al. Ankle ligament healing after an acute ankle sprain: an evidence-based approach. J Athlet Train [Review] 2008;43(5):523–9.
18. Richie D. Functional instability of the ankle and the role of neuromuscular control: a comprehensive review. J Foot Ankle Surg 2001;43(4):240–51.
19. Hertel J. Functional instability following lateral ankle sprain. Sports Med (Auckland) 2000;29(5): 361–71.
20. Malliaropoulos N, Ntessalen M, Papacostas E, et al. Reinjury after acute lateral ankle sprains in elite track and field athletes. Am J Sports Med 2009; 37(9):1755–61.
21. Tsai C, Chang W, Lee J. Effects of short-term treatment with kinesiotaping for plantar fasciitis. J Musculoskelet Pain 2010;18(1):71–80.

Specific client groups 21

The content of this chapter relates to the following Unit of Competency:
HLTREM510B Provide specialised remedial massage

Health Training Package HLT07

Learning Outcomes

- Assess suitability of clients from specific client groups (children and adolescents, women, men, geriatric clients and clients with a mental illness) for remedial massage.
- Describe the current evidence for the effectiveness of massage for these clients.
- Manage specialised remedial massage treatments, including obtaining informed consent and selecting appropriate techniques and duration of treatment, for these clients.
- Provide specialised remedial massage treatment for these clients.

INTRODUCTION

Contraindications and precautions for the remedial massage techniques described in this book have been discussed in each chapter. This chapter brings together special considerations for the following remedial massage clients:

- children and adolescents
- women
- men
- geriatric clients
- clients with a mental illness.

In the following sections special considerations for both assessing and treating these specific client groups are discussed.

CHILDREN AND ADOLESCENTS

Childhood is the period of life between infancy and the onset of puberty. The importance of cultivating a practice of paediatric clients lies in the long-term benefits of prevention and early intervention of many musculoskeletal conditions. Any trauma has the potential to disrupt normal musculoskeletal development, and the longer excessive stresses and strains persist in the body, the greater the potential disturbance to a developing skeleton. Physical therapy interventions should be commenced as soon as possible following major trauma. Children often respond well to treatment and can make sustained recoveries. Left untreated, compensations to musculoskeletal distortions can become entrenched and more difficult to treat over time. Remedial massage therapy may also be beneficial in management of such conditions as Osgood-Schlatter's disease, adolescent idiopathic scoliosis and slipped capital femoral epiphysis, often when used to support chiropractic, osteopathy and physiotherapy care.

IMPORTANT CONSIDERATIONS FOR ASSESSING AND TREATING CHILDREN

- A parent or guardian is required to give informed consent for all children under 18 years of age and must be present throughout the consultation.
- It is every practitioner's responsibility to report any suspected case of child abuse to the statutory child protection service in their jurisdiction. In New South Wales it is mandatory for 'a person who in the course of his or her work or other paid employment delivers health care, welfare, education, children's services, residential services or law enforcement, wholly or partly to children' to report suspected cases of child abuse and neglect.[1]
- Be vigilant during assessment for conditions requiring referral, such as trauma to growth plates and other vulnerable areas (e.g. condylar process of the temporomandibular joint, which consists of thin cartilage).
- Be vigilant during assessment for musculoskeletal conditions affecting children that require referral to a medical practitioner, chiropractor, osteopath or physiotherapist. Such conditions include congenital foot problems, congenital hip dysplasia, Osgood-Schlatter's disease, Perthes' disease, capital femoral slipped epiphysis and adolescent idiopathic scoliosis (see Table 21.1).
- A guideline for deciding when to refer a client with congenital foot problems is to determine if the deviation is passively over-correctable (i.e. can the foot be passively moved slightly beyond the correcting position?). If the foot can be passively over-corrected, referral is not usually required.
- Modify treatment to suit the age, size and personality of the child. Young children require short consultations to

Table 21.1 Some musculoskeletal conditions affecting children requiring referral[2]

Condition	Description
Congenital foot problems	Check the borders of the foot. Many foot problems arise from in utero positioning and will be self-limiting. Refer all conditions that are not passively over-correctable, such as: • metatarsus adductus (lateral border of foot is convex and the medial border concave). If the adducted forefoot is not passively overcorrectable refer for further investigation; • metatarsus primus varus (adduction of hallux, i.e. the hallux points inwards and there is a large space between the first and second metatarsals). Avoid narrow shoes to prevent the development of bunions; • clubfoot (equinovarus or calcaneovalgus). Foot problem is not passively over-correctable.
Pronated foot	An infant's foot looks flat because of a fat pad under the longitudinal arch. If the foot is inflexible (i.e. unable to be passively over-corrected) refer for further examination. Pronation observed when the child begins to take weight on their lower limbs could be the result of a short Achilles tendon (refer for further examination if the foot cannot be passively dorsiflexed past neutral), an in-toeing gait (refer for further examination if the foot does not assume the normal position when non-weight bearing) or rigid flat foot (refer for further examination if the pronation does not disappear when non-weight bearing and can't be passively over-corrected). Flexible pronated feet (flat feet) are common and do not require treatment in children up to 3 years of age. Pronated feet due to wide-based gait will correct after the first year of weight bearing. Pronating feet in children over 3 years of age suggests ligament laxity. Refer for treatment including a corrective exercise program.
Achilles tendon pain	If obvious causes like pressure from shoes have been ruled out, Achilles tendon pain in adolescents and pre-adolescents suggests Sever's disease which is an uncommon traction-type injury. There may be fragmentation at the calcaneal apophysis. Treatment usually involves wearing shoes with a small heel, decreasing activity to reduce pain, anti-inflammatory medication and ice/heat. Symptoms usually disappear when the apophysis closes.
Genu valgus	May be present until 5 to 7 years of age. Refer if severe, unilateral or not resolving by 7 years of age.
Genu varum	Genu varum is normal until about 18 months of age. Refer if severe, unilateral or not decreasing by 2 years of age.
Genu recurvatum	Congenital genu recurvatum is usually due to interuterine positioning. Refer if persisting more than a few weeks.
Tibial torsion	Tibial torsion is evaluated by measuring the thigh-foot angle (client prone, knee flexed to 90°, measure the angle between the longitudinal axis of the foot and the midline of the thigh). The thigh-foot angle is usually 0° at birth and 20° by the time the child is walking. Client should avoid sitting and sleeping positions which perpetuate the torsion.
Osgood-Schlatter's disease	Symptoms include pain and tenderness, often bilateral, over the tibial tubercule in a rapidly growing adolescent, especially in athletic boys. The child is often limping. This is a traction-type injury of the apophysis of the tibial tuberosity. Treatment involves decreasing activity to reduce pain, anti-inflammatory medication and ice/heat (see Chapter 19). Symptoms usually resolve when the apophysis closes.
Recurrent patella subluxation	This is characterised by episodes of knee collapse associated with lateral displacement of the patella due to a congenitally flat femoral condyle, shallow patellar ridge, tibial torsion or previous acute patella dislocation. Refer for taping and a quadriceps strengthening program (see Chapter 19).
In-toeing gait (excessive femoral anteversion)	Femoral anteversion is the angle between the femoral neck and a line between the distal femoral condyles. Normally children have 40° of femoral anteversion at birth which decreases to 10° by about 8 years of age. The normal course of excessive femoral anteversion is to decrease over time. Referral is not required unless femoral anterversion is severe by 8 years of age.
Congenital hip dysplasia	Ortolani's test assesses abduction of the flexed hip. It is performed on newborns and repeated at six weeks and three months. A child with limited hip abduction at any time must be referred for further investigation (see Chapter 18).
Transient synovitis of the hip	Pain and limp of sudden onset or developing gradually over 1 to 2 weeks due to trauma or viral infection. The child is usually 3 to 6 years of age but can be up to 12 years. The child has a toe-walking gait and holds the hip in flexion. Hip range of motion is limited and painful. Symptoms usually resolve in several days. Nevertheless, the child should be referred to rule out Perthes' disease.
Legg-Perthes' disease (avascular necrosis of the femoral head)	Perthes' disease affects children 3–12 years, boys more than girls. Groin pain and limp may begin abruptly or develop over months. Symptoms are aggravated by activity and relieved by rest. Examination reveals a flexion contraction of the hip, painful and limited range of motion and causes pain. Refer for further examination (see Chapter 18).
Slipped capital femoral epiphysis	This condition occurs in 10–17-year-old children, especially tall thin boys and obese boys. One in four cases is bilateral. Symptoms include groin pain, often referred to the knee, and a limp. Note that hip pain sometimes presents as knee, abdomen or back pain instead of the expected groin pain or limp. Onset may be sudden after trauma or gradual over weeks to months. Examination reveals a flexion contraction and marked restriction of internal rotation of the hip. Hormonal factors are thought to weaken the epiphyseal plate, allowing the head of the femur to slip posteriorly and inferiorly. Refer for surgical intervention (see Chapter 18).

Table 21.1 Some musculoskeletal conditions affecting children requiring referral—cont'd

Scheuermann's disease	Symptoms include tiredness or pain in the back from an idiopathic breakdown of the developing vertebral endplate (see Chapter 11). Sometimes increased kyphosis is observed. Refer for postural advice, osseous manipulation and extension exercises.
Structural scoliosis	Scoliosis or lateral curvature of the spine is observed on postural observation (see Chapter 11). Adam's test is positive (i.e. lateral curvature persists on forward flexion of the trunk). Refer for further investigation if moderate or severe.
Torticollis	Sudden onset of unilateral neck pain. It is managed as for adults (see Chapter 12).
Radial head subluxation (pulled elbow in a toddler)	The head of the radius subluxes through the annular ligament, which normally holds it in place. Refer for reduction.
Little league elbow	This is an uncommon condition that results from excessive throwing. Elbow pain results from traction apophysitis of the medical epicondyle. Avoid throwing activities until the symptoms resolve.
Juvenile rheumatoid arthritis	Polyarticular joint pain associated with systemic illness (e.g. fever, rash, lymphadenopathy). Refer for further examination.
Rheumatic fever	This is a rare condition following streptococcal infection. Symptoms include migratory arthritis involving several joints. Refer for further examination.

accommodate their characteristic inability to lie still on a treatment table for prolonged periods. A parent or guardian may be recruited to distract the child or assist by holding them. Apply techniques lightly and slowly. A reward system (e.g. balloons and stickers) is a useful strategy for establishing a child-friendly practice.

- Adolescence is the period between childhood and adulthood. It is marked by the onset of puberty and involves both biological and psychosocial changes. In this period of rapid transition from childhood to physical and sexual maturity, many adolescents are very shy about their bodies and remedial massage therapists need to be particularly careful to respect the client's modesty. Some adolescents become stressed and anxious as they deal with their body's physical and emotional changes. Stress is further compounded when students are preparing for important school exams. Remedial massage may also be part of a range of treatment strategies for adolescents dealing with more serious mental health issues such as depression and eating disorders. Liaise with the client's medical or other health practitioner wherever possible.

EVIDENCE FOR THE EFFECTIVENESS OF MASSAGE FOR CHILDREN

Research into the effectiveness of massage therapy for children and pregnancy is dominated by the work of Tiffany Field. Her studies have investigated the benefits of massage for infants, children and pregnant women over a range of conditions including childhood leukaemia, asthma, depression and anxiety. According to the Touch Research Institute (established by Tiffany Field in 1992) massage therapy enhances attentiveness, alleviates depressive symptoms, reduces pain, reduces stress hormones, improves immune function and facilitates weight gain in preterm infants.[3] A Cochrane review examined infant massage using 14 randomised controlled trials where babies were stroked for about 15 minutes, three or four times a day, usually for five or ten days. On average, the studies found that when compared to babies who were not touched, babies receiving massage gained more weight each day (about 5 grams), spent less time in hospital, had slightly better scores on developmental tests and had slightly fewer postnatal complications, although there were problems with the reliability of the findings. The studies did not show any negative effects of massage. The authors concluded that the evidence for the use of massage to promote growth and development of preterm and low birth weight infants was weak and suggested that wider use of preterm infant massage was unwarranted.[4]

Massage therapy shows promising results in treatment of childhood asthma. In one study parents of children with asthma were trained to administer a daily 20-minute massage for 30 days. Results for the 6–8-year-olds showed reduced behaviour anxiety and cortisol levels directly after massage but these were not maintained after the series of treatments. Lung function tests had significantly improved after 30 days of regular massage. The 9–16-year-olds experienced considerably less benefit.[5]

The role of massage in immunity has been investigated in a number of studies. A study by Zhu et al[6], for example, found that massage was helpful in enhancing immune function in children with recurrent respiratory tract infection. In another study a group of 2–8-year-old Dominican children infected with HIV-1 received massage twice weekly for 12 weeks.[7] The findings of this study supported the use of massage to preserve immunity in HIV-1 infected children.

A number of studies has examined the effect of massage on children with cancer. Field et al[8] reported increases in white blood cell and neutrophil counts in 20 children with leukaemia following daily massage by their parents for one month. Massage is well known for its positive effect on reducing stress and anxiety. A pilot study by Post-White et al[9] found that massage was more effective than quiet time for reducing heart rate and anxiety in children with cancer under 14 years of age. There were no significant changes in blood pressure, cortisol, pain, nausea or fatigue.

A systematic review was conducted into the effectiveness of abdominal massage for treating constipation and cautiously concluded that massage could be a useful treatment.[10]

WOMEN

Health issues specifically related to women are largely concerned with the physical and emotional responses to the hormonal changes that occur from the onset of puberty, throughout the monthly menstrual cycle, during pregnancy and childbirth, to menopause and the post-menopausal period. Social changes associated with child rearing (women still outnumber men in this role), including pressures on relationships and balancing child rearing and work, may also affect women's health.

IMPORTANT CONSIDERATIONS FOR ASSESSING AND TREATING WOMEN

- Always consider the influence of hormone fluctuations during assessment. For example, headaches are often associated with pre-menstrual syndrome and menopause.
- Breast cancer is the most common cause of cancer-related death in women in Australia. In Australia in 2006 a total of 12,614 women and 102 men were diagnosed with breast cancer and there were 2643 deaths.[11] The incidence of breast cancer rose over 20% from 1996 to 2006 although the mortality rate remained constant in that time. Risk factors for developing breast cancer include older age and family history of breast cancer. A common site of metastasis is bone. One of the first symptoms of cancer in the bone is a constant ache or pain in the bone which is aggravated by movement and interferes with sleep.
- Ovarian cancer was the sixth most common cause of cancer-related death among Australian women in 2006.[12] It is mainly a disease of post-menopausal women, with 60% of cases diagnosed in women 60 years and over. As in breast cancer, risk factors include older age and family history of ovarian cancer. Metastases may be found in the peritoneal cavity or in the liver, lungs or other organs. The prognosis for women with ovarian cancer is often poorer than that for women diagnosed with other common cancers. This may be attributable partly to the non-specific nature of symptoms, which often leads to diagnosis at a relatively advanced stage of the disease.
- Normal menstruation is associated with a range of symptoms such as bloating, breast tenderness, irritability, anxiety, insomnia, headache, fatigue, mood swings, abdominal cramps, constipation and occasionally joint or muscle pain. Premenstrual syndrome (PMS) refers to those symptoms occurring during the luteal phase of the cycle (10 days before the menstrual period) that interfere with daily life. PMS symptoms disappear when menses begins. Dysmenorrhoea refers to painful or difficult menstruation. In primary dysmenorrhoea, pain is most severe on the first two days of bleeding; in congestive dysmenorrhoea pain commences a few days before bleeding and is relieved by the onset of bleeding; in endometriosis pain commences a few days before bleeding and increases to a maximum within 3 days of onset of bleeding.[13]
- Abdominal massage and deep remedial techniques for the lumbar spine are contraindicated during pregnancy. Many women may not know they are pregnant in the first few weeks. Early symptoms of pregnancy include nausea, vomiting, taste and smell sensitivities, exhaustion, constipation and mood swings. In the first few months of pregnancy the massage client may be comfortable lying prone with pillows under the chest and pelvis. Relaxin, which increases ligament laxity, peaks during the first trimester and at delivery. Later in pregnancy side-lying or seated positions are preferred. In the second trimester, clients may experience shortness of breath, heartburn, frequent urination and backache, and may develop varicose veins and haemorrhoids.[14] Oedema can occur from the pressure of the growing fetus on the large lymphatic vessels of the abdomen and pelvis. In the second trimester fluid retention can cause carpal tunnel syndrome. Although oedema is common during pregnancy, generalised oedema associated with high blood pressure suggests pre-eclampsia and requires medical referral. In the third trimester, oedema may be present in the lower limbs, forearms and hands. Muscle cramps, incontinence, sacroiliac joint pain, indigestion, frequent urination and sleeplessness can continue. In addition to the usual contraindications for massage, those for massage during pregnancy include acupressure and reflexology to the areas associated with the ovaries and uterus, presence of cramping, bleeding or pelvic pain and massage on varicose veins. Vigorous techniques and over-stretching should be avoided.[15]
- Women are at risk of injury to the lower back in the weeks and months following childbirth, when they not only have weakened abdominal and pelvic floor muscles but are also required to undertake many unaccustomed lifting and bending tasks to care for the newborn. As children grow so do physical demands on new parents (e.g. carrying infants, chasing toddlers, bathing children). Advise new mothers of the importance of muscle-strengthening exercises and of postures for breastfeeding, bathing, lifting and carrying their babies that minimise the risk of injury. Relaxation massage is a good remedy for sleep-deprived and physically exhausted mothers.
- Women may bring their young children with them when they are having remedial massage. In the interest of safety, keep children in the consultation room during their mother's treatment.
- Hormone fluctuations during the menstrual cycle may affect anterior cruciate ligament laxity. The anterior cruciate ligaments may become increasingly lax throughout the menstrual cycle.[16]
- Declining oestrogen levels in menopause increase visceral fat mass and decrease bone mass density, muscle mass and strength.[17] This has important consequences for the musculoskeletal system, such as an increased risk of osteoporosis and fracture. Weight gain after menopause increases the load on the low back and lower limbs and aggravates pre-existing conditions. Muscle and joint pain is also associated with menopause, along with an increased incidence of muscle injury and slower recovery times.[18, 19] Oestrogen is thought to have a protective effect: (i) it acts as an antioxidant, (ii) it is a membrane stabiliser, and (iii) it binds to oestrogen receptors, thereby regulating the expression of a number of genes.

EVIDENCE FOR THE EFFECTIVENESS OF MASSAGE FOR WOMEN'S HEALTH

Several studies have examined the effects of massage therapy for breast cancer patients. A qualitative study into the experience of massage for 10 breast cancer patients found that massage offered a retreat from uneasy, unwanted, negative feelings connected with chemotherapy treatment. The authors suggested that massage can be added to the treatment choices available to oncology staff.[20] Another study examining the effect of massage on 39 breast cancer patients undergoing chemotherapy found that massage treatment significantly reduced nausea compared with control treatment when improvement was measured as a percentage of the five treatment periods.[21] Post-operative arm massage was also found to decrease pain in the immediate post-operative period in 59 women with lymph node dissection.[22] Another study found improved immune and neuroendocrine function in breast cancer patients following massage.[23]

A number of studies has examined the effectiveness of massage during pregnancy and childbirth. Field et al[24] compared two groups of women diagnosed with prenatal depression. One group received one session of interpersonal psychotherapy per week for 6 weeks and the other received a combination of interpersonal psychotherapy and massage therapy once a week for the same period. The authors concluded that interpersonal psychotherapy was particularly effective when combined with massage therapy in reducing prenatal depression. Another randomised controlled trial reported some positive effects of massage on anxiety during labour.[25] There is strong evidence supporting the use of perineal massage to reduce the incidence of perineal trauma although such massage is outside the boundaries of remedial massage practice.[26–28]

Evidence for the influence of hormonal fluctuations during the menstrual cycle on anterior cruciate ligament laxity is controversial. A number of studies both confirm and refute the claim.[16, 29, 30]

Studies of the effect of aromatherapy and reflexology on the symptoms of menopause, particularly psychological symptoms, have found encouraging results.[31, 32]

MEN

Chronic conditions like obesity, cancer, diabetes and cardiovascular disease are more common in men than women and yet for many men visiting the doctor for a health check-up is a last resort. As a result many health conditions among men go untreated until they become serious, more difficult to treat and/or life-threatening. In recognition of the need to improve men's physical and mental health the Australian government developed the National Male Health Policy 2010, which nominated six priority areas for action.[33] These are to promote:

1. Optimal health outcomes for males – to promote recognition of the valuable roles males play in family and community life, develop policies that specifically consider male health and modify health programs to improve the health and wellbeing of males and particularly those with the poorest health outcomes.
2. Health equity between population groups of males – to give policy priority to males who experience the highest health disadvantage, promote health messages in a way that males can relate to, and encourage health services for Aboriginal and Torres Strait Islander males to have a positive, family-oriented approach.
3. Improved health for males at different life stages – to promote the role of males as fathers, recognise the roles of Aboriginal and Torres Strait Islander men in traditional practices and parenting, encourage a focus on transition points in male lives (for example, leaving school, relationship breakdown), develop practical health promotion materials and promote male adolescent health through schools and other avenues.
4. A focus on preventive health for males – to encourage employers to deliver health checks and programs for males, fund health promotion materials, encourage health promotion activities to have a specific focus on males, raise awareness on chronic diseases among males deliver evidence-based health promotion messages to males, and monitor workplace hazards and environmental toxins.
5. Building a strong evidence base for male health – to fund a national longitudinal study on male health, commission regular statistical bulletins on male health, give priority to research focusing on male health, routinely collect and report data on male health, explore the potential for surveys on male health and monitor scientific developments relating to male health.
6. Improved access to healthcare for males – to encourage health services to be responsive to male needs and aware of health barriers they face, encourage culturally appropriate services for Aboriginal and Torres Strait Islander males and encourage medical practitioners to take up government incentives to engage Australians in prevention of chronic disease.

IMPORTANT CONSIDERATIONS FOR ASSESSING AND TREATING MEN

- Men are less likely to use health services than are females. Encourage male clients to see their doctors and other healthcare practitioners when required.
- Approximately 18,700 new cases of prostate cancer are diagnosed in Australia every year and approximately 3000 Australian men die from the disease each year. When assessing older males, be mindful that 50% of males over 50 years have a carcinomatous change in their prostate. Most of these changes are benign (e.g. benign prostatic hypertrophy); nevertheless, it is important to refer all males over 50 years who report urinary symptoms (such as frequency, urgency, nocturia or hesitancy) associated with back, hip or rib pain. Risk factors for prostate cancer include age and family history of prostate, breast or ovarian cancer.[34] Be vigilant for young men with a family history of prostate cancer and older men with urinary symptoms.
- Refer clients who are demonstrating signs of mental illnesses like depression or substance abuse to their medical practitioners. Depression in men may manifest as fatigue, irritability, difficulty sleeping and loss of interest in work and hobbies. It some cases signs of depression include anger, aggression, violence, reckless behaviour and substance abuse. Men, especially older men, are at a higher suicide risk than women.[35]

GERIATRIC CLIENTS

Projections for Australia's population place the proportion of people aged over 65 between 21% and 22% by 2031. This raises particular concerns about the projected healthcare needs of this ageing population, concerns which include the treatment and management of chronic conditions and the costs required to meet these needs.[36, 37] Remedial massage clients are likely to be called upon to treat an increasing number of geriatric clients in their clinics and in aged care facilities and in clients' homes. Particular concerns associated with massaging older clients include increased risk of osteoporosis, fragile and sensitive skin, arthritic joints and decreased muscle tone. Circulation, particularly to extremities, decreases in older clients. Clients are often taking prescribed medication and may have side-effects associated with their medication use. Moreover, many aged clients live alone and have limited incomes.

IMPORTANT CONSIDERATIONS FOR ASSESSING AND TREATING GERIATRIC CLIENTS

- Extra time may be needed for older clients to complete administration requirements, to complete case histories and other assessments, to dress and undress and to get on and off the treatment table. Speak slowly and allow time for the client to respond.
- Many older clients have more than one pathology occurring simultaneously.
- Many older clients are taking prescription medication. Always consider side-effects of medication when assessing clients and negotiating treatment plans.
- Clients may have hearing problems. Speak slowly and clearly. Minimise background noise.
- Older clients appear to benefit from the psychosocial aspects of treatment.
- Adjust techniques to suit the individual client's needs. In general, techniques are applied lightly because of skin fragility, the risk of fracture in osteoporotic clients and the risk of bruising in clients taking blood-thinning medication.
- Treatments are often short, at least initially, until the client's response to treatment has been assessed.
- Clients may require help getting on and off the treatment table.
- Clients with cardiovascular or respiratory conditions, or clients who are obese, require extra pillows to elevate their head when lying supine.
- Frail aged clients are often treated in chairs or beds. Massage may be confined to hands and feet.
- Do not cover hearing aids with hands during face, neck and head massage.
- Massage may be performed without oils or creams because of skin sensitivities and allergies. If lubricant can be tolerated, use easily absorbed creams.
- Psychosocial benefits may outweigh physical advantages of massage therapy.

EVIDENCE FOR THE EFFECTIVENESS OF MASSAGE FOR OLDER CLIENTS

There is much anecdotal evidence about the perceived physical and psychosocial benefits of massage for older clients, particularly those who are isolated. Several studies have examined the benefits of massage therapy for elderly clients. For example, self-reported health outcomes in older adults suggested better health outcomes in emotional wellbeing but also limitations due to physical and/or emotional issues.[38] Another randomised controlled trial found that a single session of plantar massage and joint mobilisation of the feet and ankles improved balance in 28 elderly patients.[39]

There have been mixed results for the effectiveness of massage for elderly clients in residential care. One study compared the level of comfort provided to 35 nursing home residents with 25 residents in a control group. The authors found no significant differences in comfort levels or satisfaction with care over time, although there were significant differences between the groups at specific time periods.[40]

Remington[41] examined the effect of calming music and hand massage with agitated nursing home residents and found that these interventions reduced agitation more than no intervention but that there was no added benefit from combining the interventions. Another study by Mok and Pang Woo[42] found that slow-stroke back massage was effective in reducing anxiety and shoulder pain in elderly stroke patients.

Although aromatherapy is often part of geriatric massage and hospice care, further research is required to substantiate its effectiveness.[43]

CLIENTS WITH A MENTAL ILLNESS

According to the Victorian Department of Health, one in five Australians will experience a mental illness at some time in their lives. Mental illnesses can come and go and most can be effectively treated.[44] Stress can trigger some mental illnesses or may prolong episodes. Through its capacity to reduce stress and enhance feelings of wellbeing, massage therapy may have a considerable role to play in management or prevention of some mental health conditions. Mental illnesses can be divided into psychotic and non-psychotic.[44]

1. Psychotic illnesses – a psychosis (e.g. schizophrenia, bipolar mood disorder) is a condition caused by any one of a group of illnesses that affects the ability to make sense of thoughts, feelings and external information. People with psychoses may develop delusions or become depressed or overly elated. Medication and support from medical health professionals can be effective treatments.
2. Non-psychotic illnesses – a non-psychotic illness involves feelings of depression, sadness, tension or fear that become so overwhelming that they interfere with normal activities like going to work and maintaining relationships. Such illnesses include phobias, anxiety, some forms of depression, eating disorders and obsessive-compulsive disorder. Most non-psychotic illnesses can be effectively treated with medication and therapy.

IMPORTANT CONSIDERATIONS FOR ASSESSING AND TREATING CLIENTS WITH A MENTAL ILLNESS

- If a client is unable to give informed consent, consent may be given by a guardian who must be present throughout the consultation.
- Remedial massage can be used as an adjunct to support primary treatments for mental illness. Effective communication among practitioners is required.
- Practitioners should be vigilant for indications of mental illness and refer clients to medical practitioners when required. People with mental disorders consult general

practitioners with physical rather than psychological complaints, including symptoms like feeling tired all the time, sleeping badly or not coping with day-to-day events.[45] Note that emotional symptoms are common but do not necessarily mean that the sufferer has a mental disorder.[45] Signs and symptoms suggesting an underlying mental health problem include:
  - seemingly inappropriate requests for urgent attention
  - increased frequency of consultation or requests for tests
  - unexpected or disproportionate outbursts during consultation (tears, anger)
  - excessive anxiety about another family member or presenting a relative as the patient
  - unstable relationships or frequent breakdowns in relationships
  - distressing or deteriorating social circumstances (eviction, redundancy, squalor).
- When assessing clients with a mental illness, consider side-effects of medication for common conditions such as depression and bipolar disease.
- Massage appears to be particularly beneficial for stress management and for treating clients with anxiety and depression.

EVIDENCE FOR THE EFFECTIVENESS OF MASSAGE FOR CLIENTS WITH A MENTAL ILLNESS

An increasing number of studies support the effectiveness of massage in reducing stress and anxiety. One meta-analysis has suggested that the most significant effects of massage are reducing anxiety and helping patients with depression.[46, 47] For example, one randomised controlled trial examined the effectiveness of a 15-minute weekly massage in nurses over a 5-week period and found statistically significant differences in State-Trait Anxiety Inventory scores between the group receiving massage and a control group who did not.[48] A study by Gurol et al[49] examined the effects of massage therapy on 63 adolescents suffering from second- and third-degree burns and found reduced measures of anxiety, pain and itching. Mok and Pang Woo[42] found that slow-stroke back massage reduced anxiety and shoulder pain in elderly stroke clients. However, when 13 complementary and alternative medicine treatments, including massage, for depression in adolescents and children were examined, the authors found insufficient evidence to draw conclusions and suggested that there is a need for further research into non-pharmaceutical management of first-time occurrences of mild to moderate depression in children and adolescents.[50]

A number of studies have been conducted into the use of massage therapy in autism. It is relevant to include autism in discussions of mental health as clients with this complex developmental disability have many behaviours and states in common with clients with mental health conditions. One study found that 13 children with autism aged between 3 and 6 years who received daily massage treatments for five months showed significant improvement of sensory impairments and demonstrated increased social skills and basic living skills on standardised measures compared with untreated children.[51] Another randomised controlled trial examined the effects of Thai traditional massage on 60 autistic children and found that Thai traditional massage over an 8-week period had a positive effect on stereotypical behaviours in autistic children.[52]

A Cochrane review into the effectiveness of massage and touch for dementia found that there was insufficient evidence to draw conclusions and that more research is needed to provide definitive evidence about the benefits of these interventions.[53]

In a preliminary study into the use of alternative healthcare practices by people with serious mental illnesses, 31% of participants reported benefit from massage therapy.[54]

KEY MESSAGES

- Informed consent must be obtained from the client, a parent or guardian (in the case of a child under 18 years of age or a client with a mental illness who is unable to provide their own informed consent). The parent or guardian is required to remain with the client throughout the consultation.
- Managing the consultation requires time management, effective communication skills and modification of techniques to suit the needs of individual clients.
- When assessing children and adolescents, consider common conditions that occur at specific ages. Treat all musculoskeletal pain as serious until proven otherwise.
- Adolescents are often particularly sensitive to their developing bodies. Careful attention is required to maintain their modesty and comfort.
- Always consider the influence of hormones on symptoms in female clients.
- Be aware that men are often reluctant to discuss health issues with their healthcare practitioners.
- When treating older males, be mindful that 50% of males over 50 years of age have a carcinomatous change in the prostate. Refer all clients with urinary symptoms (frequency, urgency, hesitancy and nocturia) for further investigation.
- Treating older clients requires time and patience. They often have several pathologies at the same time, take prescribed medication and suffer from chronic conditions. Psychological benefits of remedial massage treatment are important.
- Massage appears to be particularly beneficial in the treatment of anxiety and depression.

Review questions

1. i) What effect does excessive femoral anteversion have on gait?
   ii) What is the normal degree of femoral anterversion in neonates and in adults?
2. Briefly describe the pathogenesis of slipped capital femoral epiphysis. What symptoms can it produce?
3. What symptoms could be used to differentiate primary dysmenorrhoea, congestive dysmenorrhoea and endometriosis?
4. What effects can declining oestrogen levels have on the musculoskeletal system?
5. List three common chronic health conditions that males are more likely to experience than females.
6. What common condition affecting older males should be considered when assessing a 60-year-old male with low back pain?
7. How is a remedial massage consultation modified for a frail aged client?
8. List four signs or symptoms that could indicate a client has a mental health problem.

Research activity

Review recent research articles (published in the past 5 years) on the effectiveness of massage for one of the specific client groups discussed in this chapter.

For example, the effect of massage on:

- childhood asthma
- adolescent idiopathic scoliosis
- depression.

Sources of information include:

- Freely available journals such as
  - *BMC complementary and alternative medicine* (peer-reviewed)
  - *Massage Australia* magazine
  - *Massage and Bodywork*
  - *Massage Today*
  - *Sport Health* (Australia)
- Freely available databases such as
  - Cochrane reviews http://www2.cochrane.org/reviews/
  - Pubmed (Medline) http://www.ncbi.nlm.nih.gov/sites/entrez

Other databases are available through libraries including EBSCOhost, AMED (Allied and Complementary Medicine), CINAHL.

- Professional association websites
- Government websites
  - Australian Institute of Health and Welfare
  - Dept of Health and Ageing, Therapeutic Goods Administration
  - NSW Health
  - WorkCover authorities in each state

The quality of research is highly variable. To guide selection of readings, choose a reputable source (e.g. a peer-reviewed journal). Systematic reviews or meta-analyses are regarded as the highest form of evidence. Prioritise the use of these when they are available.

REFERENCES

1. Australian Institute of Family Studies. Mandatory reporting of child abuse. Online. Available: www.aifs.gov.au/nch/pubs/sheets/rs3/rs3.html; 2010.
2. Birnbaum J. The musculoskeletal manual. 2nd rev edn. Philadelphia: Grune and Stratton; 1986.
3. Touch Research Institute. About us. Miami, FL: Touch Research Institute; 2010. Online. Available: http://www6.miami.edu/touch-research/About.html.
4. Vickers A, Ohlsson A, Lacy JB, et al. Massage for promoting growth and development of preterm and/ or low birth-weight infants. Cochrane Database Syst Rev 2004;4.
5. Ernst E. Massage therapy is promising for childhood asthma. Focus on Alternative and Complementary Therapies 1999;4(1):30–1.
6. Zhu S, Wang N, Wang D, et al. A clinical investigation on massage for prevention and treatment of recurrent respiratory tract infection in children. J Tradit Chin Med 1998;18(4):285–91.
7. Shor-Posner G, Hernandez-Reif M, Miguez M, et al. Impact of a massage therapy clinical trial on immune status in young Dominican children infected with HIV-1. J Altern Complement Med 2006;12(6):511–16.
8. Field T, Cullen C, Diego M, et al. Leukemia immune changes following massage therapy. J Bodyw Mov Ther 2001;5(4):271–4.
9. Post-White J, Fitzgerald M, Savik K, et al. Massage therapy for children with cancer. J Pediatr Oncol Nurs 2009;26(1):16–28.
10. Ernst E. Abdominal massage therapy for chronic constipation: a systematic review of controlled clinical trials. Forsch Komplementarmed 1999;6(3): 149–51.
11. Breast Cancer Australia. Breast cancer: awareness and prevention. Online. Available: www.breastcanceraustralia.org.au; 2010.
12. Australian Institute of Health and Welfare. Ovarian cancer in Australia: an overview. Canberra: Australian Institute of Health and Welfare; 2010. Online. Available: http://www.aihw.gov.au/ publications/index.cfm/title/11158.
13. Beirman R. Handbook of clinical diagnosis: A guide for students and practitioners in the health professions. Sydney: R. Beirman; 2003.
14. Braun M, Simonson S. Introduction to massage therapy. Baltimore, MD: Lippincott Williams and Wilkins; 2005.
15. Fritz S. Mosby's fundamentals of therapeutic massage. 4th edn. St Louis, MI: Mosby Elsevier, 2009.
16. Heitz N, Eisenman P, Beck C, et al. Hormonal changes throughout the menstrual cycle and increased anterior cruciate ligament laxity in females. J Athlet Train. 1999;34(2):144–9.
17. Maltais ML, Desroches J, Dionne IJ. Changes in muscle mass and strength after menopause. J Musculoskelet Neuronal Interact [Research Support, Non-U.S. Gov't Review] 2009;9(4): 186–97.
18. Faria A, Gabriel R, Abrantes J, et al. Ankle stiffness in postmenopausal women: influence of hormone therapy and menopause nature. Climacteric [Research Support, Non-U.S. Gov't] 2009;13(3):265–70.
19. Enns DL, Tiidus PM, Enns DL, et al. The influence of estrogen on skeletal muscle: sex matters. Sports Med 2010;40(1):41–58.
20. Billhult A, Stener-Victorin E, Bergbom I. The experience of massage during chemotherapy treatment in breast cancer patients. Clin Nurs Res 2007;16(2):85–9.
21. Billhult A, Bergbom I, Stener-Victorin E. Massage relieves nausea in women with breast cancer who are undergoing chemotherapy. J Altern Complement Med – New York 2007;13(1):53–7.
22. Forchuk C, Baruth P, Prendergast M, et al. Postoperative arm massage: a support for women with lymph node dissection. Cancer Nurs. 2004;27(1):25–33.
23. Hernandez-Reif M, Ironson G, Field T. Breast cancer patients have improved immune and neuroendocrine functions following massage therapy. J Psychosom Res 2004;57:45–52.
24. Field T, Deeds O, Diego M, et al. Benefits of combining massage therapy with group interpersonal psychotherapy in prenatally depressed women. J Bodyw Mov Ther 2009;13(4):297–303.
25. Chang M, Wang S, Chen C. Effects of massage on pain and anxiety during labour: a randomised controlled trial in Taiwan. J Adv Nurs 2002;38: 68–73.
26. Beckmann MM, Garrett AJ. Antenatal perineal massage for reducing perineal trauma. Cochrane Database Syst Rev 2006;4.
27. Avery M, Arsdale L. Perineal massage. Effect on the incidence of episiotomy and laceration in a nulliparous population. J Nurse Midwifery 1987;32(3):181–4.
28. Eason E, Labrecque M, Wells G, et al. Preventing perineal trauma during childbirth: a systematic review. Obstet Gynecol 2000;95(3):464–71.

29. Deie M, Sakamaki Y, Sumen Y, et al. Anterior knee laxity in young women varies with their menstrual cycle. Int Orthop 2002;26(3):154–6.
30. Van Lunen B, Roberts J, Branch J, et al. Association of menstrual-cycle hormone change with anterior cruciate ligament laxity measurements. J Athlet Train 2003;38(4):298–303.
31. Murakami S, Shirota T, Hayashi S, Ishizuka B. Aromatherapy for outpatients with menopausal symptoms in obstetrics and gynecology. J Altern Complement Med – New York 2005;11(3):491–4.
32. Williamson J, White A, Hart A, et al. Randomised controlled trial of reflexology for menopausal symptoms. Bjog. [Clinical Trial Randomized Controlled Trial Research Support, Non-U.S. Gov't] 2002;109(9):1050–5.
33. Ageing AGDoHa. National Male Health Policy: building on the strengths of Australian males. Online. Available: http://www.health.gov.au/internet/main/publishing.nsf/content/0547F4712F6AB5D3CA257457001D4ECF/$File/MainDocument.pdf; 2010.
34. Prostate Cancer Foundation of Australia. What is prostate cancer? Online. Available: http://www.prostate.org.au/articleLive/pages/What-is-Prostate-Cancer.html; 2010
35. Helpguide.org. Depression in men. Helpguide.org. Online. Available: http://helpguide.org/mental/depression_signs_types_diagnosis_treatment.htm; 2010
36. Abbott T. What if we could start again? elements of an ideal health system. [Lecture]. Sydney; 2006.
37. Vario Health Institute. The growth of modern chronic diseases. Online. Available: www.varioinstitute.com/rationale.php; 2006.
38. Munk N, Zanjani F. Relationship between massage therapy usage and health outcomes in older adults. J Bodywork Mov Ther 2011;15(2):177–85.
39. Vaillant J, Rouland A, Martigné P, et al. Massage and mobilization of the feet and ankles in elderly adults: effect on clinical balance performance. Man Ther 2009;14(6):661–4.
40. Kolcaba K, Schirm V, Steiner R. Effects of hand massage on comfort of nursing home residents. Geriatr Nurs 2006;27(2):85–91.
41. Remington R. Calming music and hand massage with agitated elderly. Nurs Res 2002;51(5):317–23.
42. Mok E, Pang Woo C. The effect of slow-stroke back massage on anxiety and shoulder pain in elderly stroke patients. Complement Ther Nurs Midwifery 2004;10(4):209–16.
43. Howdyshell C. Complementary therapy: aromatherapy with massage for geriatric and hospice care – a call for an holistic approach. Hosp J 1998;13(3):69–75.
44. State Government of Victoria Australia. Department of Health. Mental illness: The facts 2009. Online. Available: http://www.health.vic.gov.au/mentalhealth/illnesses/facts.htm.
45. Craig T, Boardman A. ABC of mental health: Common mental health problems in primary care. BMJ 1997;314:1609–12.
46. Moyer CA, Rounds J, Hannum JW. A meta-analysis of massage therapy research. Psychol Bull 2004;130(1):3–18.
47. Muller-Oerlinghausen B, Berg C, Scherer P, Mackert A, Moestl H, Wolf J. Effects of slow-stroke massage as complementary treatment of depressed hospitalized patients. Dtsch Med Wochenschr 2004;129:1363–8.
48. Bost N, Wallis M. The effectiveness of a 15 minute weekly massage in reducing physical and pyschological stress in nurses. Aust J Adv Nurs 2006;23(4):28–33.
49. Gurol A, Polat S, Akcay M. Itching, pain, and anxiety levels are reduced with massage therapy in burned adolescents. J Care Res 2010;31(3):429–32.
50. Jorm A, Allen N, O'Donnell C, et al. Effectiveness of complementary and self-help treatments for depression in children and adolescents. Med J Aust 2006;185(7):368.
51. Silva L, Cignlini A, Warren R, et al. Improvement in Sensory Impairment and Social Interaction in Young Children with Autism Following Treatment with an Original Qigong Massage Methodology. Am J Chin Med 2007;35(3):393–406.
52. Piravej K, Tangtrongchitr P, Chandarasiri P, et al. Effects of Thai traditional massage on autistic children's behavior. J Altern Complement Med – New York 2009;15(12):1355–61.
53. Hansen N, Jorgensen T, Ortenblad L. Massage and touch for dementia. Cochrane Database Syst Rev 2006;(4).
54. Russinova Z, Wewiorski N, Cash D. Use of alternative health care practices by persons with serious mental illness: perceived benefits. Am J Public Health 2002;92(10):1600–3.

Index

Page numbers followed by "f" indicate figures, "t" indicate tables, and "b" indicate boxes.

T

U

V

W

Y